Quantum FOURTH EDITION

Leadership

Building Better Partnerships for Sustainable Health

Tim Porter-O'Grady, DM, EdD, ScD(h), APRN, FAAN, FACCWS
Senior Partner, Tim Porter-O'Grady Associates, Inc., Atlanta, Georgia
Professor of Practice, Arizona State University College of Nursing and
    Health Innovation, Phoenix, Arizona
Clinical Professor, Leadership Scholar, Ohio State University College of Nursing, Columbus, Ohio

Kathy Malloch, PhD, MBA, RN, FAAN
President Kathy Malloch Leadership Systems, LLC, Glendale, Arizona
Professor of Practice, Arizona State University College of Nursing and
    Health Innovation, Phoenix, Arizona
Clinical Professor, Ohio State University College of Nursing, Columbus, Ohio
Clinical Consultant, API Healthcare, Inc., Hartford, Wisconsin

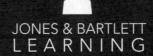

JONES & BARTLETT
LEARNING

World Headquarters
Jones & Bartlett Learning
5 Wall Street
Burlington, MA 01803
978-443-5000
info@jblearning.com
www.jblearning.com

Jones & Bartlett Learning books and products are available through most bookstores and online booksellers. To contact Jones & Bartlett Learning directly, call 800-832-0034, fax 978-443-8000, or visit our website, www.jblearning.com.

Substantial discounts on bulk quantities of Jones & Bartlett Learning publications are available to corporations, professional associations, and other qualified organizations. For details and specific discount information, contact the special sales department at Jones & Bartlett Learning via the above contact information or send an email to specialsales@jblearning.com.

The content, statements, views, and opinions herein are the sole expression of the respective authors and not that of Jones & Bartlett Learning, LLC. Reference herein to any specific commercial product, process, or service by trade name, trademark, manufacturer, or otherwise does not constitute or imply its endorsement or recommendation by Jones & Bartlett Learning, LLC and such reference shall not be used for advertising or product endorsement purposes. All trademarks displayed are the trademarks of the parties noted herein. *Quantum Leadership: Building Better Partnerships for Sustainable Health, Fourth Edition* is an independent publication and has not been authorized, sponsored, or otherwise approved by the owners of the trademarks or service marks referenced in this product.

There may be images in this book that feature models; these models do not necessarily endorse, represent, or participate in the activities represented in the images. Any screenshots in this product are for educational and instructive purposes only. Any individuals and scenarios featured in the case studies throughout this product may be real or fictitious, but are used for instructional purposes only.

The authors, editor, and publisher have made every effort to provide accurate information. However, they are not responsible for errors, omissions, or for any outcomes related to the use of the contents of this book and take no responsibility for the use of the products and procedures described. Treatments and side effects described in this book may not be applicable to all people; likewise, some people may require a dose or experience a side effect that is not described herein. Drugs and medical devices are discussed that may have limited availability controlled by the Food and Drug Administration (FDA) for use only in a research study or clinical trial. Research, clinical practice, and government regulations often change the accepted standard in this field. When consideration is being given to use of any drug in the clinical setting, the health care provider or reader is responsible for determining FDA status of the drug, reading the package insert, and reviewing prescribing information for the most up-to-date recommendations on dose, precautions, and contraindications, and determining the appropriate usage for the product. This is especially important in the case of drugs that are new or seldom used.

Production Credits
Executive Publisher: William Brottmiller
Senior Editor: Amanda Martin
Editorial Assistant: Rebecca Myrick
Production Editor: Amanda Clerkin
Senior Marketing Manager: Jennifer Stiles
VP, Manufacturing and Inventory Control: Therese Connell
Composition: Aptara®, Inc.
Cover Design: Kristin E. Parker
Rights Clearance Editor: Maria Leon Maimone
Cover Image: © Taras Kushnir/Shutterstock, Inc.
Printing and Binding: Edwards Brothers Malloy
Cover Printing: Edwards Brothers Malloy

To order this product, use ISBN: 978-1-284-05068-4

Library of Congress Cataloging-in-Publication Data
Porter-O'Grady, Timothy, author.
    Quantum leadership : building better partnerships for sustainable health / Tim Porter-O'Grady and Kathy Malloch.—Fourth edition.
        p. ; cm.
    Includes bibliographical references and index.
    ISBN 978-1-284-03428-8
    I. Malloch, Kathy, author. II. Title.
    [DNLM: 1. Health Services Administration. 2. Leadership. 3. Organizational Innovation. W 84.1]
    HD57.7
    658.4'092—dc23
                                2013047577
6048

Printed in the United States of America
18 17 16 15 14   10 9 8 7 6 5 4 3 2

CONTENTS

Chapter Three   Evidentiary Leadership: An Expanded Lens to Determine Healthcare Value 99

Chapter Four   Innovation as a Way of Life: Leading Through the White Water of Change 127

Chapter Five   Innovation Leadership 173

Chapter Six   **Leadership and Normative Conflict: Managing the Diversity of a Multifocal Workplace** **203**

Chapter Seven   **Leading Constant Movement: Managing Crisis and Change** **255**

Chapter Eight   **Living Leadership: Vulnerability, Risk Taking, and Stretching** **307**

DEDICATION

We dedicate this book to Cathleen Krueger Wilson, PhD, RN, nurse, therapist, consultant, colleague, and friend, who first conceived the possibility of this kind of book on leadership. Her creativity and imagination in applying leadership to all venues of health service were an inspiration and a joy to all who knew her. Cathleen was a role model as nurse, mother, spouse, and friend and brought the full weight and energy of her person to her work and relationships. In death, as in life, she still serves to stimulate and encourage the best in all whose lives she touched.

PREFACE

Writing a book on leadership in a time of healthcare transformation is almost a futile exercise—not that writing any book isn't difficult. Building on the previous three editions of this text and updating content remind us of both the degree and the pace of changing knowledge and insight on leadership as we move deeper into a complexity-grounded digital age. Because of our dedication to ensuring that the most current and relevant information is contained in this text, we have committed to updating its contents every 2 years. The peculiarity of books on leadership is that they can never be truly finished. Leadership is essentially a work in progress—a never-ending journey with facets and elements that add up to a broad and complex mosaic. Embedded in the leadership role is a host of behavioral, relational, interactional, and structural considerations that give form to the activity of leading. Research in each of these areas could line the shelves of libraries for generations. We submit that no one person could comprehend all that has been said and written about leadership or all the actions that have been done in its name.

Furthermore, as the world changes, new notions of how to advance the work of organizations and people emerge, new patterns of behavior develop, and these demand some level of explication and understanding. In fact, just like other segments of society, health care is going through the drama and trauma of reconceptualizing its work and priorities to take into account the new global reality, real health reform, value-driven care models, and the most recent advances in therapeutics and clinical technology. These advances are already bearing fruit and radically altering both the quantity and quality of life. And the changes yet to come will have an even greater impact than did those that have already occurred. We hope this fourth edition has kept up with the changes and reflects the best thinking on the state of the art of contemporary leadership.

An example of this is the ever-increasing digitalization and mobility of health services, creating a need to reconfigure these services and change the relationship between providers and those they serve. Accountability for choice and proper action are coming to rest more in the hands of the "users," and healthcare leaders have the important job of enabling providers to alter their practices accordingly and to prepare these users to assume the accountability that is being transferred legitimately to them. Furthermore, technology is making it not only possible but necessary to build evidence that clinical work is truly making a difference in the lives of those we serve and in the health of our communities.

A leadership book like this one serves as a dynamic snapshot, if you will, of the leadership role at a particular moment in time. In our attempt to identify and describe the correct behaviors and strategies for the role, we focus on the issues that are most representative of the current era. One of the earmarks of our era, of course, is the accelerating rate of change in the substantive reformatting of the delivery of health care. Another is the obvious challenges of ensuring access, availability, and payment for health care for all Americans. All of these issues provide unique opportunities for the effective exercise of contemporary leadership.

Healthcare leaders must push their organizations into this fray. They must be able not only to see into the darkness of the future but also to live comfortably inside the potential—that risky, unsettled space between the present and the future. And because leaders cannot pull people into a future that only they have conceived of, they must bring everyone to the table to shape the future through collective dialogue and concerted action.

In this fourth edition, we try to conceptualize the newer complexity-based realities in health care and use the emerging foundations as a template to prioritize leadership skills and behaviors—those skills and behaviors that leaders need to use to ensure that their organizations are guided accurately and effectively. Our strategy is first to provide a glimpse into the future and then to present some of the implications of the maturing sciences of complexity and chaos, thereby delineating the context of the leadership role at the outset of this new century as leaders work to make sense of this continuously emergent sociotechnical world.

Anticipating change requires the ability to predict and adapt to transformation and the crisis that both stimulates it and represents the appropriate response. Leaders must now recognize the ever-constant company of the serendipitous and the unplanned occurrences that are reflected in a fast-paced and highly changing environment. Leaders must model and inculcate a predictive and adaptive capacity into the life of their organizations and into the skills of the staff at every place in the organization. There is simply no way that reforming and advancing health care can unfold without a great deal of conflict. Most people assume that conflict in the workplace is bad and should be avoided. Nothing could be further from the truth. Conflict is a normal element of all interaction. Leaders must understand this and acquire the necessary skills to manage conflict in a way that yields the benefits that it is capable of delivering. By handling conflict appropriately, leaders also are better positioned to create a healing environment for providers as well as consumers of health care and to undertake the healing of a wide variety of emotional and spiritual injuries suffered by people as they struggle with the work of transforming the healthcare system. Building a healthy environment by being fully present and demonstrating compassion and accountability is a fundamental responsibility of the contemporary leader.

Not only is it necessary to handle conflict effectively, it is necessary to see organizations as being in constant flux and subject to continuous change. Leaders now must both predict and adapt to the patterns of change that affect their people and their organizations. This adaptive and predictive capacity is no longer an option for good leaders if their organizations are going to continue to thrive and change as new conditions and technology demand. Developing these insights and the skill of predictive and adaptive capacity provides a good skill foundation to ensure the organizations of the future continue to change and sustain themselves.

Over the previous decade, a host of authors and researchers reminded us that leaders must possess not just intellectual ability but also emotional competence. After all, establishing and maintaining relationships are essential parts of leadership, and all relationships have an emotional component. To ensure that their relationships exhibit emotional maturity, leaders need to understand the nature of emotional competence and thus touch the emotional center in themselves and others. The value of emotional maturity for leadership is just beginning to be understood.

Behavior does not exist in a vacuum, and thus the context within which people interact and work together requires as much consideration as what they do. The enormous changes that are occurring, some of them very traumatic, cause people to see themselves awash in a sea of movement that does not make much sense. Staff members often fail to understand the direction in which their leaders are taking them and begin to lose hope and any sense that their work is meaningful. Leaders, in their actions, need to provide the foundations for hope and meaning and value. They must first find these things for themselves and then translate them into a language that others can comprehend and own.

Why are some leaders more successful than others at leading an organization through transformational change? Why do some create an environment of hope and calm despite difficult or even desperate circumstances? The answers can be found in the notion of personal willingness. Willing leaders are the co-creators of change. They recognize that no one person or situation can take away their personal peace, joy, or sense of competence. They transmit these feelings to others in a way that encourages and enables them to embrace the new script and share in the writing of it.

Whether we like it or not we now live in a value-driven age. As professionals, it is becoming increasingly important to build an evidentiary foundation that provides a clear demonstration of the relationship between the processes and the impact of our work. For too long, the focus of professional work has been on the work itself: the quality of that work, the content of the work, and how well the work was done. Increasingly, the challenges between appropriate resource use and the outcomes of clinical work have raised the specter of incongruity and our often frequent failure to advance the health status of those we serve. Value now calls for health professionals to make a strong case for practice and establish a firm foundation that demonstrates a goodness of fit between the action of clinical practice and the impact of advancing social health. And now, this must be done within the context of equity-based provider teams committed to advancing the health of those they serve. Evidentiary dynamics is now a fundamental subset of both leadership and clinical work. Improvement sciences and value-based practices and payment now require both technological and practice frames that elicit best practices and advance the user experience. Ultimately, leaders have an obligation to ensure that there is a tight relationship between the aggregated net health status of the community and the resources used to obtain and sustain it.

In the contemporary context for health care, a capacity for innovation is no longer optional. Every leader now must operate within an innovation mental model. Leaders now need to demonstrate an availability to the inventive and the creative so much a part of our fast-paced sociotechnical existence. Innovation is more than a process. It is increasingly evident that there is a science that drives it. As we become more aware of the action of complexity and its consonance with the movement of systems, the role of the emergent and transformational substrate of existence becomes more definitive. It is the role of a leader to create both context and conditions that harness this energy and facilitate the discourse, discovery, and application of this knowledge in advancing the quality of life and our human experience. Creating the context for the dynamics of innovation is now a central role of leadership capacity and is essential to the ability to be sustained and to thrive.

Coaching people into the future they must live in requires special skills. Unlike in the past, leaders cannot simply force people into a mold or into compliance with demands that they played no part in setting. Allowing people to be investors, partners, and stakeholders in their own processes is a talent necessary in the new leader. Leading workers out of a toxic and perennially sick or stuck work environment is a part of this process. It requires the leader to understand the characteristics of neurotic and pathological organizations and those behaviors that prevent people and their organizations from embracing the changes they must adapt to in order to thrive in the new world of health care.

Finally, leaders must focus on the energy and spirit within to be innovative and grow and thereby act as models for others in their own search for meaning and value in what they do. But the ability to exhibit creativity, self-understanding, and personal growth is not obtained accidentally or without effort; it requires regular mental and spiritual exercise, including periods of reflection, to refine it. In the future, leaders, to sustain their effectiveness in the leadership role, will need to engage in reflective personal work and increase their level of creativity.

Like others of its kind, this book is always a work in progress. It is necessarily and forever incomplete. There is already a host of good books on contemporary leadership, with more arriving on the bookshelves every day. They too are incomplete. What individuals who want to learn about leadership must do is see the myriad available resources on the topic as making up a single dynamic and growing body of knowledge. Thus, if they want to improve their leadership skills, they should use this book as one resource along with others, understanding at the same time that the theories of leadership and their application will advance as more information becomes available.

We hope that the contents of this fourth edition of *Quantum Leadership* stimulate reflection and discussion. We believe that this book extrapolates, in a defensible manner, from current research and practices newer ways of conceiving and exercising the leadership role. At this time, leaders are challenged to take the next step in the journey toward better and more relevant methods of leadership. Those whose lives they affect have a right to expect the best that the leaders have to offer, especially as more is demanded of professionals than ever before. We hope this fourth edition plays some small role in ensuring that those who provide healthcare services get from their leaders what they have every right to expect and as a result the health of our nation is advanced.

—Tim Porter-O'Grady and Kathy Malloch

ACKNOWLEDGMENTS

We wish to acknowledge and thank our leadership colleague Jaynelle Stichler, DNSc, RN, FAAN, for her excellent contribution of chapter-based case studies for each of the topical chapters in this text. Dr. Stichler serves as an exemplar of nursing leadership and leadership practice excellence, as clearly demonstrated in the quality of cases contained in this text.

This fourth edition of *Quantum Leadership* could not have been completed without the support of a good number of people. First, I thank my coauthor, Kathy Malloch, who committed full time and energy to this book and whose collaboration continually encourages me. I also acknowledge the many colleagues in nursing and health care who were both the subject source and the motivation for this book and have much to do with its content. Their encouragement kept us focused on writing a text that is both relevant and useful. Finally, I thank Mark Ponder, RN, for his 38 years of support and partnership, and for being a sign to me that caring, loving, and nursing have nothing to do with gender.

—Tim Porter-O'Grady

The fourth edition of *Quantum Leadership* is the result of insights garnered from our many dedicated readers, and for this we are grateful. We acknowledge and thank our colleagues for their undying dedication to lifelong learning so they can influence and empower others to be the best they can be.

Thank you, Tim, for your friendship and unquestionable support—you are one very special person: a leader, a healer, a thinker, a visionary, and a great colleague. Finally, my greatest thanks and recognition go to my husband, Bryan "Mallotchi," my very best friend and confidant, always encouraging me and tolerating my inconsistencies. Without his unconditional support, my work as a leadership advocate and healer would not be nearly as meaningful.

—Kathy Malloch

CASE STUDY INSTRUCTIONS

The use of case studies in education provides a rich opportunity for students to employ situated cognition in the application of new knowledge when analyzing the case situations in a low-stakes environment. Case study analysis as a teaching method uses abstract conceptualization with active participation and experimentation as the students reflect on each case scenario, applying experiential knowledge learned from personal experience and the new cognitive knowledge from content read in the textbook chapters (Kolb, Boyatzis, & Mainemelis, 2000).

In each chapter, two case studies related to the material are provided. These can be used to facilitate classroom discussion or can be assigned for individual student learning beyond reading the chapter content. Each case study presents real-life situations, complete with complexity, structured controversy, extraneous and pertinent information, emotion, and decisions that need to be made by weighing all possible options and using the new knowledge gained from reading the chapter.

In reviewing each case, students should use critical thinking and problem-solving skills to analyze the case. They can apply principles from the chapter content to identify possible methods to resolve the case or to reflect on personal insights to enrich class discussion.

Students should be encouraged to (1) identify the stakeholders in each case; (2) describe the case situation from the perspective of each stakeholder; (3) apply the chapter's content as a framework for analyzing the case; and (4) determine a course of action to resolve the case, recognizing that there is not one correct answer or best way to resolve each case.

The case studies can be assigned as reflective essays or they can be applied as a framework that students can use to write a case from their own experience. They can present their cases to the class or demonstrate knowledge and application of the chapter's content in class discussion.

The case study analyses amplify the chapter content and engage students in applying the principles to real organizational situations.

References

Kolb, D. A., Boyatzis, R. E., & Mainemelis, C. (2000). Experiential learning theory: Previous research and new directions. In R. J. Sternberg & L. F. Zhang (Eds.), *Perspectives on cognitive, learning and thinking styles*. Hillsdale, NJ: Erlbaum.

CHAPTER ONE

A New Vessel for Leadership: Changing the Health Landscape in an Age of Reform

> The hardest thing is not to get people to accept new ideas; it is to get them to forget old ones.
>
> —*John Maynard Keynes*

Chapter Objectives

www

At the completion of this chapter, the reader will be able to

- Compare the characteristics of the Industrial Age with those of the twenty-first century.
- Enumerate the elements of quantum thinking and explain how quantum thinking has influenced the journey into the Age of Technology and the Age of Health Reform.
- Assess the impact of quantum science and recent advances in technology on health care and clinical practice.
- Describe the implications of Age of Technology thinking on the exercise of leadership in a time of reformatting health care.
- Identify the different skill sets for leaders in contemporary complex organizations.

Transformation continues to be the centerpiece of the future of health care. Ours is an ever-evolving transformative age, filled with a host of inspiring and challenging opportunities that, just a decade ago, were the stuff of science fiction. Who would have thought that this generation would see the advent of fiber optics, satellite-based universities, cloning, customized DNA-based treatment modalities, genomics, lasers, and a myriad of technological innovations that boggle the mind and enthrall the imagination? And who could have imagined that, after an intense, decades-long political and social debate, we would be confronting the vagaries and challenges of implementing significant national health reform?

Along with these many innovations come the challenging adjustments we must make to live in this increasingly digital universe. Instant communication, boundary-less relationships, the globalization of economics and politics, Internet interaction, virtual communication, knowledge that exceeds our capacity to assimilate it—all have a dramatic impact on our ability to thrive in the twenty-first century. For most of us, the changes have come so fast that we don't fully comprehend how they will affect us, and we are hard pressed to cope with their implications.

> ### Key Point
> Communication technology has created a world without boundaries. We now must create our own boundaries in a way that produces a balance among the conflicting demands of our lives.

The pace of change alone—a pace simply unheard of in the last century—is enough to overwhelm even the most energized. As soon as we have the time to consider the particulars of the most recent changes, new changes are upon us and insinuating themselves into our culture. We do not even have the luxury of identifying their advantages and disadvantages and of considering their potential influence on our lives.

Our society, for instance, is just beginning to understand the impact the Web has had and will continue to have on communication, business, and politics. Further, new elements of the Internet already alter how we live our lives and change the questions we ask about what is passing before our very eyes. Yesterday's questions will not be answered because tomorrow has become today sooner than we ever could have imagined.

Leading in a Fluid World

Fluidity has become a characteristic of doing business and managing life in every human arena. Because of the prevalence of accommodating change initiatives, the ability to adjust course has become a necessity. In this context, leadership cannot be the same. Just as the underpinnings of our society, including how we deliver health care, are being radically transformed, so must the leadership necessary to guide people through life. The old models of leadership are no longer adequate to meet the demands of the times. When the world was slower paced and systems theory, complexity theory, and quantum theory were not as well formed or as influential, the nature and role of leadership were different. Even the operational realities of the workplace have changed to the point that work itself requires different skills and a different ethos (**Exhibit 1-1**).

Exhibit 1-1   New Versus Old Skill Sets

Knowledge Worker	Employee (Former Type)
• Conceptual synthesis	• Functional analysis
• Competent care	• Manual dexterity
• Multiple "intelligences"	• Fixed skill set
• Mobile skill set	• Process value
• Outcome practice	• Process practice
• Team performance	• Unilateral performance

The stable institutions of the twentieth century have been supplanted as we more deeply understand the framework for the twenty-first century. The brick-and-mortar empires of the past are breaking up, replaced by a growing digital architecture as work moves away from institutions altogether. The infrastructure of society is becoming less institutional and more information based, and the architecture of our places of work, service, and business is changing dramatically. Information structures are primarily relational and function collaterally and in multimodal ways, whereas most of our business structures have historically functioned vertically. Leading in a complex multimodal work culture is radically different from leading in a predominantly vertical or linear work culture.

In the Industrial Age, organizations were primarily fixed, finite, and functional. Work in the Industrial Age was based on Newtonian principles, and from the beginning of the twentieth century, when Frederick Taylor laid down the foundations of scientific management, to the late 1960s, business organizations were structured mechanistically and hierarchically. Even the management theorists of the 1930s, 1940s, and 1950s did not radically alter basic organizational design. Historically, the worker has mostly been considered a subset of the work. Most training was gained on the job, and the apprenticeship model used for training was essentially hierarchical as well. The organization owned the work and set the rules. Communication and decision making traveled up and down the corporate ladder: The higher up the ladder, the greater a person's authority and autonomy. At the bottom were the workers who performed most of the functions—under the control of those who had moved "upward." Although attention was paid to both the work and the worker, this attention was barely reflected in the management structure and the application of leadership in organizations.

> **Point to Ponder**
>
> The worker is increasingly in control. The knowledge necessary to get work done is now mostly in the hands of those who do the work. Because the workplace is becoming more dependent on knowledgeable workers, a major shift in power and control has occurred, and the old structures are now in conflict with this new type of worker.

But this is no longer the case in contemporary work systems. In the current world of work, it is not the organization but the worker who owns the work. The character of work changed substantially at the end of the twentieth century—it became increasingly technical and complex, often called "knowledge work"—and now individuals usually need to be trained for jobs before they become eligible for them. Indeed, they are expected to arrive "on the run" and start contributing from the outset. Further, organizations' increased dependence on knowledge workers has created a new power equation, shifting the locus of control from the organization to the worker.

In the Industrial Age, leadership (Murphy & Riggio, 2003) meant being a good manager, guiding one's subordinates like a good parent, and directing their activities in the interests of the organization. The critical skills were those required for planning, organizing, leading, implementing, controlling, and evaluating (note the acronym constructed from these six words: POLICE). The ability to function well and undertake well-defined processes was the basis of every role. Good performance and a sense of responsibility were highly valued, strongly encouraged, and heavily rewarded.

Exhibit 1-2   Work Life Reality Shift

Old Reality	New Reality
• Scripted lives	• Own your script
• Unlimited resources	• Finite resources
• Fixed functions	• Tightness of fit
• Employee	• Stakeholder/member
• Fixed jobs	• Fluid roles
• Promotion	• Mobility

So was compliance with the expectations of the workplace. Organizational leaders used vertical communication and command strategies exclusively to ensure that the workplace stayed focused and orderly and that the work was performed efficiently. They also refined hierarchical mechanisms and fostered congruence of workplace behavior in whatever way they could.

In this industrial context the first contemporary notions of leadership developed. A whole host of approaches to understanding leadership and acting as a leader emerged during the past century, and each one reflected prevailing notions of work and workplace organization (**Exhibit 1-2**). These various approaches helped to create the current framework for leadership, both in the realms of action and decision making.

Newton and Organizational Design

Newtonian mechanics had a tremendous influence on twentieth-century science and business. In particular, Newton's model of the physical universe influenced social theorists to view social relationships, roles, and work as highly mechanistic. The reason that this mechanistic framework was so pervasive was its clarity and simplicity, linear structure and coherence, and its generalized agreement with people's notions of common sense. Especially appealing was its dependence on reductionism, the tenet that any complex phenomenon could be understood simply by reducing it to its smallest components and analyzing it compartmentally. This linear simplicity was especially appealing to business and organizational leaders and was embraced by them with great veracity in ways that would define the structure of work to this very day. As a result, entrepreneurs and organizational gurus constructed models of work in which work activities were highly compartmentalized, and they succeeded in spreading the use of these models throughout the world. Subsequently, work was generally designed with efficiency and effectiveness in mind, and special attention was paid to individual performance as a means of ensuring that the work was done as planned.

> ### Key Point
> In the twentieth century the focus of work was on performing the right processes. In the twenty-first century the focus is on obtaining the right outcomes.

Also, twentieth-century organizations focused on the assumption that by constructing work processes properly, they would produce products and services of consistently good quality. Here again, the organizational literature of

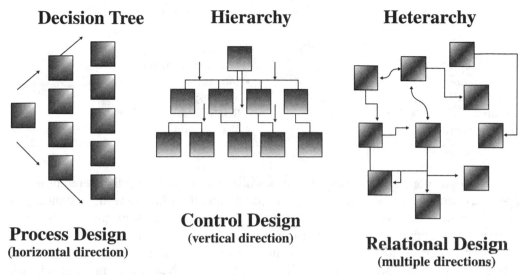

Figure 1-1 Changing Organizational Models.

the time reflected a reductionist model. The organizational gurus viewed organizations as being essentially the same as always, although differing in structure in minor ways and characterized by an increased degree of control over employees. As Peter Drucker pointed out, the cornerstone of most twentieth-century organizations was control, as indicated by the "line and box" approach to configuring the workplace (Edersheim & Drucker, 2007) (see **Figure 1-1**).

Group Discussion

We are living on the cusp of the transition between two health systems, and life in the Age of Health Reform will differ substantially from life in the traditional tertiary care system. The changes that will occur include changes in clinical work and leadership. Brainstorm at least 10 changes that will occur in health reform (under the Patient Protection and Affordable Care Act [PPACA]) over this next decade and discuss their implications for leaders.

Eclipsing the Industrial Age

For the past 30 years or so, the standard models of work and the underpinnings of society have been shifting radically. The impact of our burgeoning technology has brought about a new construct for social structures and relationships across the whole human landscape. Quantum theory, refined and applied since the middle of the twentieth century, has helped to create newer technologies that affect life from the molecular to the global levels (Sreekantan & National Institute of Advanced Studies, 2009).

Exhibit 1-3   Conceptual Foundations

Newtonian
- Mass production
- Compartmentalism
- Reductionism
- Analysis
- Discrete action

Quantum
- Envision the whole
- Integration
- Synthesis
- Relatedness
- Team action

For example, consider the computer chip, which has single-handedly altered human experience forever. Among other things, it brought about a whole new understanding of quantum principles and changed the very foundations of social life by connecting people in a new way. Further, we now live with the knowledge that everything is linked and that events in one part of the universe have some kind of impact on events in other parts. Our understanding of the linkages among all experiences is the basis for complexity science and has led to changes in the conceptual foundations of the sciences and their social application (**Exhibit 1-3**).

In turn, these changes have raised the level of conflict surrounding basic issues, ranging from the existence and nature of God to ethical and social norms. Claims that once seemed beyond question are now open to investigation and continuous challenge. New scientific discoveries have substantial religious, philosophical, and ethical implications and have caused social discomfort among those holding more traditional beliefs (Volti, 2010).

It is into this equation that organizational leaders are now thrust. The problem is that they too are experiencing the conflict endemic to the times. Most leaders have spent the majority of their lives leading in Industrial Age models, just as everyone else has. They too are confronting newer realities with beliefs and practices acquired in the past. They too are struggling to make sense of the changes occurring globally. As an additional challenge to adapting to these changes, they must also lead others to adapt successfully to a whole new model guiding human organization, relationship, and behavior. Furthermore, the related discoveries and innovations are occurring faster than the rate of adaptation. As soon as one change is accommodated, another occurs, requiring a different response (Nickerson, 2010).

Group Discussion

Healthcare providers at the beginning of the Age of Health Reform (PPACA) must be willing to leave some things behind (because they will cease to have value) and to take on some new things. List some of the practices, habits, rituals, or routines that need to be left behind, and discuss symbolic acts or events that could be used to help let go of these formally. What replaces some of these "old" practices?

Change Is

Quantum theory has taught us that change is not a thing or an event but rather a dynamic that is constitutive of the universe. Change cannot be avoided because it is everywhere, but we can influence its circumstances and consequences. In short, we can give it direction. This notion of constant change reflects foundations in quantum mechanics that suggest that matter is constantly moving in the universe and can even be in more than one place at one time while taking different forms. Quantumness is almost counterintuitive and reflects characteristics and dynamics of matter and energy that don't fit any logical, ordered, structured understanding of them.

Schrödinger, a mid-twentieth-century physicist, used his famous "Schrödinger's Box" thought experiment to show two prevailing realities operating at any given time, actual reality and potential reality. Actual reality is that which currently occupies our immediate attention. Potential reality, on the other hand, although current and present, is not yet experienced. Being still potential, it is waiting for the right moment to become expressed and thus actual.

Potential reality is the realm in which leadership takes form. The leader's role is to engage with the unfolding reality, perceive it, even predict it, note its demands and implications, translate it for others, and finally guide others into actions to meet the demands of a reality not quite present. This leader must be comfortable with the ambiguity of the "in between," that is, living in two realities, that which is ending and that which is emerg-

> ### Point to Ponder
>
> A stop sign can be used to illustrate potential reality. When first seen, it notifies a driver to stop—but not immediately. The sign is a real object, a reality, and it does require a real response. The driver's preparation to stop is the first in the chain of actions, and it is this action that links the actual to the potential.

ing. Demonstrating this comfort with the journey provides a frame for leading others through the chaos and uncertainty of constant change.

In this transformational time between two paradigms, the leader's primary role is to live fully in the realm of potential reality. The leader is not so much an operational expert and problem solver as a good "signpost reader." To be effective, the leader must anticipate the path of change and then spell it out for those who are moving their own activities, knowingly or unknowingly, in the same direction as the change is taking form (Yang & Shan, 2008).

The Transition Between Ages

Age changes do not occur quickly. Such changes generally occur over two or three decades. The challenge is not to become "stuck" in the no-man's-land between an extinguishing life script and an emerging one. The dynamics of a substantive change are moving in concert to create the underpinnings for a comprehensive transition (Bridges, 2002) from one way of living to another. This has occurred several times in human history. From the Middle Ages through the Age of Enlightenment and the Industrial Age

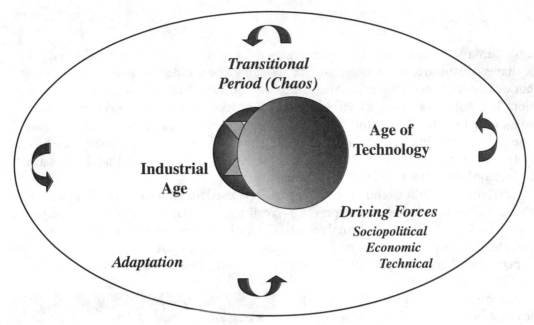

Figure 1-2 The Universal Cycle of Transformation.

and up to the current era, which we might dub the Digital Age (or the Information Age), historic indicators have presaged major shifts in human experience (**Figure 1-2**).

There is an important difference, though, between previous shifts and the one that is now occurring. In hindsight, the significance of previous shifts quickly became clear, even if it was rarely apparent during the critical transition points. Today, on the other hand, the period between predicting future changes and confronting their unfolding is too brief to allow plans to be made to accommodate them. Indeed, today's leaders act as agents of change, but, like everyone else, they must also undergo the changes themselves virtually at the same time as they perceive them. Wholly new leadership skills are required to manage in this kind of a world.

Think for a moment about some of the ways in which the script of life is being rewritten for all of us:

- The Web is now a primary business tool, and it is fundamentally altering how business gets done.
- Fiber optics, in conjunction with satellite technology, has connected the world into a seamless communications network in which information can be transmitted instantly from any place on the globe to any other place.
- Information has thus become highly portable, and, given the developments in shipping, everyone has access to almost anything they want or need from anywhere in the world.
- Technology has enabled communication and interaction to become increasingly more portable as chips have become smaller and digital devices have become packed with technology and applications in lighter, smaller, more portable hardware.

- Each person has control over any relationship, personal or business, and can personalize any interaction within any context at any time and in any way he or she desires.
- Miniaturization has made it possible for people to be mobile and still remain connected to everything and everyone. Furthermore, it has made innovations in service, communication, information, and health care faster, easier, and less expensive to implement than ever before.
- Globalization has created a world community and removed traditional boundaries between people, be they political, social, or physical. The recognition of the mobility of human experience and of work has created a new virtual and global landscape for human action.

These are just a very small sample of the transformations that are occurring. And these transformations are only the beginning. Even so, they have a major impact on our understanding, on the way we live and relate, and, of course, on the way we work.

Imagine the lives of our great-grandparents or even our grandparents and how different our lives are from theirs as a result of these technologies (keep in mind, for example, there were no cell phones before 1986). Then, consider the possibility that the children of current teenagers might never write or read as we have, interact and play as we have, relate to each other or travel as we have. And remember, this generation is currently ushering in a new way of living and working as the baby boom generation begins to retire.

In short, our generation is a transitional generation—the last generation of the Industrial Age and the generation on the cusp of the Digital Age. We are in essence the bridge between two ways of experiencing the world (compare digital immigrants to digital natives). What we do now lays the groundwork for a future that will look nothing like the world most of us have known.

Group Discussion

List dramatic discoveries and inventions that occurred during the past century and compare the way life changed as a consequence with the way life changed during the preceding millennium. Then, discuss the technological changes occurring in the first decades of the twenty-first century that affect the future of health reform and care delivery.

Leading Change

It is important that leaders be aware of the transformative work that defines their role. The Digital Age now calls for leaders to perceive their role differently and to express it in ways that best fit the characteristics of emerging sociotechnical culture (**Figure 1-3**).

The role of today's leaders is to encourage this transformation. Indeed, they must make a commitment to the journey and work hard to incorporate the changes in their lives in a very personal way. In other words, rather than simply suggesting that everyone and

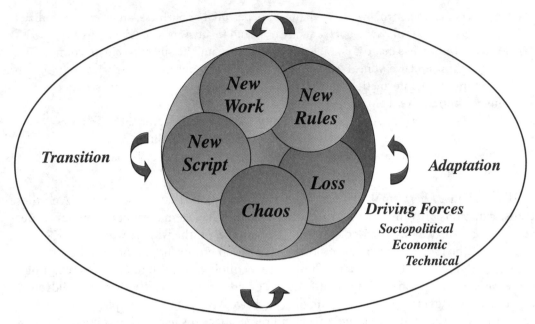

Figure 1-3 Universal Dynamics of Transformation.

Point to Ponder

The behavior of leaders must exemplify their commitment to sustain their own journey and to coordinate and facilitate the efforts of others to build a desired future.

everything must change, they must lead by example. They must serve as witnesses to the changes and show others how to adapt to the changes in their own lives.

In the initial stage of this transformation, leaders must be able to show that the coming changes represent a critical shift and must, through their passion for movement, inspire responses from others. This is not the time for complacency but for truth telling and confrontation. In short, it is a time to inform people how the changes make a substantial difference in their lives and in their work. Advancing people's awareness of this requires a level of honesty and directness once thought to be confrontational.

In the case of health care, the major reforms under way will lead to the end of the hospital-based sickness-oriented model of service delivery. Our technologies enable us to treat illnesses at an earlier stage and reduce the need for costly surgical interventions. As a consequence, not only physicians but also nurses and other health professionals must make substantial changes in the way they practice their professions and provide services. The introduction of value-driven approaches that focus on early engagement, attaining the highest level of personal health, prevention rather than treatment, and designing the system to provide a continuum of health services represents an effective model of health service (Birk, 2013).

Leaders in health care must help people sever their attachment to the kind of health-care system with which they have become comfortable. Health reform calls us all to focus on accountability, early engagement, prevention, cost-effectiveness, and a higher level of aggregate health for all citizens. So many health professionals are mourning the loss of what is passing away or has passed away. In some cases, their sense of loss is understandable, but most of what they mourn for *should not* be retained or brought back. That was then; this is now. Some of the factors that attracted many of us to health care have vanished for good. The question is not whether they will return, but how to adapt to the new circumstances and new models of health service.

Healthcare leaders must try to engage others in the process of making their own changes. They must take whatever action is necessary to impress upon health professionals that this is a time of great mobility and of shifting foundations. In particular, they must call all stakeholders to the table to work out what must be altered and what must be introduced to fashion a new healthcare delivery system. A great tragedy will occur if healthcare leaders are unsuccessful in this task and allow stakeholders simply to react to changes long since past. Complacency guarantees failure.

Leaders may be victims of their own insights and past successes, which can cause them to use an outdated recipe for success as well as misleading measures of success. They must see the approaching challenges within the context of their becoming, not through the eyes of past triumphs.

Not only must leaders close the door on the old models of health delivery and clinical work, but they must turn around and face the future, viewing the entire landscape to develop a workable vision. Often, healthcare leaders are too shortsighted, and their vision too tenuous. The conditions that determine the future of health care are vastly different from anything that we have experienced to date, and thus leaders must construct a radical vision of how services will be provided in the new healthcare landscape. The

> **Key Point**
>
> Moving into a reformed health system does not mean leaving everything behind. It does mean thinking about what needs to be left behind and reflecting on what should go with us as we move into an age with a different set of parameters.

impact of micronization, genomics, biotherapeutics, chemotherapeutics, and new economic and service delivery models is forever altering Western medicine (**Exhibit 1-4**), and so the structures that support the provision of Western medicine also need to change. The brick-and-mortar infrastructure and the current administrative and operational

---

Exhibit 1-4   Changing Medical Therapies

Old Therapies	New Therapies
• Surgery	• Lasers
• Salves and creams, drugs	• Microsurgery
• Accommodation	• Genomics
• Nothing can be done	• Pharmaceuticals
• Treatments	• Chemotherapy
• Enemas	• Radiotherapy
• Bloodletting	• Synthetic products
• General supplements	• Specified supplements

---

frameworks are no longer entirely relevant, and they must be adjusted in response to financial, political, and technological pressures of a changing healthcare system. Imagine how painful that message is for the serious and talented men and women who have devoted their lives to building their image of the healthcare system. The requirement to tear it apart and begin anew is overwhelming to them, but they are called to this task by the changes that have already occurred and those anticipated as we refine and unfold health reform over the next two decades.

> **Key Point**
>
> The greatest impediment to future success is past success.

Healthcare leaders must be able to communicate to others their vision of the future and bring as much energy and commitment to the reformation of the healthcare system as possible. They need to capture the hearts and minds of all health professionals and other stakeholders in the healthcare system by being relentless communicators and forever challenging current ways of thinking and doing. They must push against the walls of thought and work to ensure that stakeholders are fully engaged in critiquing what they do, building sustainable service partnerships, assessing the product of their work, and questioning whether what they are doing is congruent with the changing demands placed on them. Every stakeholder must continually examine the appropriateness of current work rituals and routines and determine what should be retained and what should be left behind as no longer relevant. The job of the leaders is to raise questions about the efficacy and effectiveness of current work processes and whether they are meeting new and emerging expectations for value-driven health care.

The most important task of healthcare leaders is to communicate their vision, not so much by their words but by their behavior. If the leaders cannot respond appropriately to the demand for change, others will not be able to either.

> **Key Point**
>
> The leader is an agent of change, responsible for providing others with a vision of change and ensuring that their response to the demand for change is appropriate.

Their next most important task is to anticipate the blocks in the way of substantive change. Implementing any planned modification requires the integration of numerous activities and people, and thus faces many embedded obstacles. The most notable are elements of the organizational structure, which itself acts as insulation from the demand for reform. One of the first jobs of a leader acting as a change agent is to diffuse the power of these elements and thus remove a large barrier to concerted and dramatic action on the part of the stakeholders.

Leaders must be aware that people have devoted their lives to avoiding the prospect of change and that one person dedicated to blocking change can bring the entire change process to a grinding halt. Change avoiders or resisters must be identified, challenged, worked with, empowered, and placed in the midst of the change process so that they do not impede the ability of the organization to thrive. The entrenchment of behavior and structures that reward these behaviors provide the greatest barriers to meaningful change in health care and contribute to the decline in the system. There is nothing more tragic for society than the desperate stranglehold on a system in need of great change by leaders who benefit by delaying or avoiding the necessary shifts. These leaders cease to be relevant or viable and actively contribute to the overwhelming onset of great decline and ultimate failure.

Because the transition from one age to another is a long-term process, leaders must continually set short-term goals to give stakeholders a sense of movement and accomplishment. The attainment of short-term goals enables stakeholders to mark their journey forward and visualize and celebrate the process of change. It also gives them a moment of respite and reflection and helps them gather the energy necessary for the next stage.

Leaders must look at change not as an event but as a journey—a never-ending journey. Every point of arrival, in other words, is also a point of departure. Therefore, leaders must carefully balance periods of effort and action with periods of rest and celebration so that stakeholders will be regularly refreshed and reenergized to meet future challenges.

Finally, change is experienced on a personal level and on a cultural level. And culture always rules. This truism must be solidly rooted in the mind of every leader engaged in transforming an organization. The task is to prove to workers that the modifications will improve their work or the workplace. Today's workers are faithful, not to the workplace, but to their work. They know they can take their skills elsewhere and be welcomed. Leaders must thus be aware of the demands regarding work that exist within the prevailing culture. Incorporating symbolic and cultural norms in the language and process of change helps cast it into a form that workers can understand and value. Every wise leader knows the political realities pertaining to a change process and adapts the process in light of them so that the needs of key stakeholders are met adequately and stakeholders can devote their efforts to implementing and sustaining the process.

Group Discussion

Along with the nature of work, the characteristics of workers are changing. Discuss how the times have an impact on the culture of the workplace and the characteristics of workers (especially knowledge workers), compare the characteristics of younger and older workers, and explore the issues that arise when both types of workers must perform together.

Quantum Age Requisites

Quantum realities are characterized by many new patterns and processes such as those described in this section.

Linear Thinking Is Now Replaced by Relational and Whole-Systems Thinking

Perhaps the most radical shift to occur is the move away from mechanistic (Newtonian) and reductionist models of thought and research. In the twentieth century, most research was based on vertical, reductionist (or linear) processes. Quantum science, in contrast,

13

has an affinity for complexity and uncertainty. The use of complex relational algorithms has lessened the former devotion to vertical and reductionist processing, and relational and whole-systems models now constitute a new foundation for scientific and business research. Because researchers can rapidly process and relate complex arrays of data, they can use different processes for making decisions and creating new products and technologies, such as computer chips, synthetics, bioceuticals and pharmaceuticals, and DNA-moderated clinical therapeutics.

Structure Is About Wholes, Not Parts

Our newly acquired capacity for discovering and understanding the critical vitality of linkages and intersections has made it clear to us that at some level everything is inter-dependent. Further, our knowledge of the interconnectedness of everything causes us to look differently not just at the physical components of the universe, but also at organiza-tions and human interactions (**Exhibit 1-5**). This is not to say, of course, that we always fully comprehend the nature of the interdependence among any particular elements, but we do recognize its significance.

Our understanding of the design of fractals, for example, is critical for comprehending the order that exists in chaos and for appreciating the impact of complexity on organi-zations and human behavior. The smallest level of a single organization and the most complex array of a large, aggregated system containing the organization are connected inexorably, as demonstrated through the power of fractals ($Z_{n+1} = Z_N^2 + C$).

If you have ever looked at a hologram, which is a three-dimensional photograph of an image, you may have noticed that no matter what size section you focus on, the entire image is present in the smaller piece. Holography thus can be used to explain the nature of fractals because in a fractal the complete pattern is present in any component regardless of the level of detail or complexity. A tree is a good example from the so-called natural world because its overall structure, including the trunk and branches, is similar to the branching pattern of each leaf (the fractal effect).

Exhibit 1-5   The Language of Complexity and Chaos

New words from the science of complex systems describe a world different from that which we have grown familiar. They express a whole set of dynamics that operate just outside our field of vision, yet they have a defining impact on our experience of life and the human journey in which we each play an important but not always known role. Some of the more unusual words include these:

- *Autopoiesis:* The process by which living systems continually seek to renew and reinvent them-selves, yet maintain their core integrity.
- *Autocatalysis:* A process in which information enters into a system in small fluctuations that continually grow in strength, interacting with the system and feeding back upon itself.
- *Dissipative structures:* Structures in which disorder is the source of order and vice versa. In this "dance" between order and disorder, old form ends and new form begins.
- *Strange attractor:* The activity of a collective chaotic system composed of interactive feedback between and among its various parts and evidencing attraction to its pattern of behavior.

Fractals have tremendous implications for organizations. From the smallest structural elements to the very complex patterns of behavior that exist throughout an organization, the same patterns appear and are played out in precise detail. This fact implies that at every level of the organization there exists a self-organizing capacity and that this capacity maintains a balance and harmony even in the midst of the most apparently chaotic processes. To the extent that the balance and harmony are sustained, the organization's life is advanced. To the extent that they are upset or cannot be well articulated, visualized, and acted on at every level of leadership, the organization's actions tend to impede its inherent integrity and effectiveness. It is important, therefore, that the leaders of the organization are aware of the continuous and dynamic action, the fractal effect, in all organizational behavior and structure so that they can advance the consonance and value of the organization members' activities and enhance the organization's ability to fulfill its mission continuously.

Perhaps it is even more important for leaders to recognize that, within the context of the fractals' dynamic action, their own actions have cascading and rippling implications throughout the organization. In fact, they should understand that no decision, action, or undertaking can occur in the organization without ultimately having an impact on every other action, decision, and undertaking. In addition, once they are cognizant of the web of interaction and interdependence that exists in the organization, leaders will approach deliberation and decision making only with extreme care, caution, and thoroughness.

Issues of relationship, interaction, empowerment, and ownership have become increasingly pertinent in our understanding of the nature of work. We now view individuals rather than organizations as owning the work processes, and this change in our understanding has altered the relationship between workplace and worker. Further, by focusing on different descriptors in portraying how human dynamic systems work and how processes get sustained, we have created a new framework for considering design and function within the workplace and within the entire human community. The new framework also enables us to consider what is and is not effective in the workplace and in relationships among people as well as issues of accountability, productivity, and value.

For example, no longer is it enough for leaders to assess the functional proficiency of individual workers as a way of determining whether a work process is fully effective and sustainable. Instead, they must also examine whether each worker's competence and efforts fit with the competence and efforts of other workers. "Goodness of fit," not the individual proficiency of any single

> ## Key Point
>
> Competence is not about having skills, but about using skills to achieve desired outcomes.

participant, leads to effectiveness and sustainability. Imagine the impact of this understanding on measures of productivity and performance.

The Value of Work Is a Function of the Outcome, Not Just the Process

In the last 30 years, our understanding of the value of work has shifted. In the past, the focus of clinical work was on the excellence of process, and the existence of a good work process was taken to indicate good service. We now recognize that process is not the only determinant of good service. Indeed, a work process derives its value from the purpose toward which it is directed (the desired outcome), and if the purpose does not inform and discipline the process, the process can lose its value (we must learn to create goodness-of-fit between process and outcome).

Work is not inherently valuable, despite the Judeo-Christian ethic. Consider how many people who say that their work provides meaning in their life find their life to be pointless when the function and content of the work shift. What they forgot is that work is not meaningful in itself but becomes meaningful when it fulfills an important purpose. People sometimes feel burned out when they seek the meaning that should drive the work inside the work activity itself. When the work changes they cannot cope because they experience the end of a way of working as well as an end of meaning. The problem is that their "how" has become their "why," and their means have become their ends.

> ### Point to Ponder
>
> Work is not inherently valuable. Instead, it is valuable to the extent it fulfills a purpose. Therefore, the main focus should be on whether the work achieves real value, not on the work itself.

Process is not always connected to outcome and hence to value. Nurses and physicians, particularly, have a hard time understanding this. Sometimes their commitment to treating patients is not disciplined by the recognition that the value of any treatment activity lies in the final outcome or impact. Indeed, they often provide health services in cases where there is little evidence that the services dependably result in a right outcome. Medical practice variance accounts for billions of dollars a year in healthcare expenditures. In the future, the connection between process and product—between particular treatments and their outcomes—will play a more significant role in the management of healthcare resources and the valuing of health services.

Technology Has Changed What People Do, How They Live, and Who They Are

When we view the technological advances of our time objectively, it is difficult not to marvel. Many inventions that first appeared in science fiction have been realized in the past few decades; obviously, many innovations are yet to come, including some that will alter the very structure of life. Frightening as it may be, for the first time in human history we can manipulate our own evolution and that of every other species on the earth.

Healthcare leaders need to realize that technology is transforming the very basis of health care for the first time since the development of germ theory. Genomics and related sciences are shifting the therapeutic framework for health care, probably for the rest of the century (Klug & Ward, 2012). How many of us can provide leadership in a postgenomic healthcare system? How many of us really know what that means?

Certainly, health care will depend less on the use of highly mechanical interventions, especially surgical interventions. The advances in bio-, chemo-, and pharmacotherapeutics enable many conditions that required traditional surgery to be handled more easily and less invasively through modern therapies. Even Alzheimer's disease will become a more treatable illness before the end of the decade. The question is, what are

---

Exhibit 1-6   Seven New Age Imperatives

1. Value-driven health service models
2. Medicine/nursing based on genomics
3. Mass-customized diagnosis and treatment
4. User-specific insurance programs
5. Integration of allopathic and alternative therapies
6. Payment incentives tied to outcomes (quality)
7. Focused service settings for specific populations

---

the implications of the switch to new therapeutic modalities, especially for the treatment of older persons and when the new modalities replace traditional institutional models of treatment (**Exhibit 1-6**)?

Leaders will have to grapple with these emerging realities and incorporate them into their own lives. Most people find it difficult, if not impossible, to imagine what the new technologies will mean for life in the second and third decades of the twenty-first century, despite wanting to embrace them. They need help in grasping how the technologies will affect them and what adjustments they must now make to thrive in the continually emerging digital reality (Brown, 2009).

New Rules Will Apply In the New Age

Imagine not just learning to live within the context of a whole new set of rules but leading others to embrace these rules in their own lives and work. This is the fundamental leadership task—dealing with the same changes as everyone while helping others thrive in a new reality. What makes this even more challenging is that people are inclined to reject the implications of the changes that are occurring.

Several late-twentieth-century innovations are still having a powerful impact on people's lives and on their relationship with health professionals and other service providers. These innovations include the Internet, wireless communication, fiber optics and lasers, the cloud (which helps manage large and dense information repositories), and technologies that enable these groups to converge around new clinical technologies, therapeutics, and drugs. The Internet, for example, not only has influenced global communications but also has altered the way business is conducted. For a couple of decades now, people shop without leaving home and even without any human contact. Using the many vehicles of social media, they can access a wide variety of people and information, including information they once needed to visit a library or a professional expert to get. When people meet with their doctors (often digitally), they might already have accessed health information from other sources, have questions and concerns they want to discuss, and can share the digital media they are accessed virtually in real time. The Internet, in other words, is helping to shift the locus of control from providers of health services to users, and it is also affects the patient–provider relationship in the following ways:

- Patients now determine the parameters of the patient–provider relationship, setting the stage for a different kind of interaction than has historically occurred.

- Patients are developing partnerships with providers to sort through the available choices and pick the best. They need providers to act as navigators and educators who are willing to assist them in making healthcare decisions.
- Patients need help from providers both in verifying the accuracy of the data they have gathered independently from a host of sources and in interpreting the data.
- Patients are interested in options, not orders to undergo particular treatments. They want to be able to consider a range of options within the context of their personal values and priorities and to choose the one option that fits best.
- Providers now need to be concerned with what patients know and can do in regard to controlling their own health decisions in a "user-driven" world. More of the responsibility for health care will be placed on patients and their loved ones. Providers must now transfer skills to others and share the ownership of care with others.

Although the locus of control has shifted to patients (users), essentially patients are undereducated about health care. Still, ready or not, they now must take command of their own care and acquire whatever skills they need to manage it. The current role of providers in a reforming health system is to ensure that patients/users not only have the proper tools and skills but actually succeed at managing their own care. Consequently, providers need to alter their priorities. Rather than intervening medically and providing care themselves, they now frequently help their patients to make proper health-related decisions and to learn how to perform necessary self-care tasks. To a certain extent, they are becoming health service agents/navigators, assisting their patients in obtaining the equipment and services they and their patients have determined are needed or desirable.

Health Care Will Be Provided Earlier Than in the Past

Over this next century bio-, chemo-, and pharmacotherapeutics will come to dominate the health services landscape. Because technology will enable healthcare providers to assess a person's DNA and physiology in ever-greater detail, diseases will be identified sooner than they are now. Diagnostics will make it possible to predict with high levels of accuracy a person's degree of risk for particular diseases and conditions. Preventive treatment will be supplied before symptoms manifest, and detailed, highly customized clinical services will be configured specifically to fit individual DNA characteristics.

Health professionals must ask, how will the improvements in diagnostics and therapeutics alter the practice of medicine? In the past, generally medical and nursing interventions required patients to be hospitalized. The therapies of the future will require much less hospitalization and will hardly impede patients' normal routines. The main goals of health professionals will be to provide the right therapy at the right time and to educate people about their life processes, their health, their choices (including medical and lifestyle choices), and the risks associated with each choice. As these become prevalent realities for service and economies of scale are reached, cost-effectiveness and value can be more adequately assessed and appropriate financial choices can be made.

The largest two groups of health professionals, nurses and physicians, have much to accomplish in the next two decades if they are to successfully make the transition to a digitally driven, value-grounded, reformed health system. Their clinical roles will change

Group Discussion

In the transition between ages, consumers' expectations regarding their role in healthcare decisions and processes are changing. Discuss the changes and describe the role of health professionals in helping consumers develop the insights and skills they need to manage their own health effectively, especially in the Age of Health Reform. Also, discuss the dangers of consumers making their own decisions, as well as the actions that healthcare leaders can take now and in the future to mitigate the dangers and ensure that consumers become accountable decision makers.

substantially during this period, and getting these groups to converge around a new way of addressing prevention, education, and service delivery will be challenging and a tumultuous experience for healthcare leaders. Leaders will require extreme diligence as well as a skill set that stretches their resources to the limit. To design the future, leaders must understand the current landscape and how it differs from the familiar territory of past experience.

The Context in Which Leadership Is Applied Is Undergoing Changes

From deconstructing infrastructure to confronting "new age" workers, leaders have a new set of tasks before them—tasks they are not fully prepared to address. For most leaders, most of the foundations of their understanding and expression of the nature of leadership were formed in the early and middle twentieth century and reflect outmoded models. During the last third of the twentieth century, newer models of leadership and its application emerged. These models are based on new ideas about organizational structure and managing people and processes (**Exhibit 1-7**).

In the past, organizations were built on the Newtonian principles of mechanistic functioning, compartmentalization, and vertical control (**Exhibit 1-8**). The dominant theme of Newtonian thinking is that the universe is simply one vast machine. In fact, Newton saw the universe as a sort of giant clock that could be explained in mechanistic terms, and he and his followers took the goal of physics to be the discovery of the laws that supposedly govern the parts of the universe (material particles and the

> **Key Point**
>
> People no longer have to undergo a hospital stay to obtain most medical services. More than 50% of medical treatments do not require hospitalization, and with health reform that figure will rise to more than 70%.

bodies of which they are constituents). Almost all scientific progress of the late nineteenth century and the first half of the twentieth century was grounded in Newtonian concepts.

The kind of mechanistic explanation favored by Newtonians has not accounted for human behavior and other patterns of activity in the universe, however. Even in the early decades of the twentieth century, questions were raised about the adequacy of Newtonian physics to explain the incongruous and apparently messy underpinnings of the universe.

Exhibit 1-7   The Major Tasks of the Twenty-First-Century Healthcare Leader

- Deconstructing the barriers and structures of the twentieth century
- Alerting staff about the implications of changing what they do
- Establishing safety around taking risks and experimenting
- Embracing new technologies as a way of doing work
- Reading the signposts along the road to the future
- Translating the emerging reality of health reform into language the staff can use
- Demonstrating personal engagement with health reform
- Helping others adapt to the demands of a value-driven health system
- Creating a safe milieu for the struggles and pain of changing practice and service
- Enumerating small successes as a basis for supporting staff
- Celebrating the journey and all progress made

Exhibit 1-8   Newtonian Characteristics

- Vertical orientation
- Hierarchical structures
- Focus on control
- Reductionistic scientific processes
- Top-down decision making
- Mechanistic models of design
- Process-driven action

Biology, perhaps, has offered the best evidence that not everything works mechanistically and that the universe is rife with chaos and incongruities.

Quantum theory and other more recent scientific theories have had a large impact on contemporary theories of leadership. Many of the elements of traditional leadership grew out of a Newtonian/industrial framework, especially those focusing on hierarchical control. Indeed, during the twentieth century organizational leaders tended to rely on vertical hierarchies and compartmentalization of activities to manage people and productivity, and the structures of their organizations reflected this tendency. The rise of quantum theory and the new appreciation of complexity and complex adaptive systems as foundational characteristics of the universe have changed our views of science and of life (**Exhibit 1-9**). Many mistakenly believe that all that has occurred has been a shift in

Group Discussion

Describe the core concepts of Newtonian thinking and how these concepts were manifested during the twentieth century. Consider, for example, how social institutions and structures reflected the commitment to Newtonian thinking and how Newtonian thinking influenced the leadership role.

Exhibit 1-9   Quantum Characteristics

- Multifocal characteristics
- Nonlinear structures
- Focus on relatedness
- Multisystems scientific processes
- Center-out decision making
- Complexity-based models of design
- Value-driven action

---

focus from physics to biology, but this way of looking at matter itself reflects a kind of compartmentalism. Rather, what people are beginning to understand is that all elements of the universe are a part of a broad system of intersections and relationships.

The major shifts in scientific thinking challenge all our current theories of leadership. What we once thought were the foundations of leadership are now being subjected to further exploration and clarification. Vertical control and managing ritual and routine, for instance, are no longer seen as effective processes for leadership, and the rules governing relationships and interactions within organizations have been forever altered. Further, we now recognize that the patterns of relationships in an organization are just as important as the relationships themselves or what lies within the related elements. Leaders must understand and apply these newer notions if their organizations are to thrive internally and externally (Tait & Richardson, 2010).

Leaders Must Replace Traditional Leadership Models with Models That Reflect the New Framework

The current literature on leadership contains a large array of concepts that suggest a whole new framework for action. Foremost among these is the concept of complexity and the view that everything is related. In this view, the interactions among the parts of a system are critical to the system's productivity and ultimately its sustainability (Yang & Shan, 2008). The main leadership task, then, is not so much to manage function or work, but instead to coordinate the elements (e.g., the workers) and facilitate the relationship between work and worker at every organizational level.

Leaders must maintain a panoramic view of the world to discern the direction their efforts should take. Their ability to see intersections, relationships, and themes ensures that the organization will undertake the activities it needs to thrive.

In the Industrial Age, leaders were concerned most of all with function and operation. The work was compartmentalized, and the focus was on the activities of the individual employee. The employee's work life was regulated by a set of job obligations, and by meeting these obligations, the employee was able to advance upward, receive better pay, or obtain other rewards. A performance evaluation system might have been in place to assess the employee's proficiency, and any rewards given to the employee were based on the quality of the work, not on whether the work made a difference to other employees or to the organization as a whole. Work processes have historically been treated as having more value than their outcomes.

Key Point

In the emerging age, a large part of the leadership role will involve facilitating the transition to a new way of living and working. Leaders will increasingly devote their energies to helping others adapt to the new rules for thriving in the world of work.

In this new age, the ordering is reversed. The most important question is not "What have you done?" but "What difference did it make?" The former question reflects the Judeo-Christian tradition that work is inherently valuable, whereas we now view work as valuable to the extent it achieves the purposes toward which it is directed. Consequently, leaders need to consider the relationships among the work, the worker, and the purpose of the work as a dynamic that continuously drives value. Further, they need to understand that the relationship is cybernetic, which means that each element supports and feeds the others in a seamless connection.

Although the relationship between process and outcome is clear, it is not always direct. Many circumstances and variables, including inherent and contextual influences, as well as unplanned factors, are embedded in the process and affect the relationship between each element of the work and the outcome of the work. These variables interact with the work process and influence both the process and the outcome. It is here that complexity plays its part.

The new age commitment to focusing on process from the perspective of outcome creates havoc among health professionals. Leaders must be fully aware of professionals' intractable attachment to process and the functional activities that make it up. People generally come to prize particular work activities once they become expert at and are rewarded for doing them. They find it a challenge to adjust or even eliminate what they do in the face of a lack of evidence that it produces anything meaningful or sustainable. Indeed, simply getting folks to the table to discuss the product of their activities can be difficult. Yet this is what leaders must do if they are to change the content of the work, make it more meaningful, and determine its essential value.

Group Discussion

Explore the notion of goodness of fit between processes and outcomes. In particular, discuss how a leader's expectations of staff would likely change if the leader looked at service and care from the perspective of achieving value. As part of this discussion, describe what steps the leader can take to get staff to focus on value rather than function (process). What changes would occur in the provision of healthcare services as a result of this focus on achieving value for the user?

Everything Is Part of One Comprehensive System

Formerly, it was believed that three types of functional relationships existed: Any two things in the universe were independent of each other, they were interdependent, or one was dependent on the other but not the reverse. In the quantum age, however, we realize

Exhibit 1-10   Interdependence

In nature everything is interdependent. There is an ebb and flow among all the elements of life. Leaders must see their role from this perspective. Most of the work of leadership will be managing the interactions and connections between people and processes. Leaders must keep aware of these truths:

- Action in one place has an effect in other places.
- Fluctuation of mutuality means authority moves between people.
- Interacting properties in systems make outcomes mobile and fluid.
- Relationship building is the primary work of leadership.
- Trusting feeling is as important as valuing thinking.
- Acknowledging in others what is unique in their contribution is vital.
- Supporting, stretching, challenging, pushing, and helping are part of being present to the process, to the players, and to the outcome.

---

that all things are interdependent (**Exhibit 1-10**). That is, all things are tied together in a wide variety of refined and sometimes inexplicable ways, some obvious and some all but invisible at any level of observation.

Leaders now must carry out their tasks with an awareness of the relatedness of processes, actions, behaviors, and functions. No act is independent, and no act adds to the viability of an organization independently. Every element interacts with every other element in some way, and all the elements together constitute a complex mosaic of movement and intersection. When looked at as a whole, the picture the elements present—and the information they impart—is entirely different from when they are viewed separately. Indeed, looking at the parts independently of each other may lead one to draw conclusions that might impede the progress of a whole process or prevent its completion, with lasting and perhaps limiting results.

> **Key Point**
>
> Chaos is an essential constituent of all change. It works to unbundle attachment to whatever is impeding movement. Chaos challenges us to simultaneously let go and to take on. It reminds us that life is a journey of constant creation.

To help readers adopt the proper perspective, this text discusses the principles of complexity and chaos theory and explains how chaos can affect work, relationships, organizations, and interactions. It also discusses many of the new skills and talents that leaders must acquire, as well as new metaphors and terminology better suited to describe work-related interactions and processes. By attaining a deeper understanding of the implications of systemness and complexity, leaders can relate to and interact with others in new ways and be challenged to develop a new foundation for their role as leaders.

A New Understanding of Planning Is Needed

In the Industrial Age, it was believed that everything should be outlined and planned down to the smallest detail. The expectation was that by planning future activities with great specificity, an organization could respond to the current situation accurately and effectively. This notion of planning to the last detail assumes much more control over cir-cumstances than, in truth, we actually have. New thinking in complex adaptive systems tells us that far more vagaries influence planned action than we can anticipate. It is wiser to understand the trajectory of change than it is to know the specifics of that change (Hazy, Goldstein, & Lichtenstein, 2007).

When a plan is constructed, the future looks a certain way at that moment in time, and the context at that moment creates the foundation for what is anticipated. However, because change is constant and the greater environment is forever in a state of chaos and creativity, the context is shifting rather than stable. The reality at the planning stage quickly gives way to a new reality that could not have been anticipated at the planning stage. And, of course, this cycle is continuous and never ending, making it impossible ever to plan with broad certainty.

Leaders now must incorporate the vagaries of complexity and chaos into the process of anticipating and planning for the future. Detailing the specifics of some future state in absolute or predictable terms is no longer a viable means of planning. Discernment and signpost reading are better skills to have than are those related to defining and direction setting. Leaders must realize that no real-time insight is sustainable, nor is it entirely ac-curate. It is simply a reflection of the particular point a person or organization is at a given moment in time in the longer, more continuous and relentless unfolding and becoming.

A good leader can read the signposts that suggest a change is imminent and can dis-cern the direction of the change and the elements indicating its fabric. The good leader synthesizes rather than analyzes and views the change thematically and/or relational-ly, drawing out of it what kind of action or strategy should be applied or trajectory embraced—that is, the response that best positions the organization to thrive in the coming circumstances. The good leader is adept at sensing changes in the external environment, indeed, even anticipating them, and using those insights to determine what adjustments or course shifts must occur in the planned trajectory to ensure the organiza-tion remains continuously relevant.

For a leader to act as a strategist today means not detailing the organization's future actions, but analyzing the relationship of the system to its external environment, deter-mining the ability of the system to respond and adapt in a sustainable way, and translating that relationship and ability into language that has meaning for those who must do the work of the organization (Watkins, 2012). Translating the signposts into understandable and inspiring language is more critical than almost any other strategic task. It is vital that a change have implications for those who are doing the work. Another way of saying this is that it must have meaning to them within the framework of their work activities so that they can commit to it, which they must do if they and the organization are to adapt to the change successfully. The leader's job is to describe the change with language that allows the workers to understand its value and how it will affect their own efforts.

In this new complexity framework, leaders need insights about contextual themes rather than step-by-step guidance on how to implement a minutely defined vision. They must understand that their organization is on a journey and that they need to peruse the landscape continuously for directional guidance rather than create a list of steps through which the organization will move on its way to a preset future. Becoming aware of the themes and undercurrents and reading the contextual signposts regularly is a wiser and more effective strategy for the new age leader than is laying out an itemized plan that may or may not correspond with future conditions.

Adaptation and Complexity

Central to the concept of adaptation is the understanding that all systems respond collectively to changes in their environment. It is important in this understanding to recognize that systems have an intelligence that reflect a con-

> **Point to Ponder**
>
> Good leaders know how to integrate the rational and the intuitive because both are equally important. They conflict with each other but also complement each other. Consequently, leaders must think clearly and rationally while remaining sensitive to the underlying flow of change.

tinual and dynamic interacting between all of the persons and processes that comprise the system. These ever-interacting change phenomena emerge and reemerge between a system and its environment and within the life of all the elements that give the system form. In fact, in all human dynamics, transformation and reproduction, and change and stability, are intrinsically intertwined. The wise leader understands this interaction and sees it as central to the effort of recognizing change and both embracing it and engaging it (Foti & Hauenstein, 2007; Miltenberger, 2013).

Historically, leadership has emphasized rational and operational science skills and functions at the expense of insight, intuition, and feeling. In most workplaces, the former, seen as more "masculine," is prized, whereas insight, intuition, and feeling, often viewed as "feminine," are taken to be less applicable in the more masculine corporate world.

Even in health care, caregiving and relational behaviors are more often viewed as OK for nurses and doctors to express but as having no place in the business end of service delivery. The principles of quantum science, chaos, and complexity theory, however, warn that failure to incorporate these behaviors into the operations of an organization—in addition to rational, hard-driving, objectified behaviors—reduces the organization's viability and sensitivity to its environment. In addition, too much of the rational and hard driving can alienate people and distance them from the work process, reducing their energy, their creativity, their commitment to the organization, and their ability to perform their jobs effectively.

Simply being capable and competent in form and function is not enough; leaders must also exhibit the ability to balance a complex range of skills and system resources to develop the employees' capabilities and grow the organization. They must know how to create a balance between means and meaning and enter into the relationships among all the elements at the personal level and at the organizational level. Incorporating their vast array of behaviors and skills into the mosaic of interactions creates resonance between the functional and the relational, both of which are essential for developing and maintaining the vitality of person and system.

Leaders Must Find the Right Balance

Weighing the various structures and influences in a work system and finding just the right mix of elements are challenging jobs. Yet that is exactly what leaders must learn to do. And they must learn to do it with a minimum of artificial supports.

Point to Ponder

Information and data are tools for decision making. Because information can be collected ad infinitum, the critical issue for a leader facing a decision at a given moment is whether there is enough information to make an informed decision. Of course, the circumstances determining the amount and type of required data can change. In other words, information needs are dynamic, not stable.

Throughout most of the healthcare system, the various infrastructures are so burdensome and complex that they actually interfere with the ability of organizations to do what they are designed to do. Because of widespread overstructuring, most organizations would not know how to live without the structural elements that encase every function and activity in the system. This is of special concern in a time of value-driven health reform. Much of the traditional tertiary care infrastructure must now give way to a more strongly developed primary health core. This requires deconstruction of the past infrastructure to make way for a more mobile and portable delivery system that responds to a stronger demand for population and community health practices.

In the new age, we must realize that there should be just enough structure to support the integrity of the organization, and not an ounce more. The more structure an organization has, the more that structure demands from the organization and the more resources are drawn away from the service system. Too much structure is actually an enemy of work and effectiveness. Under the rubric of "good order," too much structure drains the energy and creativity from a system and obstructs relationships and interactions necessary for the system's functioning. It ends up crippling the system's ability to do its work and to fulfill its purposes. The goal of an organization's leadership should be to reduce structure to only that required to advance the purposes of the systems and the essential processes of work.

Information, like structure, can easily be overvalued. Clearly, information should play a role in decision making. Yet there is never enough information to guarantee a decision is the right one in given circumstances. Furthermore, an organization can strangle itself with data in an effort to know everything pertinent to a critical decision before making the decision. Leaders need to accept that they will never know enough to guarantee the correctness of their decisions and that information is simply a tool that offers a glimpse of relevant factors at a given point in time. Because conditions are constantly changing, too much dependence on information can lead to poor decisions just as easily as a total lack of information can.

For information to be valuable, its quantity is not as important as its relevance and its volume is not as important as its timeliness. Leaders must know how much information is enough, what its focus is, what it indicates, and what its bearing is on the decisions that need to be made. They also must know when the limits of information have been reached and when its application requires discernment, deliberation, and judgment. The similarity between information and structure is obvious: The right amount of the right kind is critical to organizational effectiveness.

At every level of activity, there is a complex recurring geometric pattern. Quantum scientists often identify this pattern in the language of fractals. Fractals are embedded in every element and process of life. Although complex, they exert an influence on order and chaos in the universe and are evident in the action of planets and stars, plants and animals, even the beat pattern of a human heart. Our understanding of fractals and their application to organizations flies in the face of every organizational model. True fractal organizations generally represent minimal and flat hierarchies and both generate and distribute accountability and performance strategically

> ## Key Point
>
> The leader is a primary facilitator of the journey to a new way of working. The leader's role is to keep people on the journey and help them understand what that means to them.

and equitably throughout the organization. In more traditional models, including the organizational charts and job descriptions associated with them, a more concerted effort is made to exclude from organizational life the normative disorder, fluidity, and chaos that lies just below the surface. Yet no matter how rigorous the structure, the turbulence, fluidity, and even chaos burst through and create creative discordance and confusion, making nonsense of efforts to control it.

It is impossible to codify all the activities in an organization. How many healthcare facilities, in an effort to truly control circumstances, implement numerous policies and procedures that then are promptly neglected until the next accreditation visit? It is simply not possible to classify all the elements, interactions, and relationships necessary for the care of human beings. The vagaries of the human condition block organizations' ability to create formats or structures that set adequate behavioral or procedural parameters for treating medical conditions. The foundations of action are rooted in the principles of care and service, but although the principles are constant, the context within which they are applied is not.

Here again, it is the relatedness among factors that should drive a leader's response in complex systems. Because the elements, behaviors, and variables affecting action are uncertain, the leader's task is to achieve as much balance as the circumstances allow. And because this balance is fluid, the leader must act to adjust it in response to changes in the circumstances, including internal and external influences. The leader is always interpreting, explaining, adjusting, and applying the issues and dynamics affecting the character of the work and the integrity of the workplace.

Group Discussion

In a fractal, the whole is replicated in each part. Each branch of a tree, for example, shows the same pattern as the whole tree, as does each leaf. The indentations and projections in a few feet of shoreline may mimic those in a 100-mile stretch of coastline. Apply the notion of a fractal to organizations, groups, and teams. For instance, how does the notion of a fractal apply to the design of an organization? To the relationship among leaders? To roles? How does it apply to the organizational chart for a healthcare system?

Besides being an explicator of complexity wherever necessary, the leader must be present to the staff in a way that assures them of positive connection, understanding, and experience. The leader must show that he or she is as vulnerable to the vagaries of circumstance as anyone and can live with chaos comfortably and knowledgeably. Still, it is difficult at best to deal with normative chaos embedded naturally yet deeply within every system. People fundamentally crave order and want their leaders to deliver a sense of stability and "normality." Despite this fact, leaders, rather than insulating people from innate complexity, uncertainty, even disorder, must instead help people to embrace these factors, understand them, harness them, and develop the personal skills necessary to positively use them to transform themselves and the systems within which they live.

Chaos and Paradox Are Always at Work

Even at the fundamental levels of life, chaos is hard at work. Creatures as small as one cell are constantly undergoing both accidental and transitional modifications that give them a better chance of thriving. It is a basic requisite of all life to adapt to changing conditions. The demise of the dinosaur is a good example of what happens when living beings fail to adapt to changes in their external environment.

The age within which we currently live is vastly different from the age we are exiting. Science and technology alter every aspect of our lives. Our challenge is to embrace the new circumstances and sort out their implications and applications as we go. For the person who says, "I don't want to learn about the digital world and how to use advanced technologies," the best response may be, "You could certainly choose to die; it is the only way to intentionally avoid your future." Although facetious, that piece of advice reflects an element of truth. Technological advances and the need and capacity to adapt to them are not going to go away.

In the coming age, leaders will be called to tell the truth, teach coping and adaptation skills, learn new skills, and apply them in new ways in new settings. The infrastructure that generated past leadership roles is disappearing, and the new circumstances demand new roles and challenge everyone to respond to an entirely new set of questions.

Furthermore, the new age will open the door to uncertainty and a general lack of "rightness." The prevailing principles will be open to interpretation and will be applicable in a host of ways. No one response to a change or answer to a question will be clearly the only one or the best one. There might be many correct responses depending on the cultural, social, economic, and intellectual context. Leaders must respect the diversity embedded in every condition or issue (**Exhibit 1-11**).

Every leader is now required to know the techniques for finding common ground, for sorting through the various landscapes representing the diversity inherent in each issue. Also required are consensus-building and group-process skills because a leader's job is to get people to come together around issues and help them determine appropriate responses within the context of their own roles. This is a challenge that cannot be met by establishing standardized job procedures or rules. Indeed, competent leaders must be able to "set tables" wisely and carefully to ensure that the right people are engaged in the right way around issues that are central to their role and essential to their adaptability and sustainability.

Exhibit 1-11   Paradox

Many paired elements of life appear contradictory but at a deeper level are in fact complementary. These include the following:

- *Chaos and order:* There is order in all chaos and vice versa.
- *Creativity and tension:* Tension leads to creativity and creativity causes tension.
- *Conflict and peace:* Conflict is necessary to peacemaking, containing in it the elements upon which peace must be built.
- *Difference and similarity:* Difference seen at a great distance appears as an integrated whole.
- *Complexity and simplicity:* Complexity is simply the visible connection between aligned simplicities.

Leaders must develop an affection for legitimate risk and for the boundaries of agreement and understanding. They must be able to "push the river" so that the mental models people bring to the resolution of concerns or the determination of strategies and actions are shifted or even fundamentally altered. There is nothing worse in deliberation than using a mental model or frame of reference that does not fit the prevailing circumstances. As we move inexorably into the new age, we must try to understand its characteristics within the context of its "becoming" rather than of the past. Peter Drucker said it best when he suggested that we must all close the door on the Industrial Age and simply turn around (Drucker, 2009).

It is in turning around to face the future that we begin to confront the inadequacies of our historic mental models. We begin to see the future unfold within its own context rather than one we bring to it from our past experience. We look over the landscape of our becoming and are stimulated to go to those places that least fit our prevailing mind set and that challenge what we understand and the language we bring to the journey.

Leaders need to be called out of certainty into experimentation. They must take smaller steps and let the measured consequences of each step suggest the best direction in which to move next. It is in the steps of experimentation—of testing and evaluating—that their direction and its appropriateness can be discerned most easily. Finally, leaders stand to gain most information about what is viable and sustainable by bringing a variety of testing procedures together and using them jointly.

Pay Attention to the Informal Network

In every organization there is a formal structure and process and an informal network. The informal network is primarily relational and carries most of the information about how people in the organization think or feel and what their sentiments are regarding almost anything in the system. It is as vital and valid a part of the

> **Key Point**
>
> All decisions and actions are rife with risk. Risk cannot be eliminated and should not necessarily be decreased because courses of action that possess great value tend to be associated with higher risk. What is important to determine is not whether the risk can be eliminated, but whether the level of risk is appropriate for the actions undertaken and, if so, what strategies can accommodate the risk.

system as any other, and it requires attention because, among other things, it typically contains essential pieces of the dynamic that have been overlooked or missed as well as the "undiscussables," issues that are too sensitive to lay on the table and opinions that do not reflect the prevailing point of view. Embedded here, too, are some of the most dynamic notions of what should happen or what should be done.

All organizations, large and small, have a small number to hundreds of informal networks that operate as peer groups, colleague networks, service teams, care communities, long-term employee groups, task forces, and so forth. Huge inflows and outflows of information, sharing, and knowledge move dynamically through these matrices and informal groups in ways that have a significant impact on organizations and systems. Indeed, much more of the real daily work, relationships, and interactions is expressed in informal networks than is seen in the more formal structures of organizations. Leaders generally fail to recognize the power and influence of these informal networks and use them far less than the capacity and value they bring to organizations warrant. Although these informal networks are powerful, they represent a level of complexity and relational density that is difficult to manage in formal and systematic ways. However, through leadership recognition, access, and interaction within the context of these informal networks, much can be accomplished and a great deal of the dynamics of change can be effectively harnessed to enhance quality and improve service.

Group Discussion

Karen Weiss, RN, is the head of the nursing department in a medical clinic. The staff members like her because she can get things done and keep things moving. Although she has a highly developed sense of order, recent changes are making it harder for her to stay "in control." She feels as though things are getting ahead of her and she is losing her touch. Others also are not as satisfied with her performance as they were. Discuss the following questions: What is the real issue in this case? How is Karen's need for control in conflict with the principles of complexity? Who is accountable for decisions? Should Karen change her manner of leading? If so, how should she change it, and what does she need to do to change it? How does Karen ensure that the staff is more involved in decisions that affect their own lives?

All elements of the system, whether formal or informal, are a part of the dynamic of change in the organization. Each can be a vehicle for action and even transformation. Leaders need to notice all the informal pathways and networks of communication and relationship, from hallway conversations to lunchtime discussions, from whispered comments to sarcastic asides—each plays a role in the complex web of interactions necessary for sustaining the organization. Taking an opportunity to hear, communicate, or interact is never inappropriate. All means are legitimate and deserve attention. Each, when joined with the others, contributes to discovering the state of the organization and determining the proper actions to take to strengthen it.

Simple Systems Are Linked to Create More Complex Systems

The universe consists of a web of simple and discrete networks that cannot survive or function without some intersection and interaction with each other. Complexity is the sum of simplicity. Each is intrinsically linked with the other. Simple systems seek each other in a mysterious dance of self-organizing and join with each other at appropriate intersections to configure a larger whole. Called *chunking*, this process is similar to fitting together pieces of a child's erector set to build a structure. Each element has its own purpose and meaning, but its purpose remains unfulfilled until it interacts with the other elements. In short, their linkage, connection, and interactions demonstrate a synergy of interfaces and relationships that can define the operation of the whole only when seen acting together.

The implication for human organizations and behaviors is that all things begin with the simple. Sustainable change rarely operates from the top of a system; instead, it usually is initiated and lives at the center and works its way outward. For instance, the purpose and meaning of a service organization are generated over the places where the staff does its work, closest to where the services are provided, which is also where the organization's value-grounded, dynamic growth, adaptability, and creativity originate and are sustained.

Leaders need to understand that sustainability comes from the places where the organization lives out its life—essentially its points of service. There, the pieces of the organization come together to fulfill the organization's purpose. Providers and clients come together to carry out the processes toward which the organization's infrastructure and operations are directed.

Although leaders profess to recognize the importance of the point of service, traditional organizational design does not reflect its key role in deciding and acting. The organizational hierarchy typically strangles the essential dynamics of the point of service and creates an artificial and unsustainable framework for decision making and action to happen at places far away from the point of service. Individuals not at the point of service take

> **Point to Ponder**
>
> Traditionally, knowledge has been viewed as something that can be possessed. Today, however, it is viewed as a utility—something not possessed, but accessed. People who want to use knowledge should know how to access it, how to apply it, and when to let it go.

responsibility for strategy, policy, and direction setting and, by so doing, exclude those whose obligation is to carry out work and actions to fulfill strategy, policy, and organizational direction. A universal principle of system effectiveness states that the farther away from the point of service a decision is made about what goes on there, the higher the risk, the greater the cost, and the less sustainable the decision. Sadly, many organizations increase their risk and their costs and fail to attain their objectives as a result of failing to incorporate this principle into their way of doing business.

Staff, in constructing the correct complex relatedness and infrastructure, must be free to "chunk" from their center and create linkages with the strategic, financial, and support structures that facilitate their work. Here again, tearing away much of the intervening infrastructure and the organizational layers and compartments serves to free the organization to enter into the more fluid and variable relationships it needs to provide stakeholder engagement in a way that advances health care. Then, those who own them can join the simple, essential components of local locus of control and systems strategy to other essential components to construct a web of intersections and resonating connections that hums with the life and meaning underpinning sustainability.

The operation of digital equipment perhaps best exemplifies these forces at work. Software code defines functions but must interact with other pieces of data before it is useful to the technology user. A certain segment of code might have application value, but it must interact with other segments before this value can be realized. In other words, each segment has value in virtue of its contribution to the whole.

Learning occurs in the same way. Simple concepts lead inexorably to understanding other simple concepts, and when they are all ultimately tied together, the learner understands the interdependence of different simple processes and thereby achieves knowledge. Furthermore, the learner recognizes that knowledge, rather than being valuable in and of itself, is valuable to the extent that it can be applied in action.

What complexity teaches us about knowledge is that it is not so much a capacity as it is a tool. It has relevance at a particular moment or in a specific situation. A shift in the context, an increase in understanding, or new information affects the elements of knowledge and challenges the person to "move on" and adjust what is known, valued, and applied. In fact, an endless dynamic is composed of the aggregation of knowledge, the letting go of what is no longer valid, and the reaching out for what is next and expands the endless journey of learning. The critical point here is that what is relevant or irrelevant, adequate or inadequate, at any given moment is not the whole of a person's knowledge but rather developing and adapting pieces or elements of knowledge (chunks). The person moves in and out of these chunks and, in so doing, alters the relationship between themselves and the whole complex of knowledge.

In systems thinking, leaders are aware of the importance of intersections. At intersections much of the work of leadership unfolds. The interface between the elements of a system is where the challenge and the work of effectiveness occur. The problems of creating good fit between the pieces of a system require focus and effort on the part of the leader and serve as the place where most of the "noise" and confrontation between people and systems unfold.

Good leaders understand this and can use it in the interests of others and the organization. They never get so attached to any specific item, process, or activity that they treat it as permanent and/or unchanging. Each item, process, or activity is part of a mosaic and comes and goes depending on demand at various times. Good leaders know to let go when that is appropriate and to take on and adjust when that becomes necessary. Furthermore, they know that the organization's complex and chaotic circumstances require them to keep an eye on the larger picture, read the changes (in the constant interface between environment and organization) that are occurring or that are about to occur, and make the necessary adjustments at the appropriate time.

Good leaders know that a complex, adaptive system works when the simple systems work. If something is wrong at the point of service, the system as a whole is affected. Because the interdependence between simple components is so tight in an effective and

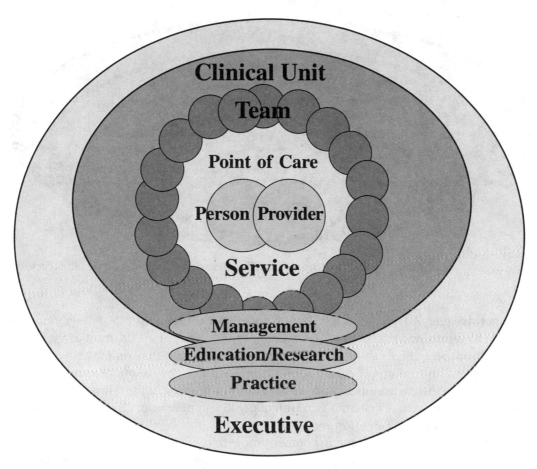

Figure 1-4 Point-of-Service Systems Design.

viable complex system, any break in the simple (or local) systems leads to breaks at all levels of the complex system. By ensuring the effectiveness of the simple systems, good leaders facilitate the integrity and efficiency of the whole system (**Figure 1-4**).

Systems Do Not Compete with Each Other, but Instead Simply Seek to Thrive

Chaos theory and quantum theory hold that competition is anomalous. Still, the current literature on organizations and their management contains numerous discussions of the viability and importance of competition. This is a simplistic and often uninformed notion of the conditions and circumstances of thriving and advancing both as individuals and. as communities. This rather antediluvian and unidimensional notion associated with thriving and advancing holds sway among the most powerful in the business and political communities to the detriment of those communities they lead.

All living systems seek to thrive. At a fundamental level, they are not concerned with each other's survival unless it is somehow related to their own need to thrive. To this end, all life has a complementary and interdependent relationship with other life rather than

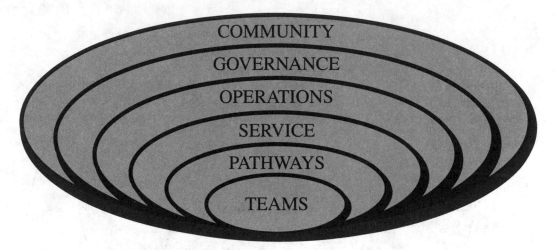

Figure 1-5 Structural Integrity and Interdependence: Functional Components of a Health Structure.

a competitive one. Adaptation is not about competition between the fittest but about survival of the fittest, and the survival of a system depends more on its inherent adaptability to its environment and its ability to build community response than on anything else. To thrive, the system must have beneficial interactions with its environment, universal internal response to the environment, and the capacity to adjust to the prevailing conditions quickly and effectively. A system is fundamentally in competition with itself to thrive, not with anyone or anything else (**Figure 1-5**).

Generally, the concept of being in competition with oneself is foreign to unilateral capitalistic ways of thinking (as opposed to collateral capitalistic notions). Still, even unilateral capitalism treats competition as fundamentally a personal exercise—a contest between oneself and others for profitability and success. What this approach fails to recognize is that success has less to do with one's competitors than with one's own adaptability, creativity, energy, and commitment to succeed. In other words, the pursuit of success should not be viewed as a contest with others but as a personal effort to give one's best and to thrive in the environment one has chosen to live in.

In the emerging age, persons and organizations will be challenged to adjust to a new context with a new set of rules. Those who thrive will be those who can read the signposts of environmental shifts quickly and effectively and apply the resulting insights to their own lives and operations. Organizational leaders need to learn the fundamentals of thriving in the new age of fast-paced technology drivers. They must make a diligent effort to keep up with the transformations in technology, global communications, information infrastructures, and social conditions and the drive for sustainable value. Here again, reading the signposts to create a tight fit between the demands of environmental changes and the system's capacity to embrace and adapt becomes a very important skill. Paying attention to indicators, monitoring innovations, experimenting with new and unfamiliar approaches, and living comfortably with ambiguity and the noise of constant change are all essential skills of good leaders of the future.

The Compression of Time Will Affect How Work Is Done

There simply cannot be a leader anywhere on the earth who has not noticed the not-so-subtle change in our sense of time and space. Most people have noticed how time has sped up and how radically its quickening has affected the content and flow of work. Leaders can turn anywhere and hear others in the organization suggest that there is insufficient time to do all that is required. Leaders themselves are aware of how very little time they seem to have to meet a growing set of demands.

Technology, including the prevailing methods for purchasing and shipping material goods, is primarily responsible for the compression of time and work. For example, LASIK surgery, a type of corrective eye surgery, takes only 7 or 8 minutes to complete; Internet grocery stores deliver groceries within 2 hours of order placement; and communication by email and text message is virtually instantaneous. Quick transmission of information and quick delivery of goods and services are increasingly normal in our global society.

> **Key Point**
>
> There is never enough time. Technology has compressed time so that what once was enough is now insufficient. Leaders must help others see their work from the perspective of compressed time. For example, now that clinical interventions require less time, practitioners and patients must shift their expectations to fit the narrowed time frame.

The need for narrow hierarchy—for many layers of decision making and management—has all but disappeared from the business world. In the late 1980s and early 1990s, business leaders reconfigured their organizations to eliminate management structures that had long been part of organizational culture. The goal for organizations was to become nimble and fluid, and whatever impeded their achievement of this goal was either cast off or reconceived.

Today, healthcare organizations are experiencing a similar crisis. The growing demands of a value-based approach to health reform and system transformation require a complete reconceptualization of the design and infrastructure of healthcare delivery. The need to move from tertiary, process-heavy health service delivery to a more nimble primary healthcare model that advances the net aggregate health of American citizens creates new pressures for deconstructing, reconceiving, and recalibrating contemporary health service designs and models. Impeding this transformation is tertiary-care-driven brick-and-mortar infrastructure that supports a delivery system that is no longer relevant (this infrastructure hinders the system's survival). Changes in technology, service structure, clinical models, consumer demand, and healthcare economics coalesce in response to the need for value-driven healthcare organizations that possess the same fluidity and nimbleness required of technology-grounded businesses.

The current chaos in the health system arises from conflict between leadership commitment to an outmoded infrastructure and a system design that reflects value. The myriad stakeholders in the healthcare industry—administrators, nurses, doctors, hospitals, pharmacists, and so on—struggle to hold on to their piece of the healthcare pie without realizing that the pie is now being sliced in an entirely different way. The

<table>
<tr><td>

Point to Ponder

Over the next decade as healthcare reform advances and services and interventions become more mobile, organizational leaders will be engaged in the deconstruction of the institutional infrastructure of health care—the bricks and mortar.

</td></tr>
</table>

emerging healthcare system demands a significant change in the intersections of professions and their relationship to the health system and the individuals and populations it serves.

The compression of time works inexorably to reconfigure the context for health care and restructure its framework—often without consent from participants. Healthcare leaders must focus on interpreting external demands and translating them into internal actions. They are being called into the chaos of creativity to produce a good fit between the new value framework and the infrastructure that must be constructed to support it.

Much of the current work of healthcare leaders involves deconstructing existing health service models. The current infrastructure must be deconstructed so that it can be replaced by newer, value-driven models of service and support. Leaders must perform a range of activities in reconfiguring health care to fit the coming age, when space and time will be even further compressed, services will be more fluid and mobile, and the locus of control will shift from the provider to the user. The changes that will occur include these:

- *The hospital bed will cease to be the main point of service.* During the next two decades, the number of hospital beds will decline by approximately 25%. Indeed, in the current healthcare paradigm, admission to hospital bed–based services is an indicator of the failure of the health system to provide health-based services that circumvent inpatient services.
- *The service structure will be decentralized.* The healthcare system will deliver small, broadly dispersed units of service across the continuum of care.
- *Increasingly, services will move out of the hospital.* By the end of the next decade, more than 70% of the medical services currently provided in hospitals will be provided in clinics, community settings, health homes, and primary care nurse practitioner and physician offices.
- *The core practices of the professions will be substantially altered.* The institution-based late-stage services that once predominated will be replaced by high-intensity primary care–based interventions that do not require hospitalization. These interventions will transform the roles of the various health professionals.
- *Users of health services will become more accountable for their own health.* Providers have the major job of helping to transfer the locus of control of medical decision making and life management to individuals, who have never had it and do not yet know what to do with it. Healthcare providers' work over the next two decades will include educating the users of health services and assisting them in acquiring the necessary skills to manage their own health through health management and preventive healthcare programs.
- *The users of health services and the technology of health care will progressively interface.* Virtual and technical interaction and communication will become the norm of health service provision. Connection between providers and patients will increasingly be virtual and seamless, with supporting technology enabling the provision of clinical services to patients remotely.

For the deconstruction of health services to be effective, leaders must know that this value-driven transformation is taking place and agree to lead the effort. The conditions are already in place, but the work of making the change meaningful and feasible has yet to be done. If a leader is opposed to the transformation or is unable to acquire the necessary skills, both the leader and the transformation will suffer.

One responsibility of leaders is to help others mourn the loss of practices and roles that are becoming irrelevant. For example, many popular reasons people have entered the health professions will no longer apply to their emerging roles. Despite this, health professionals continue to believe that their initial intent for entering their profession is still valid. Or they simply refuse to acknowledge that their idealization of the past might be keeping them from embracing the emerging and far different future of health service, to their own detriment.

One way to aid health professionals in mourning their losses is to help them enumerate these losses and determine what they must let go to obtain the skills and master the roles they need to function in the emerging reformed and transformed healthcare system. Each person must voice his or her losses and symbolically let them go to turn in the direction of change and meet the coming challenges. By doing this, a person becomes free to explore the innovations and ultimately design a personal strategy to accommodate his or her profession and its role in transforming health care and improving the experience for people and communities.

Death is part of the cycle of life and is a requisite of all change. Not everything in the universe that thrives will always do so. When circumstances change radically, some formerly vigorous systems fail. In some cases, the demands are beyond the system's capacity to adapt; in other cases, the changes call for a new work format that cannot be achieved simply by altering some of the characteristics of the workplace.

Leaders are obligated to help those that should diminish or die do so quickly. They are expected to make it clear to the staff that the process of bringing something to an end is as necessary as any other organizational process. A part of the tough work of facilitating necessary change is altering staff attitudes about the permanence of work. Employees do get stuck in their rituals and routines. Their attachment to these routines may be the only point of security they have in this quickly changing world. What they might not know is that holding onto practices that are no longer relevant endangers their ability to succeed in the future. Leaders must "truth tell" to keep staff in mind of the fact that work effort and function are transitory and that a mindless attachment to the work itself may be the greatest impediment to their own success and that of the system.

Group Discussion

Twenty years ago the average length of stay in a hospital was 5.7 days. In the coming decade, the average procedure will require a stay of only 4.5 hours or fewer. These two facts indicate the extreme shift in the nature of clinical services. Discuss how the new service model will change the way healthcare providers work. What tasks will cease to possess value? How can leaders convince staff to abandon old practices that are no longer relevant? And what are the implications for patients?

Leaders must keep their eyes fixed on the work and on how changes might affect the ability of staff members to do the work. The function of work continually changes, and attachment to work routines simply slows individuals' adaptation. A refusal to adapt does not diminish the demand for change; it just makes the adjustment to the change increasingly more difficult for the individual.

All Change Ultimately Makes Good Sense

As Stephen Hawking has so many times eloquently stated, "Change is." Chaos, complexity, and change are not things but forms of dynamic activity. According to Hawking, they are the only constants in the universe (Hawking & Mlodinow, 2009). They will never cease because their end would be the end of everything. Perpetual dynamic movement is what underpins every action and process. This aspect of reality is less understood and less often made use of than physical laws, but it exists nonetheless.

Leadership is mainly concerned with adapting to change, and all the leadership functions and activities outlined in this and other contemporary leadership texts are informed by this understanding. In fact, theorists are inclined to be less definitive than formerly in their statements about the attributes of leadership and in their recipes for leadership success. Instead of being guided by an unchanging set of principles, leaders need to be fluid and adaptable because their role changes in concert with the changing conditions.

Leaders are aware that it is in the pursuit of meaning that the direction of a change can best be discerned. They continually look past the real and the present toward the unformed and potential to better evaluate the present and the direction of transformation (assessing how changes in the external environment create a demand for personal and organizational change). The subtle themes and ebbs and flows that lie just beneath the surface of events and experiences have more to say to leaders than do the events themselves.

Leaders know that much of what is seen and experienced is a metaphor for the operation of the infrastructure of change. The chaos so often represented in the change process is a cover for an explicit and elegant order that can be perceived only by focusing on the whole rather than on the parts. Indeed, looking at only the individual parts makes it almost impossible to see the integrity, order, and beauty embedded in an elegant web of flow and linkage. Staff is hungry to obtain from the leader this insight about the operation of the whole and how changes at this level of the system affect the choices and actions of persons at the system's points of service.

Leaders are motivated by the connections that give meaning and value to the current and the real (**Exhibit 1-12**). The rules that guide the journey of change are both simple and complex, and the full set is not fully comprehensible all at once. An important task for any leader is to discern the predominant operating variable(s) affecting the journey at any given moment. Using insight, the leader can apply the value the predominantly operating variable(s) represents and use it as a window for viewing the next

---

Exhibit 1-12   Unmotivated Versus Motivated Leaders

Unmotivated	Motivated
• Focus on the present	• Focus on the potential
• No time for the work	• New kind of work
• Things are getting worse	• Things are different
• Cannot do the work any more	• New mental model for work
• No one knows . . .	• How can I get to know . . . ?
• It is too much for one person	• Share the work
• This too shall pass	• It is a journey I lead
• Doing more with less	• Doing different work differently

---

factors, principles, or interacting forces pushing toward the changing next steps in any transformation.

Leaders are forever caught in the potential. The ability to thrive in this potential distinguishes good leaders from the rest. Good leaders are always on the edge of chaos, looking over the horizon, looking just beyond the precipice. Located there, they can read, interpret, and express what they discern. Their real gift is their ability to backtrack to where those they lead are living and working and translate what they have seen into a language that has force and meaning for those who can hear it. They then have the job of getting behind the staff and pushing them into their own conceptualization and definition of response to the emerging reality, allowing the staff to own what they see and act on it in a responsive and viable way.

Conclusion

Leadership skills are learned skills, and their mastery requires neither magic nor a high level of intellectual capacity. Leaders emerge in a wide variety of circumstances and reflect a broad range of talents and personalities. There is no one pattern of behavior or personality type that is most suitable for the leadership role. In short, leaders come in every size and shape.

What leaders must possess is the ability to understand the vagaries and complexities of human interactions and relationships. In their role as leaders, they must take into account chaos and complexity as these do their work and create their inimitable patterns of adaptation and growth. Good leaders live in the edge land between now and the very next thing and can engage folks in the journey of the whole across the landscape of a preferred and optimistic future.

Leaders in the coming age will need new skills and new insights about leadership and the preferred methods of "journeying." These skills and insights can be learned, adapted to current conditions, and applied in a variety of ways to meet the demands of the journey. In their application, an individual may come to discover the leader in him- or herself, feel the excitement of leadership work, and inspire others in the journey of discovery and advancement.

Case Study 1-1

Transforming Leaders

Cameryn is the vice president for professional development at a large metropolitan hospital in the Midwest. She has been in her role for 6 years and has accepted new responsibilities over the years, widening her scope of work to include the direction of all of the clinical nurse specialists (CNSs), the new graduate residency program, and the research- and evidence-based practice initiatives. She also oversees the Magnet program, which strives for continual readiness for redesignation.

Cameryn and some of the other leaders in the organization have become concerned about the competence level of some of the nurse managers and their assistant managers, clinical leads, and shift supervisors. The managers and others "get the job done," but they do not seem to be focused on inspiring the workforce to achieve excellence in their work or preparing potential leaders for succession. In fact, some of the managers seem to be threatened by informal leaders who excel in the clinical setting rather than encouraging them to develop their skills and competencies so as to assume direct leadership roles in the future.

For all in manager and supervisory roles, the hospital provides a quarterly leadership educational event with motivational speakers. The feedback regarding the leadership event is positive, and it is expected that the managers share with their staff the new knowledge gained from the motivational speakers and presentations. How this new knowledge is shared and disseminated is not assessed. Cameryn wonders whether it is shared at all and questions how well the leadership messages are integrated into the daily behaviors and activities of the managers.

Cameryn has been reading about transformational leadership and how one of the characteristics of a transformational leader is to inspire others to achieve what they previously thought was impossible. Cameryn reflects on those in her own career who inspired her to return to school for further education and ultimately to seek roles where she could influence nursing practice and patient care. In her heart, she wants to provide the same experience for all developing nurse leaders in the clinical setting and also in beginning-level management positions. She believes that management is far more than "getting the job done and completing tasks" and needs to include behaviors that transform individuals into those who have a thirst for new knowledge and quest to constantly change the status quo to achieve excellence in their work.

Cameryn is inspired to do something about the development of the nurse managers. She realizes that the first step would be to inspire her colleagues to embrace the same vision for nursing leadership at all levels within the organization, especially with their focus on managing budgets and meeting organizational priorities. Cameryn is convinced that with better prepared frontline managers, many of the organizational priorities could be achieved more expediently. She wants the group to examine the current roles expected of clinical leads, shift supervisors, nurse managers, and their assistants and the personal and experience requirements for the roles. She also wants to impress upon her colleagues that their own behaviors strongly influence those who are watching their interactions with others and daily behaviors in their roles. She realizes that this is a sensitive subject, and she decides to develop a strategy to informally lead her colleagues on a journey for their own improvement and to influence them to improve the experience of their direct reports. She realizes that the interconnection between her colleagues and their direct reports is critical for the changes that she envisions to transform every nurse manager and supervisor into true inspirational leaders.

Cameryn decides to move beyond the occasional inspirational speaker and elects to empower the management team at all levels with as much information as possible about transformational leadership, workplace empowerment, healthy work environment, and nursing excellence. She works with the Collaborative Governance Council for Professional Development to initiate a leadership journal club for clinical leaders and all levels of management. The journal club is led by the members of the Professional Development Council who choose the journal articles to read and review. The council also establishes group meeting norms, leads the discussions about the articles, and creates a short summary of the articles for all of the nursing staff to read in the *Magnet Nursing Newsletter*.

Cameryn also decides that it is important to determine the actual learning needs of those in management positions, so she develops a self-assessment tool using the leadership domains outlined by the American Organization of Nurse Executives and the Benner levels of competency as the response set. The new assessment tool provides information as to how each manager, assistant manager, clinical lead, and shift supervisor perceives his or her level of competence in each of the leadership domains. From that information, Cameryn plans to develop educational content and experiences that are targeted to areas where managers perceive themselves to be least competent. She also meets with those who are more expert in the leadership domains and discusses their mentoring those who are less experienced and competent and presenting some of the formal content needed for development of the frontline leadership team.

Recognizing that professional development is a very complex and multileveled task, Cameryn also plans to develop educational content and experiences for the more expert group to teach them how to mentor others and how to prepare and present educational content using teaching methods that are innovative, engaging, and inspiring to the learners. Cameryn realizes how interconnected each level of the plan is and how necessary it is to create a fluid and adaptable project management plan to guide the various stages of development to transform nurse managers into true leaders.

She soon realizes that in her work with the collaborative governance councils to develop an educational intervention for the frontline managers, she has forgotten to engage the Human Resources department, which is also responsible for leadership development. There are many indications of their discontent with her new leadership development program. When Cameryn recognizes their concern, she meets with them to discuss ways that Human Resources could be instrumental in the assessment and development of frontline managers.

Needless to say, not all of her colleagues embrace her vision to transform the leaders in the organization. Many barriers emerge that would dissuade most from continuing to achieve their vision, and Cameryn is disappointed at times and must continually refocus her energies to remain on course despite the barriers. When she recognizes that one of her colleagues or one of the nurse managers is not "on board," she spends personal time talking with that person and helping to translate the vision so that it could become his or her reality as well. She is continually engaged in dialogue with others to support the change effort, and she formally recognizes the actions and efforts of those who are involved in mentoring less experienced nurse leaders and those who are involved in the educational activities.

The transformational process has taken several years, but reflecting on the progress, Cameryn and her colleagues believe that significant changes have occurred in the organization and that all of the nurse leaders at every level have benefited from the efforts to enhance the competencies and skills of the frontline managers. The benefits of the program are validated with significant improvements in the employee opinion surveys and in surveys to assess the healthy work environment.

Questions

1. How do you think that complexity science and quantum leadership provide a framework for an initiative to advance the competencies and skills of frontline managers and to change the management culture to a leadership culture in an organization?
2. How effective do you think that Cameryn was in transforming the leadership culture in her organization? What might she have done differently to facilitate the change process?
3. One of the roles of the quantum leader is to read the signposts that give direction and feedback regarding the change process. What were some of the signposts that Cameryn encountered during the development of the frontline manager group, interactions with her colleagues, and the encounter with the Human Resources department?
4. In your opinion, what effect will advancing the frontline managers, her own colleagues' competence, and transformational leadership culture have on the organizational climate, nursing satisfaction, and even patient outcomes?

Case Study 1-2

Inspiring Greatness

Lynn has been the dean of the College of Nursing at a prestigious university for the past 2 years. Others describe Lynn as having incredible energy and vision, and being someone who is in constant motion, leading and transforming the college into a powerhouse among the other colleges at the university. It would seem that Lynn knows no limitations or boundaries to her visions. She is recognized as an extraordinary leader by her colleagues at the university, and she is known as a national and international expert in her clinical area of expertise as well as in her direction for the development of many interdisciplinary programs within the College of Nursing. Lynn has multiple appointments to national advisory boards and is a fellow in the American Academy of Nursing as well as a number of other nursing practice academies. She sits on several interdisciplinary strategic planning expert panels for national healthcare reform and other health initiatives. Clearly, she is recognized as one of the top leaders in nursing and health care.

Lynn is the first to recognize and acknowledge that being a national expert does not make it any easier to initiate and execute change within one's own organization. Even though Lynn is acknowledged as an external leader, she's continually challenged internally with the same barriers of resistance that less recognized experts encounter when they try to initiate change within their organization. Although Lynn has boundless energy and is motivated to help others make a significant difference in their work and contributions, she also struggles with how to manage those who do not embrace her vision or have the same passion for accelerated change. When asked how she manages her feelings related to the naysayers in her life, she states that she seeks to listen carefully to the message that they are trying to impart and understand their perspective on the matter and their concerns and fears. From that framework, she tries to find a connection between her own vision and the vision of those who oppose her, realizing that a shared vision is the beginning of all successful change. She then seeks to find a way to focus their attention on what is shared in common in their visions and highlights areas where they are interdependent or mutually dependent on one another to achieve their visions.

The nursing and healthcare literature is replete with evidence and opinions about the need for interdisciplinary collaboration to ensure optimal patient outcomes, professional role satisfaction, and healthcare excellence. With this in mind, Lynn proposes to develop an interprofessional curriculum for the colleges of nursing, medicine, pharmacy, and social services. Lynn develops a proposal for the intercollege planning committee and the provost that outlines a number of courses that could be taught with an integrated curriculum to students from each of the colleges. She also includes how the proposed integrated curriculum could be budget neutral or actually realize a cost savings because classes presented to each college in duplicate would be eliminated and integrative classes would be developed using fewer faculty and facility resources. Lynn supports the proposal with evidence about the positive effects of an interdisciplinary approach in improving relationships among professionals and the recommendation from the Institute of Medicine and Robert Wood Johnson Foundation report on the future of nursing.

Lynn is not an inexperienced leader, so she anticipates that there will be resistance to her proposal. She tries to prepare herself for all the voices that will say, "It can't be done. We've never done it before. We are successful with the current curriculum structure," and offer a host of other objections. Some of the loudest voices of opposition justify their position by stating that the social power imbalance between nursing and the other healthcare professions is a reason why the integrated curriculum should not be implemented. Some mention that the intellectual level of the medical and pharmacy students is far different from that of the nursing and social work students and that the nursing and social work students would not be able to manage the rigor of the courses needed to educate future physicians and pharmacists.

Some of the meetings are intense, chaotic, and filled with motion as the curriculum committee discusses the pros and cons of having an integrated curriculum. At times Lynn is very discouraged with the progress, but she keeps focused with positive energy and strong belief that her proposal is critical to improving patient care. She recognizes that the simple proposal is loaded with complexity and the discord that is happening is an important part of the process as participants reflect on their beliefs and values. At times Lynn wishes that the provost would simply step up and direct the group to develop an integrated curriculum because Lynn realizes that the provost supports the proposal. On the other hand, she realizes the value of the change process and how the participants' values and beliefs will morph over time as a result of the discussions, readings, and continual analysis of the pros and cons of the proposal.

Lynn recognizes the need to be patient and not to push the change, but rather to quietly influence the others on the merits of interprofessional education. She provides a number of articles from reputable journals, arranges for speakers on the topic, and even creates an all-day workshop to bring in national speakers and participants to discuss strategies to develop interprofessional curricula. Of course, she arranges the workshop around the availability of the other deans so that they can attend the workshop as well. She even arranges for a few of the more forward-thinking deans to present at the workshop. She invites one of the other deans to copresent with her at an international conference focused on interprofessional education. Lynn acts as if they have already accepted the idea even though she knows that part of her strategy is to convince them to accept the proposal.

Within the year the curriculum committee not only accepts the proposal for an interprofessional curriculum to begin the next year, but actually acts as if the notion was their idea to begin with. At this point, Lynn realizes that she has successfully managed the change.

Questions

1. Identify the elements of complexity in this case study.
2. How effective do you think Lynn is in managing the conflict, complexity, and the chaos that emerges around her proposal to develop an interprofessional curriculum?
3. How well does Lynn read the signposts and develop strategies to manage her vision?
4. What processes might have been used to help the curriculum committee to accept the proposal and move beyond their personal agendas, values, fears, and doubts about the importance of interprofessional education?
5. What role do you feel that a quantum leader needs to play in developing consensus around decision making?
6. What quantum leader characteristics does Lynn portray in leading the group to embrace her vision and to change and adapt the curriculum to an interprofessional focus?

References

Birk, S. (2013). The future of physician leadership: Physician leaders and the changing healthcare landscape. *Healthcare Executive, 28*(1), 8–10, 12–14, 16.

Bridges, W. (2002). *Way of transition.* New York, NY: Perseus.

Brown, S. M. (2009). *Essentials of medical genomics.* Hoboken, NJ: Wiley-Blackwell.

Drucker, P. (2009). *Management.* New York, NY: Harper Collins.

Edersheim, E. H., & Drucker, P. F. (2007). *The definitive Drucker.* New York, NY: McGraw-Hill.

Foti, R., & Hauenstein, N. (2007). Pattern and variable approaches in leadership emergence and effectiveness. *Journal of Applied Psychology, 92*(2), 347–355.

Hawking, S., & Mlodinow, L. (2009). *A briefer history of time.* New York, NY: Bantam.

Hazy, J., Goldstein, J., & Lichtenstein, B. (2007). *Complex systems leadership theory: New perspectives from complexity science on social and organizational effectiveness.* New York, NY: Vintage Press.

Klug, W. S., & Ward, S. M. (2012). *Essentials of genetics.* Boston, MA: Pearson.

Miltenberger, L. (2013). Pathways to effective collaboration: A dialogue on the new competencies required for the nonprofit leader. *Journal of Leadership Studies, 7*(1), 46–47.

Murphy, S. E., & Riggio, R. E. (2003). *The future of leadership development.* Mahwah, NJ: Erlbaum.

Nickerson, J. A. (2010). *Leading change in a Web 2.1 world: How ChangeCasting builds trust, creates understanding, and accelerates organizational change.* Washington, DC: Brookings Institution Press.

Sreekantan, B. V., & National Institute of Advanced Studies (Bangalore, India). (2009). *Science, technology, and society.* Shimla, India: Indian Institute of Advanced Study.

Tait, A., & Richardson, K. A. (2010). *Complexity and knowledge management: Understanding the role of knowledge in the management of social networks.* Charlotte, NC: Information Age.

Volti, R. (2010). *Society and technological change.* St. Louis, MO: Worth.

Watkins, M. D. (2012). How managers become leaders. The seven seismic shifts of perspective and responsibility. *Harvard Business Review, 90*(6), 64–72, 144.

Yang, A., & Shan, Y. (2008). *Intelligent complex adaptive systems.* Chicago, IL: IGI.

Suggested Readings

Barrow, J. D., Davies, P. C. W., & Harper, C. L. (2004). *Science and ultimate reality: Quantum theory, cosmology, and complexity.* Cambridge, United Kingdom: Cambridge University Press.

Basole, R., & Rouse, W. (2008). Complexity of service value networks: Conceptualization and empirical investigation. *IBM Systems Journal, 47*(1), 53–70.

Best, A., Greenhalgh, T., et al. (2012). Large-system transformation in health care: A realist review. *Milbank Quarterly, 90*(3), 421–456.

Bryman, A. (2011). *The SAGE handbook of leadership.* Thousand Oaks, CA: Sage.

Busch, M., & Hostetter, C. (2009). Examining organizational learning for application and human service organizations. *Administration and Social Work, 33*(3), 297–318.

Erickson, J. I. (2013). Reflections on leadership talent: A void or an opportunity? *Nursing Administration Quarterly, 37*(1), 44–51.

Everett, L. Q., & Sitterding, M. C. (2013). Building a culture of innovation by maximizing the role of the RN. *Nursing Administration Quarterly, 37*(3), 194–202.

Fine, M. (2009). Women leaders' discursive constructions of leadership. *Women's Studies in Communication, 32*(2), 180–202.

Malik, P. (2009). *Connecting inner power with global change: The fractal ladder.* New Delhi, India: Response Books.

Malloch, K., & Porter-O'Grady, T. (2009). *The quantum leader: Applications for the new world of work.* Sudbury, MA: Jones and Bartlett.

Nelson, M. (2009). A cloud, the crowd, and public policy. *Issues in Science and Technology, 25*(4), 71–76.

Orlando, R. 3rd, & Haytaian, M. (2012). Physician leadership: A health-care system's investment in the future of quality care. *Connecticut Medicine, 76*(7), 417–420.

Pati, S., Reum, J., Conant, E., Tuton, L., Scott, P., & Abbuhl, S. (2013). Tradition meets innovation: Transforming academic medical culture at the University of Pennsylvania's Perelman School of Medicine. *Academic Medicine, 88*(4), 461–464.

Porter-O'Grady, T., & Malloch, K. (2009). *Innovation leadership.* Sudbury, MA: Jones and Bartlett.

Ross, Y. (2012). Nurses can lead on implementing healthcare reforms. *Nursing Management, 19*(7), 9.

Song, Z., & Lee, T. H. (2013). The era of delivery system reform begins. *Journal of the American Medical Association, 309*(1), 35–36.

Starr, P. (2011). *Remedy and reaction: The peculiar American struggle over health care reform.* Hartford, CT: Yale University Press.

Zimmerman, B., Lindberg, C., & Plsek, P. (1998). *Edgeware.* Irving, TX: VHA.

Quiz Questions

Select the best answer for each of the following questions.

1. For the past 30 years we have been leaving which age?
   a. The Middle Ages
   b. The Age of Technology
   c. The Information Age
   d. The Industrial Age

2. What is the primary vehicle moving us out of the past age?
   a. Economics
   b. Technology
   c. Satellites
   d. Politics

3. As we get closer to fully living in the new age, the pace of change _____.
   a. Quickens
   b. Slows
   c. Becomes unstable
   d. Stays about the same

4. Adaptation means _____.
   a. Adjusting to the current reality
   b. Accommodating the emerging reality
   c. Bringing the past reality forward
   d. Living fully for today

5. What happens in the process of autopoiesis?
   a. Living systems seek to continually reinvent themselves.
   b. Living systems leave behind forms they do not like.
   c. Living systems maintain their stability throughout each change.
   d. Living systems end themselves because they have no other role.

6. What is accountability a matter of?
   a. Using good work processes
   b. Acting responsibly
   c. Performing efficiently
   d. Achieving desired work outcomes

7. Systems thinking identifies which of the following as an essential characteristic of all systems?
   a. Codependence
   b. Predictability
   c. Interdependence
   d. Incrementalism

8. Chaos is essential to all change. What is the primary purpose of chaos?
   a. To confuse people enough to make them change
   b. To challenge people to see the changes that are coming clearly
   c. To cut people's attachment to the past and engage them in the "noise" of change
   d. To get people to identify the characteristics of a particular change and to respond specifically to those characteristics

9. What is the primary role of the leader during a time of great change?
   a. To help people embrace change and engage with the change efforts of others
   b. To explain the kinds of changes people can expect
   c. To keep people from experiencing too much pain during the change process
   d. To push people into necessary changes and help them cope

10. Chaos theory and complexity science require leaders to alter their understanding of how change works. To develop a new understanding of change, leaders must first see their role in relationship to which of the following?
    a. The changes that are occurring in the workplace
    b. The whole system and its place in the change process
    c. The staff's issues and their responses to the demands of change
    d. The challenges that lie ahead in implementing new changes

Ten Complexity Principles for Leaders for Thriving in the Quantum Age

Do not go where the path may lead, go instead where there is no path and leave a trail.

—*Ralph Waldo Emerson*

Chapter Objectives

At the completion of this chapter, the reader will be able to

- Analyze the key characteristics of complexity and their impact on the leadership role.
- Evaluate personal characteristics and their fit with the leadership skills needed in the sociotechnical age.
- Formulate personal goals for adapting to the leadership role in the presence of chaos and complexity.
- Summarize the principles of complexity and describe their practical implications for the leadership role.
- Apply the principles of complexity theory to the personal exercise of leadership.

Ours is a time of significant social, cultural, and economic transformation (Brewer & Sanford, 2011). New scientific foundations grounded in the concept of complexity and its impact at every level of existence have altered our understanding of the leadership and management of change. The growing understanding and explication of quantum theory and the subsequent application of complexity and chaos theory to human organizations have altered the nature of leadership forever. Leaders must now more deeply understand the implications of complexity theory for the leadership role and for the processes associated with transforming work and the workplace. The principles of complexity theory largely determine how best to help others own their own change, undertake the right change processes, and understand the new rules of engagement in this postindustrial age.

Throughout the world, people are being overwhelmed by their work, the pace of change, the limitations on their time, and the endless advance of technology and the related social changes (Nelson, 2009). Especially now, health care is experiencing severely increased demand for transformation in an environment of severely diminished resources. Reflecting the many demands of health reform, the pace of change is so rapid that many healthcare leaders have left the field and many health professionals are considering whether to follow. Several factors operate to create this situation:

- *Change is endless.* In the "good old days," it seemed as though changes came in an ordered fashion and with enough time between them to allow people to adjust to the new demands. Indeed, because changes came so rarely and moved so slowly, people almost believed they created them rather than responded to them. Today, changes come so quickly that it is difficult to know when one change ends and another begins. Further, five or more changes may be unfolding at one time, and because people must deal with these changes simultaneously, they often do not know how they are doing or if any of the changes are sustainable. They may be confronted by so many changes and may be making so many changes that they wind up changing the changes. Stephen Hawking stated, "Change is," by which he means that change is a constant. Change is not a thing, but a dynamic, a context for everything that happens in the universe. During a time of transition, forces converge to make it possible for many changes to occur simultaneously. What is most striking about the nature of change today is the large number of forces converging and the large number of changes unfolding at the same time.

- *The growing social, political, and economic forces driving contemporary health reform and transformation to reflect a stronger value orientation accelerate the requirement to embrace and engage entirely new notions of healthcare service and value.* The transformation of the healthcare system requires movement out of a predominantly tertiary care model of service delivery toward more general use of value-driven models of episodic, population, and continua of care services. Approaches to accountability, value, and affordability require a new level of consciousness between provider and user and significantly different approaches to designing health care, providing service, advancing health-based outcomes, and creating a sustainable and affordable framework for health delivery in the United States. All of this requires the capacity to reconceptualize approaches; define new methods and models of care delivery; evaluate effectiveness, value, and sustainable health outcomes; and reduce the untenable cost of health service. When linked and integrated, the degree of complexity and intensity invested at every level of leadership and service in health care has few historic parallels. Challenges associated with this major transformation are constant and operate at both the collective and individual levels of leadership.

- *Information is remarkably more available than in the past.* Previously, the amount and kind of information needed at work were rarely readily available. Today, the vast amount of data on hand makes it very difficult to distinguish what is relevant and valuable. The goal is not simply to find the right information, but to find it at the right time in the right form. Indeed, too much information is just as much a hindrance as too little.

Making good decisions is still a matter of choosing data carefully. Further, this is the Information Age, which means that information is the key to sustaining integrated activities and assessing their value and impact. The importance of information has in turn affected the content and manner of decision making. Clinicians, for example, rather than depending solely on traditional medical principles and human judgment, now must draw from increasingly complex categories of evidence-grounded information in their decision making.

- *Knowledge is more a utility than a capacity.* In the twentieth century, knowledge was treated as a possession: One had knowledge or gained knowledge. The process of learning was essentially a process of "stuffing" facts into one's head. As a result of this process, the knowledgeable person possessed knowledge and could draw from it when necessary. Today, however, from the quantum perspective we see knowledge as a utility. Because so much information is available, no one has sufficient capacity to acquire all the knowledge he or she will need. Thus, the focus has shifted from possession to access. To use knowledge appropriately, people must be able to access the right knowledge at the right time in the right way for the right purpose, apply the knowledge wisely and well, and then let the knowledge go when it is no longer relevant (Hildreth & Kimble, 2004). The current challenge for leaders is to recognize that knowledge is a utility and to develop the skills needed to access knowledge in the fundamentally new context for knowledge management (Maliszewska, 2013).

- *Technology is changing the character and content of the service relationship.* Virtually nothing has changed the circumstances of life as radically as the application of new technologies. Most of us confront technologies that we read about in science fiction novels and assumed we would never live to see. Twenty years ago, the average length of stay for hospital services (the only healthcare services available) was 5.7 days. Today, the average length of stay for many high-tech services is 4.5 hours. What a dramatic change for the providers and users! Technology affects all the elements of service. Procedures once done only in a hospital under close supervision can now be done in a clinic or even at home. Laser therapy, CT scanners, nanotherapy, DNA-moderated interventions, and micro therapeutics, to name a few, are signs of the radical shift occurring in the delivery of services. The shift is still in its formative stages, with much more to come as a result of improvements in pharmaceuticals, technotherapeutics, and the application of genomics.

- *Wireless technologies now operate in a way that defies boundaries.* We live in a boundary-less world, with all that that implies. This sense of universal collectivity changes the perceptions of differences, boundaries, and barriers and allows each of us to remain connected to anyone, no matter where in the world we live. We can take our technology into any location, no matter how isolated, and still be connected to every other part of the world. This sense of the world and our connection to it has led to global communities of work, entrepreneurship, innovation, communication, and social enterprise (Marshall, 2009). New kinds of international partnerships and models that connect people and systems and challenge old constructs of boundary, be they national, regional, work related, organizational, or social, are emerging.

The preceding list merely indicates the dramatic changes that affect health care and other arenas of social existence. Further, the pace of these and other evolving and revolutionary changes is not likely to slow any time soon. The quantum, complex, even chaotic nature of change as the convergence of forces periodically brings about an age of transition, and that is exactly what we are living through now.

Chaos and Complexity and the Dance of Change

The interacting and intersecting character of complexity draws us into a web of relationships and understanding that will ultimately change our way of living. From strange attractors to webs of influence and relatedness, the elements of complexity theory alter the rules of work and interaction by giving us a deeper understanding of the relatedness of things and the role of change and discernment in human progress.

The strange characteristics of complexity are embedded in human activities as well as physical processes. An item at one level of reality is affected by everything else at all other levels. Sometimes we can see and understand the causal process. In most cases, however, the cause is not transparent and requires special knowledge to be understood. In addition, because of the connection of all elements of any process, the observation of the process affects what takes place, as evidenced by the wave–particle duality of electrons, which explains how electrons exhibit wave characteristics or particle characteristics depending on the experimental arrangement.

> **Key Point**
>
> Understanding complexity is requisite for understanding relationships. Complexity science teaches us that everything is related at some level.

The impact of leadership often depends on the amount of time the leader spends living in the potential. Schrödinger's cat, a famous thought experiment intended to illuminate the difference between actuality and potentiality, helps us understand the importance of leaders applying the principle of the potential to their own role. In 1935, Schrödinger used an imaginary scenario to illustrate a quantum mechanics problem. He posited that a cat might at one time be both alive and dead depending on an earlier random event. In the experiment, a cat, a flask of poison, and a radioactive substance are placed in a sealed box. If an internal monitor detects radioactivity, the flask is shattered, releasing the poison that ultimately kills the cat. Schrödinger's interpretation of quantum mechanics implies that, after a while, the cat is simultaneously alive and dead, yet when we look in the box, we see the cat either as alive or dead, not both. The question is: When exactly does quantum supposition end and reality collapse into one possibility or the other? These rather complex notions indicate that things are not always what they appear to be. In a state of quantum

> **Point to Ponder**
>
> How many leaders realize that their primary work is to help others deal with the changes that affect their lives and their work? Living in the potential for change is focusing on the "journey" of work rather than on the "events" of work. This journey should be a leader's primary focus.

Exhibit 2-1   Actual Versus Potential Reality

Living in the Actual	Living in the Potential
• Focus on the present	• Inclusion of coming events
• Living the experience now	• Seeing the work as journey
• Focus on good process	• Focus on good outcomes
• Key is work quality	• Key is right results
• Emphasis on current activity	• Read "signposts" of change
• People focus on their own work	• People focus on team

entanglement, the states of two systems that once interacted and then separated may not be divided each into their own definitive state. This interpretation of quantum mechanics implies that the states of two systems collapse into a definite state when either one of the systems is measured.

Actual reality is the state in which most of us live; it is where we perform our actions out of awareness of the present. We live actively in the present and attempt to meet the demands that lie right in front of us and that define our experience in current time and space. Potential reality, though just as real and current as actual reality, has different characteristics (**Exhibit 2-1**). Living in the potential means being aware of a reality that is not present but that is inevitable because of the prevailing circumstances or the force of its trajectory. A good example is the standard stop sign placed at intersections. When a driver sees the sign, he or she understands what it means and is willing to respond to it appropriately. However, the driver does not stop immediately because that would be an inappropriate (or untimely) response. The sign is a symbol of potential reality in play; action is inevitable but does not occur instantly.

Group Discussion

Sue Craft loves the details of managing her department and tends to focus on the staff issues of the day. There does not seem to be a problem beyond her abilities, and follow-up is her specialty. Sue has noticed, however, that more problems than usual are emerging. Although she is not certain where all of them are coming from, a lot more changes are originating "up there" than usual, creating more daily problems. She is beginning to feel overwhelmed. Discuss the options available to Sue for dealing with the increase in problems. Consider the following questions: Is her focus on the problems that arise daily appropriate for someone managing a department? How might her leadership role be altered to help her handle the large number of changes being handed down by the higher levels of management? How might Sue change her orientation to be better in touch with future issues?

Leaders are good signpost readers. They understand what the signposts indicate about the journey and act on them only as the circumstances dictate. Good leaders have what

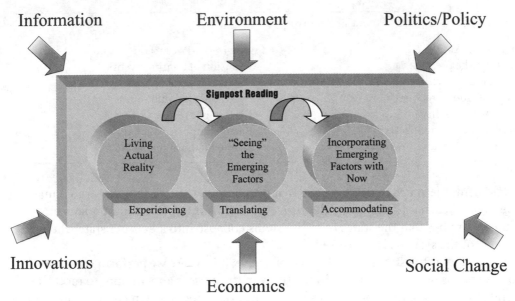

Figure 2-1 Seeing the Journey into the Future.

is called predictive and adaptive capacity. This is the ability to see and understand the interface between environment, organization, and persons and to predict the impact that interface has on action. From the perspective of action, the leader can predict the trajectory that lies ahead and adapt practices and behaviors that best demonstrate the convergence between the demands of the environment and the trajectory of the journey. Leaders' ability to anticipate which actions will be needed, through accurate reading of the signposts (predictive and adaptive), is one of the keys to good leadership. It also demonstrates living in the potential (**Figure 2-1**).

How many organizations have been led by people who live so thoroughly in the actual that they are unable to anticipate events far enough ahead of time to allow for an effective response? How many organizations merely react to one crisis after another because the power of the potential is not incorporated into the leadership role in a way that enables it to be applied properly and at the right time?

Living in the potential requires leaders to recognize that they are managing a journey and thus need a specific set of predictive and adaptive skills. Leaders who have been raised on the twentieth-century model of leadership tend to focus on the goal or end-point and implement activities that will get people to that goal. In a chaotic period, when deconstruction occurs at the same rate as construction, or even faster, the dust of change makes it difficult for leaders even to see the goal. Instead, they must read the signposts of change, understand how they indicate the trajectory of decisions and actions, explain to others what they mean, and engage others in activities that move the organization in the direction indicated (Heifetz & Linksy, 2002). Two skills are critical here: the ability to read where the change is occurring and determine the right responses, and the ability to anticipate the next signpost early enough to evaluate current progress and determine one signpost's relationship to the next one (adaptation). In short, leaders need to respond fluidly to current demands and changing circumstances, remain open to the messages carried by longer term indicators, and act in accordance with these messages (Das, 2013).

Many leaders get sucked into the concerns of daily work (actual reality) to such an extent that they lose sight of the potential. When leaders focus their energies on daily activities, they are not able to discipline these activities in the light of imminent influences or circumstances. In many, if not most, organizations, the ability of leaders to engage their own future at the right time is frequently compromised by the fact that they never saw it coming. All eyes are on the activities of the moment, which consume everyone's attention and prevent anyone from seeing the emerging shifts and circumstances that will ultimately affect the organization's ability to thrive.

Many authors, from Nicholas Negroponte (1995) to Kevin Kelly (1995), have delved into the dynamic of complexity to make it understandable and applicable to human enterprises. They have derived certain principles for and a number of insights about the coming age and how to navigate it. The remainder of this chapter presents rules that can help leaders consider the leadership role and separate out the activities that best match the demands of the new world of work (Crowell, 2011; Uhl-Bien & Marion, 2008).

Principle 1: Wholes Are Not Just the Sum of Their Parts

Wholes are made up of smaller units that interact with each other to sustain the whole.

In the twentieth century, managers believed they had to focus simply on the units of work for which they were responsible. They were evaluated within the context of their own units of service, and if they did well in those units, managed the workforce well, and advanced productivity and profitability, they were rewarded and sometimes even promoted.

In a systems mind-set, any service unit is looked at as a part of a broader context that gives the unit direction and purpose. A unit does not simply provide services independently of its relationship to other parts of the organization. Each unit, at some level, is required to ensure that what it does fits well with the activities of the other units. According to systems theory, the fit between the components of a system is as critical as the work of any one component. This notion of goodness-of-fit is what drives the understanding of the relationship between the whole and its parts. The whole is not simply the sum of its parts; it is instead the representation of the interface and coordinated interaction and integration of all of the parts in a synergy and fluidity of relationship, interdependence, and collective support.

> **Key Point**
>
> Leaders need to focus on issues of "fit." They live in the "white space," the connections, most of the time and must constantly attempt to see where the intersections are and how they facilitate the work of the system.

The most common problem in systems is that a unit and the people that make it up get co-opted by their work and their intentions. Because they leave their work and relationships within the context of the unit, they forget that whatever they do has a broader frame of reference that must be taken into account in assessing the viability of their work.

An organizational leader must always keep the focus on the organization's broader purpose. The leader's role is to ensure that there is a goodness of fit between the activities of those at the point of service and the overall work of the organization. This takes considerable doing, especially when the leader also must pay attention to the kind and quality of work done at the point of service. Being present at the point of service can cause the leader to get caught up in the day-to-day activities of the service and to forget the ultimate goals toward which these activities are directed.

Group Discussion

Systems are different from institutions. Systems thrive on relationships and intersections, and models of systems reflect relationships rather than control. Discuss the effect that a systems orientation would have on the design of a healthcare facility. Draw an organizational chart to reflect relationships instead of functions, including relationships to the community, other services, other health systems, and so on. Finally, discuss the differences between leading a facility that is a system and leading a facility that is an institution.

Leaders are responsible for seeing and living "systemness." The differences between institutions and systems are significant (**Exhibit 2-2**). In institutions, most of the work is compartmentalized and organized vertically, which, together with the focus on process, creates a clear separation among the various loci of work. Because the focus is on results at the point of productivity, special roles are created to address the issue of fit. Yet those responsible, from managers to specialty engineers, are not located where most of the work is done, and those who do the work are instead engaged in the tasks to be done and the processes to be undertaken.

Point to Ponder

Everything in our society reflects a vertical orientation, including organizational hierarchies. Leaders now must complement vertical thinking, which is about control, with horizontal thinking, which is about relatedness. Both are necessary, yet leaders, because of the prevalence of vertical thinking, must at this time concentrate on building horizontal connections.

In most organizations, the organizational chart speaks volumes about the structuring of work and the value placed on it. Lines and boxes enumerate the various functional capacities expected within the context of each role. The reporting infrastructure is critical to the structuring of work, and clear lines and patterns of interaction are important—but only with regard to communication about work activities.

Workers at the point of service generally are not concerned with value, linkage, and integration. Instead, they are busy performing the routines of daily work and perfecting these routines so that the work gets done effectively and within the allotted timeframe. As a result, they often view the work as more important than its purpose and become caught up in the politics and process of work, which impairs their ability to embrace change and adjust their activities in response to new demands.

Exhibit 2-2   Institutions Versus Systems

Institutions	Systems
• Unilateral interests/goals	• Multifocal interests/goals/values
• Nonaligned	• Strong alignment of stakeholders
• Driven by self-interest	• Collateral interests
• Focus on structure/function	• Focus on relatedness
• Highly competitive	• Outcomes driven
• Survival focused	• Centered on thriving
• Vertically integrated	• Horizontal/vertical linkage

In systems, on the other hand, the real work of management and leadership is to refocus work and place it into its appropriate context. To do this, however, leaders must avoid being equally co-opted by the work and thereby prevented from identifying its relationship to other factors that influence it. Imagine, for example, how challenging it is for leadership and staff to reconfigure the work they do and the service they deliver within the context of a value-driven framework for health care. Different from functional and process-based focuses, where the emphasis is on the quality of the work, value-based practices center on the intensity and integrity of the relationship between the work, its purpose, and the achievement of a sustainable health outcome.

Many of the problems in organizations arise from the inability of leaders to think and act horizontally or collaterally. In other words, leaders must be able to see the whole and characterize each of the units of work within the context of its contribution to the whole. They must also be able to see how the units work together to advance the purpose and value of the whole. The interface and the intersection of work in all the various locations in a system are as critical to the success of the system as is the quality of any individual effort in the system.

In essence, leaders, regardless of their location, see all work from the perspective of the whole system. Indeed, they analyze each work activity in terms of the function it plays in achieving the purpose of the whole. The leader's role is based on the system's imperatives and how the individual and collective work activities operate in concert to achieve them. At the same time, the structure of the system enables the leaders to see and act out of systemness and keep in touch with the demands of the whole. A part of constructing more effective organizations is the consideration that the compartmentalization and isolation of leader and staff action in departments, services, and units limit their ability to connect. More value must be attached to individual effort to seamlessly connect it to the purposes of the system. The reverse is also true: Infinitely challenging for executive leaders is the capacity of leadership to connect the strategic imperatives of the system in a meaningful way to the individual work activities unfolding in departments, services, and units.

Systems operate more as biological units than as mechanical structures. They are the sum of all the dynamics that drive them. Therefore, they are best viewed as a set of relationships and intersections rather than as a mere collection of components. In systems, the intersections between the elements are as critical as what goes on within any single element. The goodness of fit between the actions and processes of a system is what ultimately creates the fluidity that is the system's essence. Goodness of fit is much more important than any element by itself. Effective leaders always examine the activities of the members to determine their goodness of fit with each other. One of the leader's challenges is to bridge the dichotomy between the workers' focus on good task and their need to focus on good fit.

Leaders and staff need to recognize that no one person can make a sustaining contribution though his or her own efforts alone. Although an individual's efforts can achieve incremental improvements, the sustainability of these improvements depends on the degree of interface between the individual's efforts and the consolidated and aggregated efforts of the whole. The ability of leaders to make this fact clear to the staff is critical to the effectiveness of their activities.

As noted previously, work is not inherently valuable. Instead, its value lies in its purpose, and the efforts of leaders should reflect this reality. Yet decades of process and functional orientation at every organizational level have made a belief in the value of work effort alone a fundamental part of every worker's belief set. Just observe the reaction of healthcare workers to the myriad work-related changes that, in their view, prevent them from effectively doing the activities with which they have become most familiar. In addition, many workers are mourning the fact that they are no longer performing the tasks they had come to know so well. What they have forgotten is that many of these tasks have been made obsolete by changes inside and outside the organization, and leaders now have the major challenge of reintroducing staff, as well as other leaders and managers, to the concept of system and then convincing them of the importance of fitting the organization's work to its changing purposes. This is especially true as leaders attempt to create the change context that translates the national imperative to move health care out of volume constructs into a much stronger value framework.

During the twentieth century, the various healthcare disciplines, out of a need to find meaning in their professional work, tried to define themselves and to devise and promulgate practice parameters. Indeed, one of that century's achievements is the contribution of the healthcare disciplines, from nursing and medicine to pharmacy and nutrition, to the improvement and elaboration of health services, leading to a broader and more complex array of services than has been available at any time in human history.

Today's challenge for the health professions is to make their boundaries more fluid and to renegotiate their roles to create a comprehensive continuum by better integrating the health services they provide. Value-based health care now demands that the professions find the interface between their roles and construct the collateral and collaborative network of relationships and interactions that best meet patients' needs and advance the quality and value of health service. The professions now must find what connects them rather than focusing on what separates them. In other words, here again the components (the professions) must converge to address the whole (the public's health). Further, technological tools now make it possible to do this—and make it necessary, at least if the health professions are to ensure the health of people over ever-increasing life spans.

Group Discussion

Discuss the healthcare professions as they are currently configured and predict their likely future. Are they going to be able to function effectively in the twenty-first century as they now exist? If not, how will they have to be revised to remain relevant in the new age of health care?

Principle 2: All Health Care Is Local

The integration and effectiveness of health services depend on local relationships, not centralized authorities.

Everyone has heard at least once that all health care is local. As Martin Buber would have said, all health services are provided within the context of the "I-Thou" relationship: In healthcare language, someone provides a service, someone receives it. Through this fundamental human equation, care and healing emerge, and everything from structure to equipment, competence to relationship, is reflected in it. When two or more parties interact, the result is always an intimate bond represented through the exchange of feelings, thoughts, expectations, conversation, and action (I-Thou). From a systems perspective, most of the other components of the system converge at some level to support this exchange, and those that do not ultimately will impede it.

The function of structure in a service system is twofold: (1) to ensure the integrity of the system and the ability of its components to work in concert to achieve its ends efficiently and effectively and (2) to facilitate the work of the system. In health care, the purpose of a health system is to address the needs of the community. The system, of course, cannot serve its community without also serving individual members of the community at the point of service; although at the governance level, the system serves the community as a whole. Both levels—the point-of-service level and the governance level—are essential, and each supports the other.

The main implication of this principle is that each element of the system must serve to empower those at the point of service and allow them to provide care to the community through their individual acts. In an effective system, 90% of the critical decisions are made at the point of service, and the life of the system is always primarily lived out there as well. At the point of service is the intersection between the purpose of the system (strategic) and the place where the meaning and the life of the system is expressed (point of service).

An effective system has no more structure than is absolutely needed for its work. When unnecessary structure exists, it tends to suck resources and work away from the point of service. The more structure a system has, the more likely the system will support its structure rather than its services, the more money the structure will

Key Point

All health care is local. A system operates from its point of service outward. If a healthcare provider is not directly giving care to a patient, he or she is serving someone who is.

cost the system, the fewer the resources the system will have available, and the less able the system will be to thrive and fulfill its purpose.

In a system, everything operates from the center out. Systems are organic in shape and design. The most obvious configuration for a system is a circle. That this is so indicates that systems are more about relationships and intersections than about anything else. Systems possess flow and fluidity and are more dynamic than static. They encompass interactions and relationships in a continuous and vibrant interplay that results in the fulfillment of their purposes. All the activities of a system work together to help the system adapt to changes, meet its goals, and ensure its survival.

Every system takes its life from the places where it intersects with the greater community. In particular, a health services system is directed toward advancing the health of the community where it is located, and there is obviously a tight relationship between the system and the receivers of its services. The system must therefore make sure that its services reflect the community's culture. The leader's role is to ensure that the purposes of the system and the needs of the community are congruent and that everything the system does is directed toward meeting those needs in a culturally appropriate manner.

All other components of a system are intimately connected to its center—the place where it carries out its mission. At this place, the point of service, the provider and the receiver of services meet, the community is served one member at a time, the life of the system is expressed, and the value of the system is realized. All the system's other components should be configured to support the activity at its center.

The point of service is also where the majority of conflicts occur and where a poor structure has the largest impact. If the processes at the point of service are not structured with goodness of fit in mind, the system will begin to break down. Eventually, its purpose will become lost and its ability to thrive will be compromised.

The vast majority of the work done by the leader of a system involves building sustainable relationships, driving innovation, and keeping the system intact and on course. Because a system is a membership community, it can easily lose sight of its purpose and forget what its real work is. The leader seeks congruence between the system's purpose and the work of its members, and in doing this the leader faces the challenge of overcoming the ever present conflict between personal and collective agendas. The leader must keep aware that the system is a membership community and remind others of this fact as well. A good leader realizes that the system's survival depends on the dance between good structure and good process, the members' focus on the product of their work, and the positive impact the system has on those it serves.

A good leader also ensures that the structure of the system does not impede the system's fluidity and flexibility—its ability to quickly adapt to changing conditions. To do this, the leader must revise the structure as the system grows to position the system to better serve the

> ### Point to Ponder
>
> Culture rules. The point of service is driven by the culture of the patient population. The system is driven by the culture of its community, which gives it purpose, and the culture of its members or workers, who give it focus. These constituencies converge to drive the system to thrive.

community. The leader also must be sensitive to the tightness of fit between the system's structure and its purposes because the structure has the potential to obstruct the work processes rather than support them. When the structure does act as an obstacle and draws to itself unnecessary resources, it must be reconfigured.

The point-of-service workers must be able to act so as to meet the demands of the culture of those they serve. For example, they should have few constraints placed on their ability to make decisions and construct appropriate service arrangements and processes. Of course, their actions should be informed by principles and practices worked out in advance by the stakeholders at the point of service.

The configuration at the point of service must, at some level, reflect the character and content of the work. Here the issue of differentiation becomes critical. Each population-based service configuration is unique because it represents the characteristics of the specific population served. The twentieth-century addiction to sameness must be overcome. The rules that govern the functioning of each service must be derived from the service's relationship to those served, not its relationship to the prevailing structure of the system. Although structure is critical at other places in the system, it is not appropriate at the point of service because there the culture of the population is more important than the needs of any other element of the system.

The notion of the point of service is dramatically changing as the various elements of health reform are translated into action in an accountable care format. Value-based care along an episodic or population continuum demands much more fluid, portable, and variable approaches to both designing and delivering healthcare services. This notion of point of service includes a stronger orientation to user-driven, home-based, community-centered approaches to service delivery that moves providers out of an institutional frame of reference into a service-based frame of reference. This shift represents a stronger grounding in community- and population-specific models of care delivery. The service provider is much more mobile and adaptable at the point of service in a clinical model that addresses the cultural and structural issues of users more than the institutional structural formats of the provider (Hines & Mercury, 2013).

Group Discussion

The point of service drives approximately 90% of the decision making in a healthy and effective system, and therefore most of the decisions should be made by the workers located there. For example, the Ritz-Carlton Hotel is well known for allowing its point-of-service workers to make service decisions to enhance guest experiences. Discuss the effects on a health system of moving 90% of the decisions made to the point of care. What impact would this have on the authority structure of the system? What changes would have to occur to make the transfer of decision-making power sustainable? How would staff have to change to manage the additional decision-making responsibilities?

The preceding makes clear the importance of the point of service and the need for structural independence and functional liberty at the point of service. Each point-of-service worker has an obligation to ensure that the decisions and activities that unfold there are congruent and that each is informed and disciplined by the system's purposes and direction as it addresses the needs of the community. Furthermore, the decisions made at the point of service should predominate because they give form to the work of serving the community one person at a time. Out of this dynamic—consisting of the interplay of the system's purposes with the worker's decisions and activities—come the seamless and symbiotic relationships between the system and the workers that create the place where the system lives out its purposes and makes a difference in the lives of those it serves.

Principle 3: Value Is Now the Centerpiece of Service Delivery

Anything that adds value to any part of a system adds value to the whole system. The sustainability of the system requires the aggregation of numerous additions of value.

In the Industrial Age, assessments of value were often based on volume. One of the most common measures of the value of work, for instance, was the quantity of work done. Even the language of health care reflected a volume orientation: Nurses, physicians, and other health professionals, as they said, wanted to do the "most" they could do for their patients. The processes associated with work were viewed as almost more important than the work's purpose, and there was a sense that the activity of providing health care was inherently valuable. The orientation toward process was almost sacrosanct, and much attention, even in the quality movement, was devoted to establishing good processes for delivering services.

Users of health service have the right to know about the services they are provided, including the quality and cost. Increasing emphasis on healthcare transparency requires that users of health care have the information necessary for good decision making and can choose health services and providers based on some objective, measurable notion of value. Providing reliable value including cost and quality information helps inform user choice. Users use this information to make particular choices in a way that is consistent with their values and their resources. Over time the use of user-modified cost and quality information informs more effective thinking and appropriate resource use.

Good value is driven by a notion of high-level interoperability. Interoperable systems (integrated or converged) are deeply embedded in the DNA of effective service systems. The integrity and integration of processes, functions, and structures necessary to support an effective service are essential. Cell phone technology is perhaps one of the best sources of evidence of interoperability: Many thousands of functions, components, and elements converge to create an instrument that can be used for multiple purposes, from grocery list making to gasoline purchases, information seeking to entertainment, access to education to services and products. Accessibility and high levels of integration and interoperability in the health system facilitate user choice, utility, effectiveness, and, ultimately, good experiences and positive health impact.

Although process integrity is vital, it does not itself create or add value. Work processes are always disciplined by and gain their meaning and value through the purposes toward which they are directed. Any activity, to be meaningful, must at some level advance some purpose; otherwise, the worker is taking value away from the enterprise. Even if the worker does nothing, the action of doing nothing is actually drawing value away because purpose could have been positively advanced by almost any activity—an activity that is not being performed. Work, then, either adds value or reduces it. It adds value when it advances the purposes of the system, and it takes value away when it fails to advance these purposes.

In a true system, all activities, roles, and functions, no matter how large or small, have value. Each, when working in concert with the others, does something to advance the system's purpose and has an impact on the system's vigor and viability. For this reason careful selection of every role in the system is essential to the system's ability to thrive. This ability depends in part on the goodness of fit between roles and functions, not simply on the roles and functions themselves.

Value, however, is not just tied to the persons who do work. Value is more closely linked to the products of that work. Increasingly, there is a demand for transparency between process and product so that this fit is continually assessed and evaluated to determine the efficacy of the relationship between process and product. Users expect to have the right and the capacity to make value decisions based on data that reflect the effectiveness of health work through the lens of its impact on health. Increasingly, government entities, insurers, and advocates require that accountability-driven evidence-based data be con-

structed and made available to enable users to make wiser health service choices. This public representation of value allows users to make effective judgments related to health service comparability, costs, quality, and sustainable impact. Through this mechanism, both the form and action of value become drivers of choice based on measures of quality, cost, and impact (Hacker & Walker, 2013).

> ## Key Point
>
> Everyone in a system is obligated to add value to the system. Everyone is doing something, even if it is negative. If someone is not adding value, he or she is taking away value.

The triadic relationship between purpose, person, and performance is the cornerstone of any measure of vitality in any kind of system. The effective leader understands this relationship almost intuitively. It is so embedded in the dynamics of the system that almost nothing can be accomplished if it is not used as a framework. The whole is a reflection of the fit between its parts—of the congruity and resonance of the many functions that make up its infrastructure. As these elements join in a seamless dance of intersection and interaction, each individual element becomes invisible, but all of them together, at least in a true system, work so harmoniously and are so tightly interwoven that they are perceivable only as a whole. In a noneffective system, the parts and pieces are easy to see because of their incongruence and lack of flow or fit and because they appear out of context. Rather than contribute to the whole, they draw resources, energy, and attention away from the whole, impairing its integrity. They can cause a system to break down and fail to achieve its purpose.

Contemporary thinking about evidence-based practice reflects this focus on essential systemness. Evidence of making a difference in the lives of those we serve cannot be determined unilaterally. Isolating individual action from the intersection with other forces and actions simply does not tell us whether any sustainable difference has been made and whether our actions had anything to do with the difference or change. Only when integrated and synthesized, if you will—with other related and connected efforts— does the convergence of the effort produce anything meaningful. The convergence of efforts, related and linked together, drives evidence of contribution and sustainability of effort and outcomes. In current efforts to establish evidence-based clinical processes as a foundation for clinical decision making, success is limited to the extent that the system connections between stakeholders are made and the interface of collaborative efforts is established. Evidence of making a difference is also evidence of collaboration, integration, and systemization of all the related contributions.

Leaders must operate out of an understanding that each component of a system is a microcosm of the system. To lead any one component, a leader must direct his or her vision from the perspective of the whole toward the part, rather than the reverse. The focus should be on the whole system and on how each component contributes to the integrity and action of the whole. From this perspective, the leader diagnoses the element and evaluates its goodness of fit with the other elements as they contribute to the whole. The leader also attempts to keep value, which depends on the congruence of work, quality, and resources, at the center of everyone's sense of relationship to his or her work and to the workplace (**Figure 2-2**).

The leader is always aware of the connection between the elements of the system and the fluidity and "tightness" of the intersections between elements, where the life of the system is most evident. Questions related to interface, connection, integration, communication, and interaction are the driving concerns of the leader. If there are problems in a system, even if they originate in inadequate or failed processes, they are ultimately expressed as brokenness between the elements and in their failure to exhibit the flow, seamlessness, and linkage essential to the system. For the system to advance, individual contributions must be woven together in a way that achieves substantive consonance.

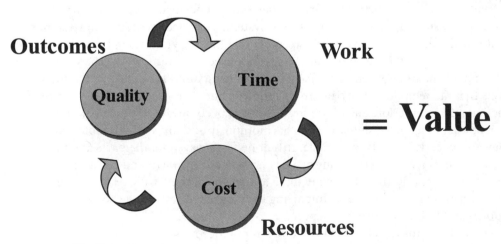

Figure 2-2 The Value Equation.

Principle 4: Simple Systems Aggregate to Complex Systems

Simple systems combine with other simple systems to form more complex systems. Complexity grows incrementally through the interconnection of smaller, simpler systems (called chunking).

To understand complexity, we need to look for the simplicity that is generated from its center. Everything is related to everything else in some way. This concept lies at the center of any understanding of how systems operate and thrive. The task of a system's leader is to delineate the linkages and intersections among all elements of the system. The leader identifies the common elements present everywhere in the system and those unique contributing elements that are located at critical places in the system and contribute to the effectiveness of the whole.

> ## Point to Ponder
>
> A leader who is head of a particular service or department must see his or her role from the perspective of the whole system. In fact, the best way for leaders to look at matters is as if the leader is leading the whole system from the perspective of the particular service or department. Each leader's commitment to the system gives the leader, no matter where he or she is located, focus and a framework for the expression of his or her role.

Every element of a larger system is a system itself. It has its own simplicity, complexity, integrity, and chaos. If the component system is viewed only as something simple, its fit and contributing purpose remain invisible. They are disclosed when the system is seen in the appropriate context (i.e., as part of the larger system).

Each component system abides by the same rules as the larger system. The component system must have fluidity, fit, and integrity, and its parts must intersect and operate in a way that advances its contribution and value to the whole system. The component systems' substantial and continuous interaction—what Kevin Kelly calls clumping—maintains the integrity of the larger system (Kelly, 2010).

With regard to component systems, there are two basic requirements. First, each must have well-integrated components and function well internally. Second, the systems must

Group Discussion

Sam Casey, as head of his department, has consistently looked out for the interests of his department and its staff. Occasionally, he has had to fight other departments to get what he wanted for his own. According to him, that is all part of being a good leader. Discuss whether he is right. Among other things, consider Sam's approach from the perspective of systems thinking. What problems is his approach likely to create? What advice could Sam be given to help him improve his leadership? How should a departmental leader balance the system's needs and the functional needs of the department?

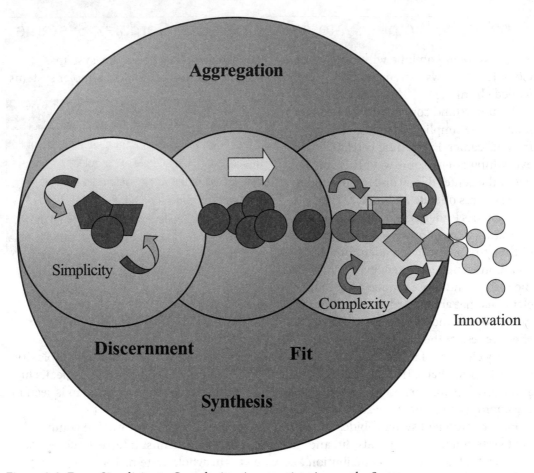

Figure 2-3 From Simplicity to Complexity: Aggregation Across the System.

intersect and interact with other related systems to make up the larger system and ensure its effectiveness (**Figure 2-3**).

In the past, leaders have not always paid attention to these requirements. Many organizations have suffered from the narrow focus of leaders who concentrate on their area of responsibility to the detriment of other component systems and the enterprise as a whole. Even reward systems sometimes encourage people to excel at the expense of others, destroying relationships, obstructing interaction, and skewing the distribution of the available resources. Whole organizations are held hostage to these highly unilateral decision makers and never fully achieve their potential. The glue of trust is never established, precluding the level of productivity that can result from a truly resonating system.

Every leader of a component of a larger system must ensure that the component operates effectively. The effectiveness of a component system, however, cannot be achieved simply through having an internal locus of control. For example, in an organization that provides health services, although the point of service drives the content and culture of the entire organization, the point of service must also reflect the obligations and operations of the entire organization. Each smaller system should mirror the larger system, although it is refined in its specific manner of representing it. Anyone who comes directly to the smaller system should see a picture of the whole system, including that system's mission, service, quality, and outcomes, all of which should be manifest in the smaller system's work.

Too often, healthcare organizations have components that do not fit together well. Think how typical it is for people seeking healthcare services to be asked the same questions over and over again as they move through the system. From admissions to treatment, a patient may face five or more points of query simply because the components do not interact seamlessly enough to eliminate the need for them. The cost of allowing simple systems not to operate smoothly together has never fully been measured. Complex systems work because they act interdependently, representing their synthesis at every point in the continuum. Without this synthesis, systems break down and ultimately fail, affecting everything within them and everything to which they are connected.

Principle 5: Diversity Is Essential to Life

Diversity is essential to life on every level. Only where diversity is present is the capacity to thrive ensured. Diversity makes chaos visible because it pushes systems to forever adapt to changes in their environment.

It is common wisdom—at least if you believe the literature on leadership—that conflict should be avoided and that processes must be in place to reduce conflict to a minimum. Unfortunately, nothing could be further from the truth.

Diversity is the visual manifestation of the chaos that exists within all systems. That chaos is the energy that arises from the confluence and conflict among the elements of a system as they intersect to create the conditions necessary for the system's adaptation. Diversity is a characteristic of the endless dance of design and configuration as the elements confront each other and sort out a way of fitting together.

In creating an effective and meaningful workplace, leaders must attend to a number of issues. First, they must understand that diversity is necessary for a system to thrive. Kelly (1995) uses *heterogeneity* to refer to the essential element in the movement and adaptation of any system. Whichever word is used, a wide range of views and roles is essential for determining the direction the system should move in and for establishing the common ground necessary for leading the participants and elements in that direction. Homogeneity is the enemy of success because it represents the unilateral, the stable, the inert. Missing from homogeneity is the contrast, conflict, and interfacing among elements and their sorting and reconfiguring around ever-changing circumstances as the system keeps rhythm with the environment within which it must thrive.

The presence of conflict indicates that a system is healthy and energetic. It enables the leader of the system to see the differences that exist and challenges the leader to sort through the differences to determine what they indicate. Embedded in these differences are the many varieties of influence that, when viewed together, tell the leader where the organization is, what the issues are, and what the organization's responses might be.

Leaders must recognize that their main work is interpreting present activities in light of their potential to create the future. The future does not simply happen. Each future moment is part of a flow of activities whose completion lays the foundation for the next set of activities arising in the next moment. Each moment encompasses indicators of the next moment and of the changes that will occur then. To influence the future, therefore, the leader must be able to see the vortex of conflicting and converging elements to get a sense of the trajectory of these forces and what their convergence tells about the context and content of potential change.

The leader must be able to harness chaos through its visible conflicts and divergences because these reveal the direction of any changes that are occurring. For this reason leadership roles in today's world are more that of gatherers than directors. In the old Newtonian model, the leader of an organization was expected to determine the organization's strategic endpoint and direct the organization toward it through personal influence. Today the leader's strategy should be to connect with the diverse components of the organization to engage the collective synergy that yields insight about the appropriate and right choices for the system's trajectory. In doing this, the leader should capitalize on the strengths, skills, insights, and wisdom that are located in these diverse participants. Only by embracing and engaging the diversities and conflicts within the organization is the leader able to discover the actions most likely to keep the organization thriving.

Group Discussion

Charles Frederick has been the chief operating officer of a health clinic for 2 years. He is nice enough but hates to have his views or leadership questioned. Therefore, although he hires bright people like himself, he tends to favor people who think like him so that he will not have to fight to achieve his goals. In time, his staff have come to understand this and have stopped offering different insights and points of view. Discuss what happens when leaders hear only what agrees with their own thinking. What is missing from the decision making in such a situation? What are some of the problems that arise? Among other issues, what are the effects on accountability?

Here both the value and the meaning of conflict become especially important. Conflict is a vehicle for discerning the proper direction for the organization to take. In particular, it is the strongest indicator of where to begin the work of determining the most appropriate actions at any given time. The leader both honors the essential differences that exist and uses them to reach clarification. These differences include cultural differences as well as the diversity of insights, opinions, and skills possessed by members of the organization. No one person has all the knowledge and abilities necessary to adequately "see" the patterns of emergence embedded in diversity, complexity, and chaos. Only through processes that actualize the disparate potentials present in the full range of participant contributions can the signs of change and its themes be found. A good leader can tap into this diversity by using effective methodologies. Through dialogue, for example, the leader pulls out the premises, themes, and signposts that indicate the best direction for the organization to move in and the actions most likely to lead it in that direction. The goal for the leader, in short, is to utilize collective wisdom and, through the coalescence of this effort, establish the foundations for organizational common ground.

Principle 6: Error Is Essential to Success

Both random error and conscious error are essential to the process of creation. In fact, error underpins all change.

Historically, leaders have been taught that error, especially in health care, is harmful and must be avoided at all costs. And of course, in the clinical sense, for the most part that is true. However, what we have now come to understand is that error is an essential constituent of all change. Further, error can be used as a measuring device to indicate where people are currently located on the pathway to some desired impact, endpoint, or outcome. Therefore, leaders must value error as a useful leadership tool.

Error is present everywhere in the universe. It is embedded within systems and contributes to their adaptation and thriving. Error indicates where a system has to adjust to new circumstances. It forces people to stop a process of change long enough to assess the situation and make the necessary modifications before resuming the process.

It informs the agents of change of where they are in the change process and what is actually happening (Erwin, 2009). It alerts them to a change in conditions or a breach in the process or a demand for a different response. Error indicates where and how the system is in relationship to a process or an initiative. It alerts people to the convergence of incongruent variables that led to the mistake or flaw and that indicate their presence or impact on the flow of events.

> **Key Point**
>
> Error is essential to all progress.
> Far from being a deficit, error indicates where someone is on the journey.
> The only unacceptable error is the error that is repeated.

Error is an essential teacher. At varying levels of complexity, error indicates a break in the confluence and congruity of processes in a way that causes participants to note the break, assess the situation, and take action. Although some errors are certainly undesirable, such as those resulting in death or severe damage, even they serve as indicators of critical problems and as incitements to action. They teach, inform, advise, warn, and alert by showing that the current circumstances vary dangerously from the norm or from expectations. They point dramatically to important lessons and ensure that these lessons are, in fact, learned.

Error plays a critical role in learning and in developmental activities. When error fails to teach the negative energy embedded deep within it begins to emerge, operate, and create problems. The only inappropriate error is the error repeated. An error's repetition indicates that the relevant lesson remained unlearned (**Exhibit 2-3**).

Leaders can use error, as a constituent of change, to evaluate a change process and determine the best activities for advancing the system and preventing the same mistakes or flaws from recurring. A leader's attitude toward error determines how he or she addresses individual errors. If leaders value errors as tools, they tend to use each individual error as

Exhibit 2-3 Mistakes Versus Errors

Mistakes	Errors
• Are nonrandom	• Are random
• Are repeated	• Are repeatable
• Do not result in learning	• Contain lessons
• Impair sustainability	• Foster sustainability

a guide to improving performance. If leaders treat errors solely as a cause for punishment, individual errors will never be able to serve as indicators of problems and as stimulators of corrective action, to the organization's detriment.

Of course, some errors must be controlled. Life-threatening or risk-intensive errors must be managed in a way that reduces their incidence and impact, even though these also have the capacity to teach. They cannot, however, be eliminated entirely. Concerted efforts to eliminate all error and strive for 100% error-free processes and environments defy reality. Error is the universe's mechanism for ensuring change, adaptation, and advancement. Error is always present at some level. The total absence of error serves as a metaphor for death. How error is managed and used, where it occurs, how risk is strategically handled, and how improvement results are the keystones for effective error management processes.

Point to Ponder

Risk can never be fully eliminated. Indeed, risk should be viewed as a resource that simply requires good management. It is inherent in all human activity and must be accommodated in any plan. Planning for error makes room for risk and provides the space to learn from it.

Leaders must remember that there is a certain randomness to error and that all the good planning and control in the world cannot eliminate every mistake and defect. Errors can be reduced by a high degree of management and control, as demonstrated in the redundancy approach: Redundancy, standard processes, protocols, routines, algorithms, and so forth compensate for inherent error by making multiple and organized options available to anticipate and respond to the errors that do occur. For example, the airline industry (and increasingly health care) is built on good error management, which accounts for the fact that the level of risk from errors in flight is lower than the risk present in almost any other business activity.

Healthcare organizations also have a large capacity for reducing risk from errors. Because of the focus on value as an outflow of health reform, more attention is being paid to risk and error systems in these organizations. Indeed, many errors and risks are still not discussed and may even be ignored or overlooked because of the legal implications of exposing clinical errors with their attendant risks. In recent years, however, the unacceptable level of risk resulting from medication and medical procedure errors has brought about a renewed emphasis on risk reduction and error management activities. Increasingly, healthcare leaders use error as a tool in managing behavior and as a vehicle for change, rather than as a cause for disciplinary action. Consequently, they and other leaders would do well to become familiar with the new science developing around the management of human error. As comparative effectiveness becomes a more important part of measuring and evaluating essential clinical value, increasingly sophisticated digital processes and tools become a common part of clinical leadership decision making.

Principle 7: Systems Thrive When All of Their Functions Intersect and Interact

Systems thrive when their functions and dynamics intersect and interact in a continual dance of relationship and transformation.

Newton once described the universe as a great machine. Einstein said it was more like one great thought; his point is that nothing in the universe is mechanical or organized in a machine-like structure. Modern notions of thinking and behavior are based on the emerging scientific principles and observations of our time and guide the management principles of the twenty-first century. An outdated Newtonian management perspective is that the purpose of workers is to accomplish the economic and production goals of the organization, generally through monetary, coercive, and control mechanisms.

More recent discussions of leadership in organizations represent later Western philosophical thought (generally that of Kant) and indicate the belief in the paradox of being subject to nature but also free from it. This move away from scientific rationalism deepens the understanding that people are both subject to the laws of nature yet free to set their own direction and goals. The product of disbelief generates a deeper understanding of self-organizing systems (instead of the notion of systems driven by an external, objective force living outside of the force's impact and therefore not influenced by it) demonstrating a growing knowledge of the action, interaction, and interdependencies of "wholes" generally understood in the concepts of formative teleology. The notion that humans are a part of nature as well as observers of nature makes them full participants in a way that cannot separate them from what they observe and participate in. Human beings essentially are free to act but are inextricably entwined with the nature of which they are a part, subject and mover at the same time (thus, human's actions have consequence and interact with other actions that also generate consequences). The contemporary struggle in this formative teleology is that the "agent" of change must use objective notions and ideas in a way that incorporates them inside of the "experience" of any change. The leader then allows this dynamic interplay to unfold in innovative and creative ways that generate new ideas, processes, and products that push the human experience continuously forward. In this scenario the effective leader is more facilitating a dance of interaction than directing a series of processes or functions.

Systems science posits that the universe operates as a set of interacting forces and interdependent relationships. Everything in the universe is in some way acting on or interacting with something else. Because interdependence is an essential characteristic of systems, the leadership role in a system is critically different from the leadership role in institutional models of organization. An essential ebb and flow enables complex interactions that flow out of a constant energy that represents an essential disequilibrium out of which streams novelty, innovation, creativity, and highly dynamic relationships and

---

Exhibit 2-4   Linear Versus Collateral Thinking

Linear Thinking (Industrial Age)
- Vertically oriented
- Hierarchical
- Mechanistic
- Reductionistic
- Compartmental
- Controlling

Collateral Thinking (Information Age)
- Multidirectional
- Horizontal
- Whole oriented
- Integrative
- Intuitive
- Relational

---

interactions. This text rests on a foundation represented by this complex, emergent, and multifocal role of leadership, which reframes a conception of leadership that can be both formal and emergent.

More traditional theories of leadership—those that informed the work of leaders and organizations in the twentieth century—reflected both linear and vertical thinking (**Exhibit 2-4**). This mechanistic and highly structured approach to leadership favored the use of compartmental, formal, structured, and definitive work formats and processes to organize and codify work and its products. Workers were considered subsets of the work and were organized and treated accordingly. Much of what defined work was both developed and owned by the organization and those who directed it.

In the latter part of the twentieth century and the beginning of the twenty-first century, the very foundations of work and the workplace began to change as a result of the emerging scholarship around complex adaptive systems and the subsequent complex responsive processes. Newer models evolved because of the advent of computers, chips, and information technology and their impact on every aspect of society. Knowledge work became increasingly important to the workplace, and organizations now require substantial knowledge capacity, most of which they could not own separate from the human beings who create it. The emergence of the knowledge worker changed the relationship between the worker and the work, and also between the worker and the workplace. In today's world, workers typically acquire the skills and knowledge needed for a certain type of work in an academic setting rather than in the workplace. In complex thinking these workers are essentially "freed" from the organization by virtue of their own knowledge creation, generation, and utilization capacity, which operates independently of the structural constraints of the organization. In fact, knowledge workers and their capacity have become an economic value center, and systems and organizations compete to access these resources that they feel they traditionally or historically "owned." This has turned the understanding of work

> **Point to Ponder**
>
> Advances in technology have made work more portable. Knowledge workers, because of their high-level skills, have gained substantial control of the work they do and have also become more mobile. Unlike the previous generation of workers, they are not faithful to the workplace. Instead, they are faithful to the work, moving anywhere the opportunity to do it appears.

and value on its head and changed the fundamental complex of relationships, interactions, intersections, and values in the social and economic enterprise.

Because of the accelerating digitalization of work and relationships, workers also have become much more mobile and portable because their skill sets have much broader utility than they did previously. Knowledge has become a resource in extreme demand, to the point where it is in essence a scarce resource, and consequently workers now are more important to the workplace than the workplace is to the workers. Because knowledge has great utility, portability, and transferability, workers have many more employment and value options.

While the worker has been changing, so has the workplace. In local enterprises as well as global entities, the organization and design of work have been radically altered. Organizations at all levels have had to create tight, efficient, nimble, and quickly adjusting work units (just-in-time models) to thrive in the more fluid, horizontal world of digital and wireless communication, fiber optics, nano structures, and other highly sophisticated technologies.

In this new world of intersections, interactions, interdependencies, and horizontal linkages, the entire infrastructure of work has been altered, as has our understanding of the mechanics necessary to facilitate effective work. The movement from institutions to systems has created a foundation for a new characterization of work and the worker.

Systems encompass closed and open components. Closed components are predictable, efficient, and ordered. They are the parts of a system that are constant and remain unaffected, at least directly, by external influences. The open components are adaptable and change in response to the constantly shifting demands of a dynamic environment. All functions and relationships in a system interact with and are dependent on the intersecting actions and processes in the system. Components such as production, service, management, governance, support, and locus of control are all included, according to common understanding, in the set of system functions. Of course, the relationship between the elements of process and outcome, as well as the relationships between structural and process components, is complex and as changing as technology and environment demand. In a complex system, no one element remains inert as other elements adapt to internal and external forces or lead the process of adapting to these forces.

This constant wave or flow of change and adaptation operates as the undercurrent of every system. The action never stops. The leader of a system, always aware of this movement and the constant exchange of energy among all the components, looks for the drivers and receivers of action and change (agents). The leader's attention must be on the ebb and flow of the cycles and the vortex of change as the system interacts with external sociopolitical, economic, and technological forces. The object is to discern the effects of these forces and to judge which actions will maintain the system's integrity, adaptability, and viability.

The leader of the system, of course, cannot perform these tasks unilaterally. All the leaders of system components must be made aware of the processes and skills necessary to manage systemness and of the interacting elements that make systems thrive. Any system is negatively affected if a single leader acts in the best interests of his or her component and without consideration for the impact of his or her behavior on the integrity of the whole. Such a leader actually holds the system "hostage" to his or her own component.

Component-centered behavior is common in traditional organizations. Various units, services, or departments of an organization might operate over long periods of time either independently or at the expense of other parts of the organization, especially if great sums of money can be produced as a result of their unilateral behavior. However, component-centered behavior is not sustainable. The dynamics of shifting information, service, and technology interacting with constantly changing demands of the environment creates the conditions that change strategy, trajectory, technology, resources, and the nature of work. Ultimately, the day always arrives when the organization has to pay substantially for its unconnected behavior, and the organization's ability to thrive will likely be threatened.

Every leader of a system component must recognize that his or her proper role is not simply to make the component thrive but to help make the whole system thrive. The leader's main attention of course is on his or her functional obligations to the component, but ensuring the fluidity, interface, connectedness, and flow of the component with the full range of system interactions (goodness of fit) is that leader's real work.

Over the years many theoretical approaches have emerged to try to define the structure and processes associated with an organization's work. From bureaucratic theory, the human relations school, the contingency and resource-dependent approaches to the strategic, population, and institutional models, theorists have written extensively on how and why organizations function as they do. According to the complexity approach, any element may act at any given time in an organization, and the interaction of forces will tell the leader how the organization is behaving and what the implications of its behavior are for its work and its transformative journey. Every system must possess structure and cultural foundations and must be able to respond flexibly to the environment and relationships, create value, improve itself, and interface directly with the external processes that influence its future. In other words, each theoretical approach contributes at some level to our understanding of how systems operate and how to make them effective (Northouse, 2012).

Biological metaphors frequently have been used to characterize the activities of systems, and each metaphor can assist leaders to focus on the functions and relationships that must work in concert. Signs point to an increase in complexity as a fundamental part of the evolutionary process. This complexity is an intrinsic force of evolution toward more complex organisms. In addition, general complexity is advanced by the astronomically large number of simple organisms that, although they are simple, establish complex interactions and relationships with each other in the larger environment. These simple organisms must work inside a complex network of interactions and partnerships in a way that facilitates balancing the whole environment, which is their medium for thriving. These multilevel, multilateral, simple organisms, when aggregated, create an integrated and collaborative collective that must maintain a tenuous balance and whole systems integrity to support the general thriving of each species and all species.

The analogy of a hologram is helpful in understanding organic complexity. In each part of a hologram, regardless of how many times it might be divided, the whole is always present. In short, the whole is always present in each of its parts. In this analogy, a whole system is reflected in each of its parts, and the relationship between the whole and each part is critical to both thriving. The role of the leader, in this perspective, is to keep focused on both the whole and the parts of the hologram—the constant interchange between the parts and the whole and the impact of the parts on each other and on the operation and integrity of the whole.

Group Discussion

The Industrial Age saw the emergence of a whole host of schools of leadership thought. Discuss the various approaches to leadership advocated by these schools (e.g., bureaucratic, human relations, behavioral, contingency, and situational). Then, reflect on the type of workplace that is emerging and discuss the implications for leadership style. As a help, consider which approaches to leadership might be appropriate or sustainable in the new age of work.

The leader must pay special attention to the points of interaction among the various components because therein lies most of the action, energy, and noise of a complex system, as well as most of the relationship, goodness-of-fit, and workflow problems. Because of the intensity of the dynamics there, sometimes problems and issues are not resolved or are "turfed" outside the locus of accountability that exists at these connective points. Examples include physicians taking their problems to the "administration," managers letting relationship problems "hang," and staff members refusing to deal with other staff members because the interactions would be too painful. Indeed, in any human system most activities, perhaps as much as 90%, reside at the point of service (the dynamic intersection) and the boundaries between the various services. Because these locations are where the applied work of a clinical system gets done, most of the issues affecting the work arise here. The problems are exacerbated if they are not resolved where they arise.

As principle 7 states, a system thrives to the extent of its intersections and interactions of its functions and actions. The best metaphor here is that of a continual, dynamic dance of interaction. The leader's role is to act as choreographer and ensure that the parties and the parts resonate with each other in a seamless contributory partnership to sustain the energy of the system.

Key Point

The primary job of a leader is to manage relationships and interactions, mostly at the intersections of the system. Seeing the organization holographically (i.e., in three dimensions) can help the leader detect the interactions and processes that occur there.

Principle 8: Equilibrium and Disequilibrium Are in Constant Tension

There is a constant and permanent tension between equilibrium (stabilizers) and disequilibrium (challenges). This tension is essential to life and reflects the fact that disequilibrium is the universe's natural state. For the leader, it is important to continually investigate and to understand how the relationships among parts of a system generate the collective behaviors of the entire system and how that whole system interacts and relates with the environment of which it is a part.

Although it is normal for the universe to live on the edge of its own chaos, a certain amount of stability is necessary for change and for undertaking action. The role of the leader in this delicate equation is to find the points of stability and use them as places where evaluation and action can occur. The notion of variation is central to the balance between stability and instability. Agents of change (e.g., individuals, families, businesses, communities, countries, and computer programs) interact continuously with the variables and elements affecting events and direction of movement. Through use of their skills, knowledge, mental and physical properties, and location, leaders, among other agents of change, can take the best path to achieving improvements.

Leaders understand the dynamic interaction between stability and change and walk the narrow way between them with consciousness and purpose. The leader is constantly opposing the normative forces of entropy and dissipation even as those forces manifest in organizations and people, to ensure that the human system remains dynamic, active, and changing positively. They understand that absolute and continuous stability is synonymous with death. Recognizing this, they know the value of chaos and the necessity of harnessing it to improve the circumstances and processes of work and productivity.

> ### Key Point
>
> In systems language, *stability* is another word for death. Absolute stability is the absence of life. The leader always walks a tightrope between stability and chaos, tending to favor the latter.

People do not make change. Instead, like disequilibrium, change is universal. This fact is at odds with the usual desire of people for stability and quiet in their personal lives. Leaders understand both the prevalent human wish for stability and the universe's tendency toward the creative and the chaotic. They know that they must develop strategies for addressing the conflict between equilibrium and disequilibrium—strategies that take into account both the environment and their own goals. Further, they know that not all strategies work as planned, and they periodically evaluate every strategy in use to make sure it is having the desired effect and revise it as necessary.

Time and shifting circumstances, often in part created by earlier strategies, have an impact on the chance of success of current strategies and on the formation of future strategies. A strategy that has stood the test of time can suddenly become unavailing. Changes in people and conditions can converge or act independently to influence what will work and what will not. Leaders must understand that wide variation in the effectiveness of a strategy over time is normal, and they must keep this fact in mind as they attempt to lead change and help people adjust to the inevitable adaptations that are a constant part of life.

The fluctuating effectiveness of strategies is one reason that measures of success are so critical to making judgments about what works. By using structured approaches to evaluating success, leaders can better determine what is working, what is not, what is shifting, what is emerging, and what adaptations need to be implemented. Measures do not have

> ## Group Discussion
>
> Margie Smith likes to have all of her ducks in a row. She believes that good order indicates good leadership. Her office is clean and orderly, and her life is highly structured. Margie hates when people clutter up their lives and are unable to think logically or act rationally. She works hard to make sure that her staff know what she expects and do everything as she thinks it should be done. Recently, though, the pace of change has picked up, and new programs and technologies are being implemented faster than Margie can handle. She has become less orderly, less comfortable, and, at times, short with staff. She occasionally speaks negatively about some of the changes, she has asked her supervisor whether the rate of change could be decreased, and she has even begun to think about looking for another job, one that would give her more control. Discuss what Margie needs to do to cope better. What changes should she make in her role as leader? What is the chaos she is experiencing trying to tell her? Is changing jobs going to be an effective solution to her current discomfort?

to be perfectly accurate; they simply have to say something about where changes are occurring and what adjustments are indicated. In a complex system, an apparently "wrong" outcome is as significant as a "right" measure might be. In other words, in the chaos of change, it is as important to know the wrongs as it is to know the rights.

Changes in people or populations may create a need for changes in process and approach. A change may alter people's circumstances, even their behavior, resulting in a need to alter the strategy or approach for the next stage of change. For example, people are affected by using the Internet, and thus those who use the Internet will likely require a process and mechanism of change that accommodates their new "position" as Internet users. For example, in pre-Internet times, "presence" meant that you were geographically located in relationship to another; in the digital experience of the Internet, "presence" has no geographical requirement. This digital notion of presence is now changing how we make and keep relationships, connect personally and emotionally, learn, communicate, and manage knowledge. If any approach to change does not accommodate or use these emerging digital realities, the adaptations implemented will have limited success. In general, the changes people undergo must inform the strategy used by leaders to guide further evolution. Here it is important to emphasize the concept of relevance and change. The relevance of a change is directly related to its timeliness and appropriateness within the context of the environment (for example, the digital universe) at any given point in time. There is nothing worse for an organization than to retain a strategy that lacks currency or to suggest a strategy that lacks timeliness and relevance.

Leaders look to people as both designers of change and vehicles of change. Although leaders are interested in changing people, they must be aware that people are a source of their own change because they are sources of learning and adaptation for each other, they act as initiators and/or recipients of change or improvement, and they are part of an environment that is itself always in transition (Chrispeels, 2004). A good leader is aware that the people with whom she or he works are virtual experts on their insights, position, and condition relative to a desired or needed adaptation. By looking at the population, the leader determines where it is in relation to any given change and uses these observations as a template for evaluating measures and indicators of the external forces of change. The general behavior of a population always influences its specific behavior, just as any specific behavior might inform the leader about the best methods for altering the population's general behavior. For example, if a population uses a specific tool, such as a handheld digital device, for managing personal information and communication, it will more easily adapt to using such a device for communication, documentation, and interaction in the clinical setting. People's individual behaviors serve as both signposts and templates for broader and further adaptation in other settings and circumstances. Thus, as noted, leaders must be good signpost readers and translators and must use their interpretive skills to facilitate further change and adaptation.

Leaders must also understand that complexity and chaos represent inherent energy. Although leaders do not generate the energy, they harness it in support of a particular form and direction. This energy is always swirling in human circumstances—it never stops. Leaders discipline the energy, driving it in a direction that results in desirable or congruent changes. The interaction between energy and effort is what gives the changes their form, and it is the substance that can be defined and measured.

A leader must be able to discern the interaction patterns in the energy and flow of a change because these patterns are most indicative of the context and content of the change. The interaction among forces, agents, and environment is the substance of the change and informs the leader about appropriate responses. The leader looks for the convergence of these forces and elements. The "story" that they contain, when well read, tells the leader what responses are likely to lead to specific outcomes or products. From this set of responses, the leader selects those that are likely to move the system in the direction that is needed or desired.

Not all selections will be correct. The leader will choose an ineffective response as often as an effective one. Here again, it is not the selection that is critical to the change process but what the effect of the selection tells the leader and what the leader's response is. When a strategy is correct and does result in a preferred behavior or condition, adaptation is said to have occurred, and this adaptation forms the foundation for the next change. For example, particle beam CT scanners were highly successful as diagnostic tools, yet they also formed a foundation for future improvements and refinements. Electron-beam whole-body CT scanners currently provide more detail and accuracy and have broader diagnostic and clinical utility, but these scanners could not have been developed until the earlier scanners had been devised and used. Adaptations often build on previous adaptations. In fact, all adaptations are temporary and merely serve as the foundation for future adaptations.

> **Key Point**
>
> The leader lives in the space between action and potential, anticipating the next step and translating the process for others.

Leaders are constantly aware of the intense interactions of complexity. These interactions are often represented in a chaotic vortex of energy that on the surface looks undecipherable. Yet when critically "read" and put into context, the vortex often reveals the "stuff" that will ultimately influence the next stage of change. Leaders are always pushing up against this potential energy, and good leaders are those who can translate it (context, systems, processes, and structure) into concerted actions. When an action joins with other related actions, the entire set creates the foundation for meaningful change. This can be viewed as a process of harnessing complexity. Through understanding and using complex interactions and intersections, through recognizing that all this is clothed in complexity and chaos, good leaders act to create the future.

Principle 9: Change Is Generated from the Center Outward

Effective change generally moves from the center of a system to all other parts, influencing everything in the system. Successful and sustainable change is rarely ever driven from the top of any system.

Every system has a unique life that defines its meaning and value and gives it an individual character. Within the system are all the activities that create balance among the work of the system, the internal demands, and the external requisites for thriving. Because every system is part of a larger system, there is an ever-evolving dance or interchange among the activities inside the system and between the system and the larger environment of which it is a part (**Figure 2-4**).

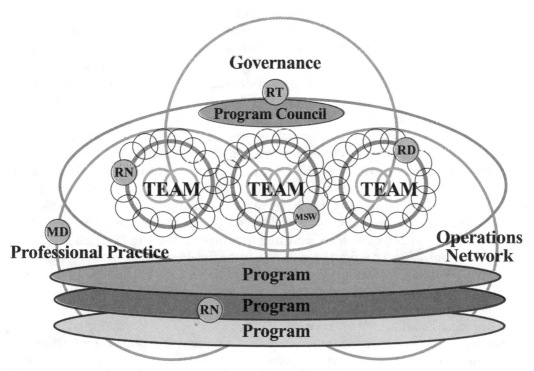

Figure 2-4 Out of Simplicity: A View of Complex Health Systems.

Key Point

A system thrives only when those at the point of service own the decisions that are made there.

The "center" (i.e., the point of service) is where the system lives the majority of its life, and the workers at the point of service are especially critical to its ability to adapt and thrive. However, many components of a system contribute to its integrity and allow it to function and adapt, and many types of personnel, from managers to staff, play a role in advancing the work of the system.

In a service system, the value of the system is determined by the character and content of the services offered. The services have value when they are provided in a manner that satisfies those who use them. In addition, the services contribute to the system's ability to thrive by demonstrating that the system provides valuable, high-quality services. Even more than the activities of marketing and business planning, the delivery of services creates the system's reputation; thus, the people who deliver the services are critical to the ability of the system to thrive. They are, in fact, much more critical to the system than any other single role or factor, although this statement should not be taken as denigrating the value of any of the intersecting roles that make up the system.

No service system can be sustained if the point of service does not deliver. Although this truth is easy to state, in many, if not most, service organizations, the power, independence, flexibility, and locus of control necessary to respond immediately and appropriately have been designed out of the system's point of service. These organizations have a vertical array of controls, hierarchical structures, and processes that obstructs decision making where the pertinent issues most often arise—at the point of service. The ascending ladder of control moves the authority for decision making away from the point of service, and the farther away the locus of authority is, the less likely the decision will meet the need that motivated it. In a typical example, a physician on a unit who has a problem with a staff member might take the issue to the administrator to make sure that the highest level of authority is brought into play. But if the problem is to be solved permanently, the solution must involve those who are located where the problem originated, and so action on the solution must ultimately be returned to the point of service.

Systems develop dynamic and cyclic patterns. In a typical pattern, there is a core or center point where the pattern either originates or culminates. The mosaic of activities ultimately builds on or supports the center point (**Exhibit 2-5**). In a service system like a healthcare organization, all structure that is sustainable builds on the service configuration, and the system's sustainability depends on the degree of congruence between the prevailing service structure and the supporting structures. If the system is well designed, most of the organizational configurations advance the freedom of activity and judgment at the center point (i.e., point of service). If they do not, they increase the chance that the supporting systems become the center point and therefore draw energy away from the proper locus of control, creating a framework that demands attention and resources that should be focused on the point of service.

The more the focus of a service system is drawn away from the point of service, the more expensive the structure of service becomes. Articulating Taguchi's rule: the farther away from the point of service a decision about what happens there is made, the higher

---

Exhibit 2-5   Mosaic of Decision Making in a System

Point-of-Service Decisions
- Individual
- Service driven
- Judgment based
- Highly variable

Unit or Service Decisions
- Coordinated
- Support based
- Standards driven
- Resource related

Team-Based Decisions
- Team defined
- Group standard
- Protocol driven
- Agreement based

System Decisions
- Integrated
- Collective
- Direction setting
- Resource generating
- Support systems based

---

the cost, the greater the risk, and the lower the sustainability of the outcome. In a system in which those responsible for structuring the system are not dedicated to enabling the locus of control to remain at the point of service, the tendency is for more and more decisions to move away from the point of service and for more infrastructure to be built to compensate for the lack of control there. In addition, the more infrastructure that is built, the more extensive (widely dispersed) the lack of control becomes. The cycle of compensation continues until there is so much infrastructure that the cost of supporting it exceeds the cost of providing services (Mori & American Society of Mechanical Engineers, 2011).

> **Key Point**
>
> When any system has too much structure, the energy of the system begins to support the structure rather than accomplish its objectives. Unnecessary structure draws resources away from the system's services and interferes with its ability to do its work. The same holds true for unnecessary management.

The leader of a service system labors to fully comprehend the essential interactions among the system elements and assess the degree to which those interactions facilitate the work going on at the center point. The leader also must assess the degree to which the system's configuration supports the openness and ownership of decisions and actions at the point of service and the amount of compensation necessitated by inappropriately made decisions. The leader judges the level of skills at the point of service and looks at the support structures necessary to ensure that the level of competence there is right and in the right configuration to meet the needs of those served. It is not just what the leader knows about the people, the services, or the system that matters, it is also what the point-of-service workers know.

The effectiveness of the system is directly related to the system's support of decision ownership and application at the point of service. In addition,

> **Point to Ponder**
>
> The only difference between revolution and evolution is the time and pain it takes to make a sustainable change.

when structure at the point of service supports decision making and action there, less infrastructure must exist at other levels of the system. Financial and professional costs accelerate when the locus of control shifts to other places in the system. To avoid fostering illegitimate loci of control leaders must ensure that most decisions and actions remain at the point of service. A shift in the locus of control away from the point of service causes a misfit between decisions and the specific situational needs of the services and their providers. It also obstructs the provision of competent, skilled, high-quality services and the workers' sense of ownership of their work.

Leader are fully involved in setting up and assessing the adequacy of the support structures of the overall system. These structures must be configured in a way that does not take from the point of service what belongs there. So also must the functions of strategic, operational, and service support be configured in a way that allows them to be understood and implemented there. The goodness of fit between the contextual activities of the strategic and support systems is vital because all the processes that unfold in the structure of the overall system must ultimately contribute to the provision of services. The leader's understanding of the impact of structure is critical to informing the database of the point-of-service workers that guides their decisions and actions. Leaders act as moderators of the relationship between those in the strategic and support systems and those at the point of service.

Principle 10: Revolution Results from the Aggregation of Local Changes

Revolution (hyperevolution) occurs when many local changes are aggregated to inexorably alter the prevailing reality, called the paradigmatic moment.

Most changes that occur are progressively evolutionary; that is, they happen in a continuous and dyanmic process over a period of time—most often over a very long period of time. Included are many iterations of evolutionary dynamics within which change can occur (co-evolution, punctuated equilibrium, mutation, adaptation, speciation, etc.), yet all of them lead to a change of some kind. As Darwin pointed out, the evolution of species is a dynamic process in which the living creatures best able to adapt to the changing environmental circumstances survive and thrive. This is no less true in the human enterprise.

A revolution, on the other hand, is a dramatic, almost instantaneous, change in conditions, and it presents living creatures with the challenge of adjusting quickly. In a revolution, many events converge to create a situation in which life can no longer be lived in the same way.

A revolution usually occurs in a system when the components converge to make enough of a demand for significant change. This demand is usually a result of the components being acted upon by the external or internal environment or by natural, sociopolitical, economic, or technical transformations. To thrive in the face of the demand for change, the system must quickly alter its structure and behavior to operate effectively under the new conditions.

Group Discussion

New sciences such as genomics and complexity science, advances in older sciences such as pharmacology, and technological developments are conspiring to change the health services format. What is currently in place will be deconstructed, and newer structures and models need to be conceived. Brainstorm the dramatic changes affecting health care at this time. Then discuss how they will alter the design of health services. What might some of the new designs be and how will they change the use and location of healthcare providers in the health system?

Much of what is happening in health care is revolutionary in nature. The very foundations of health care are being transformed by the impact of new technologies, in the realm of computers and the Internet, robotics, pharmaceuticals, and genomics, and sociopolitical and economic reforms. Technological advancements are so pervasive and influential that, in concert, they are fundamentally altering health therapeutics as well as the delivery of health services. The same can be said for the sociopolitical and economic forces. In particular, health services are less "bed based" than they were previously, the structures of hospitals and other healthcare organizations are being radically transformed, and providers must seek new ways of offering services that demonstrate effective health outcomes within a cost- and service-value chain.

The role of healthcare leaders is to focus on the implications of the revolutionary changes of health reform, including the implications for the behavior of those who work in the healthcare fields. Leaders must help other healthcare professionals to adapt to the changes and must position healthcare organizations to continue to thrive in an emerging value paradigm. They must discern the new roles, processes, and behaviors that will be necessary for future success.

The current transformation in health care is attended by changes in other conditions that challenge healthcare organizations to alter their way of business. For instance, the environment will require these organizations to reconfigure supporting structures and finances because the older configurations have become severely stressed in a way that threatens them. A further threat is presented by the fact that while the supporting infrastructure of economics, policy, and work is being reformed, the existing structures and behaviors will be even less effective than they were previously.

Here again, the leader of a healthcare organization must recognize the critical nature of the shift and undertake the dramatic and sometimes perilous process of quickly revising structure, processes, and behaviors to become more congruent with the emerging demand for sustainable health value (**Figure 2-5**). Besides reading the signposts of the change accurately, the leader must begin to create a sense of urgency about the change in the minds of those who will live in this new world. The issue that creates the drama and suspense is whether everyone's responses will be timely and appropriate. The leader must move people quickly through mourning the loss of established rituals and routines and raise the stakes for thriving and advancing the work in the context of a new set of reforms.

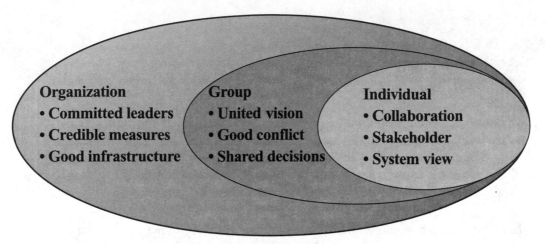

Organization
- **Committed leaders**
- **Credible measures**
- **Good infrastructure**

Group
- **United vision**
- **Good conflict**
- **Shared decisions**

Individual
- **Collaboration**
- **Stakeholder**
- **System view**

Figure 2-5 Organizational Levels and Associated New Age Characteristics.

Key Point

Leaders are agents of change. They bring the vision and context of change to the stakeholders so that the latter can develop the content of change.

In a time of revolution, all the principles of adaptation and complexity management come into play. The leader's ability to apply these principles and bring the elements of complexity and chaos together determines whether the organization thrives. As an agent of change, the leader knows that a variety of "agents" in a system can stimulate action or change. The leader is always looking for how these agents act to create the critical events that lead to an adjustment or a transformation.

The leader also knows that there is a variety of choices and strategies that can create a good fit between the demand for reform and our response. The leader looks for the relationships in the demand for change. By paying attention to the themes and mosaic that best demonstrate the flow and impact of the patterns, the leader can facilitate the making of good decisions and the undertaking of effective actions.

There is both substance and artifact in all change. The leader's role is to sort through the options and determine which elements are evidentiary and which are simply "noise" representing the change itself. The leader does not discard the artifacts of change but instead determines their value and uses them either as tools of change or symbols of the journey itself. These artifacts may tell the participants where they are in the journey and may also provide help in getting through the journey's various stages (Boje, Burnes, & Hassard, 2012).

Testing the way of the transformation is as important as any other activity. Although many things that occur during a revolution are important, equal amounts of "stuff" are unhelpful or even obstructive. Furthermore, it is important to determine where the system is in the process of change—what has been accomplished and what has yet to be done, what the deviations are, and what the successes are. Consequently, a means of measurement is needed so that the agents and strategies selected can be validated against the distance traveled and so that the expectations can be compared with the reality (**Figure 2-6**).

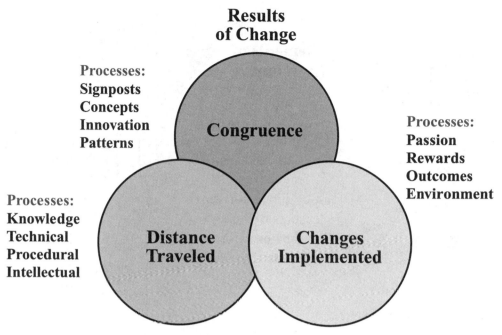

Processes:
Signposts
Concepts
Innovation
Patterns

Processes:
Passion
Rewards
Outcomes
Environment

Processes:
Knowledge
Technical
Procedural
Intellectual

Figure 2-6 Evaluating Transformation.

Exploration and experimentation are essential elements of any major change. The context is often significantly different from what was previously experienced or lived, and as the context changes, so too do the rules. Both the journey and the way of living that results from the journey are so different from the past that previous experience is inadequate to meet the new demands. The script gets written as part of the journey itself. This means that most of the change agents are learning about the change at the same time as they are leading the adaptation to it. This is especially true during a postparadigmatic change where the script is essentially new to all the players. Here leaders must successfully demonstrate their own capacity to learn, predict, and adapt as discernment, experimentation, application, and short-term evaluation yield data not previously available. When the script is written as it is lived, the collective wisdom garnered from the active engagement of all participants is critical to the assessment of effective progress.

Choosing strategies that fit the circumstances is not always easy to do. Because the ground shifts as people try to learn to live on it, the leader must have an open attitude regarding what is to be discovered. Leaders must understand what is meaningful and sustainable on the journey thus far and how it has been experienced. A leader's experience forms the database for the next stage of the journey.

At the same time, the leader experiments with actions. Because the leader does not know what the sustainable or valuable actions are until they are applied, the leader recognizes that there is an element of risk that must be embraced. All actions are prone to error. Indeed, the very risk of error advances the opportunity for learning and adaptation. Any particular error may contain the answer to a problem or at least be a signpost that could not be discerned in any other way, making the error a tool for the evaluation of direction and goodness of fit.

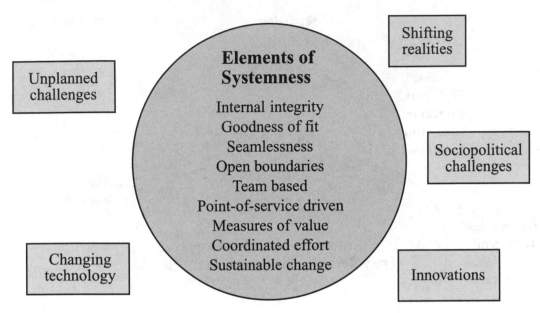

Figure 2-7 A System and Its Context.

In short, the leader sees everything within the context of systemness. All elements of a dynamic system are related and interact with each other, and the interactions, when aggregated, are what create the conditions for the system's adaptation and ability to thrive. When internal need and external conditions converge, they create the demand for change and adaptation.

Leaders see systemness everywhere and recognize that they can play a major role in the system's ability to adapt and improve (**Figure 2-7**). Whether a leader plays such a role largely depends on the leader's ability to anticipate, live in the potential of, and embrace each change at the right time. In addition, the leader must realize that he or she is an important change agent and must always act out of that understanding.

To ensure that the system adapts appropriately to changes and continues to thrive, the leader needs to keep in mind the following:

- The leader must apply the skills of exploration and those of exploitation, and know when to apply each skill set.
- Throughout a period of change, the leader must know which processes accommodate and use inherent variation and which processes maintain stability and good order, and then use these processes appropriately. Some level of inherent stability and some normative forces help to reinforce adaptation, and yet innovative and creative solutions and strategies often are embedded in the chaos and variance. In other words, both stability and variability are essential for adapting to change.
- Knowledge of the inherent interactions of elements in the system can direct the leader to build on those intersections that bring coherence, integrity, and trust into the system. These features of systemness can enhance people's ability to change and adapt quickly and well.

- All strategies have consequences. The leader must determine the appropriate strategies for guiding the system in the right direction. The implementation of these strategies must take into account that random influences may lead to valuable insights not available in any other way.
- Systems are membership communities. They operate through the consent of their members. The relationships among the members, including their communication with and support of each other, are as critical as any other factor for ensuring sustainable adaptation.
- Failure can be an important measure of direction and change. It should not, however, be an uncontrollable factor and should operate within the context from which it emerges. Small changes should not contain large failures. If they do, that indicates that the associated strategies are ineffective or misconceived.
- The team is the basic unit of work, and the relationships among the core members drives all successful change. Here is where change gets lived out and applied. The interaction, relationship, and competence of the team members are essential to the viability of the team's work and the sustainability of the system. In human systems, all else exists to support the work of this unit.
- Small changes lead to big changes. Further, all changes affect the system as a whole, either individually (evolutionary change) or in the aggregate (revolutionary change). It is not possible to affect any part of a system without ultimately affecting the whole system.

Crisis and creativity frequently emerge in unanticipated places and ways. Often in the act of achieving something else the creative and innovative arise. Leaders must always be open to serendipitous and emergent forces that arrive unexpectedly.

Conclusion

The presentation of principles in this text is neither exhaustive nor fully developed. This chapter serves merely as an introduction to concepts important to leaders in the Information Age, who must operate using different ideas than those common in the Newtonian-inspired Industrial Age. Leaders must review the adequacy of their skill sets in light of the realization that the era of unilateral and vertical orientation of functions is quickly passing.

Dramatic and dynamic changes continue to affect the leadership role. To understand this role in the new age of work and reform, leaders must learn about quantum principles and how they are to be applied. They must also become adept at understanding biologic metaphors, which are much stranger tools of thought than the old machine- and building-based metaphors. Permanent structures are no longer good models for work, especially in health care, and the architectural infrastructure characteristic of the coming age has a value-based format within an information infrastructure. Leaders must devote their full energy to pulling people out of work and service models that no longer operate efficiently and placing them in a context that demands thinking and acting in radically new ways.

It is interesting to note that, in recent times, people have not become more isolated. In fact, the opposite has occurred. Human beings have more potential for relationship and connectivity than at any time in history. The tools of connection and communication are creating linkages that were once only dreams. Living in this kind of a world, however, brings its own set of challenges and requires a different way of relating and behaving.

Leaders have an obligation to move people and structures into the new framework for work and leisure. To do this, they need a different mental model, new tools and skills, and a genuine desire to move both themselves and others into the new age. They need new knowledge, true enough, but they also need excitement so encompassing that others can see it and feel it, be energized by it, and develop the hope and enthusiasm necessary for creating a sustainable future.

When all is said and done about leadership—and these days much is said about it—it is important for every leader is to engage with and embrace the script of life and to get others to do the same so that the conditions of life are improved. Through discernment and exploration, design and formation, experimentation and application, leaders can help foster the richness of experience that enhances the quality of life for all. The effort to make life better and the chaos out of which improvements emerge give form to the leadership role. The process of discerning and drawing from the complexity of all systems the simplicity that lies at their center and applying that simplicity to the lives of others gives critical substance to the work of every leader.

Case Study 2-1

Creating Change in the Midst of Chaos

Nancy has been the CNO at Shady Point Hospital for 15 years, but this last year has been the most difficult for her. It seems as if there has been one change after another this year, and Nancy is tired of trying to lead the nursing staff through the changes, making sure the physicians are satisfied, and ensuring that the patients receive the best possible care. It seems that the staff are fatigued with all the changes and meetings as well, and some have said, "We just want to be nurses and take care of patients." It was easier in the past—the hierarchy and structure of the hospital seemed to provide some stability. Nurses were content to work at Shady Point for their entire careers, and nearly 50% of the nurses had been there 15 years or longer. Some of the nurses actually had trained at Shady Point's nursing school, a diploma school that closed 25 years ago.

Feeling the pressure from other hospitals' CNOs in the Northwest Healthcare System, Nancy has been investigating what it will take to commence the Magnet journey. In preparation, she has hired a director of professional development and research who has a doctoral degree from a respected university. Although it seemed like a great idea in the beginning, she notices now that the nonproductive education hours are completely over budget and the CFO is pressuring her to correct the problem. The new director of professional development is encouraging the nurses to develop career plans, return to school, and to become certified. Now, many of the nurses who feel like they should return to school to get a bachelor's degree or certified in their specialty are demanding more support for tuition reimbursement, increased pay after they obtain their specialty education, and some paid hours for attending classes. Nancy is overwhelmed with all the demands and changes and the pressures she feels from the rest of the executive team to stay in budget and to improve the nurses' satisfaction levels. The entire organization seems to be in a state of chaos under demands to reduce operating expenses while the staff and physicians are demanding more and more. Nancy typically holds things "pretty close to her chest" and tries to manage the nursing department on her own without sharing many of the details with her team of directors.

At wit's end, Nancy seeks the counsel of a colleague in a neighboring state who has led his hospital through complex times and even led the nursing staff to Magnet designation. He advises her to reach out to her colleagues on the executive team because the nursing department is core to the business of the hospital. He thinks that she needs to create a shared sense of responsibility for the changes that are occurring in the hospital and in nursing and to work toward a better understanding of how a satisfied nursing staff influences patient outcomes, physician satisfaction, and departmental relationships. He also advises her to develop her own directors to work together as a high-performing team and to be more transparent about the pressures she feels to meet operating targets. They talk about her adjusting her own attitude to the job with a goal of creating new mental models about the demands. Perhaps she could consider them more as challenges that need to be solved rather than impossible situations.

Just talking about all that she has faced seems cathartic and speaking out loud about the problems seems to give her new direction. She realizes that some people would have simply entered into her negative feelings and either advised her to seek a different job or pitied her situation. Nancy is grateful for her colleague's honesty, and she tells him how much she appreciates his boldness and encouragement of her reaching her full potential. They agree that she will keep in touch with him and that he will mentor her over the next few months. She takes some time off to relax and think things through, and she is actually surprised to feel excited to return to work again.

Nancy arrives at work with a new sense of commitment and resolve. She calls together the directors of the various nursing departments and the director of professional development and research and talks with them about her vision to transform the nursing division. She shares her concern that obtaining Magnet designation will be a huge challenge in the economic climate of the hospital. She is very frank with the directors about all that needs to occur and asks them to join her in this endeavor. Some of the directors are very excited about the possibilities of changes in organizational structure, advancement of the staff capabilities, and transformation of the organization to a high-performing one. Nancy asks the director of professional development and research to do a gap analysis of the organization's current capabilities in comparison to the Magnet requirements. She also asks that the directors work together as a team to identify strong nurse leaders among the staff who can compose a new Magnet steering committee. Nancy shares her vision that the Magnet steering committee should design the collaborative governance structure for the nursing division, and that the directors should act in roles as consultants instead of designing the structure themselves. The director group soon realizes that Nancy's style of leadership has changed dramatically since her vacation, and they are excited and uneasy about the changes she outlines.

Nancy also meets individually with the COO, CFO, and her CEO to share her concerns about the across-the-board budget cuts that negatively affect the nursing division and, ultimately, patient care quality. She shares a plan of how to reduce expenses while preserving the professional role of the nurse as the team leader in the planning and implementation of patient care. She tries to develop a shared vision among her colleagues so they will be invested in her plan to develop and advance the nursing division, but also see her as responsible and accountable for the financial integrity of the overall organization. Nancy also meets with the other divisional leaders to discuss how their roles intersect in meeting the organization's goals and financial targets.

As part of the transformation of the nursing division, Nancy works with her direct reports to discuss different leadership styles and leadership theories. She introduces them to concepts such as the servant leader, transformational leadership, and motivation and change theories. She recommends that the directors who do not have master's degrees in nursing leadership consider returning to school, and she offers them one day off per week to attend classes. She still expects them to meet their productivity and financial targets and other quality indicators, but she sees the potential in each individual and is confident that the directors will be able to accomplish their roles at the hospital and their new student roles. All the while she is speaking, she is constantly observing the directors' body language, facial expressions, and reactions to her thoughts on expanding their knowledge, skills, and capabilities in leading high-performing teams. Although she realizes that there is some risk in asking her direct reports to return to school while working full-time, she is confident that their exposure to new knowledge will also expand their success at work. She reassures them and lets them know that she is available at any time to talk with them about their fears and concerns. She also encourages them and particularly the director of professional development research to motivate the staff nurses with diploma and associate degrees to also continue their education toward the bachelor's degree. Nancy indicates that she is in negotiation with one of the local universities to provide some of the education on site at the hospital to facilitate the nursing staff and directors furthering their education. She shares that she is also working with Human Resources, her executive colleagues, and the Shady Point Foundation to develop nursing scholarships and tuition reimbursement up to $1,000 per person per year.

After a few months, Nancy reflects on all the changes that are occurring at Shady Point Hospital and the pressures she continues to feel to be a good steward of the hospital's resources. She feels excited about the transformation she is witnessing in her directors and the staff as a whole. She also feels more connected with other divisional leaders and the executive team, and although they don't always agree on solutions to problems, they do agree to work as a team to accomplish their shared goals. Changes are coming fast, but Nancy has found strength within herself and her director team that she never dreamed possible.

Questions

1. Who are the stakeholders in this case? Analyze the case by taking on the role and perspective of each stakeholder.
2. How can Nancy possibly lead Shady Point to thrive in the face of the organizational chaos and complexity?

3. What strategies would you use to prepare the nursing team for a Magnet application?
4. What should Nancy do to sustain the gains she has seen in teams at Shady Point?
5. What strategies can a leader employ to create a shared vision?

Case Study 2-2

Developing Service Lines in a Healthcare System

Ella has been the executive director of the Women's and Children's Hospital for the past 10 years at Best Health Memorial Hospital, which is the flagship hospital in a major healthcare system. Five other hospitals in the healthcare system are located within a 50-mile radius of Best Health Memorial Hospital. As executive director, Ella provides leadership to approximately 600 professional staff members who report directly to 12 different managers. The managers also report to 5 directors who provide leadership for the women's surgical areas; labor, delivery, recovery, and prenatal services; maternal and infant services, and neonatal intensive care services. In addition, one director is responsible for professional development and research and supervises the clinical nurse specialists who are assigned to each of the clinical areas.

Ella reports directly to the CNO, who also is responsible for executive directors of other major divisions including acute care (including oncology, orthopaedics, and general medical-surgical care), critical care and emergency services, rehabilitative services, and home health and hospice services. Ella is one of four nurse leaders who direct women's and children's services for the hospital in the Western Regional Health System. The Women's and Children's Hospital at Best Health is the largest in the healthcare system, and the other hospitals include the following: (1) one suburban hospital with a small delivery rate of approximately 900 annual deliveries; (2) one urban hospital with an annual delivery rate of approximately 1,500; (3) an urban hospital with an annual delivery rate of approximately 3,500 and a level II neonatal intermediate intensive care nursery; and (4) one suburban hospital located approximately 50 miles from Best Health with a strategic plan to develop a new maternity service line with a level II neonatal intermediate intensive care nursery. All of the other hospitals have transfer agreements with Best Health's Women's and Children's Hospital for high-risk perinatal and neonatal transports for tertiary care. Beyond the transfer agreements, there is very little coordination of efforts or sharing of resources among the five hospitals.

Ella has assumed the informal leadership among the other directors of maternity and newborn services at the other hospitals, and she is respected for her national reputation as a leader in women's and children's services. Ella is a frequent speaker at the national conferences associated with maternal newborn health and children's health services. She has recently attained her PhD in nursing with an emphasis on nursing leadership, is certified by the American Nurses Credentialing Center (ANCC) and the American Organization of Nurse Executives (AONE) in nursing leadership, and is certified in high-risk perinatal services by the Association of Women's Health, Obstetric and Neonatal Nurses (AWHONN). Ella is also a frequent contributor to journals specific to maternity, newborn, and women's services.

The president of Western Regional Health System and his executive team have decided to develop specialty-focused service lines for women's and children's services, cardiac services, orthopaedic services, and cancer services. Other service lines will be developed in the future depending on the effectiveness of these four service lines in reducing variation in care, redundancy of services, and costs associated with patient care protocols. It is also hoped that the service-line structure will improve market share and recognition for excellence with improvements in quality outcome indicators, physician and patient satisfaction, and coordination of care across both inpatient and outpatient services related to each of the specialties. To initiate the vision for service-line integration, four corporate vice president positions are announced with star performers in each of the service lines selected for the new role.

Ella, the star performer for women's and children's services, was appointed as the corporate vice president (VP) for women's and children's services. Although surprised and excited about this new role, Ella had mixed feelings about leaving her executive director position at Best Health Memorial Hospital's Women's and Children's Hospital. She and the other newly appointed corporate vice presidents will be relocated to the corporate offices rather than having an office at any one of the five health system hospitals. A new executive director will be recruited for Best Health's Women's and Children's Hospital. The president of Western Regional Health System announced the new organizational structure, vision for system integration, and a newly appointed senior vice president for Service-Line Integration position. The new senior VP is a physician who was recruited from an academic position on the East Coast and who has some experience with a large healthcare system developing a service-line structure. All of the new corporate VPs report directly to Dr. Thomas, the new senior VP.

Needless to say, these organizational changes create absolute chaos among each of the entity hospitals' executive and leadership teams because they are uncertain how the new system structure will affect their strategies and decisions related to the service lines within their own entities. Some of the executive and leadership teams are fearful that they will lose autonomy in decision making related to the service lines. The leaders of the smaller hospitals are pleased that they might have more resources allocated to them as a result of the system change because they often did not receive as many resources as were allocated to the larger hospitals in the system.

There is significant scuttlebutt around the organization as to how the corporate VPs were chosen independent of the usual process of opening positions and allowing inside and outside applicants to be considered. The unilateral decision by the president and his executive team upset many of the leaders in the healthcare system, who voiced concern that this same process might be used for other key positions in the future. Several are concerned that their own power and authority base will be undermined by these newly appointed corporate VPs and ultimately by the senior VP for Service-Line Integration. The entity leaders are also concerned that their roles and responsibilities in physician recruitment, program development, financial management, and philanthropy will be minimized with the new service-line structure.

The chaos and confusion regarding the new organizational structure are often blatantly apparent at the system-wide executive meetings chaired by the president of Western

Regional Medical Center. He finally informs the CEOs of each of the entities that they must put a positive spin on their communication to their leadership teams as well as the staff at each of their hospitals. He provides as much information as possible regarding the position descriptions for the senior VP and the corporate VPs and has several open discussions about his vision for service-line integration across the system. He also suggests that the CEOs read several articles written by national leaders in healthcare integration and authors of books on "systemness." Over the next months, the president invites national speakers to present at Western Regional Healthcare System's corporate offices with invitations for the entity leaders to attend and discuss system integration that has been successfully implemented at other major healthcare systems throughout the United States.

Ella becomes excited about her new role, and she reads everything possible about vertical and horizontal integration of healthcare systems. She begins to meet with the new senior VP and the other corporate VPs who are now her peers. Her position description includes service-line development, integration, and innovation with an emphasis on improving quality and financial indicators by reducing variation and redundancy. She also meets with data analysts to assess the volume, financial, and quality outcome data for each of the entities. Because she had enjoyed a very positive relationship with each of the entity's directors of Women's and Children's Services, she expects to continue this positive relationship in her new role. She also meets with the CNO who was involved in the development of new women's and children's services at the outlying hospital.

When she meets with each of the directors at the respective entities, she is surprised to receive a less than positive reception. Suddenly, her colleagues who had worked with her so well in the past seem distant and negative in their interaction toward her and her ideas related to service-line integration of women's and children's services. With the exception of the CNO who was developing women's and children's services from scratch, the others strongly emphasize their desire to maintain their autonomy in the direction of their services instead of centralizing decision making related to women's and children's services. It seems to Ella that they have no concept of the president's vision for service-line integration or what systemness would look like. Despite her frequent meetings with them and developing an organizational structure for women's and children's services with them, she seems to receive only cordial and superficial coordination of services rather than a commitment to true integration.

Ella's experience is not unique, and the other corporate VPs report similar reactions with the exception of the orthopaedic service line. In one of the service-line meetings, Ella mentions that the hospitals are acting more as a confederation of hospitals rather than as a healthcare system. Each of the entity hospitals struggles to maintain as much autonomy in decision making as possible while the corporate system leaders attempt to integrate service lines to create a total and comprehensive system of care for the community with branding of the Western Regional Healthcare System as a name for healthcare excellence.

The orthopaedic service line seems to be more advanced in its integration of services because there are few threats among the orthopaedic surgeons and nursing leadership at each of the entity hospitals. They see system integration as an opportunity to obtain more resources for capital equipment, marketing and promotional services, and specific leadership for the specialty beyond the current immersion in general acute care services at each of the entities. The cardiac service line struggles with the system integration initiative because each of the entities desires to be named the premier cardiac center within the healthcare system, and several of the interventional cardiologists are direct competitors for market share within the region. Because there are two cancer centers in the healthcare system, the cancer service line also struggles with how to manage competing centers of excellence with physicians and leaders who have no incentive to integrate their services or referral systems. In fact, physician and entity leaders for the cancer service line voice their discontent with the system initiative, stating that it reduces their ability to enhance their market share coming from the smaller hospitals within the system.

Ella continues to review the literature related to the development of systems in general and healthcare systems specifically. She realizes that for the women's and children's service line, she needs to demonstrate the value that could be added by the integration of services across the entities in contrast to each entity acting alone. She also realizes that it is important to identify areas where autonomy in decision making is legitimate and to support each of the entity leaders in their efforts to maintain entity autonomy in their specific region within the city. She recognizes that it will be difficult for each of the entities to give up its respective individual branding within its community, so she advocates at the system meetings for the development of a system brand that also allows for entity branding as a developmental step in the overall goal of system integration. Because each of the entities also provides services to different cultural groups, Ella suggests that these diverse cultures be highlighted in the branding of each of the entity's programs and services. This action recognizes each of the entities for a unique contribution to the system as a whole.

Several different actions and initiatives to develop system integration are tried, and many succeed, whereas others are not so successful. Ella tries to analyze the forces at play in each of the successes and failures. One area that is very successful is the development of a system organizational structure for women's and children's services for the service line that was designed by the entire group of entity leaders. System-wide councils were developed using successful models of shared governance reported in the literature. The following councils were developed: (1) Operations Council, which focused on financial and productivity goals and supply and capital acquisitions; (2) Quality Council, which focused on nurse-sensitive indicators and other quality outcome indicators; (3) Professional Development and Education Council, which focused on integrating orientation and on-boarding, professional development courses, and preparation for specialty certifications; (4) Research and Innovation Council, which focused on developing system-wide research projects, evidence-based practice projects, and new innovations that could be shared among the entities; and (5) Patient and Family Education Council, which focused on the integration of all educational materials for patients and families and the standardization of clinical protocols for patient education across the system.

Ella led the process of developing each of the councils with respective charters, deliverables, and reporting structure to a system-wide steering council composed of physician leaders in women's and children's services and the entity directors at each of the hospitals. It seems that over time the entity directors moved from simply coordinating efforts at each of the hospitals to actually working toward integrating some of their professional education offerings and patient education materials and activities. They also began to assume responsibility in developing a new women's and children's service program at the outlying hospital. Ella begins to realize that system integration could not simply be mandated by system leaders but rather that systemness is a developmental process. Reflecting over the past few months, Ella notes that moving toward systemness has several identifiable steps that include developing trust among the service-line and entity leaders, sharing information and resources across the hospitals, coordinating services and programs across the system, and, finally, developing strategic thinking from a systems perspective instead of the individual entity level.

Questions

1. How do you think that the president's announcement to move to a service-line platform and the centralized decision to appoint service-line vice presidents in contrast to an open recruitment process affected the system service-line initiative?
2. What do you perceive the differences are between a confederation of hospitals and a fully integrated healthcare system?
3. How would you strategize to minimize the fears and anxiety of entity leaders in the development of a system-wide service line?
4. In this case, what are the apparent barriers and contributors to system integration for the service lines?
5. In your opinion, how much autonomy in decision making and marketing and promotions should each entity have in an integrated healthcare system?
6. What are the factors that might affect the decision to honor entity autonomy in contrast to system integration and centralization of decision making and marketing and promotional activities?

References

Boje, D. M., Burnes, B., & Hassard, J. (2012). *The Routledge companion to organizational change*. Oxon, NY: Routledge.

Brewer, G., & Sanford, B. (2011). *Decade of change: Managing in times of uncertainty*. New York, NY: Gallup Press.

Chrispeels, J. H. (2004). *Learning to lead together: The promise and challenge of sharing leadership*. Thousand Oaks, CA: Sage.

Crowell, D. M. (2011). *Complexity leadership: Nursing's role in health care delivery*. Philadelphia, PA: F. A. Davis.

Das, T. K. (2013). *Managing knowledge in strategic alliances*. Charlotte, NC: Information Age.

Erwin, D. (2009). Changing organizational performance: Examining the change process. *Hospital Topics*, 87(3), 28–40.

Hacker, K., & Walker, D. K. (2013). Achieving population health in accountable care organizations. *American Journal of Public Health*, 103(7), 1163–1167.

Heifetz, R., & Linsky, M. (2002). *Leadership on the line*. Boston, MA: Harvard Business School Press.

Hildreth, P. M., & Kimble, C. (2004). *Knowledge networks: Innovation through communities of practice*. Hershey, PA: Idea Group.

Hines, P., & Mercury, M. (2013). Designing the role of the embedded care manager. *Professional Case Management*, 18(4), 182–187.

Kelly, K. (1995). *Out of control: The new biology of machines, social systems and the economic world*. New York, NY: Perseus.

Kelly, K. (2010). *What technology wants*. New York, NY: Viking.

Maliszewska, J. P. (2013). *Managing knowledge workers: Value assessment, methods, and application tools*. New York, NY: Springer.

Malloch, K., & Porter-O'Grady, T. (2009). *The quantum leader: Applications for the new world of work*. Sudbury, MA: Jones and Bartlett.

Marshall, J. (2009). Jeff Immelt and the new GE Way: Innovation, transformation and winning in the 21st century. *Financial Executive*, 25(5), 13.

Mori, T., & American Society of Mechanical Engineers. (2011). *Taguchi methods: Benefits, impacts, mathematics, statistics, and applications*. New York, NY: ASME Press.

Negroponte, N. (1995). *Being digital*. New York, NY: Knopf.

Nelson, M. (2009). A cloud, the crowd, and public policy. *Issues in Science and Technology*, 25(4), 71–76.

Northouse, P. G. (2012). *Leadership: Theory and practice*. Thousand Oaks, CA: Sage.

Uhl-Bien, M., & Marion, R. (2008). *Complexity leadership*. Charlotte, NC: Information Age.

Suggested Readings

Berwick, D., Nolan, T., & Whittington, J. (2008). The triple aim: Care, health, and cost. *Health Affairs*, 27(3), 759–769.

Boleman, L., & Deal, T. (2008). *Reframing organizations: Artistry, choice and leadership*. San Francisco, CA: Jossey-Bass.

Foti, R., & Hauenstein, N. (2007). Pattern and variable approaches in leadership emergence and effectiveness. *Journal of Applied Psychology*, 92(2), 347–355.

Hawking, S., & Mlodinow, L. (2009). *A brief history of time*. New York, NY: Bantam.

Hazy, J., Goldstein, J., & Lichtenstein, B. (2007). *Complex systems leadership theory: New perspectives from complexity science on social and organizational effectiveness*. New York, NY: Vintage.

Juarrero, A., & Rubino, C. (2010). *Emergence, complexity, and self-organization*. Litchfield Park, AZ: Emergent Publications.

Krames, J. A. (2008). *Inside Drucker's brain*. New York, NY: Portfolio.

Malloch, K., & Porter-O'Grady, T. (2009). *The quantum leader: Applications for the new world of work*. Sudbury, MA: Jones and Bartlett.

Miller, J., & Scott, P. (2007). *Complex adaptive systems: An introduction to computational models of social life*. Princeton, NJ: Princeton University Press.

Yang, A., & Shan, Y. (2008). *Intelligent complex adaptive systems*. Chicago, IL: IGI.

Quiz Questions

Select the best answer for each of the following questions.

1. Change can be defined as a dynamic rather than as an event. This means that change is _____.
   a. Cyclical
   b. Periodic
   c. Timely
   d. Continuous

2. Complexity science is based on a new understanding of the operation of the physical world. What is this understanding referred to as?
   a. Newtonian physics
   b. Quantum mechanics
   c. Universal science
   d. The Einstein principle

3. A number of converging forces have ushered in the new age. The three main forces converging are sociopolitical, economic, and _____.
   a. Technological
   b. International
   c. Scientific
   d. Commercial

4. Systems are dynamic entities driven more by relational elements than by functional processes. In this way, which of the following do they resemble?
   a. Biological structures
   b. Business structures
   c. Social structures
   d. Information structures

5. In a healthy system, 90% of decisions are driven by which of the following?
   a. The top of the system
   b. The bottom of the system
   c. The point of service
   d. The managers

6. According to complexity theory, anything that adds value to a part of the system adds value to the whole system. Which of the following is an implication of this principle?
   a. Each part of the system drives the work of the whole system.
   b. The whole system is the only legitimate source of sustainable value.
   c. All real value derives from the work of the people in the system.
   d. Every component of a system contributes to the integrity of the whole system.

7. In complexity theory, how is chunking defined?
   a. It is the support provided to a complex system by the operation of simple systems.
   b. It is the formation of a complex system by the incremental aggregation of interacting and interdependent simple systems.
   c. It is the operation of a complex system consisting of independent parts.
   d. It is the dynamic relationship between independent simple systems.

8. Diversity is essential to change for which reason?
   a. It creates the variety required by change.
   b. It accentuates the similarities that exist through change.
   c. It makes chaos visible and underscores the need for adaptation.
   d. It highlights the difficulty of reconciling differences.

9. Error is also essential to change. Not all errors are acceptable, however. Which of the following errors are to be avoided?
   a. System-based errors
   b. Errors in judgment
   c. Repeated errors
   d. Human errors

10. Systems are driven by different rules than are functional institutions. Which of the following are the cornerstones of systems design?
    a. Relationships and intersections
    b. Functions and actions
    c. Policies and processes
    d. Rules and regulations

11. To ensure the system's vitality, the leader of a system must pay special attention to which of the following?
    a. Stability
    b. Chaos
    c. Form
    d. Function

12. When does revolution in a system occur?
    a. When the pace of evolution is insufficient for the necessary changes
    b. When things cannot continue to operate in the same way
    c. When violence is introduced into the system
    d. When many local changes occur at once

CHAPTER THREE

Evidentiary Leadership: An Expanded Lens to Determine Healthcare Value

We cannot deny our connectedness while we build our separateness.
—*M. J. Wheatley and M. Kellner-Rogers,* A Simpler Way

Chapter Objectives

WWW

At the completion of this chapter, the reader will be able to

· List five major drivers for documentation of value-based outcomes.
· Discuss the leadership challenges in selecting metrics for healthcare organizational evaluation.
· Describe innovative leadership strategies for measurement in complex social systems.
· Gain an appreciation of the realities and challenges of creating more robust measurement models reflecting the complexity of health care.

There is a great and pressing need to reformulate the way in which health care is valued, measured, and reimbursed. Quantum leaders have experienced both the challenges of linear measurement models and the potential for integration of complexity principles into the healthcare system measurement models. Further, quantum leaders are well positioned to lead initiatives that challenge current measurement assumptions and to create models more reflective of the complex nature of healthcare work.

The purpose of this chapter is not to provide a template for measurement, but rather to offer a new lens for healthcare leaders to consider, compile, synthesize, and evaluate the multiple variables of the healthcare experience. Necessarily, each organization must customize its measurement model to include industry standards and facility-specific measures reflective of the mission and vision. Leaders can create revitalized measurement templates specific to their organizational context. Also in this chapter, the challenges of measuring health care and suggestions for reconceptualizing healthcare measurement using the characteristics of complexity are presented.

Key Drivers for Change

The need to challenge current assumptions and create more robust models emanates from multiple sources and issues. Five major issues are discussed in this section and serve to stimulate action. The Points to Ponder included challenge each of us to think differently and consider new strategies that can be useful to reach effective measurement and valuing of health care in the United States. The Points to Ponder comments include explorative ideas, challenges, and thoughts about the assumptions that currently drive the healthcare system. The first issue, not surprisingly, is the belief that health care is too costly.

Issue: Cost

The general notion is that health care in the United States is too costly and the quality outcomes are less than desirable. The U.S. system–nonsystem of health care continues to be too costly and too unsafe. Patient safety is not viewed as having substantially improved following the release of the landmark 1999 Institute of Medicine (IOM) report announcing 48,000–98,000 deaths yearly from medical misadventures (Altman, Clancy, & Blendon, 2004; Committee on Quality of Health Care in America, 2000; Minot, 2009). In addition, the Affordable Care Act requirements to achieve fully or nearly full access for Americans presents new challenges for managing the cost–quality equation.

Issue: Cost Shifting

The cost of health care is affected not only by the actual services provided and supporting technologies, but also by numerous well-intended initiatives designed to control those costs. Regulations, both national and local, are in place to control and monitor costs and quality. Price adjustments and cost shifting serve to "even the playing field" for payers, providers, and patients. Sophisticated mechanisms to control access to care and payment for services further complicate the system. Not surprisingly, there is an unending quest to reduce the disparity between the costs and quality and ultimately to achieve the highest quality health care at the lowest cost. Unfortunately, achievement of this admirable goal has eluded

> **Points to Ponder**
>
> If we are spending too much, how much are we willing to spend? And what level of quality are we willing to fund? Perhaps the issue is not how much we spend; rather, the issue is the quality and consistency of outcomes. The common understanding is that health care is too costly. Given that healthcare expenditures in 2011 were at 17.9% of the Gross Domestic Product (GDP), should there be a different question or many different questions that would inform us what the dollars should achieve and how much the United States is willing to spend (Centers for Medicare and Medicaid Services, 2008; Fleming, 2013)? What kind of health care could we have if the expenditures were at 10% of the GDP? What services at what level of quality are we willing to pay for? If healthcare reform efforts were based on a defined amount of expenditure, level of quality, and defined access, would the recommendations be different or more acceptable? Perhaps a new valuation process that integrates the costs and value of innovation should be considered.

the U.S. healthcare system. Shifting costs between payers has become normative; however, the fairness of this practice is seldom fully supported. Incredible attempts are made to level the payment structure in a social system that is multi-tiered and based on individual values and rights.

Issue: Demand Without Accountability

Citizens of the United States believe there are no limits to treatment access. Health care is believed to be an inherent right for every individual to have access to every available treatment. Further, the health-care system has yet to create expectations or boundaries for those receiving care. There is no accountability for healthy behaviors as the requirement for receiving healthcare service funding. Funding continues to be provided to both individuals who actively engage in healthy behaviors and those who repetitively engage in unhealthy behaviors that exacerbate existing conditions. Healthcare funding is based on a one-way model: presence of illness or disease. There is no expectation that healthcare prescriptions will be attended to or followed.

Issue: Partial Measurement and Avoidance of Ambiguous Evidence

Measuring the empirical or observable and easily quantifiable variables has dominated the healthcare system. Traditional finance references identify metrics for returns on

> **Points to Ponder**
>
> In a free and democratic society, will the more successful and more fortunate individuals always need to subsidize those less fortunate? Or is there a better way to support those less fortunate? Is a national health plan the only way to eliminate or control cost shifting? The greater challenge for the people of the United States is to determine and acknowledge whether health care is a right or a privilege. Currently, our rhetoric espouses health care as an individual right while our financial system funds health care as a privilege on the basis of those who have resources for payment.

> **Points to Ponder**
>
> It would seem that both the desire to have all health care without personal accountability and the propensity of providers to overhelp others have rendered the current system to be disastrously dysfunctional. Why is it so difficult for Americans to say no when there are not enough available resources to match the demand? Will changing spending behaviors change the state of the U.S. healthcare system? Will changing our expectations become the best first step to reform? Is it possible to change this behavior, to change the expectations of all citizens? Can we work to guarantee a level of basic services? Should U.S. citizens bite the bullet and continue to give more dollars to the healthcare system? Should every available healthcare service be available to every citizen regardless of the cost?
>
> Can we really afford one-way health care? Is the best practice to give and give and give without the expectation for healthy behaviors? The failure of fully engaged patient–provider relationships unnecessarily increases the cost of healthcare services. How do we engage patients in the healthcare process to ensure full-circle accountability within the system?

TABLE 3-1   Complexity and Healthcare Measurement Implications

Property Complexity Description	Implication for Healthcare Measurement
Connectivity	• One standard metric is seldom adequate to tell the story. When measuring, ask the question, "Did the results affect any other metrics?" If hours of care were decreased, were the necessary services provided to ensure the desired level of quality?
Interdependence	• Reliance on other elements of the healthcare system is the norm.
	• There's more to consider than the financial return on investment. Utility, effectiveness, health, and functionality must also be considered.
Emergence	• Be available for unpredictable results/outcomes/events.
	• Unintended and unanticipated consequences often occur after implementation of correction of another problem, creating the need to consider other information.
	• Highly structured forecasting and planning may be of limited value.
	• Identify "anticipatory metrics"—what could happen with this decision?
	• Examine the traditional metrics and at least three additional sequential evolving metrics to increase awareness of the impact of emergence.
	• When measuring, focus on principles rather than specific goals and targets.
	• Be open and available to reconsider existing opinions.

investment, ratios for cash management, and allocation percentages for expense categories (**Table 3-1**). The use of mathematical tools such as graphs, charts, and statistical formulas provides important data that are easily understood. Unfortunately, measurement of selected healthcare elements is often used to inform the totality of the system. In general, they are insufficient to capture the complexity of healthcare work. Although these tools have value, they also have limitations when applied to the nonlinear and multidimensional processes of health care. In the current model, reimbursement is provided for selected and discrete clinical interventions or procedures regardless of the surrounding circumstances and patient status or values.

The ambiguous or qualitative information such as patient–provider relationships, effectiveness of the procedure, patient satisfaction, and healthy behaviors practiced is not considered in the reimbursement categories. Further, the highly regarded five categories of outcomes reflective of quality (achievement of appropriate self-care, demonstration of health-promoting behaviors, health-related quality of life, the perception of being well cared for, and symptom management to criterion) are not considered in the current payment model (Mitchell & Lang, 2004).

There is more to the healthcare experience than net income margins, cost per case, and hours per patient day. Every metric has a story connected to interdependent measures of quality and quantity. Historically, ambiguous evidence such as relationship effectiveness, surveillance work, and team collaboration measurement has been avoided. The adage that you cannot manage what you do not measure has been used in healthcare quality and measurement discussions, and this idea further challenges us to develop systems that do measure and account for what is valued and managed (Minot, 2009). Documentation and accounting for the relational and qualitative aspects of patient care in the healthcare model need to be identified and connected to the system. To begin, the antecedents, concurrent processes or interventions, and unplanned outcomes need to be identified and linked to each financial metric.

> ### Points to Ponder
>
> Errol Morris (2008), documentary maker, described as "an individual with a forensic mind with painter's eyes," noted in the *Harvard Business Review* that few people really know how to get an accurate read on situations. Information is filtered, unpopular opinions are avoided, and partisan views are veiled as objective arguments. The same can be said for getting an accurate accounting on healthcare services. Too often, the challenges in selecting the most appropriate groupings of financial and quality metrics are insurmountable, and leaders settle on financial and volume measures because they become the only thing a leadership team can agree on.

Group Discussion

Foolproof Elasticity

The foolproof elasticity formula is believed by some to be critical to successful operations and management. For example, if the cost of care for 5 patients is $50,000, then the elasticity formula dictates that the cost of care for 10 patients would be $100,000 and the cost of care for 20 patients would be $200,000 and so on. Unfortunately, the complexity of the processes and resources involved in patient care render this formula invalid and unreliable. In your discussion group, identify a list of variations that would occur in patient care and invalidate the elasticity formula.

Interestingly, the healthcare system is working desperately to improve the quality of health care, to manage relationships, to consider the impact of the context in which health care occurs, and to integrate patient personal values into care processes. Unfortunately, the emphasis is on creating more discrete and isolated measures rather than inclusion of measures reflective of these variables. The formation of relationships, the work of clinical surveillance and oversight, the engagement of team members and patients, and the perceptions of quality and respect are but a few of the important

Key Point

Unraveling Ambiguous Evidence

1. Scrutinize and unravel preconceptions. Identify at least three preconceptions that might get in your way.
2. Let the evidence be your guide.
3. Focus on the source (point of care or intersection between patient and caregiver) not the second- or third-hand interpretation. Minimize filters of information or interpretations by those removed from the actual situation.
4. Look around the event. Examine and integrate the connections, antecedents, and subsequent events of healthcare work.
5. Tell the story using measurement language and concepts.

concepts to which it is difficult to assign quantifiable metrics and dollars. Patient satisfaction measures are increasingly rigorous for what they measure. What does not occur regularly is documentation of the story they tell—the connections and interdependencies between providers, patient care processes, values, and the context of care. For example, the events and resources required to achieve levels of patient satisfaction are seldom if ever identified and at best are only inferred.

The pathway to a meaningful measurement system is not found in magical analyses of costs, charges, and profits. Despite the quest for a foolproof elasticity formula (see the preceding Group Discussion), a formula in which changes are predictable based on past experiences, is at best incomplete. With such formulas, there is always a clarification, an exception, or a confounding variable that marginalizes the value of the formulation. At best these formulas are a beginning, not the final word.

As previously noted, avoiding inclusion of the contextual information (environment, resources, etc.) can be disastrous and costly. Single-source financial metrics can lead to decisions that are short sighted and incomplete. Further, when one entity tries to improve its fitness or position, this may result in a worsening condition for others. Each "improvement" in one entity therefore may impose associated costs on other entities, either within the same system or on other related systems.

Issue: Using Evidence Is Optional

Evidentiary information is inconsistently identified and applied in patient care. The source of the inconsistency is widespread and ranges from lack of knowledge or access to current evidence to personal practice preferences. National studies have documented the significance of evidence-based practice and its relationship to higher quality of care, improved patient outcomes, decreased geographic variations in the delivery of care, reduced healthcare costs, and greater job satisfaction (Heater,

Key Point

Focus on principles versus specific actions or rules. It may feel comfortable to develop an annual quality plan with sharply defined strategies and targets, but a better approach is to outline general goals and boundaries for improvement through which the organization moves toward the desired emergence.

Becker, & Olson, 1988; McGinty & Anderson, 2008; Shortell, Rundall, & Hsu, 2007; Williams, 2004). The current adoption rates for the provision of care based on evidence, caregiver expertise, and patient values is unconscionably slow.

Perhaps greater accountability should be placed on the providers and caregivers in addition to organizational leadership. Given the clearly defined scopes of practice, licensing regulations, and independent practice models, it would seem that more emphasis should be placed on the source of the practice. This is not to minimize the role of the organization and leadership in creating the appropriate context for evidence-based practice, rather it is shifting the accountability to the locus of practice. It is about shifting from being rule or policy driven to principle driven. The principle of patient safety that is adopted by every employee should negate the need for innumerable policies and procedures telling individuals how to be safe!

> ## Key Point
>
> **Be wary of root cause solutions . . .**
> An example of selecting and analyzing an isolated component is the root cause analysis model. Organizations have typically approached complex problems from the angle of ferreting out and eliminating specific factors (root causes) thought to be responsible for undesired results. In fact, targeting precise improvement strategies toward singular root causes may result in the unpleasant and unexpected emergence of new problem-laden systems. The key to mastering desired change begins with a focus on holistic systems and the relationships among components in those systems.

These six major issues of high cost, low quality, cost shifting, demand without account-ability, partial measurement, and the inconsistent use of evidence provide significant incentives for us to consider the healthcare system in a different way. Given the current state of disarray and dysfunction in our system, continuing with the same practices and valuation model can only perpetuate more of the same. A measurement system that reflects the complexity of health care is desperately needed; a system that provides evidence to assist individuals to address these issues and improve the allocation of healthcare resources more effectively is desperately needed.

Points to Ponder

Using available evidence seems so logical. The increasing availability of computerized systems and availability of the Internet to most providers and patients strongly support the use of evidence in practice. Such strategies as linking the use of federal or state funds to evidence-based practice and penalties for failure to use state-of-the-art practices deserve careful consideration. With the Institute of Medicine goal to have 90% of clinical decisions based on evidence by 2020, a different approach may be in order (McClellan, McGinnis, Nabel, & Olsen, 2007). Further, the leadership role in the facilitation and translation of evidence is to more actively and assertively ensure that contemporary evidence is considered and integrated to achieve optimal outcomes.

A Very Complex System

There are other healthcare challenges that could be added to this list; however, these issues describe the major problems emanating from the complexity of the healthcare system and serve as the foundation for the creation of a contemporary healthcare valuation model. In this section, a discussion of the phenomena of complex systems—connectedness, interdependence, and emergence—is provided to further inform the new valuation model.

Complexity science rejects the belief that systems and processes are like machines with parts that can be separated, analyzed, and modified or replaced. All healthcare organizations are complex and evolving social systems with innumerable behaviors, not mechanical assembly-line models. The realities of complexity are evident in nearly every aspect of the healthcare system and can better inform how healthcare value can be determined and documented more effectively. What is not evident or understandable is the continuing reliance on mechanistic models of thinking and measurement; thus, these principles are discussed as impetus to rethink the current model.

Connectivity and Interdependence

In complex systems, all things intersect and interact with each other and necessarily provide the energy to sustain and enhance the life of the system. No person, event, or process is ever fully isolated or immune from influences of other persons, events, or processes. Intuitively and intellectually, leaders recognize this reality, yet they operate on the premise that events and individuals are isolated and processes are linear. Table 3-1 includes a description of complexity principles and the implications for healthcare measurement.

The implications for the healthcare system are significant. Connectivity means that a decision or action by any individual (group, organization, institution, or human system) affects other individuals and systems. That effect may not have equal or uniform impact and will vary with the "state" of each related individual and system at the time. The connections or relationships between events provide the essential information to create an accurate representation of what needs to be considered for valuation. Documenting and determining value in an organization necessarily include valuing of the relationships and interdependencies among components in a system and the impact of those relationships as an essential part of the value statement. For example, the trajectory of communication is seldom linear or unidirectional. Communication may emanate from one individual and ultimately connect to numerous other individuals. The interactions and interdependencies in the worlds of patients, families, visitors, and healthcare professionals result in innumerable communication pathways and variables.

Beyond simple connectivity of elements of a system, relationships and dependence among elements quickly emerge as entities collaborate and support each other. This interdependence occurs among individuals within a system and between systems. Individual components in a process or system are not independent of other factors of the environment, technology, or political influence. Interdependence assumes mutual reliance on individuals and entities of a system. The behaviors and systems in which health care

Group Discussion

Emergence and the Electronic Health Record
From the implementation of the electronic medical record, new challenges and opportunities emerge. Brainstorm with your team members a list of positive emergent events and negative emergent events.
- Were these events anticipated?
- What is the cost of the events?
- Finally, create a mind map of all of the emergent events that occurred to further illuminate the concepts of connectivity and interdependence.

occurs are multidimensional with multiple dimensions interacting and influencing each other. The social, cultural, technical, economic, and global dimensions continually interact and intertwine in the creation of healthcare outcomes.

Emergence

In a complex and highly interconnected system, the future is rarely known and only somewhat predictable. Beyond our connections and interdependencies, systems offer us the possibility of becoming something different: the possibility to emerge into entirely new ways of being. Emergence or the evolution of new behaviors, relationships, processes, and products is the result of our interdependencies. This reality requires recognition of these phenomena and accounting for the management of the uncertainty or essential course corrections that must continually occur. Emergence is evident in the basic nature of patient care. To illustrate further, patient care is often guided by standards of care and algorithms for evidence-driven practices; however, despite the best map for care, the actual care is determined when all of the information and conditions connect. In essence, patient care is underdetermined until the situation is at hand and the caregiver and patient are engaged. The time of day, presence of family, mental and emotional status of the patient, and level of pain all converge to determine what and how care will actually happen.

Although glaringly obvious, these fundamental characteristics of our healthcare systems are not central to mainstream business management and leadership, where the focus is largely on measuring and controlling certain system components, discrete financial indicators, and specific performance goals.

Key Point

We witness emergence any time individuals come together and accomplish more than what was thought possible. The collective wisdom and creativity of individuals seldom disappoint us.

Key Point

No metric, such as hours per patient day (HPPD) or salary expense, should ever stand alone. Each metric has an important and essential story that cannot be isolated and considered as representative of work.

The driving assumptions for a new model focus on addressing current issues and recognizing the complexity of the work and expectations for ongoing evolution and course corrections as the future unfolds. Quantum leaders can now guide their organizations in the development of more robust models for the valuation of health care. The goal is to measure the reality as completely and accurately as possible. A new model for healthcare valuation must necessarily serve to document traditional financial data as well as the value of teamwork, patient provider engagement, and the degree of evidence integration.

New Healthcare Valuation Model

Given the complex nature of the healthcare experience, traditional metrics viewed in isolation are limiting and short sighted for effective decision making in health care. Financial metrics should be the beginning and not the end for measurement of healthcare effectiveness. Evaluation should occur in light of multiple, interconnected variables rather than a single traditional financial metric. Multiple metrics and information are needed specific to the achievement of goals and patient experiences as well as financial resources in the determination of healthcare value (Gold, Helms, & Guterman, 2011). No metric should ever stand alone for decision making without a supporting story. The following strategies are presented to begin the value transformation.

Strategy 1: Document the Story

A healthcare system driven by cure of disease, promotion of health, and prevention of disease is not sustainable if the context is not considered in every step of the process and evaluation. Anderson and McDaniel (2000) caution against assuming that practices that work well in one place can simply be transplanted elsewhere. This logic, though alluring, ignores the fact that even systems that appear analogous often have underlying differences. Kiel (1994) offers a similar assessment, noting

Group Discussion

Create a story or narrative that identifies connections, interdependencies, accountability, evidence, and evolving conditions. Describe both the realized past scenario and the desired future(s). Narratives include the individuals, their roles and motives, relationships between the individuals, the activities, and the potential outcomes. The narrative of what actually occurred serves to document the connections, interdependencies, and emerging events. The desired narrative serves to document how patient needs are evolving, which new provider services are being offered, and the challenges occurring in the environment.

that "two systems with very similar starting points may evolve along very different trajectories" (p. 5). This is not to say that healthcare quality's current emphasis on transplanting best practices is ill placed, but rather that common sense, flexibility, and a smattering of creativity must accompany the introduction of any new practice into an organization. Fraser and Greenhalgh (2001) recommend nonlinear approaches such as storytelling, case studies, role-playing, and simulations to illicit the essence of complex situations. An insightful leader encourages his or her organization to consider how the organization's unique norms, histories, values, and processes may impede or facilitate adoption of guidelines, recommendations, and other improvement strategies.

Consider the ever present expectation to increase profitability (see the following Group Discussion). A long-held assumption is that the profit margin can be controlled by clearly defined and discrete actions or individuals. Mandating a change in financial processes or expenditures is believed to be the requisite for success. The reality is that the profit margin is affected by many unknown and evolving influences and is connected to and intertwined with nearly every variable within the healthcare system. The traditional model with its well-intentioned steps to cut expenses at believed intervention points requires serious reconsideration. Consider the following two scenarios in which two approaches were used: (1) the traditional mandate for expense reductions (Story A) and (2) the more contemporary shared leadership approach to increasing revenues (Story B). The process focus begins with decreasing expenses by selected percentages. However, the trajectory and interdependence of the impact of this action are seldom articulated. A decrease in labor hours affects far more than the individual whose hours are reduced.

The outcomes from the Group Discussion of Story A and Story B are successful from the perspective of the target goal; however, the connecting variables were affected quite differently. In Story A, the effect on staff and patient satisfaction was decidedly negative. Patient safety and quality were also negatively affected, as was long-term caregiver turnover. The results in Story B are quite different. This approach sought to engage caregivers and support staff in addressing the challenge to increase the profit margin. Not only did the revenues increase with minimal increases in expenses, but the approach also increased caregiver satisfaction and long-term tenure. No negative impacts on patient satisfaction were identified.

The challenges of measuring health care are the result of the limitations of traditional analyses and measurement tools as well as many firmly entrenched practices believed acceptable.

Rarely, if ever, can a single metric such as net income or profit margin reflect the totality and reality of the situation, namely, an effective healthcare system. A profitable enterprise may in fact have delivered substandard care, alienated caregivers, and created negative relationships within the community. Traditional measurement approaches, though vital, do not hold all the answers. Most measures are limiting and may be deceptive because of the hidden variables contributing to the single metric. Antecedent and concurrent events affect outcomes in multiple ways.

Group Discussion

A 15 percent increase in profitability was the target for two facilities in a large healthcare system. Both facilities achieved the goal.

Story A.
To achieve this increase in profitability, the facility implemented an initiative to decrease expenses beginning with labor hours. All staff hours were decreased by 20 percent to achieve the desired increase in profitability. To achieve the decrease in labor hours, nurses increased the number of patients cared for, decreased hourly rounds to twice a shift, and decreased discussion of medications with patients during medication administration. As a result, patient satisfaction decreased specific to response time to call lights, understanding of medications decreased, and the number of falls with injury increased. Further, nurse turnover increased and job satisfaction decreased.

Story B.
To achieve the increase in profitability, the facility engaged the shared leadership councils to develop innovative ways to increase revenue. Three creative online projects were developed to package the facility's unique clinical standards and practices for clinical simulation, technology adoption, and transplant services to other organizations. Marketing staff assisted with both national and international advertising for Asia, Japan, and Australia. A total of 160 staff hours were required to create the new revenue center and begin generating revenue. Specific metrics that were affected include caregiver satisfaction, labor hours for creation of the new center, and Internet support for the service.

Measurement Category	Story A	Story B
Revenue	Unchanged	↑3%
Expenses	↓15%	↑0.5%
Labor hours	↓15%	↑0.5%
Nurse-to-patient ratio	↑25%	Unchanged
Patient satisfaction with response for call light	↓10%	Unchanged
Patient satisfaction with education regarding medications	↓15%	Unchanged
Patient falls	↑15% (2 falls with injury	Unchanged
Caregiver satisfaction and perceptions of quality patient care	↓20%	↑5%
Caregiver perceptions of involvement in decision making	↓15%	↑10%
Caregiver turnover	↑7%	↓5%

Group Discussion

A Clock-Out Survey?

Very specific information from caregivers can be obtained at the end of the shift. In light of the increasing computerization resources associated with time and attendance systems, discuss the value of a quick yes/no survey from every caregiver at the time of clock out. The questions, limited to three or four, could be:

1. I provided quality patient care today.
2. My team worked well together.
3. I had the supplies I needed to do my work well and in a timely manner.

Strategy 2: Extend Traditional Tools to Manage and Oversee Complexity

In light of the limitations of traditional financial measurement methodologies, quantum leaders need to explore and develop new tools to illuminate connectedness, interdependence, and emergence as the means to better understand system complexities and nuances. Often, leaders wonder if new roles or support staff are needed to advance this measurement and data analysis work. Some organizations have created Chief Data Officer (CDO) positions to assist with this work. What is especially important is for leaders to focus on the work to be done rather than the title of a position. Managing and analyzing large data sets are an emerging discipline and require high-level analytical competencies (Mauboussin, 2012; McAfee & Brynjolfsson, 2012; Thurston, 2012).

Moving beyond the emphasis on the selection of appropriate quantitative variables for value determination such as net profit, revenues, expenses, and return on investment is the beginning. This is not to say that these metrics are not important; rather, they are incomplete when disconnected from the totality of the variables representing the healthcare situation. Complex quality problems within complex systems rarely have one root cause or a single solution. Tools and methods that identify multiple aspects and relationships are needed for complex valuation. Although it is impossible to predict the unpredictable

Group Discussion

Consider the persistent and unresolved issue of patient medical errors. An organization may monitor medication error data over time, using measurement tools such as run charts and control charts. Unfortunately, these tools do not include the antecedents and concurrent events that influence the outcomes on the run or control chart. Use a mind map to describe and display the same situation. What are the advantages and disadvantages of each tool?

Key Point

Measurement Missteps

· *Measuring against yourself:* Both internal and external benchmarks are important to recognize available resources and the potential in the industry.

· *Looking backward:* Historical performance occurred under a different set of circumstances, for example, patient types, caregiver skills, physical settings, regulations.

· *Putting your faith in numbers:* Return on investment is only one of the variables for evaluation; cost-effectiveness, cost utility, and so forth add information to the analysis. Further, the story associated with the numbers is of equal importance.

· *Gaming your metrics:* Some metrics result in users "manipulating" numbers to meet targets. Moving expenses to different categories to avoid inclusion defeats the purpose.

· *Sticking to your numbers too long:* Metrics can lose their essence as the business evolves. The use of hours per patient day has long been seen as an incomplete metric given that the associated costs of support staff, education time, and patient engagement are not included in this metric.

· *Not enough metrics:* Single-minded metrics can lead to focusing on the wrong priorities.

· *Focusing on inputs over outcomes:* Although the processes and inputs of work are important, the results or outcomes are the real measure of organizational success.

Adapted from: Anthony, S. D., Johnson, M. W., Sinfield, J. V., & Altman, E. J. (2008). *Innovator's guide to growth: Putting disruptive innovation to work.* Boston, MA: Harvard Business Press.

and to design solutions for every potential scenario, three contemporary tools provide new insight into valuation: mind maps, the geographical information system (GIS), and scenario planning.

Mind Mapping

The mind map tool has become a powerful vehicle for collecting, organizing, and synthesizing large amounts of information. Although initially developed by Tony Buzan (Buzan & Buzan, 1993) to improve memory of content, his brother Barry integrated the creativity aspect of the tool, thus creating an incredibly robust method for increasing understanding of complex phenomena. The use of diagrams, shapes, and colors provides individuals with the means to expand and explore ideas, creating linkages between elements while maintaining focus on the central theme. The mind map is a very useful tool for documenting connectivity, interdependencies, and emerging phenomena in health care. When a particular healthcare scenario is mapped, the identified elements, linkages, and pathways become the essential elements for consideration in valuing health care more accurately and completely.

GIS Model

A geographical interface system integrates hardware, software, and data as the means to capture, manage, analyze, and display multiple forms of geographic reference information (Bolsted, 2005). The unique feature of this model is the display of multi-dimensional, multilayered aspects of complex situations. This approach provides for unique views of complex situations as the means to question, interpret, and better understand the phenomenon of interest. In addition, this model provides a means to solve problems by looking at data in a way that is quickly understood. The utility of GIS in healthcare analyses is that perspectives from point of care, local communities, regional areas, and national impact can be viewed and analyzed quickly and expertly.

Scenario Planning

Scenario planning is the third tool that provides a unique way to capture the essential elements for valuing healthcare situations. Scenario planning is especially useful in creating capacity for the unknown future. Participants in a workgroup are challenged to think more broadly and more creatively in addressing an unknown or extremely outrageous problem. The purpose is to move out of traditional thinking patterns and develop creative solutions not previously considered. This information now becomes available to teams as they confront uncertainty and embark on course corrections. The outrageous scenarios provide background ideas and potential solutions for consideration.

Strategy 3: Quantify the Value of Teamwork

It is no secret that expertly functioning teams are more likely to achieve excellent results and have minimal or no errors as a result of their effective collaboration. The financial value of expert teamwork and the cost of poorly functioning teams are not traditionally integrated into value formulations. Teamwork across disciplines is critical and at the same time very difficult to monitor and quantify. The increasingly complex nature of health care and the complex issues that caregivers face require a unique balance of responsibility and freedom to do the right work. The conditions for teamwork where issues are complex—namely, an environment that supports involvement in decision making, professional autonomy, and creativity in ensuring achievement of patient goals—are supporting variables that are linked to positive patient outcomes.

Measurement strategies to identify levels or degrees of teamwork contributing to patient care processes and outcomes begin with qualitative assessments, quantification of the specific cost of labor hours associated with the identified work, and examination of outcomes. The unit of analysis best begins with the shift of work or the patient event. **Exhibit 3-1** identifies the group of metrics that integrates expert functioning teamwork. Once the variables are identified, comparisons can be made to identify best practices among optimally functioning teams.

Exhibit 3-1 Measures of Teamwork

1. Hours of work
2. Skill mix
3. Levels of education of members
4. Years of experience of members
5. Overtime hours
6. Patient complaints
7. Patient satisfaction
8. Caregiver feedback
9. Negative patient outcomes

Strategy 4: Focus on Engagement of Providers and Patients

The need for full engagement of patient and provider has never been more important as the resources for

Group Discussion

System components depend on each other for their success. For example, a nurse depends on the presence of patients to provide care, a place to provide that care, supplies, medication, and support staff. For the care of your assigned patients for one shift, create a mind map that identifies the components required for patient care, the sequence of events, and the factors affecting patient outcomes.

- How many relationships did you identify?
- Which elements are working well together?
- Are there areas of congestion or dysfunction that are not working?

health care become scarcer. Creating and supporting accountability for evidence-driven interventions and patient behaviors that support healing and healthy behaviors can be some of the most cost-effective behaviors in this time of resource crises. The coordination of care processes, collaborative care planning that fully engages patients and their families to commit to healthy behaviors, and following agreed-to evidence-driven plans require skilled dialogue that creates both accountability for progress and sharing of information when plans are not working. The relationship between patients and caregivers is best supported with integrated, computerized electronic record keeping that can be accessed by both patient and caregivers. It is no longer acceptable for records to be provider contained and not accessible by patients.

Group Discussion

When organizations are attempting to empower staff and the point of service, the hard part is not getting caregivers engaged. The hard part is that the senior people get scared. It is usually the senior leaders who pull the rug out with the belief that the work is disturbing the system, not directing it. The lack of clear knowledge of what the outcomes are going to be is unacceptable and a threat to patient safety. To prevent a premature death of point-of-care creativity and innovation work, it is important to communicate regularly, understand the complexity system mental model, and realize the need for continuing growth.

Consider a unit in your organization that has many opportunities for improvement. Design a plan to empower staff to identify the issues, prioritize the challenges, select the tools of innovation to address issues, communicate progress to key stakeholders, and evaluate progress.

Strategy 5: Begin Locally with Change

Changing a long-standing culture of single financial measurements requires courage, persistence, and a plan that begins at the point of service, not in the boardroom. Kiel (1994) noted quite some time ago that often the best results come not from large-scale efforts, but from small, well-focused actions. Given the challenges at the unit level specific to medication administration, safe environments, teamwork, nurse–physician collaboration, and retention of competent staff, the opportunities are available for unit-driven activities to begin the processes working from the inside out.

The work of leadership is not to direct this work; rather, it is to empower staff at the point of care to be aware of the challenges and expect staff to use the tools of innovation to create better processes and outcomes. Leaders need to provide the infrastructure specific to time, role expectations, and resources to test new models. It is especially difficult for senior leaders to let go and empower direct caregivers to operate within loose boundaries and be creative in finding better solutions. Indeed, this is reflective of the transformation of cultures from a controlling, mechanical model to a shared leadership model that embraces the complex nature of human systems.

Strategy 6: Plan and Budget for Course Correction Work

In light of the reality of complex systems interactions and uncertainty, the work of course corrections must become recognized as normative and part of the work of adapting and growing; thus, mechanisms and measures for this work need to be included in the budgeting process. Specifically, it is important to at least determine a percentage of resources that will be needed for course correction. Developing expertise in quantifying course correction resources requires creativity and persistence. Beginning with comparisons of planned work and actual work is the optimal starting point. Using the pre- and post-analysis of events, or the variance data, becomes informative for more accurate resource planning. To be sure, no leader ever believes that 100% of work will be perfect and not need revisions or modifications to achieve goals. The work for each organization is to determine a percentage of resources that needs to be allocated for course corrections.

Strategy 7: Create the Business Case for the Healthcare Story and Course Corrections

Building the business case for new work is essential. Although there is not experience or history to rely on, there is an expectation for certain processes, certain outcomes, and the expected value to be achieved (Business link, 2005). This information needs to be systematically collected and integrated into a plan that serves as the road map for managing new ideas.

The following steps are essential components of the innovation business case:

1. Create the narrative for the product or service.
2. Identify the goal or purpose of the product or service. Include the relationship to mission-driven and financial goals, patient care quality, and patient safety.
3. Determine projected costs, course correction costs, and excluded costs. Be sure to include the rationale for each category, namely, why costs were included or excluded.

4. Project benefits for this work. Examples include meeting quality and safety goals, increasing profitability, and enhancing the organization's reputation.
5. Target levels of performance goals. Ideally, the goals should be 100% satisfaction and zero errors.
6. Anticipate profit or loss.
7. Nonfinancial benefits are expected. This includes information related to ambiguous evidence or evidence that has not traditionally been quantified such as degrees of patient–caregiver engagement, effect on reputation, or recruitment potential.
8. Determine key stakeholders, namely, those individuals who have a significant influence on success of this work.
9. Anticipate risks and plan to mediate risks or unexpected results.
10. Create an overall summary of long-term and short-term value to the organization and community.

The following exemplar is provided to share the creation of a business case for the healthcare story. Each leader and organization has different experiences and information that can further enhance this important work. A story from a very satisfied patient serves as the foundation for determination of value.

1. The healthcare story: My neighbor's mother died recently and left this story in her will with directions to donate a specified amount to the healthcare system.

    My last year of life has been blessed with incredible support from the healthcare system for my aging body and the realities of the end of life. During this time, my hypertension, diabetes, and irregular heart rhythm required routine monitoring and evaluation. My chronic constipation has been a problem for years; however, I am willing to live with it with the occasional oral remedies to manage it. I never felt like I was overtreated or asked to have tests or studies that I did not understand or for which there was an expectation that a positive change could be made. My healthcare providers and coaches, Dr. Karen (physician), Dr. Michael (nurse practitioner), and Mary (office receptionist), consistently assured me that my records were complete and shared appropriately with other providers as needed. Getting an appointment with my providers was handled efficiently and effectively—I never waited when I thought I needed to be seen—or at least got a call from Karen or Michael to discuss my questions and concerns.

    One short episode in the hospital was incredible—my blood sugars were out of control and the members of the healthcare team quickly reviewed my records and worked diligently to stabilize me. There was very little paperwork and interviewing—the only questions were about updates and new events in my life. I felt like I was one very special person and recovered quickly and went home within two days. I am now able to read again, watch TV, and walk to the mailbox. I am thrilled to be able to do these things without shortness of breath or anxiety.

    Charges, billing, and payment for my care were always clear. Before I left the office or hospital, my bill was presented and the exact amount Medicare would cover was identified as well as the amount I would need to pay. I never received bills for things I had not been advised about.

I know this is special health care because my neighbor didn't have the same experiences that I did. She, too, had many illnesses associated with aging. She was seldom able to get an appointment with her provider in less than a month. She went to the emergency department several times last year for things that she was waiting to see the provider about. In addition, she had two colonoscopies in the last two years—she didn't know why but thought it had something to do with her constipation.

The metrics or measures for this story offer the beginnings of a new mental model for health care: Begin with a successful story and identify the associated metrics to support similar care. In this story, metrics are extracted to identify the meaningful variables that are not often identified with traditional measurement approaches. These metrics contribute to the business case for complex patient care and provide for a more complete measurement picture of the healthcare experience.

Within this story, there is an incredible amount of information that can serve to illuminate new strategies for healthcare measurement. Multiple categories of value that reflect traditional metrics and those reflecting the complexities of health care are embedded in the story. The following can be learned from this story:

- *Patients can be realistic and do not want every symptom managed aggressively.* Living with chronic constipation, although uncomfortable, is tolerable for many individuals. They are not looking for the miracle cure (or multiple colonoscopies) to a chronic problem.
- *Understand and integrate the patient values; age does matter.*
- *A complete and integrated patient medical record reduces redundancy and the chance for errors.*
- *Access to care providers in a timely manner is important because it can avoid unnecessary stress for the patient and unneeded visits to the emergency department.*
- *Teamwork and communication make a positive difference.*
- *Clarity and communication of charges and patient accountability for co-pays are essential parts of the service of health care that needs to be addressed along with the service rather than months after the event.*
- *Single-source billing is possible.* It's like a Visa bill: all charges on one simple statement.

2. Goals and purpose of this story: The expectations from this story are multifocal and relate to the patient, the caregivers, and the organization. Examples of expectations are as follows:
   - *Integrated and accessible medical record available 24/7 to enable communication among providers and caregivers specific to patient's multiple diagnoses of hypertension, diabetes, and heart disease.*
   - *No redundancy of services or requests for information already provided.*
   - *Access to providers and feedback within 24 hours.* Providers are accessible for unanticipated needs as well as every 3 months for monitoring of diabetes and hypertension. No visits to the emergency room.
   - *Respectful and meaningful relationships with providers.* Patient is elderly, hard of hearing, and has some vision impairment. Decisions for care are made by the patient

with full information from providers and supporting evidence. Patient does not want unnecessary diagnostic testing or medications unless they will support or enhance current quality of life.

- *Personal level of independence and functionality includes limited ambulation with a cane and limited driving to church, bank, and grocery story.*
- *Payment and billing of healthcare services are fully understood at the time of treatment.* At the time of service, all charges and costs to the patient are known and discussed. There are no unanticipated charges to the payer or the patient.

3. Cost of care is identified as office visits, medications, blood glucose monitoring equipment, and +10% allocations for course corrections should the patient need to visit the emergency room.
4. The benefits of this coordinated and respectful plan of care include sustained quality of life for the patient, a high degree of patient satisfaction, and a positive community reputation for the healthcare system.
5. Anticipated levels of performance are 100% patient satisfaction and zero medical errors. Also, zero visits to the emergency room are the goal.
6. The anticipated profit for these services is 2%.
7. The stakeholders include the patient, providers, office staff, and the local pharmacy.
8. The anticipated risks in this plan are the potential emergency room visits for unexpected emergencies or unavailability of office staff.
9. The short-term and long-term benefits of this model of patient care include health maintenance and functionality for the patient, financial viability of the organization, and a positive community reputation for the organization as a resource for quality healthcare services.

Case Study 3-1

Are We a System or a Confederation of Hospitals?

Pacific Grove Healthcare System comprises six community hospitals located in a 100-mile radius, two major integrated physician organizations (IPOs), a healthcare plan, a hospice and home health service, and a freestanding rehabilitation center. The corporate executives have recently hired a chief nursing executive (CNE) to simplify the reporting structure for all of the CNOs at each hospital and IPO. The new CNE has a PhD in nursing and is nationally recognized for his success in developing integrated systems for health care. The new CNE has just completed a 10-year engagement at another large healthcare system that made dramatic changes in nursing services resulting in a system-wide Magnet designation by the American Nurses Credentialing Center (ANCC). The CNE has published many papers and spoken at national conferences about the challenges and successes of integrating nursing services across a multihospital system.

One of the first changes that the CNE made was to develop a new structure for nursing services that included several system-wide councils for (1) operations, (2) research and innovation, (3) professional development and scholarship, and (4) clinical excellence. The CNE announced that the intent and purpose of these system-wide councils were to facilitate planning, implementation of programs and services, and evaluation of the effectiveness of nursing services across the system. The CNE emphasized the importance and value of creating the system-wide councils and the need to lead the system effort and let go of the traditional unilateral decision making by inviting others in the organization to participate in decisions that affected patient care and nursing practice.

At first the CNOs at each hospital resisted reporting to the system CNE and the expansion of membership on the various system councils to individuals other than the CNOs. They viewed this structure change as marginalization of their roles and power structure. The CNE met with them individually and as a group in a planning retreat to address their concerns and shared stories and case studies from his previous organization that illustrated the benefits and outcomes of integrating nursing across the system. As a group they developed a list of attributes that they believed essential for a fully functioning system and the strategic actions that would need to take place before nursing in the system could be completely integrated. They also discussed the benefits and barriers to system work. The CNE led them through a mind mapping experience to expand their thinking about the challenges and opportunities in leading system work. From the mind map bubbles, the CNOs explored scenarios that would illustrate some of the situations that they might be facing in the future. The group discussed possible leaders and the membership for each of the councils and decided to invite some of the top leaders in each of the hospitals' Magnet council structure to participate in the system-wide councils.

To facilitate the effectiveness of this change, the CNE also engaged the services of an academic partner from one of the local universities to facilitate a professional development curriculum focused on leading group meetings, building consensus, managing conflict, managing change, financial planning and management, and system integration. Once the membership was decided and the leadership selected for each of the system-wide councils, each of the members was invited to participate in the learning experiences to build their skills and competencies in system work.

The CNE invited all of the system council members and the CNOs to participate in a retreat where he presented his vision for an integrated nursing service line across all system entities. He shared that "success" would have many definitions, but one measure of success would be system-wide Magnet designation. He presented the characteristics of a high-performing system with examples of cost savings, financial gains, and program and service expansions from other system organizations that had achieved integration of patient care and nursing services across their systems. He outlined several measures that would guide the evaluation of their work including financial, quality, satisfaction, work environment, and patient outcome metrics. He indicated that each hospital would continue to report their individual progress on these metrics, but the aggregate of all of the system entities was a better measure of system performance. Each of them would also be evaluated on system metrics in addition to their individual entity goals. Each of the councils would include clinical nurses who were active in their unit practice councils and their entity's collaborative governance councils.

Bolstering his vision for integrated patient care and nursing services, the CNE mentioned several business partners whose companies were interested in funding and involvement in the Research and Innovation Council, which was a tremendous opportunity to expand patient care and nursing research efforts. Academic partners representing the local colleges would also participate in the Professional Development and Scholarship Council in an effort to provide additional opportunities and resources to advance the education level and leadership skills of clinical nurses and frontline managers. It was also suggested that patient representatives be selected to participate in the Clinical Excellence Council to ensure that the "voice of the customer" was heard as a focus area for planning. Clinical nurses and interprofessional partners would be invited to participate on the Operations Council to integrate efforts of nursing and other professional providers.

At the end of the planning retreats, the CNOs and others who had participated were excited but a bit overwhelmed at the layers of change that were planned for each of their entities and for the entire system for patient care and nursing services. Some had doubts about the value of such a change, but most trusted that the new CNE would be able to direct and facilitate such a change because of his experience and reputation for accomplishing a similar process in another organization. Most were eager and pleased to be empowered to participate in such a lofty goal of integrating nursing services across the entire organization.

Questions

1. What is your impression of the new CNE's plans for a layered change process to integrate patient care and nursing services across the healthcare system?
2. What barriers do you think will challenge the efforts toward system integration?
3. How do you think that the CNE can ensure accountability of his CNOs to support such change and promote systemness in their own organization as opposed to promoting their own entity's interests?
4. What other metrics or measures would you recommend to assess the success of the integration process?
5. Describe the attributes that you think would be essential for a fully integrated nursing system.
6. To achieve the attributes that you outlined in question 5, what developmental elements would be needed to achieve an integrated nursing system?

Case Study 3-2

It's That Time of the Year Again!

"Good grief, it's that time of year again!" This seemed to be the mantra of the entire group of nurse directors at St. Thomas Hospital as budget season approached. There seemed to be a spirit of quiet anticipation and resignation to the fact that each of them would be spending the next 6 weeks reviewing operational and financial data, planning unit budgets, negotiating for changes in financial and productivity targets based on last year's information, and presenting the final budget to their direct reports once they were approved by the finance department. There never seemed to be enough financial resources to support all of the proposed initiatives, planned volume for the future, and changes that seemed essential, causing great conflict among the various layers of management in the organization as they competed for a greater "piece of the pie" for their respective departments. The finance department disseminated the budget forms and the operational and productivity data trended over the past 3 years.

Irene, one of the department directors commented, "It's like planning the future looking in the rearview mirror!" Irene was particularly sensitive to using the past data for staffing projections because her department had experienced significant changes affecting staffing, productivity, and expenses. The entire department had moved into a new building with a completely different configuration of the nursing units, all private rooms, and centralized nursing station that increased distances that nurses had to walk when providing patient care and retrieving supplies and equipment. The new unit configuration completely changed the way that nurses practiced, making the past 3 years of data ineffective for planning the future. Irene realized that she would have difficulty convincing the CFO of this fact because the goal of the hospital was to have a budget-neutral plan for the next year to accommodate major changes in reimbursement methodologies proposed by the new Affordable Care Act. It had been clearly announced that none of the departments would receive more money for staffing than they had been allocated in the past, making Irene a bit nervous about how she would justify the need for additional dollars needed because of the unit configuration change in the new building.

To prepare her case for presentation to the CFO, Irene benchmarked her units with other hospitals of similar size, complexity, and configuration. She had asked the architectural firm that designed the new unit for names of other hospitals so that she could interface with their nursing directors. She had many questions about how they allocated staffing in the new configuration and particularly with a remote centralized nursing station. Irene had hoped for a design that would allow for a documentation area between every two private rooms, locating the nurses closer to the patients, but space constraints prevented the achievement of this design; at least this is what Irene had been told by the architects and the hospital's executive team. Now Irene was accountable to staff the unit with the same resources that had been used in a more compact semiprivate configuration with the same number of patient beds. Therefore, Irene felt that it was essential that she gather evidence from directors at other hospitals who had also made the change to a new unit configuration.

Irene also needed to add additional money for cross training the staff to the new computerized documentation and medication administration systems, and these expenses would not have been realized in the budget snapshots for the past 3 years. It seemed that all of these changes not only affected the budgetary expenses, but also the staff morale on the unit because they were becoming "change fatigued." Irene was certain that any budgetary restraints on staffing levels would tip the staff into becoming more negative about the organization. She did all possible to make her staff aware that she was advocating for their needs and included some of the clinical nurses in the budget planning meetings so that they could share information from a clinical perspective and provide input to their colleagues as well. Irene included representation from pharmacy, dietary, and the therapies because their workload had also changed with the new unit configuration. Irene's intent was to develop a comprehensive proposal making the business case for her additional needs with the input of her interprofessional partners. Together they created a narrative that would support the new budget and developed two separate budgets that would illustrate how the unit configuration changed the resource needs for each of their respective departments. One of the proposals reflected the resource needs that would have been budgeted for the previous unit configuration and compared that with a second budget developed for the new unit configuration, which demonstrated the incremental increases resultant from changes in the physical design. Irene realized this was an important step in presenting her case to the CFO because patient type, acuity, and volume did not change appreciably over the past 3 years, but rather the physical design affected nursing care hours needed for the same projected volume and acuity.

Questions

1. If you were Irene, how would you present your business case to the CFO requesting additional nursing care hours and staffing dollars for the new budget?
2. What are the benefits of an interprofessional approach in supporting Irene's proposal to the CFO?
3. What evidence does Irene need to acquire to support her budget proposal?

Conclusion

In summary, this healthcare valuation model is innovative and requires courage to be tested and implemented. What is most important for the healthcare leader is the recognition of the unresolved issues in our current system, the adoption of healthcare reform, and the ever-increasing complexity of the system. To be sure the system will not improve with waiting and thinking; action is required to begin remodeling and testing new ideas that reflect the complexity of the healthcare system.

References

Altman, D. E., Clancy, C., & Blendon, R. J. (2004). Improving patient safety—five years after the IOM report. *New England Journal of Medicine, 351*(20), 2041–2043.

Anderson, R. A., & McDaniel, R. R. (2000). Managing health care organizations: Where professionalism meets complexity science. *Health Care Management Review, 25*(1), 83–92.

Anthony, S. D., Johnson, M. W., Sinfield, J. V., & Altman, E. J. (2008). *Innovator's guide to growth: Putting disruptive innovation to work.* Boston, MA: Harvard Business School Press.

Bolsted, P. (2005). *GIS fundamentals: A first text on geographic information systems* (2nd ed.). White Bear Lake, MN: Eider Press.

Business link. (2005). The business case for innovation. Retrieved from http://www.nibusinessinfo.co.uk/content/business-case-innovation

Buzan, T., & Buzan, B. (1993). *The mind map book: Radiant thinking.* London, England: BBC Books.

Centers for Medicare and Medicaid Services. (2008). National health expenditure projections 2008–2018. Retrieved from http://www.cms.gov/Research-Statistics-Data-and-Systems/Statistics-Trends-and-Reports/NationalHealthExpendData/downloads/proj2008.pdf

Committee on Quality of Health Care in America. (2000). *Crossing the quality chasm: A new health system for the 21st century*. Washington, DC: National Academies Press.

Fleming, C. (2013). US health spending growth projected to average 5.8 percent annually through 2022. Health Affairs Blog. Retrieved from http://healthaffairs.org/blog/2013/09/18/us-health-spending-growth-projected-to-average-5-8-percent-annually-through-2022/

Fraser, S., & Greenhalgh, T. (2001). Coping with complexity: Education for capability. *British Medical Journal, 323*, 799–803.

Gold, M., Helms, D., & Guterman, S. (2011). *Identifying, monitoring, and assessing promising innovations: Using evaluation to support rapid-cycle change*. Commonwealth Fund Pub. No. 1512. Retrieved from http://www.commonwealthfund.org/~/media/Files/Publications/Issue%20Brief/2011/Jun/1512_Gold_promising_innovations_rapid_cycle_change_ib_FINAL.pdf

Heater, B., Becker, A., & Olson, R. (1988). Nursing intervention and patient outcomes: A meta-analysis of studies. *Nursing Research, 37*, 303–307.

Kiel, L. D. (1994). *Managing chaos and complexity in government*. San Francisco, CA: Jossey-Bass.

Mauboussin, M. J. (2012). The true measures of success. *Harvard Business Review, 92*(10), 46–56.

McAfee, A., & Brynjolfsson, E. (2012). Big data: The management revolution. *Harvard Business Review, 92*(10), 59–68.

McClellan, M. B., McGinnis, J. M., Nabel, E. G., & Olsen, L. M. (2007). *Evidence-based medicine and the changing nature of healthcare*. Washington, DC: National Academies Press.

McGinty, J., & Anderson, G. (2008). Predictors of physician compliance with American Heart Association guidelines for acute myocardial infarction. *Critical Care Nursing Quarterly, 31*(2), 161–172.

Minot, J. (2009). Geographic variation and health care cost growth: Research to inform a complex diagnosis. Retrieved from http://www.rwjf.org/en/research-publications/find-rwjf-research/2009/10/geographic-variation-and-health-care-cost-growth.html

Mitchell, P. H., & Lang, N. M. (2004). Framing the problem of measuring and improving healthcare quality: Has the quality health outcomes model been useful? *Medical Care, 42*(2), II4–11.

Morris, E. (2008). Making sense of ambiguous evidence. *Harvard Business Review, 88*(9), 53–57.

Priesmeyer, H. R. (1992). *Organizations and chaos: Defining the methods of nonlinear management*. Westport, CT: Quorum.

Shortell, S. M., Rundall, T. G., & Hsu, J. (2007). Improving patient care by linking evidence-based medicine and evidence-based management. *Journal of the American Medical Association, 298*(6), 673–676.

Thurston, B. (2012, December). Data is the new language. *FastCompany*, 136.

Wheatley, M. J., & Kellner-Rogers, M. (1996). *A simpler way*. San Francisco, CA: Berrett-Koehler.

Wikipedia. (n.d.). Geographic information system. Retrieved from http://en.wikipedia.org/wiki/Geographic_information_system

Williams, D. O. (2004). Treatment delayed is treatment denied. *Circulation, 109*, 1806–1808.

Suggested Readings

Anthony, S. D., Johnson, M. W., Sinfield, J. V., & Altman, E. J. (2008). *Innovator's guide to growth: Putting disruptive innovation to work*. Boston, MA: Harvard Business Press.

Christensen, C., Kaufman, S. P., & Shih, W. C. (2008). Innovation killers: How financial tools destroy your capacity to do new things. *Harvard Business Review, 87*(1), 98–105.

Jacobides, M. G. (2010). Strategy tools for a shifting landscape. *Harvard Business Review, 89*(1), 77–84.

Kohn, L. T., Corrigan, J. M., & Donaldson, M. S. (2000). *To err is human: Building a safer health system.* Washington, DC: National Academies Press.

Likierman, A. (2009). The five traps of performance measurement. *Harvard Business Review, 87*(10), 96–101.

Wheatley, M. J. (1999). *Leadership and the new science: Discovering order in a chaotic world.* San Francisco, CA: Berrett-Koehler.

Quiz Questions

Select the best answer for each of the following questions.

1. Which of the following statements characterizes customizing measurement in health care?
   a. It is necessary to integrate local facility resources to identify the most accurate use of resources.
   b. It makes it difficult to compare healthcare practices across the country.
   c. It is irresponsible given the need to develop safe and reliable systems that can be replicated.
   d. It is important to all leaders to be creative and support individual goals.

2. Why does cost continue to be an issue in health care?
   a. Healthcare reform is too costly.
   b. Cost shifting is a reality that legislators do not want to address.
   c. The overall system is fragmented and inconsistent.
   d. Most citizens do not know how much they really want to spend on healthcare services.

3. Which of the following statements characterizes cost savings in health care?
   a. Cost savings are possible if patient accountability for provider instructions is required.
   b. Cost savings are difficult to determine in light of system complexity and current inefficiencies.
   c. Cost savings are possible if patients would practice healthy behaviors.
   d. Cost savings are most likely if the private sector assumed control of the healthcare system.

4. Which of the following statements characterizes personal patient accountability?
   a. It is important but does not really affect the cost of health care.
   b. It could significantly affect the demand for services.
   c. It is an untapped component of the healthcare equation for rational spending and allocation of resources.
   d. It is a violation of individual rights and should not be considered in the healthcare model.

5. Which of the following does complexity theory do?
   a. Illuminates the challenges of valuation in the healthcare system
   b. Introduces unnecessary information into the system
   c. Is limiting in that it is not applicable to all healthcare interactions and relationships
   d. Is an outdated paradigm that further complicates healthcare issues

6. Which of the following statements characterizes ambiguous evidence?

   a. Ambiguous evidence is a reality that should not be considered in healthcare valuation because of its subjectivity.

   b. Ambiguous evidence provides an opportunity for manipulation of the reimbursement system.

   c. Ambiguous evidence is a reality of the healthcare experience and system complexity that needs to be considered.

   d. Ambiguous evidence should be discounted in financial analyses.

7. What does emergence, a reality of human relationships, require of leaders?

   a. To plan for eventual conflict between providers and patients

   b. To be sure there is a well-planned patient care plan

   c. To identify the budgeting implications for unanticipated changes

   d. To recognize and plan for course corrections because no plans ever emerge completely as planned

8. Which of the following statements characterizes documenting the story?

   a. Documenting the story is interesting however nearly impossible to integrate into a measurement system.

   b. Documenting the story requires skilled clinicians to interpret the information.

   c. Documenting the story is not accepted by financial experts.

   d. Documenting the story is a robust method to illicit as much information as possible about the patient care experience.

9. Which of the following statements characterizes traditional measurement tools?

   a. They continue to be adequate for complex measurement.

   b. They require supplementation with more comprehensive models of measurement.

   c. They should be minimized to decrease the complexity in the current system.

   d. They have some limitations; however, they are usually accepted by legislators and financial experts.

10. What is the business case for the healthcare story?

   a. It is another iteration of a strategic plan.

   b. It requires additional resources and does not provide additional information.

   c. It integrates the elements of a healthcare situation, comprehensive information, and the challenges of valuing new models.

   d. It is an excellent model to support national healthcare reform.

CHAPTER FOUR

Innovation as a Way of Life: Leading Through the White Water of Change

The great use of life is to spend it on something that will outlast it.
—*William James*

Chapter Objectives

At the completion of this chapter, the reader will be able to

· Identify three key contextual characteristics necessary to create an organizational frame for innovation.
· Name the central obligation of the critical roles of leadership in creating a context for innovation.
· Outline the various role obligations of leadership in building a structure of innovation across the network.
· List the components and elements of the innovative infrastructure of the organization that supports the activities of innovation at every place in the organization.

We are in an age of major transformation, change, and innovation. The postdigital and postreform age increases the demands on organizations and systems to engage and embrace essential structural and technological shifts that alter the foundation of their design and work. The leader now must create both a strategic and structural imperative that incorporates new and emerging technologies and innovations in the evolving "way of doing business" (McCarthy, 2011). The almost daily impact of emerging and new technological applications makes it nearly impossible to conceptualize or even afford all of them. Technological applications today are continuously altering the delivery of healthcare services (Cassey, 2007). Technological innovations have become their own "disruptive technologies" insofar as each succeeding generation of clinical technology makes the preceding generation obsolete (**Exhibit 4-1**). This is the state and these are the conditions that healthcare leaders and providers must function in every day.

Exhibit 4-1   Disruptive Technologies

- Innovations
- Unanticipated
- Threaten existing products/realities

- Represent unexpected competition
- Fills roles unfilled previously
- Revolutionary and often destructive

Driving the Culture of Innovation

The elements and requisites of innovation require an entirely different cultural context from the one that has been in existence in health care for the past 100 years. The compartmentalized, hierarchical, rigidly ordered, unilaterally medically controlled hospital and healthcare service model is no longer relevant as a frame for sustainability in contemporary healthcare service structures (Porter-O'Grady & Malloch, 2010a). The complexity and breadth of knowledge that are now inculcated within a wide variety of clinical practices in health care call for reconceptualization of the infrastructure and framework that have historically defined and directed the actions and relationships between and among the various key players in health service delivery. In addition, the demands of health reform require a total reconceptualization of health care, the way it is offered, and the way it is funded. The introduction of value-driven financial and service models for health care and the requisite that citizens' health be the ultimate attainment change both the configuration and trajectory of health services.

The historical culture of medical subsidiary and subordinateness that has driven health care for the past 100 years clearly delineated the primacy of the physician's role and both legally and functionally limited the role of other provider disciplines. Although this did much to strengthen the scientific and academic bases of clinical practice, creating a positive trajectory for clinical science, invention, and applied technology, it has also had negative side effects. Three major negatives persist: (1) a lack of interdisciplinary collaboration, linkage, and interaction; (2) unilateral educational pathways for each discipline that duplicate content and resources; (3) social, cultural, and professional barriers and boundaries between disciplines that result in both identity and relational conflicts. Each negative is a precise social and cultural constraint that impedes the creation of a dynamic and responsive organization available and ready for innovation (Hall, 1993).

The historical culture of functionalism and process-fixed notions of work has also created an existing frame that makes it virtually impossible to embed a dynamic of innovation that is represented by high levels of integration, interaction, and relationship. Collateral and interactional collaboration among disciplines based on equity and value is now a fundamental centerpiece essential to the success of health reform. Indeed, the historical focus on functionalism and work processes actually removes the more professionally driven urge toward sustainable impact, outcome, and evidence of making a difference so important in reform (**Exhibit 4-2**). These latter characteristics are more commonly associated with the social mandate of professionals rather than the functional processes of an "employee workgroup" orientation. The historically delineated "external" (independent) role of the physician and the predominantly "internal" (employed) orientation of other developing disciplines have created a significant wall between them.

Exhibit 4-2   Historic Focus of Work

- Emphasis on function
- Policy and procedurally driven
- Characterized by control

- "Employee" oriented and managed
- Active, not reflective

By maintaining its independence and unilateral locus of control, the medical profession has been able to develop based on the separate and unique needs of its members (Moore, 2005). The nursing profession and other emerging disciplines, on the other hand, have not had the same opportunity by virtue of their more dependent location as both subordinates and employees (Baer, 2001). Although the nursing profession has led the way in creating a unique body of knowledge and an academic frame for knowledge creation, generation, and utility, it has not moved with the same degree of dispatch toward professional independence by virtue of its two historically subordinating factors: that it is predominately composed of women, and that it has been historically employee based (Porter-O'Grady, 1990). Both of these circumstances have been well documented, and the conditions parallel the historic journey to equity of women and of the profession of nursing (Ashley, 1976; Porter-O'Grady & Malloch, 2010b; Rounds, McGrath, & Walsh, 2013).

Equity

Creating a culture amenable to innovation is necessarily based on the relative understanding and application of equity within an organizational framework. Equity is a statement of value and suggests to all the specificity and clarity of value that each role plays in contributing to the life and integrity of an organization. Equity assumes equality, but it bases that assumption on notions of value. Equity suggests that in any membership community, the members are there because of their unique capacity to contribute to the effort of the community as a whole (**Exhibit 4-3**). Indeed, the whole community is defined by the aggregate contribution of each of its members. In the case of professionals, it is not the obligation of the community to demonstrate unilateral value for the member. It is, instead, the obligation of individuals to demonstrate their specific and unique contribution to the aggregate contribution of the whole. This classic interdependence between members of the community sums the value of this contribution in a way that demonstrates the significance of the community. In short, the professional community represents the sum of the value of the contributions of each member. It is vital for professional communities to recognize the centrality of value to the life of the profession (Porter-O'Grady & Malloch, 2010a).

Exhibit 4-3   Equity

- Value-based
- Reflects accountability
- Characterized by equality

- Horizontal relationships
- Inclusive, suggesting ownership

Further, it is important for each profession to recognize its unique and significant contribution to the life of the system in concert with other disciplines and workgroups. Sustainability depends on the notion of value between disciplines as much as within them. Equity suggests that each discipline represents its essential interdependence with the other disciplines necessary to the achievement of impact and outcome (Mazur, 2003; Porter-O'Grady & Malloch, 2010a). In contemporary health care, no single discipline can operate effectively and achieve sustainable value independent of its relationship with other disciplines, which it depends on for its own contribution or success (Rapport, McWilliam, & Smith, 2004). This intensity of interface and degree of interdependence are the earmarks of contemporary healthcare service. However, to make these essential principles live in current healthcare service systems and networks, the organizational infrastructure and leadership capacity must be constructed to reflect these more relevant tenets.

Equity therefore suggests that the following considerations be reflected in the organizational constructs necessary to establishing a creative and innovative organizational infrastructure:

1. Each discipline makes an intentionally equal and unique contribution to the work of other disciplines and to the evidence and impact of patient care.
2. Accountability is the centerpiece of the role and obligation of each discipline and demands clarity of understanding regarding ownership and expression of it.
3. Partnership, not subordination, represents the essential character of horizontal connection necessary to determining and obtaining value and for the synthesis of effort necessary to sustain it.
4. The fact that nursing as a discipline is located at the center (nodal point) of the clinical network is a statement of location, not of control. However, the centrality of the nursing role in coordinating, integrating, and facilitating both the structure and the continuum of care within the organized healthcare system must be acknowledged.
5. Each discipline must know the contribution it makes in relation to other disciplines and its contribution to equity. It is the aggregation and mutuality of the unique contribution of each discipline that create the aggregate of effort that is ultimately more viable and sustainable.
6. Contemporary health systems are networks, not hierarchies. They are successful to the extent that relational clarity is established between them. Positional control (lines and boxes on organizational charts) no longer adequately describe the nature of the relationship or the interaction among elements of the network and players in the system.
7. Evidentiary dynamics drive clinical actions and relationships and demand the synthesis and integration of interdisciplinary effort to legitimately define and sustain clinical value and viability.

Creating an equitable clinical infrastructure demands an understanding of how networked professional organizations operate and function effectively (**Exhibit 4-4**). By using shared decision-making principles and practices, the organization must reject approaches based on positional control and build instead on decisional locus of control

---

Exhibit 4-4   The Professional Mandate

For the professions, the direction of obligation is from the professional to the professional community. The profession is not obligated to the member. It is the members who owe obligation to the profession, enabling and sustaining it in its value and work. The profession is defined by the collective action of each member, committed in his or her own life to represent its values and social mandate in every thought, action, and impact.

(Porter-O'Grady, 2007). For the foundations enumerated here to become a normative part of the organizational dynamics, the healthcare system must confront, resolve, and better identify a structural frame based on decisions rather than positions (Porter-O'Grady, 2009a).

Decisional Structures

One of the first steps necessary to building a context that truly stimulates and sustains innovation is the reconfiguration of infrastructure based on decisional accountability rather than positional authority (**Exhibit 4-5**). The traditional hierarchical organizational structure created positional management structures that authorized the manager to control and administer components of the organizational structure. Although that traditional business construct brought order and form to the delivery of healthcare services, it did so at the expense of staff decisional ownership, investment, and appropriate locus of control. It invested in the manager accountabilities that rightfully belong to the disciplines; when the disciplines surrendered them, the ownership necessary to achieve and sustain value disappeared. Indeed, it created an illegitimate locus of control for authority and autonomy that should rest with the professions who own it. Once divorced from this accountability, the professions lost legitimacy (some suggest they may have never obtained it), and the managers to whom these accountabilities had been assigned could never achieve legitimacy because their role could not obtain or sustain the outcomes attendant to legitimate ownership. Such outcomes could only be achieved and sustained by the disciplines that owned these accountabilities (Alberto & Colacino, 2008).

This management-driven illegitimate locus of control is evident in the endless cycles of new initiatives that become necessary to engage workers. Because of the intense effort of managers to obtain ownership from staff in the interests of the organization, managers must create a culture of "buy-in" both to get and keep workers interested in the goals and

---

Exhibit 4-5   From Position to Decision

Positional Control
- Hierarchal
- Reductionistic
- Vertical
- Locational
- Directive

Decisional Control
- Relational
- Multilateral
- "User driven"
- Value centric
- Direct impact

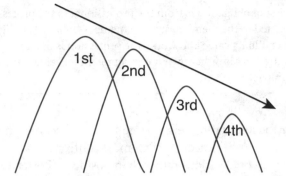

Figure 4-1 Trajectory of Diminishing Successive Initiative Efforts

initiatives of the organization as defined, directed, and controlled by the management structure. The problem with these initiative-driven activities is that they become increasingly more difficult as more effort is directed to them. Staff demonstrate decreasing interest in investing in an endless array of new initiatives and become less excited and interested the more of these initiatives are created for them (**Figure 4-1**). Buy-in is not ownership. Investment is not simply engaging staff in issues with which they do not personally identify. Engagement means enrolling people by incorporating their perspectives and personal values in decisions and actions that affect their lives (Nohra, Groysbery, & Lee, 2008; Walker, 2012).

Personal value means more than the hygienic factors of pay and benefits. Pay and benefits certainly are addressed through the foundations and basics of work activity. Beyond that, there is no evidence to suggest that interest, ownership, or investment can be obtained or sustained through those same means (Nohra et al., 2008). A stronger connection between personal values and goals and those of the organization must be made in a manner that evidences and represents a convergence of meaning and value between the organization and those who compose it. This is especially true for professionals. Because professionals see their work as a social mandate rather than as an employee-driven activity, the kind of engagement necessary to sustain them cannot be obtained simply by initiative and hygienic incentives (Gkorezis & Petridou, 2008). As indicated earlier, if professionals are seen and treated simply as an employee workgroup, their commitment to the values of the profession as well as their interest in the external goals of the organization will diminish. This loss of professional identity has a great impact in ways other than the fact that they are simply becoming another employee workgroup. This loss of professional attachment and value is accompanied by a loss of meaning, commitment, and purpose—a loss that ultimately affects their relationship to the workplace, to each other, and to the work of the profession (Bahuth, Blum, & Simone, 2013).

This focus on alignment of decisional structures with appropriate locus of control for the decisions is a critical element in the configuration of structure in a way that supports creativity, innovation, and professional commitment (Porter-O'Grady, 2009b). Locating decisions in the places where they are most effectively exercised and configuring them in a way that represents the expectations and activities unfolding at that place in the organization are critical pieces in the alignment of structure and process with work systems. Some of the greatest impediments to creativity and innovation are the organizational and structural barriers that limit this sense of ownership and that have control over decisions that directly affect what people do (Humphrey, 2008).

In relating to professionals, this notion of locus of control is a critical factor for leaders. *Locus of control* simply means that decision and action are located at the most legitimate place, where information can most effectively be deliberated, decided, and acted on in a way that specifically advances purpose and, ultimately, success. One of the greatest problems in complex organizations is related to decisions being made by people and in places where they cannot most effectively be acted on in an efficient and effective way. Perhaps one of the greatest errors in organizational leadership is exemplified by decisions made by leaders who are not positioned appropriately to make such decisions or who do not demonstrate the relevant content competence necessary to make those decisions effectively and to translate them into viable and sustainable implementation processes for those who must both implement them and live with the consequences. Innovation demands the kind of infrastructure support that allows ownership, freedom, and investment on the part of innovators. Innovators must be allowed to control their circumstances, undertake creative processing, and maintain dynamic interaction in ways that can yield genuine benefits unconstrained by illegitimate control that is exercised from outside the immediate "circle of innovation" (Pink, 2009).

Group Discussion

Differentiating professions from employee workgroups is an important consideration for leaders as they work to more clearly establish the relationship between the organization and the professional. Professionals are driven by accountability, which incorporates the elements of autonomy, authority, and competence. As you refine your understanding of the role of the professional, consider and discuss the following key questions:

- What do professionals need that is different from the needs of employee workgroups?
- Name at least two leadership behaviors that are essential to lead professionals versus employee workgroups.
- Identify at least two structural changes in the organization necessary to adapt to the needs of professionals as differentiated from employee workgroups.
- Is it possible to be both employed and professional in the contemporary healthcare workplace? What might have to change to make the organization more supportive of the life and action of a professional?

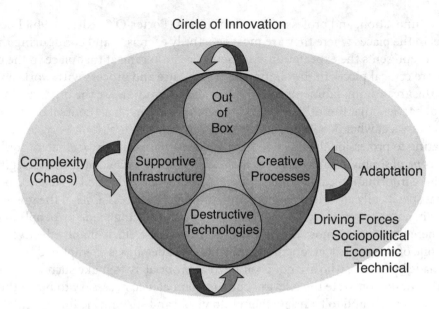

Figure 4-2 Circle of Innovation

The circle of innovation simply is a context in which the innovative dynamic unfolds in a way that eliminates the traditional structural impediments, operational practices, traditional processes, and operating role expectations that preclude the necessary flow of interactions that feed the innovation process (**Figure 4-2**). Line controls and positional decisional authority and expression do little to facilitate the out-of-the-box constituents necessary to innovation and do much to shut down those very processes. Certainly, leaders must be aware of the necessary constraints and parameters that influence the dynamic of creativity and innovation. However, these realities are incorporated into the innovation process itself and are not successfully managed in an innovative organization outside the circle of innovation. When exercised outside the circle of innovation, the only outcome is to shut down the innovative process, turn off the innovators, and reestablish rote, ritual, and routine (Coyne, Clifford, & Dye, 2007).

Innovation is by definition unsafe. Not unsafe in the traditional sense, but in the sense of being willing to undertake risk, to open doors not previously opened, to threaten processes hanging on the edge of irrelevance, and to create possibilities not previously perceived as a part of the emergent reality of the organization. To address these characteristics, the historical and traditional structural frames need to be seen as a part of the control mechanisms of the traditional system. A more effective perspective representing the networked mosaic of intersections and interactions that sustain a dynamic and responsive human system (organization) needs to emerge (Malloch, 2010).

Driving from the Point of Service

Networked organizations and systems constructs are more relational entities and less organizational hierarchies. Hierarchies are always present, and their value should not be diminished: They represent breadth of relationship rather than intensity of control.

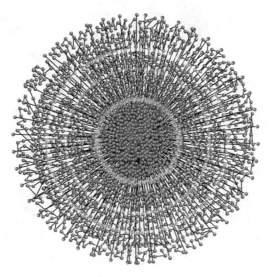

Figure 4-3 Network of Intersecting Nodes and Links

In all living systems, homeostatic mechanisms represent and demonstrate the essential linkage between smaller elements and larger systems elements to which the interaction and convergence of the smaller elements contribute (Yang & Shan, 2008). This hierarchy is a representation of relatedness, interdependence, and synthesis rather than compartmentalization and control, as has been evident in traditional organizational structure. The control in networks is exemplified by the enumeration of their points of intersection and the nature of their interdependence (**Figure 4-3**). These factors contribute to each element's definition of its value and significance as well as its specific role in contributing to the accelerating value of the whole as visualized in the integrity and operation of the network. The saying "a brokenness in any part of a network is a brokenness in the entire network" is the best definition of this principle of synthesis. All networks and organizations represent the sum of the integration and synthesis of the efforts of each of their parts and their convergence, where individual contribution joins with the whole to create truly symphonic action (Anderson & Willson, 2008; Shultz et al., 2013).

This notion of the centrality of value out of the point of service or point of productivity is critical to understanding the distribution of decision making in a way that best exemplifies both the kinds of decisions that need to be made and the nature of the resulting actions that need to be taken. Seen from the perspective of the whole (the network), each point of action recognizes its unique function and contribution within the mental model of the whole (**Figure 4-4**). In this way, no compartments, departments, services, or local actions can ever be undertaken without a clear sense of the effect such action will have on the integrity of the network. This perspective sees decisions distributed in a way that represents the appropriate loci of control so that people at key "nodes" or locations in the system know what decisions belong to them and the effect those decisions have on the network. Part of the real work of leadership, therefore, is to clearly and appropriately delineate a "grid of accountability" that carefully enumerates the location of specified decisions in

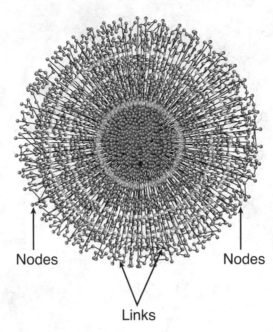

Nodes   Nodes

Links

Figure 4-4 Network of Intersecting Nodes and Links

a way that creates a mind map of the decisional loci of the network (Nelson, 2009). In this way, leadership creates a view of the mosaic of decision points across the network that represents the relational, interactional, and synthesis dynamics of the system; best shows the integrity of the system; and demonstrates the concert of actions converging to meet goals, advance purpose, and strive to succeed in the larger environment.

Wise executive leaders understand that human systems operate in this manner, and they recognize the importance of creating the structural configurations within the context of the dynamic vision of a network. The executive, rather than looking for control or to manage organizational ego (line hierarchy), seeks integrity, convergence, and synthesis of the entities of the network around mission, vision, purpose, and strategy—all of the components necessary for the system (network) to thrive in the larger, ever-changing environment. In such an organizational view, those in the executive suite effectively see themselves as purveyors of the goodness of fit between the ever-moving demands of the external environment and the operating and internal dynamics of the organization. The innovative element embedded in this scenario is demonstrated in the organization's ability to create new responses, processes, and products when innovators challenge the realities of the external environment and create conditions and configurations that can push the edges of new thinking and generate opportunities to redefine action and outcome by what they create from within (Erwin, 2009).

The effective and wise leader of innovation recognizes that the life of the system operates predominantly from its point of service. At the heart of the system is where the intensity of the life of the organization is best visualized. It is here that the executive recognizes that all prevailing structure and support converge either to advance or impede life lived at

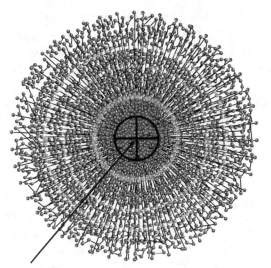

Core of the network: The point of service where all structure and effort converge to fulfill the purposes of the system.

Figure 4-5 Network Convergence at the Point of Service

the point of service and system effectiveness. This leader recognizes that purpose and organizational life are not sustained at the top or at the periphery of an organization. Certainly, the goodness of fit between the internal life and dynamics of the organization and its appropriate and sustainable interface with the external environment is managed, facilitated, and refined in the executive suite. However, if the system is to live and be sustained, the determining factor is demonstrated by how well strategy is transformed into action at the point of service and lived out by those who work there and how this action drives the tactics and actions that lead to organizational thriving (**Figure 4-5**).

Alignment, Not Motivation

The leader of innovation sees the critical value of good alignment between the various loci of control and decisions in the organization. This leader seeks to ensure that the greatest degree of empowerment is enabled close to the various points of service so that as much freedom, ownership, and investment in the life and work of the system can unfold in those places. This leader sees the organization as a membership community and has a high level of understanding of the rights of membership and the obligations of ownership. In this frame, the

> **Key Point**
>
> Alignment is the key element in the leader's role in motivation. Aligning staff motivation with organizational goals is the only sustainable way of ensuring staff investment and ownership. It is more work, but motivation lasts longer.

leader of innovation is constantly building partnerships, interfaces, relationships, and points of convergence in the network that, when aggregated, move the system effectively in a direction that ensures its long-term viability (Busch & Hostetter, 2009).

Alignment is a critical element of creating context for innovation (Fine, 2009). The alignment of motives is a much more powerful and viable strategy for engagement than is the constant leadership emphasis on motivation. Much has been written about motivation, very little of it factual. Often, when one reads and researches motivation, a heavy emotional overlay begins to appear. Usually, the suggestion is that if leaders can only help staff feel more excited, energized, and spirited, these workers would demonstrate more investment, engagement, and commitment. If leaders could only make workers feel better, they could make them produce more. Although it is important that workers feel good and be happy, much of what produces those feelings comes from them, not from leaders or the workplace. It is the height of hubris to suggest that the leader is so influential and demonstrates such exceptional persuasiveness that he or she can permanently excite and motivate others by force of personal charisma. These perspectives that underpin much of what is written on motivation remain essentially invalidated by any real, disciplined, or formal research. In fact, research demonstrates that motivation is internally generated (intrinsic), controlled by the individual, and reflected by personal perspectives, experiences, challenges, and opportunities. Motivation externally mandated is simply not possible; it must be generated from within, connected with a set of values and intentions derived from an individual's life and linked and connected to organizational life.

> ### Key Point
>
> Leaders cannot motivate anyone to do anything. Motivation is always internally generated. The role of a leader is to create congruence between external realities and internal motivation. To do this, the leader focuses on creating good alignment between personal motives and organizational goals.

Simply said, it is not possible to externally motivate anyone to do anything in the long term. In organizations enamored with the idealization of motivation, so many organizational resources, such as time and effort, are wasted on motivating individuals to undertake activities that these organizational members have no interest or investment in or ownership of. Each time an organization attempts to stimulate worker excitement over a new initiative that was originated with little investment or participation from the staff, workers demonstrate decreasing interest, involvement, and excitement. More often than not, many of these ideas intended to motivate staff originate in the minds of those who don't have to implement them, add them to their own workload, or even devote the necessary time and energy to them. Adding a new initiative is like grinding salt into the open wounds of failed past initiatives from which workers have not yet fully recovered. Clearly, it is no wonder that so many initiatives are either short lived or fall short: They fail to understand the real elements of engagement and use the mechanics of motivation inappropriately (**Exhibit 4-6**).

Alignment, on the other hand, is an entirely different leadership skill that yields infinitely more viable outcomes and value. Leadership alignment creates a context for

---

Exhibit 4-6   Elements of Motivation

- Internally generated
- Must be consistent with personal values
- Characterized by engagement

- Connects with personal ownership
- Gains are mutually advantageous

---

innovation by suggesting the necessary configuration of personal response to the demands of the external environment and the need for personal ownership of that response. In the process of alignment, the leader sees the demand for change through the perspective of ownership and engagement. The leader recognizes that any demand for change has a dramatic and immediate impact on all elements of the organizational network and requires the configuration of response that integrates and links every component of the network in a consonant and collaborative process that adequately addresses the challenges and growing demand of the change process.

For the leader, the much harder work of sustaining organizational effectiveness and integrity is looking from the perspective of goodness of fit between the demand for significant change and the responses necessary to address it effectively. In the management discipline of alignment, the leader constantly looks at issues of impact and effects of the change on the community and individuals. Here, the leader looks at the change from the perspective of the various constituents by asking such questions as the following: How does this change affect them, inform them, challenge their current circumstances and conditions, and call them to action in a way that has meaning for them? Furthermore, the leader is concerned with using the most appropriate language to present the issue and the need for response that reflects the values of those who must respond.

When alignment has been established, the leader becomes concerned with how the language of the issue driving change best fits the involved constituents. The leader then uses a frame of reference that the involved community or individuals can identify with and personalize. Within this frame of reference, the leader, having established alignment, can engage those who feel the impact in a way that challenges them to reflect, respond, and act (Colbert & Witt, 2009).

In creating alignment, the leader never divests ownership and partnership in change issues or events from any member of the community affected by the change. The assumption of alignment doesn't reflect divorce of ownership from stakeholders in the network (organization). This basic understanding of membership in the work community drives the leadership mental model and expression in a way that includes all members of the community sharing a stake in its life, direction, and decisions. Although decisions are differentiated by their characteristics—strategic, tactical, process, and personal—the leader recognizes that every member of the community has a stake in all decisions and, ultimately, plays some meaningful role in the exercise of any of them. In the process of alignment, the leader understands that participation in decisions is differentiated by role, not by position. Each player in the membership community (network) plays some role in relationship to every decision.

Through this application of alignment, differentiation in role and decision making requires a different set of competencies, not a different level of engagement and ownership. In creating a context for innovation, the leader in this set of circumstances recognizes community ownership of the work of the system and further acknowledges the need to clearly delineate the attributes, skills, content, processes, and actions of the various stakeholders based on the expression of their stakeholding represented by their locus of control. The leader understands it is appropriate for the board to make decisions about strategy; it is necessary for executives to make decisions about priority; it is essential for managers to make decisions about tactics and budget; it is required for staff to make decisions about process and action. Each has his or her role, yet, in a network, the role of each is cross-referenced and intersects with others' roles. Each informs the role of others and is represented in others' decision making so that the decisions are fully informed in regard to their impact on the system, including the effective challenges and opportunities related to successful implementation. This is especially true in organizations predominated by professional workers (knowledge workers), where every decision at any place in the system has an impact on the integration and activity of each discipline. This understanding of alignment of stakeholders drives many of the principles and structures of shared governance that have been detailed and articulated in other works (Porter-O'Grady, 2007, 2009b). Although creating structures and processes that represent the principle of alignment requires organizational competence and management talent, it yields relevant and sustainable results.

To create a context for an energizing and innovative workplace, leaders need to articulate the foundational principles that guide the constructs necessary to point-of-service ownership and investment in the innovation process. Not considering the principles associated with good alignment considerably challenges the leader's ability to create a context for innovation and to sustain the innovation dynamic as a way of doing business in any setting. The following are the key foundational principles related to creating this framework:

1. It is virtually impossible to undertake the activities of innovation in a "closed" environment with rigid hierarchy, tight control, compartmentalized structure, and narrowly vertical organizational structures.
2. Creativity and innovation are stimulated and encouraged in environments where network configurations predominate, reflecting strong horizontal alignment, relational configurations, decisional synthesis, and a highly collaborative organizational construct.
3. In work environments predominately composed of professionals (knowledge workers), shared governance structures that ensure that stakeholders are represented and engaged in decision making provide the strongest opportunity for involvement, creativity, and innovation.
4. Effective innovation occurs closest to its point of impact. The context for innovation reflects this understanding and makes it possible for the structural elements that support innovation to operate effectively in the places where innovations are created.
5. Innovation is a dynamic with clear components and processes. Leaders must understand the elements necessary to advance innovation and competently create conditions that make the innovation dynamic possible in their settings.
6. Motivation occurs where good alignment is established. Leaders, therefore, must focus on creating an understanding of alignment between required change

and appropriate response to it. Ownership of the response to change is directly related to the perceived value of that change and the effect it has on the life of the community and its individual members.

7. Successful alignment occurs when individuals, struck by change, can demonstrate their ownership of change with language and action that reflect the personal impact of the change and their engagement.

8. Innovation is also a discipline. It is important that innovation be appropriately supported with sufficient resources, time, technique, and focus in a way that ensures that the activities of innovation have a place in the work of the organization. Innovation is not just a process; it produces a product, change, outcome.

9. Sustainable innovation demands good leadership. Every leadership role in the organization should have as a part of its performance expectations the facilitation, coordination, and integration of innovation processes at every point of decision making in the system.

10. Innovation is driven from every place in the organization. The organization's contextual framework for innovation must be reflected in the decisions made and processes implemented, from the board room to the patient. Every stakeholder in the organization must see him- or herself as a part of the dynamic of innovation that defines the organization.

These foundational principles provide the content and contextual frame necessary for innovation to become a way of life in the organization. Each comprises a portion of the elements necessary to attain and sustain an innovation framework that leads to a

Group Discussion

If motivation primarily comes from within and is generated by individuals, leaders must use different strategies for engaging staff. The leader's charisma and personality are not sufficient to create the context for consistent and constant staff engagement. Aligning staff's personal motivation with organizational goals is critical to generating investment and ownership by the staff. It is important for the leader to take time to delineate the drivers of staff self-motivation to help staff align their personal drives, insights, and goals with the goals of the organization. As a group, discuss how some of that can occur as you respond to the following questions:

1. What techniques might the leader use to get a sense of individual staff members' personal work motivation?
2. How might the leader determine what themes or consistency exists between individual motivators and the capacity to align staff motivation as a group?
3. What information must the leader delineate or make available to staff about the organization and organizational decisions as a first step in engaging with them in both responding to the organization and advancing personal and organizational agendas?

continuum of successful responses to the demand for innovation. What is important for leaders to keep in mind is that innovation is merely the response to the constant demand for adjustment and reconfiguration of the relationship between the eternally changing external environment and the organizational and human response to this demand for change.

Creating Stakeholder Value

As health reform leads us into a deeper understanding of the demand for value, the leader must now be aware of the need to emphasize value-driven processes at every level of the system. The traditional, all-encompassing volume-based approaches to care and service delivery in the health sector have created a mental model at every level of delivery that is difficult to dismantle. The notion of value is a critical element in the consideration of innovation. Stakeholder value is of special concern. Organizations are made up of structures, processes, and persons in a networked mosaic of interdynamics that operate in a way that sustains the action of each element and the synthesis of the whole (Basole & Rouse, 2008). This reality provides the frame for understanding the operation of value in the organization. A fundamental underpinning of the notion of value is the reality that each element of the enterprise must be a part of both the experience and the expression of value. People especially look for meaning in what they do as a reflection of their place in the world. This need for value operates in every individual and therefore is present at every place in the organization.

The central tenet of value recognizes that every human being is involved in personal activity that seeks to validate and even extend his or her value in the world. In the search for personal meaning, individuals seek a means of expression of who they are or what they do. This, of course, is no less important in the workplace. The historical and industrialized notion that workers are subsets of the work and therefore either do not reflect or give up their personal identification of value when they walk through the workplace doors is simply unsupportable. The basic need for meaning and its expression and value exist in the hearts and minds of people regardless of where they may be located and is simply not surrendered when they enter the organization. Furthermore, the idea that individuals surrender personal identity, desires, and goals and subordinate them to the externally determined values, strategies, and actions of the organization as defined by selective others is also invalid. It is simply not possible to give up personal identity, meaning, and value and mindlessly subordinate them to those constructed by others. Yet, in the vast majority of work organizations in the United States, this has been precisely the expectation and framework on which workplaces have been traditionally organized (Gkorezis & Petridou, 2008; Hertzberg, 1991; Lynch & Verner, 2013). The idea that organizations are membership communities made up of a diversity of individuals, each with a unique set of values, has simply been a foreign notion in the traditional construct of organizations.

The wise leader understands that the individual needs to find meaning and express value, even in the workplace. This leader knows that relationship at work is a constant and dynamic negotiation between individual values and choices and the strategic imperatives of the organization. In this regard, good leadership is simply a successful effort to

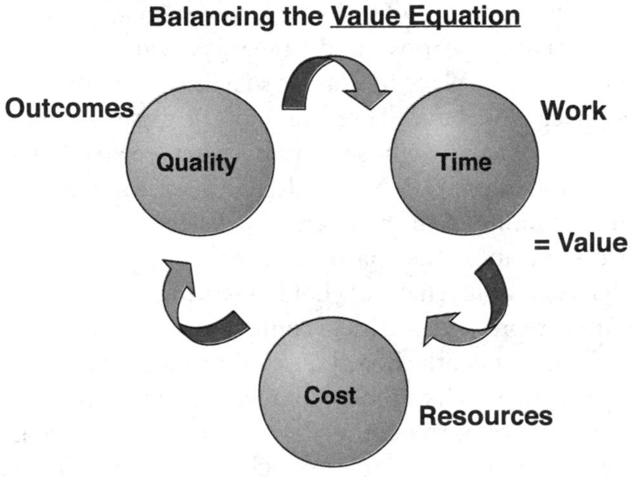

Balancing the Value Equation

Figure 4-6 Creating Sustainable Value

converge these forces into a synthesis that represents organizational mission and strategy and individual value and purpose. This "dance" between the individual and the organization reflects the essential skill sets of alignment that are critical to the success and sustenance of an entrepreneurial and innovative organization. In short, the leader works to create equilibrium, a "value equation" that represents the effort to coherently link and integrate the personal and organizational variables in a way that sustains both organization and individual (**Figure 4-6**).

The Contextual Role of the Board

Each role in the organizational network is a unique set of characteristics and functions that must be performed effectively to create a sustainable context for innovation. As previously stated, every level of the organization is required to demonstrate its obligation of creating a context sufficient to support and sustain innovation throughout the organization. The role of the organization's board is unique in this regard because it must not only be responsive to the external demand for creativity and innovation but must also make that demand operate as a key component of organizational life (Colley, 2005; Haffeld, 2012).

The board is obligated to create the strategic fit between the external demand for change and the internal organizational response (Kuratko, Goldsby, & Hornsby, 2012; Nadler, Behan, & Nadler, 2006). Here, leadership makes decisions about the unique characteristics of the

> **Key Point**
>
> The innovative board recognizes its central role in linking the system or organization to the external environment, which influences its ability to thrive and sustain. The board constantly works to translate circumstance into action through its capacity to predict environmental changes, directly confronting challenges with a carefully constructed and relevant response.

organization, its mission, purpose, and strategic response to its place in the broader social context. This focus on mission, purpose, and strategy provides the peripheral frame of the organization in regard to its place in a larger social and economic context. Through the strategic process, decisions about the response of the organization to collaboration and compatibility with external demands versus decisions related to stretching the mission and parameters of the organization to push into unexplored territory fall under the capacity for innovation coming from the board.

In the innovative organization, the board ensures that its members have access to and are aligned with external and internal stakeholders. At the board level, alignment with appropriate stakeholders represents a critical contextual accountability within an innovation framework. In this dynamic, the board seeks to include members and stakeholders from the larger community as well as those from within the membership community. Effective, innovative boards create a fluid relationship between board membership and other stakeholders within the organization. An effective, innovative board seeks to create a dynamic connection between the point-of-service stakeholders and those operating at the governance level. Innovative boards recognize the need to be informed from a variety of real perspectives: those that reflect environmental concerns and the internal responses to them related to social, economic, budgetary, and process realities. In addition, the board recognizes the need for interaction and communication with those from the points of service who share the board's perspectives with an eye to translation, design, processes, and application realities that can only be articulated from their perspective.

Those composing the board must be able to evaluate environmental indicators and benchmarks that inform them of particular and significant changes in the environment. This environmental awareness of significant contextual changes creates a requisite for the board to respond in a timely fashion in a way that best informs strategic decisions and guides organizational direction. The innovative capacity embedded in this role is exemplified by the board's ability to predict changing environmental conditions and their impact on the organization far enough in advance so that the organization can competently and comprehensively respond.

The effective, innovative board overcomes the historical isolation of board members and the practice of decision making referencing only the most senior levels of the organization. The historical justification for this has been to maintain the board focus on governance, not operations, as though exposure to other members of the organization would somehow taint their ability to uphold this obligation and diminish its "purity." Of course, nothing could be further from the truth. Exposure to essential stakeholders who share information that cannot be as effectively communicated through other means does not diminish the obligation of the board to act in the strategic best interests of the organization. In fact, it emphasizes that obligation while making it imperative to design mechanisms that communicate information to the board that it needs to hear in a language that represents the people and places in the organization where strategy formation becomes real, is translated, and either succeeds or fails. As Chris Argyris once indicated, many American organizations falter strategically simply because the "designers were rarely the implementers and the implementers were rarely the designers" (Argyris, 1999).

Group Discussion

There is always much discussion regarding nursing membership on organizational or systems boards of trustees. Much of this discussion reflects the historical perception and relationship of nurses to the healthcare organization, a frame of reference that challenges notions of nurses at the governance table. Yet nurses are more than 60% of patient care providers in healthcare organizations, representing the largest single stakeholder group offering healthcare services. Tradition allows that physicians are at the governance table, yet nurses are excluded. As a group, and in recognition of the significance of the profession of nursing in healthcare organizations, it is now time for you to make the argument for nursing representation on your healthcare system's board of trustees. Respond to the following questions to help construct your argument:

1. What unique value does the nurse representative bring to the board different from what is already present?
2. What area of expertise would you expect the nurse to contribute as a member of the board?
3. What skills and credentials would you suggest the nursing board member bring, and how would you make sure this nurse represents the larger community?

Innovative organizations are well recognized by the ease of access to information, individuals, and ideas. This fluidity is represented in a strongly horizontally oriented organizational construct that diminishes the impact of positional hierarchy and extends the exposure to broad-based role differentiation and accountability. In horizontal constructs, power is differentiated by roles, not by positions. Relational power and access to power in innovative organizations are more highly valued than positional or control power. Here again, in the innovative organization this effort to build and extend relationships and access represents the struggle to create stronger role accountability, impact and intersection, and ready access to people and processes that facilitate both creativity and work effectiveness.

Because the board creates the contextual framework for innovation, the board needs the opportunity to consider strategy and the organizational constructs necessary to support dynamic innovation. If the board is to make accurate and appropriate strategic and directional decisions, it should understand the management approach to building in organizational and resource supports for innovation in a way that exemplifies innovation as a mechanism that stimulates creativity in health service provision. There has to be some assurance at the board level that the approaches and processes used in the organization make it possible for those strategies to succeed. Connecting board strategic initiatives to point-of-service processes and actions helps more strongly ensure a positive outcome, one that advances the organization with congruence between board direction setting and point-of-service design and implementation.

At the governance level of the organization construct and context for innovation originate. Through defining expectations of relationship and access and setting the decision-making table to include relevant stakeholders prior to making strategic decisions, the board creates both the frame and the behavioral pattern for an innovation that can be replicated throughout the organization. The board simply sets the tone for both the expectations and the behavior of the organization it governs. As it demonstrates the creative and innovative in its own structure and processes, the board serves to evaluate its effectiveness and efficacy through the strategic lens.

The C-Suite and the Context for Innovation

Senior executives must lead the translation of strategic imperatives into tactical obligations. Officers and agents of the board link strategic decision making with tactical response and join strategy with the operating life of the organization. Senior executives are uniquely located between governance and function to ensure effective translation of strategy and incorporation of strategy into the life of the organization so that the organization can meet external demands for continuous change and relevance and implement an internal design that ultimately ensures alignment between strategy and action.

In the preparation of strategy, the senior team informs the board of the external and internal factors influencing priority setting and decision making, helping to guide decision makers with information and tools that represent the most accurate and relevant data available (Marshall, 2009). Once strategic decisions are made, the senior team is obligated to connect the links and nodes in the network in a way that effectively and successfully translates strategy into decisions and actions that move the organization toward a positive and successful response to strategic choices (**Exhibit 4-7**).

The senior team is the first link in the chain connecting organizational alignment to the strategic goals. Executive leaders focus specifically on the linkage and connections between key stakeholders and the nodes and networks in the system. These leaders seek to "set the table" and connect key stakeholders whose role is to engage particular strategic goals and translate them into operational decisions and actions (Goodman, 2009). In the innovative organization, executive leaders primarily provide access, linkage, forums, and format for connecting critical stakeholders in a way that invests ownership at the appropriate locus of control and engagement with the various decisions and actions necessary to successful design and implementation.

Unlike traditional allocations of executive skills, in the innovative organization, executives are primarily seen as points of linkage, intersection, and connection between the

---

Exhibit 4-7   Central Role of C-Suite Leaders

- Link and bridge between board and staff
- Informs the board and translates strategy to the system
- Provides good linkage between the "nodal" loci of control

- Creates a positive context for worker relationships
- Builds the infrastructure for decisions and action

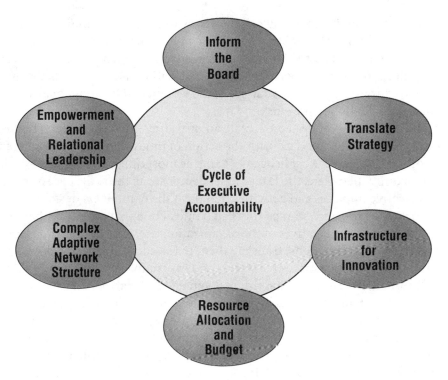

Figure 4-7 C-Suite Roles

various constituencies and nodes of the network. They ensure that the essential and appropriate stakeholder structures, resources, and processes are aligned so that the strategic effort is both in the right hands and has what it needs to succeed. The oversight role at the executive level is responsible for determining and evaluating whether the right focus, relationships, infrastructure, resources, and processes have aligned appropriately to ensure that the elements necessary for successfully translating strategy into action are in place and operating effectively. In the innovative organization, the executive continually asks the following question: Is the right decision being made by the right person in the right place at the right time, and is it fulfilling the right purpose? From a quantum systems perspective, the senior executive is interested in the effectiveness of the system of decision making and action, not the decisions and actions themselves (that is a first-line leader role). From the executive perspective, if there is alignment between the infrastructure and systems supporting effective translation of strategy into action, the outcomes of innovation should be evidenced in the successful products of innovation (**Figure 4-7**).

First-Line Leaders: The Pivot Point of Innovation

The most important and most highly skilled management leader lives at the intersection of the system and its point of service. Here, translation meets reality and the critical interface between design and action occurs. Here, the most dynamic evidence of lived innovation must be most visible, and here the skill sets necessary to ensure that innovation occurs are most apparent. From a quantum systems and innovation perspective, the first-line leader is often the unsung hero. The need for effective and successful management skills is most critically evidenced in this role. This role defines the location that represents the interface between the structural and process dynamics of the system and the functional and action dynamics of those who do its core work.

The first-line manager is obligated to create an operating milieu, a context, that most evidences the frame and its interface with the action of innovation. It is here where the dance of stability, risk, and the challenge of change is most difficult, yet it is here where the most opportunity lies. Here, the leader must demonstrate the skills necessary to facilitate the creative impulses and activities that push the parameters of stability, yet still ensure that those processes can be translated into action that makes a difference and gives life to the strategic imperatives of the organization. Here, the leader can ask the strategic and the tactical questions, translate them to the actionable, and help ensure that the translation works, demonstrates real value, and is sustainable.

The first-line manager needs to establish real and effective partnerships between the stakeholders; set the right table for deliberation and design; ensure the right configuration and mix of stakeholders at the table; and determine appropriate human dynamics and group processes are used to move innovation from table to workspace. Ultimately, these elements ensure that timely, appropriate, effective, and viable outcomes are achieved (Carey & Von Weichs, 2003; King, Conrad, & Ahmed, 2013). This leader is most fully connected to the points of service and, horizontally, to the nodes and networks in the system that reflect the points of reference and intersection necessary to creating the linkages and partnerships essential to successful design and action. The first-line manager must demonstrate the ability to manage uncertainty, diversity, and differing degrees of stakeholder diligence.

> ## Key Point
>
> The first-line leader is the key leadership role on which the organization or system most depends. In this role the strategic, tactical, and actionable converge. Here, the symphony of the organization and its members is constructed and conducted by the only leader who has both place and capacity to ensure its success.

Especially important to the first-line leader is the talent associated with selecting and setting the deliberative table where stakeholder partners will engage each other in the innovative process, using a discipline that guarantees results. Skill sets related to strategic translation, group construction, deliberative dynamics, the creative use of the tools of innovation, and the disciplines of decision making are all essential to the role of the first-line leader.

All too often in traditional healthcare organizations, this role has been understated and underresourced. Often the most skilled clinical provider, without the requisites to excel, has been appointed to this role. The results of this rather serendipitous and relaxed selection process have been disastrous to both the advancement of the role of leader and the competencies necessary for engagement and innovation. The truth is, this is perhaps the most important role in the organization and demands the greatest skill capacity and maturity. Selection here cannot be incidental or accidental. Preparation for this role should include the most critical elements of skill development and the greatest focus of succession planning. In an innovative organization, this role becomes critical to the vitality and the success of the innovation process.

In addition to basic skill, development of the following additional requisites of the role of the first-line leader in the innovative organization is mandatory:

- The first-line leader has an ability to identify the creative in others and to recognize the unique characteristics of the out-of-the-box thinkers, those who challenge current notions: the idea generators, the tinkerers, the first engagers, and the persons who seem to live in the question "why?"
- The first-line leader possesses leadership skills of curiosity and information gathering that are reflected in the ability and willingness to read broadly, listen carefully, perceive subtleties in the changing environment, recognize and take advantage of good timing, challenge and raise questions that generate new insights, and willingly engage others who do the same.
- The first-line leader is able to set aside real time for conversation and exploration that challenge ritual and routine, barriers, inadequate or unnecessary processes, and ideas that raise issues about being or doing differently.
- The first-line leader can create a safe space for debate and dialogue to engage differences in insight and align differing notions in a way that both translates and transforms them into positive and actionable items.
- The first-line leader is determined and focused on pursuing the innovation process through its various stages, helping stakeholders successfully move idea to action and process to outcome.
- The first-line leader recognizes the value of incremental failure in any innovation undertaking. Innovation is a nonlinear process, and the opportunity for ultimate success is moderated by the number of failures necessary to arriving at a viable outcome. Making space for failure and defending the processes that inevitably include failure are part of the leadership requisite to advocate for, defend, and articulate the value of innovation and the vagaries it incorporates.

An important part of creating a context for innovation at the point of service is the character and behavior of the first-line leader. Leaders, by virtue of their role, create the context for worker experience. The leader can either make it exciting, interesting, and challenging work or simply represent and reflect operational focus and the status quo. In a time of great change such as currently occurring in health care, the status quo—although all too common—is not sustainable. Each category of leader must do his or her part in creating context for innovation, from the places where strategies are formed to the places where they are transformed into action and outcome. In a networked organization, each player must do her or his part to fulfill the accountabilities of each role, creating the interfaces and synthesis in roles that are necessary to generate a living and sustainable context for the innovation dynamic (**Exhibit 4-8**).

Exhibit 4-8   Creating a Context for Innovation

Old Models of Work	New Models of Work
• Passive	• Ownership
• Obedient	• Participation
• Compliant	• Challenged
• Ritual	• Engaged
• Routine	• Experimental
• Policy	• Seeking evidence
• Process driven	• Inquiring
• Manager dominated	• Relating
• Job oriented	• Stretching

Creating a Context That Supports the Innovator

Innovation is essentially a point-of-service activity. Everyone has a role to play in the processes associated with successful innovation. Although the innovator is often perceived as a person who stands out by demonstrating a unique personality, role characteristics, and patterns of behavior, this is rarely correct. Invention is often mundane and serendipitous. Invention most frequently generates out of frustration, the unworkable, and barriers to successfully doing what one thinks is necessary. The notion of the innovator and inventor as a dreamer or mad scientist working alone in some dark and chaotic space creating something out of nothing is more myth than reality.

Innovation is ultimately a collaborative effort. The vast majority of innovations are the products of the collective wisdom and effort of many stakeholders gathered together around the commitment to produce something new or different (Estrin, 2009). It takes a community of diverse and committed individuals to create a truly viable innovation. This reality is what most drives the demand for effective leadership and coordination of stakeholders in both the creation of a context that makes it safe for innovation and the generation of a process that actually produces innovations. The leader's ability to obtain the best thinking and most committed processes within an innovation dynamic is the best indicator of the existence of an appropriate process supporting innovation in the workplace.

Innovators must have a sense that it is safe to innovate. *Safety*, in this case, means that the environment for work reflects an abiding respect for the individual and an opportunity for individuals to hear and fully engage in the decisions and actions of the unit or service. In creating a context for innovation, the importance of engagement cannot be understated. The leader's ability to shape an environment of ownership and investment in the decisions and actions of the workplace lays the critical foundation upon which safety and openness depend.

This is especially true in working with professional and knowledge workers. These individuals already have a sense of ownership with regard to their knowledge and the work they do. If the workplace environment and the leader behaviors understate or undervalue that sense of ownership, the knowledge, energy, and commitment necessary to translate that into deliverables are simply missing. If they are missing long enough, both

Group Discussion

Building a community of innovation requires significant talent on the part of the leader. Creating a context that makes innovation possible involves a great deal of work in transforming the system in a way that values innovation. Every member of the work community brings something to the innovative process. Leadership is required to determine the particular and unique characteristics of individuals, discern the contribution these characteristics can make to the innovation process, and build a community of innovators that balances the skills and talents in a way that makes the innovation process work.

As a group, think of a specific innovation that would improve the life of practice in your department, service, or unit. After having identified a specific innovation, reflect together on the staff that makes up the service; list their unique attributes and characteristics with a mind to what role they would play in innovation. Place this information on a flip chart using a mind mapping or concept mapping approach. Think about how each might contribute, the role he or she might play, and the manner in which you might organize the innovation initiative to best make use of member skills and to serve and advance the innovation idea. Once the design is concluded, test it out and see where it takes you.

the creativity and inventiveness associated with them go missing as well. And once lost, it takes a great deal of effort to reengage ownership and to generate the potential value embedded in it. This is one of the classic challenges of contemporary clinical organizations. Many clinical professionals do not have a sense of partnership, engagement, and ownership sufficient to respond with enthusiasm, interest, and creativity to the huge number of initiatives generated by organizations without their consent, involvement in design, and commitment to the additional activities necessary to obtain the outcome.

It is incumbent upon the leader to create a context for creativity and innovation that reflects more horizontal and adult-to-adult relationships among all members of the service and unit. The challenge for the effective leader is to confront existing boundaries of roles that reflect a more parent–child, superior–subordinate, manager–staff, boss–employee set of relationship parameters that result in prescribed perceptions and role interactions. Breaking past these highly vertical patterns of behavior is essential to effective leadership of professionals.

> **Key Point**
>
> The leader of innovation must see staff as partners. This is especially true in the professional organization where knowledge work is the center of the profession's activities. Here, the leader engages the staff as peers, as owners of their practice. Out of this sense of ownership and the obligations associated with it the professional demonstrates commitment to advancing care and the innovations necessary to make the processes associated with it better, more effective, and more sustainable.

If the leader can effectively translate his or her role of manager to partner with staff colleagues and clarify expectations of the role in a way that reflects specific accountabilities embedded in that role, a more normative relationship can be generated in a way that supports the requisites of innovation. Here, the leader generates a clear understanding of the accountabilities of the role in delineating the frame for those accountabilities in the requisites associated with the management of human, physical, material, support, and system resources. These management definitions and the roles and decisions associated with them need to be as clear to staff partners as they are to the manager. Some of the greatest impediments to developing the partnership role between management and staff are the ambiguity around issues of locus of control and the possibility that legitimate locus-of-control is malleable, personality dependent, and can change at a moment's notice, totally based on the feeling and temperament of the manager at any given time. Clarity around manager role expectations and patterns of behavior creates a level of consistency and trust in the role so that stakeholders have an accurate perception of expectations and actions upon which they can both depend and build real partnership.

Innovation and the Membership Community

Innovation is essentially a collateral process that engages a number of interested stake-holders. Once the foundations of manager consistency and role expectation are well established and clearly performed, the expectations of staff member roles in an innovative organization can be explored and clarified. Sustainable organizational innovation depends on the ability of leaders in the system to create a heightened awareness of the system as a membership community made up of the individual relationships and networks of relationships necessary to advance the purposes of the organization (Day, 2008; Dickinson & Mannion, 2012). It needs to be understood and embedded in organizational culture such that when a new member comes on board with the organization, the obligations and expectations of membership form the foundation of role value, performance, and behavior.

Just as there can be no ambiguity about the parameters of the manager/leader role, ambiguity about the membership in the organization must also be eliminated. This is especially true in professional and knowledge worker–driven organizations. Managing professional and knowledge workers requires a significantly different leadership frame of reference and capacity (**Exhibit 4-9**). These expectations must be clearly prescribed and described upon an individual's entry into the organization in a way that signifies an adult contract between the individual and the organization. Associated with the idea of membership are two elements: rights and obligations. Both must be enumerated clearly. The rights of membership are the personal benefits and recognition that comes with engaging other members in the system in a way that advances the net advantage of each and of all. Obligations are the individual's requisites for contributing to the mission and purposes of the community, the work expectations necessary to obtain outcomes and sustain the community, and the performance and behavioral expectations that reflect the actions of membership and the functions that contribute to it.

The assumption that underpins the context for innovation is that each member of the organization plays a role in the innovative dynamic embedded in the culture of the

Exhibit 4-9   Creating a Professional Practice Community

Employee Workgroup	Professional Community
• Vertical relations	• Horizontal relations
• Manager driven	• Expectation driven
• Function focused	• Partnered
• Process oriented	• Engaged
• Time bound	• Invested in impact
• Work is central	• Making a difference
• Getting work done	• Community member
• Check-off tasks	• Focus on value
• Job oriented	• Role oriented

system (Heskett, 2012; Kalisch, 2008). This allays the idea that innovation is a special talent or unique capacity of a very few individuals with distinct personal characteristics. In an organizational culture of innovation, the expectation is that all members of the network are full participants in the organization's processes of innovation and that each member contributes to sustaining the dynamic of innovation embedded in the character of the organization (Porter-O'Grady, 2013). As a result, the following fundamental role expectations are embedded in each member's participation in the innovative life of the organization:

- Membership in the work community is not simply a job. From the outset, membership implies commitment and alignment of personal goals and actions with those of the organization and an agreement to fully participate in advancing them.
- Each individual recognizes the unique skills and talents he or she contributes to the community and can articulate precisely what these are along with a commitment to fully access and use them in the best interest of the community.
- Mechanisms in the organization clearly articulate processes that assess, value, and evaluate the goodness of fit between the personal characteristics of the individual and the collective values of the community. Creating goodness of fit is the critical first-stage emphasis of developing a value-based relationship between the individual member and the membership community in which members seek to participate.
- Policy and documentation of the system clearly state membership rights and obligations as well as expectations for participation and engagement in the creative and inventive processes of the innovative organization. These foundations present a clear position for the new member regarding the organization's expectations that members will be creative and fully participate in activities that advance the viability of the system in a constantly changing external environment.
- A full and clear explanation and demonstration of the processes and activities associated with the innovation role of the individual in the system are detailed at the outset of the relationship and incorporated into the fundamental orientation experience of new members.
- Mentorship of new members includes activities associated with the innovation dynamic and the member's participation in it, along with an evaluation and a plan for developing and refining individual members skills and competencies associated with fully participating in the activities of innovation.

Creating a culture of innovation is purposeful work. Both the infrastructure and the processes of the organization must reflect the characteristics of innovation, and these must be fully embedded in the expectations, operations, and functions of every place in the organizational network. Skill development and innovation attributes are neither obtained by nature nor accident. This deliberate work must be reflected in every level of the network in a way that can be seen from governance to service, from policy to practice, from decision to action, and from person to product. Creating a context for innovation means creating the culture within which innovation is a normative behavioral expectation, not the exceptional gift of the relative few (Hickey & Kritec, 2012; Viney & Rivers, 2007).

Balancing Innovation with Value

Creating a culture for innovation requires more than simply creating an environment where innovative processes can freely unfold. It is equally important to ensure that the focus on innovation connectivity actually advance the interests of the organization. The organizational network, the actions and coalitions converging around the purposes and goals of the organization, must reflect a consistency of focus and energy directed to truly meeting the interests of the organizational community as a whole. From the strategic imperatives established through the governance process for the focused activities of delivering outcomes directed by those at the point of service, each component of the organization must demonstrate the convergence of plans and actions around those priorities that represent significant value for the organization.

Value now has larger implications for healthcare leaders. In health reform, value is a national strategic goal for the delivery of health services. Focus is on the value of creating truly healthy outcomes where the health of the nation is advanced and the cost of ensuring that health is controlled. The move from volume-based to value-driven health care now calls for a major shift in the mental model of care delivery and in the structure of organizations and leadership in ensuring that the health of the nation is advanced. Real value must now be clearly enumerated, defined, delivered, and measured in ways that represent effectiveness, efficiency, efficacy, and good use of available resources. Value implies stewardship of both services and resources in a convergence that ultimately positively affects service, outcome, and national health.

While leaders are creating the infrastructure and conditions that make the creative processes an operational characteristic of the work of the organization, they must discipline this creativity with the value creation process, which is just as essential to the dynamic integrity and sustenance of the organization and to those it serves. Developing in the system and individuals the creative processes associated with idea generation, valuing experimentation, developing good predictive capacity and intuition, building processes that move people and systems out of the box, implementing innovative group dynamic processes, and translating idea into action are the critical factors of innovation as a way of life at each and every node and network interface in the organization. Each factor must be valued, developed, and refined as the foundational skill sets of the innovative organization that are truly reflected in the operation of the organization. And value demands that they make a difference.

At the same time, these creative and innovative elements need the discipline of direction. All innovative processes and organizational systems should respond to the organization's relationship with its external communities and the strategic demand of the organization to excel and to thrive (Salge & Vera, 2009). This means that leadership and staff must be as cognizant of and as fully engaged in the value creation processes that bring form and substance to innovation and the creative frame within which the creative endeavors unfold. Although this is a delicate dance, viability requires insightful balance and continual review of the components of value creation: mission, vision, value, trade-offs, priorities, resources, risks, markets, margins, and outcomes. Leaders, therefore, have the obligation to continually and carefully balance the vagaries of the innovation process against the discipline of organizational direction and goals.

> ### Key Point
>
> Innovation is not merely a process. It is a dynamic. Innovation gives new meaning and direction and challenges the historic, the expected, and the routine. It calls innovators to adopt an attitude that reflects that all work processes and activities are subject to the discipline of constant inquiry and reassessment.

The innovation dynamic should be as much a part of ensuring the integrity and sustainability of the system as it is part of responding to the ever-challenging and changing demands of the external environment. No system can be all things at all times; this is why systems are disciplined by mission and purpose. Although mission and purpose may be altered over time as the organization is reviewed in the context of a changing environment, they do give the organization a sense of self and place, and they call members to more clearly see themselves in that place. Mission and purpose further call leaders to raise the questions of innovation in light of how it advances the integrity and sustainability of the system given its position and role in the greater social, political, and economic contexts. Leaders of innovation remain constantly aware of this strategic balancing act and deal with the ambiguities and vagaries inherent in innovation. This is reflected in the struggle between operations and innovation and the ever present potential of self-transformation in an ever-changing environment (**Figure 4-8**).

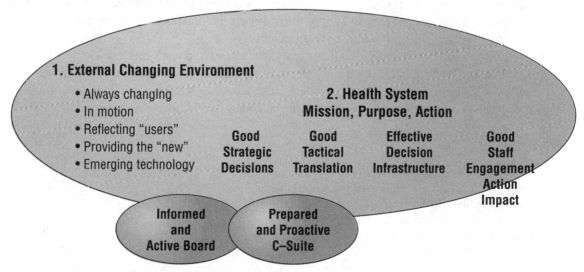

Figure 4-8 External "Fit" and Role of Mission

Differentiating Roles in Innovation

Different locations in the organization or system focus on different kinds of innovation. Clearly, leadership does not want administration to undertake activities associated with clinical innovation and neither does it expect clinical leaders to lead physical plant innovations. Although there must be a point in the organization where a range of innovations undertaken by the system is assessed and determined, specific innovations should reflect the content and character of the innovators who will lead them. At the same time, "setting the table" for specific innovations may necessarily include interdisciplinary and multifocal membership at the table to address the full range of elements associated with a particular innovation. Whatever the case, the infrastructure and construction of models and processes of innovation should be located and reflect the character of the obligation of those to whom the innovation is related. Providing leadership opportunities in innovation at the places in the organization and with the people located there is a centerpiece of structuring effective innovation.

A part of creating the structure and context for innovation is the development of an interdisciplinary forum whose primary obligation is to act as a clearinghouse for establishing innovation priorities and the linkage of those priorities with the strategic imperatives and direction of the organization. The primary purpose of this group is to help discipline and direct the innovation process in the organization in ways that prevent the organization from dissipating its energy and resources and, instead, help focus resources and processes on those innovations that most likely address the strategic and directional priorities of the system (**Exhibit 4-10**). The infrastructure for this process should be as important and central as any decisional process in place in the organization. Here, the integration of strategic choices and innovation priorities takes place and the challenges of ambiguity, external driving forces, and internal service demands, as well as the interface of mission, operations, and practice, are deliberated and delineated. Also, this forum serves as a centerpiece for evaluating the various elements of innovation and innovation projects in the system to determine their continuing viability, progress, and efficacy in light of the changing circumstances and conditions that drive the need for innovation in the organization.

Important also is a clear delineation of role expectations and work processes with regard to innovation. Although it is the role of governance to establish a firm strategy, that process cannot be successful if it is not appropriately informed. Clearly, the work of being fully and appropriately informed cannot be thoroughly and adequately undertaken unilaterally by the

---

Exhibit 4-10   Forum for Innovation Priority Management

- Tie innovation initiatives to strategic priorities
- Represent organizational arenas and stakeholders
- Create format, structure, process, and evaluation
- Integrate innovation activities to advance system's viability
- Assess process, competence, progress, and impact
- Champion innovation structure, learning, and action
- Communicate all innovation progress to system

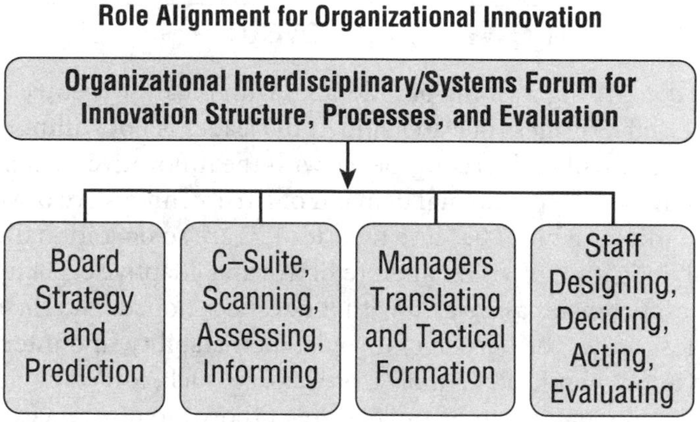

Role Alignment for Organizational Innovation

Figure 4-9 Role Alignment for Organizational Innovation

board. The officers of the corporation, those that occupy the C-suite, have a significant role to play in ensuring that the board is appropriately informed regarding the conditions and circumstances that influence decision making around strategy. With regard to the innovation process in the organization, the interdisciplinary forum whose obligation is to coordinate, integrate, and facilitate the various innovation tactics and processes in the organization informs senior leadership and the board. They do this by providing them accurate and up-to-date information about the place, progress, and impact of current innovations. Furthermore, they share information they have garnered about issues of organizational fit with the external environment, potential challenges to organizational integrity, and predictive-adaptive indicators of a shift in the external environment. Finally, they articulate the resource implications and demands affecting innovative choices and the potential for future innovations.

Consistent with these contextual accountabilities are the activities associated with the various innovation projects enumerated in the organization. Incorporated into the innovation process and the activities located in these places are mechanisms that define methodology, decision making, work process, design progress, and the activities associated with successful implementation. Equally important are the evaluations that determine whether particular innovations and the processes associated with them are making progress or are stalled or even blocked. Activities and progress with regard to these local innovation processes need to be reported back to the network innovation forum for review and decision making. The forum needs to indicate their continuing support or a need for altering processes, direction, or goals for the innovation (**Figure 4-9**).

Creating a culture of innovation is both easier and wiser than simply attempting to change culture as a way of responding to external demands. If the infrastructure and the culture of the organization are grounded in innovation and innovation is a part of the operation and functional mechanics of the system, adaptation to change becomes incorporated into the DNA of the system. Whereas the processes, mechanics, and techniques of innovation can be found in other resources, it is important here to emphasize innovation as a way of doing business. If innovation is seen as a role obligation of each member of the network community, it is easier to actualize the processes associated with innovation and to build them into the organization's work processes (Perel, 2005; Webb, 2011).

Leadership and the Will to Innovate

If we've learned anything over the past decades with regard to people at work, it is the centrality of the effectiveness of leadership. If the leader is not willing, neither is the staff. This notion of will and its congruence with the innovative dynamic is critical to the understanding of the contextual demand of a truly innovative organization. Many organizations "miss the boat" because their leaders are so operationally and functionally fixed. The real obligation of vision and predictive and adaptive capacity is often simply ignored, the competencies associated with it never developed, and the readiness of the organization lost under the burden of myopia, inert stability, and internal fixation.

Innovation is a dynamic, not simply a process. As such, innovation demands leaders and organizational members to be fully aware of those circumstances and conditions that call each to discern the reality of their work, the challenges associated with doing it, and the changes necessary to sustain it. Interestingly, though, individuals bring to organizations a whole range of cognitive, behavioral, and perceptive skills that, when appropriately and successfully converged, create the very synergy necessary to respond appropriately to shifting demands that affect person and organization. The issues related to this understanding frequently have to do with the capacity of the leader to engage human diversity, the organization's continuing challenge to respond to an ever-shifting environment, and the competencies necessary to implement processes that effectively address and appropriately respond to the convergence of these forces in a way that ensures individual and community thriving.

Human systems have a natural tendency to stability and rigidity. Human organizations tend to work diligently to control the ambiguities and vagaries of the internal environment as a way of advancing normative and stable work processes, relationships, and organizational routines. Through such mechanisms, people and organizations determine that they can better handle the stressors of permanent "white water" by eliminating all risk associated with it. The problem with this perspective is that the chaos, complexity, and uncertainty of organizational life in the larger context of reality are normatively uncertain. Attempting to eliminate the uncertainty and to create stability as the prevailing mechanism for organizational integrity and viability is both inadequate and inappropriate as a strategic, organizational, or operational activity (Walumbwa, Lawler, Aviolo, Wang, & Kan, 2005; Weberg, 2012).

Truly innovative organizations fully understand the inability to create any sense of permanent contextual frame for their work and life. These organizations seek to harness

> ### Key Point
>
> Innovation is a skill set and a contemporary capacity for the leadership role. Innovation is no longer an option with regard to organizational vitality and the construction of the future. Innovation is now a way of life for organizations that seek to advance and to be sustained. The ability to both understand and express predictive and adaptive capacity has become a subset of leadership competence and can no longer be optional if the role and the organization to which it relates seek to be successful.

these dynamics and create the processes of response to them as the normative vehicle for organizational life. Chaos, complexity, and uncertainty need not be permanently accompanied by stress, reaction, and the feeling of being continuously overwhelmed. Once leaders recognize the constituents of the dynamic context of change, they begin to discern and to articulate the appropriate mechanisms that harness this energy and give insights into the behavioral modalities that best inform the life of the organization and its response to these prevailing circumstances. Once this is understood, the organization becomes imbued with the very life that it represents and incorporates in it the energy that reflects the congruence between its internal life and the external conditions and circumstances to which it must always respond if it seeks to continually thrive.

The leader seeks both to meet this challenge and to address it within structure and role. Leaders at all places in the organizational network seeking to create the innovative dynamic are a part of the construct of the network's operation and pattern of behavior. These leaders seek to align the innovation dynamics with the operational processes of the organization. Here, leaders construct the organizational framework, the operational

Group Discussion

You are leaders of innovation. As a leadership group, you are charged with developing a program of learning for all of the management leadership in your health system regarding value-driven health care. As a part of its vision and leadership expectation, the health system has committed to constructing a strategic imperative and an infrastructure for innovative value-based care delivery to help transform the organization into a truly health-based, population designed, and innovative enterprise.

Your group has been charged with helping to develop leaders with the innovative insights and capacity necessary to build a truly patient-centered, value-driven health service enterprise. You are putting together a 12-month education program that will ensure that each level of leadership understands its role and that each leader has the capacity to fully engage and express confidence in the exercise of his or her leadership role in the movement to value-based health care.

Respond to the following questions about how you might structure this innovative value-based care delivery system:

1. Based on this chapter, what are the various role expectations for value-based innovation of board members, C-suite members, managers, and professional staff?
2. What might the content of the program be if emphasis must reflect the construction of policy, principles, protocols, structures, and processes associated with making the organization a patient-centered value driven enterprise?
3. In your attempt to be innovative in the design of leadership development for value-based patient care, what innovative learning dynamics and processes might you incorporate into this learning program as a mechanism for more deeply embedding this new innovation into the patterns of leadership in the system?

modalities, and the decision and action processes in a way that reflects creativity and innovation as the normative response to the organization's place in the larger culture. In doing so, leaders heighten the awareness of the organization as a system and its individual members about the fundamental necessity to be fully engaged in the life of the organization and involved in the work process in ways that are inherently innovative and creative (Hildreth & Kimble, 2004; Leong & Anderson, 2012). In these organizations, leaders and members are constantly looking for the challenges to historical and current ways of being and doing, seeking to inform organizational action in a way that alerts them early enough in the dynamic to respond to these challenges appropriately. In this way, they avoid the critical reaction that comes from late awareness, inadequate response, and an existing infrastructure that narrows people's focus to function and action rather than to purpose, value, and outcome.

Conclusion

We are now in a value-driven age. The question of this age is no longer, "What are you doing?" The real question of the time is, "What difference are you making?" The answers to these questions are as different as the questions themselves. The innovative organization asks the questions related to whether the organization matters, has value and impact, and, indeed, makes a difference sustainably. A system's sustainability and continuing need to make a difference define the relationship and the synergy between the external environment that constantly grows, adapts, and changes and an internal environment that accepts the challenge of change, creates modalities that incorporate change into its way of life, and creates structure, process, and relationships that embrace its own becoming. In this way, both the person and the collective of the organization advance the life of the system, its purposes, and the integrity and synergy between the innovative work of the organization and the creation of its own future.

Case Study 4-1

Developing a Culture of Interprofessional Collaboration

As the CNO a large metropolitan hospital, Jesse has established a strong reputation as a "mover and shaker" in nursing leadership circles. He is greatly admired by his colleagues who are CNOs at other hospitals in the region. For the most part Jesse is proud of his many accomplishments and very satisfied in his current role at the hospital, but lately he has been feeling restless and is concerned that the entire organization could do a better job of creative thinking to address needed changes to ensure excellence in patient care, excellence in the work environment, and excellence in individual professionalism.

Jesse shares his concerns with his colleagues on the hospital executive team, and they all reassure him that he should simply be satisfied with the hospital's reputation as a premier place to work, receive care, and practice professionally. Despite his colleagues' opinions, Jesse feels that there is an opportunity to make the best even better. He feels that there are a number of age-old issues confronting nursing that never seem to be completely addressed or resolved. The notion of interprofessional practice and collaboration is one example. Jesse realizes that the nursing profession has talked about the importance of interprofessional practice for at least 4 decades, and most recently interprofessional practice was cited as critical for optimal patient outcomes in the Robert Wood Johnson Foundation's *Future of Nursing* report, the Institute of Healthcare Improvement's report, and the Agency for Healthcare Research and Quality's report.

Jesse realized that the healthcare literature is replete with articles citing the benefits of interprofessional collaboration and its importance in enhancing job satisfaction, organizational commitment, and professionalism and for minimizing job stress and interprofessional conflicts. In spite of all of the evidence and rhetoric about interprofessional collaboration, Jesse realized that the hospital had not achieved interprofessional collaboration or practice. Although the hospital had made great strides in improving the organizational culture by addressing behavioral standards and values that were to be the norm for every employee and every physician affiliated with the hospital, there were many instances when physicians practiced very independently from the nurses caring for their patients.

Both nurses and physicians were frustrated, feeling that they were not valued or respected by the other party for their knowledge and skills in caring for patients and families. Several particular situations triggered Jesse's concern about the subject, and he felt that there was an underlying tension that could be a platform upon which to initiate some creative dialogue and ideas for changing the culture to support and encourage interprofessional collaboration and practice. He realized, however, that it was impossible to motivate others to make a change in their relationships and interactions with others, but he considered his options for developing some internal motivation that would spur individuals to take the lead in championing such a change. Jesse wanted to ensure that there was alignment among the nurses and physicians with the hospital's behavioral standards and values, which were widely accepted by employees and physicians throughout the organization. It seemed, however, that some physicians and nurses felt that collaboration was not a part of the accepted values. Jesse wanted to change this perception so that interprofessional collaboration would be a valued behavior among all disciplines and specifically between nurses and physicians.

After much thought Jesse decided to form an interprofessional task force composed of nurses, physicians, and key individuals from other divisions such as radiology, dietary, surgery, and laboratory services. In choosing individuals to be a part of the task force, he invited individuals who were exemplar collaborators and some who were referred to as "problem" individuals. He also identified a group of individuals who could be champion leaders on each of the nursing units from the recommendations of the directors of the respective nursing services. The plan was to roll down the work of the task force to the point of service and to bubble up ideas from the point of service to the task force.

One of the directors suggested that all newly hired nurses and nurses in the Nurse Residency Program be rotated for a day or more in each of the ancillary departments, which would give the orienting nurses the opportunity to see the internal workings of each of the departments and how they interfaced with the respective nursing units.

All of the directors felt that this was a very worthwhile plan, although there were some front-end investment costs because the on-boarding of new nurses would take at least an extra week. They all believed that this action would create a better understanding of the intersections between the nursing departments and the ancillary support departments.

The first meeting of the interprofessional task force was very introductory in nature, and most of the participants were a bit skeptical about the efficacy of such an initiative. The "problem" physicians and nurses were the most skeptical, and their body language spoke loudly that they didn't value this new initiative nor did they value the notion of collaboration. Some of the more skeptical physicians were of the belief that the physicians were the authority for the patient plan of care and that nurses were simply to follow physician orders. A few nurses on the team were quite content simply to follow physician orders and had no need for any further interaction to discuss a patient's condition, needs, or plan of care. On the other hand, a few very progressive physicians and nurses were excited about an initiative to improve communication and collaboration among all team members for the benefit of the patients and families. Fortunately, Jesse noticed that these individuals were more vocal in the task force, and he hoped that they would create the context for an innovative strategy to improve point-of-service interprofessional collaboration and provide some peer pressure for the others to follow. Jesse realized that this entire initiative was a cultural change and that it would need time to be formulated, implemented, and solidified in the minds of individuals for collaboration to become a new value and behavior.

The interprofessional task force convened a number of meetings, and the group brought forth many ideas. Part of the process included presentations of studies in both the medical and nursing literature that demonstrated the importance of interprofessional collaboration in ensuring optimal patient outcomes. Most of the participants on the task force were very engaged in the process, inquired as to how certain actions might be initiated at the unit level, and asked how they might ensure that the nurses and physicians at the unit level could take ownership of the change. Jesse and the rest of the executive team reviewed the progress of the task force and attended many of meetings to assure the team that they were supportive of their work. The executive team also brought in an industrial organizational psychologist who was a noted specialist in organizational change to facilitate the team meetings and discussions. The group was quite energized with this external consultant, who brought a new perspective and fresh ideas to the table.

After several months of meetings, the task force was finally ready to roll out an innovative strategy to promote interprofessional collaboration at the unit level. Jesse and the rest of the executive team were amazed at the ownership that the team had taken and how enthusiastic they were to launch the initiative. One of the physician leaders offered to be the physician champion, and the group planned that she would present the initiative and plan at each of the specialty physician meetings and to the medical executive committee. Similarly, a clinical nurse offered to be the spokesperson for nursing because it was hoped that the initiative would quickly be embraced by nurses at the point of service if the initiative came from a clinical nurse rather than a line manager or director.

Because competency of the bedside nurse is one of the most important attributes of collaboration, emphasis on knowledge and skill development of all nurses was a component part of the initiative. As a part of the nursing competency skill list, communication, conflict management, crucial conversations, and the art of collaboration were added as learning modules that would be included in nursing orientation, on-boarding to the hospital, and annual competency checks. These same modules were added to the on-boarding orientation program for physicians as well, and the group planned that topics of interprofessional collaboration, teamwork, and conflict management would be added to medical staff education. The hospital elected to add collaboration to its list of values and behavioral standards, and statements related to collaboration were added to every employee's annual performance appraisal form.

Although a number of different initiatives were used to facilitate building the culture of collaboration, there was a belief that nurses and physicians interacting together at hospital-based celebrations, social gatherings, educational venues, and on the unit would build the trust level necessary in collaborative relationships. Clinical nurses and clinical nurse specialists were frequently invited as participants in the medical staff education programs to present the nursing perspective on topics. Physicians were also invited to be speakers at the quarterly leadership meetings and other nursing education venues.

Jesse suggested that the director of research conduct a formal study to evaluate nurse and physician perspectives on the level of collaborative behavior existing before and after the rollout of the task force initiatives. The director of research invited the chief of the medical staff to join her in preparing an institutional review board (IRB) proposal for such a study, and when the IRB gave approval, the current baseline level of collaborative behavior of both nurses and physicians was evaluated. The director of research and the chief of the medical staff presented these initial findings together at the medical staff meetings and to clinical nurses at the unit level. The year after some of the task force initiatives had been implemented at the unit level, the two research partners surveyed the nursing staff and physicians again to determine whether any changes in perception of the level of collaborative behavior between nurses and physicians could be measured. After analyzing the data, they were surprised to see that a small improvement in the level of collaboration had occurred. They decided to make the study a longitudinal study and agreed that they would survey the staff and physicians every year as part of the employee opinion survey and the physicians' satisfaction survey.

Approximately 5 years after the first interprofessional task force meeting, Jesse proudly sat in the audience as the director of research and the chief of the medical staff presented 5 years' worth of data demonstrating constant improvement in the perceptions of nurses and physicians about their collaborative behaviors. Over time, nurse–physician collaboration became the norm and was highly valued by both nurses and physicians. In the nurse and physician satisfaction surveys, the engagement of nurses and physicians rounding together to patient bedsides was cited as one of the most appreciated factors.

While reflecting on the past 5 years in progress toward this cultural change, Jesse realized that he had simply set the stage for the change to occur, chose individuals who were passionate about the topic (both positively and negatively), identified champions who would lead the change process, and was available to provide support as necessary.

Questions

1. How would you consider Jesse's vision for a cultural change to normalize interprofessional collaboration as an expected behavioral standard and personal value as an innovation?
2. How did Jesse and the rest of the executive team create the context for an innovative solution to this age-old problem in health care?
3. In what ways did Jesse and his directors create the context and expectation of new employees and new physicians for collaborative behaviors?
4. How did Jesse and the executive team create alignment with this organizational goal and the overarching behavioral standards in the value statements?
5. What were some of the initiatives that motivated the interprofessional task force to become engaged in the process and to become owners of the solution?
6. How would you have handled the dissenting physicians and nurses who did not recognize the importance of collaborative behavior and who held on to past values of hierarchy, authority, and submissive, task-based nursing?
7. Although all of the initiatives were not described in this case study, if you were Jesse, what might you have done or suggested to set the context for such an important cultural change?
8. Describe what you might do as an innovation leader to ensure point-of-service engagement and ownership in creating a culture of collaboration? How would you ensure the support of other executives who might not be familiar with nor value the benefits of collaborative relationships among healthcare team members?

Case Study 4-2

Creating a Culture of Innovation

Fred is the president of a large multihospital healthcare system that is nationally recognized as one of the most successful vertically integrated healthcare systems in the nation. The organization was recently designated as one of the first providers in a statewide accountable care contract because of its organizational structure, which supports community-wide point-of-service care, holds exemplar quality standards, and is a positive workplace for healthcare providers.

Even though he holds a lofty position in the organization, Fred often interacts with individuals at all levels of the organization. He makes a point of visiting each of the hospital campuses and talking with gardeners, nurses, dietary aides, physicians, and, of course, patients and their families. Fred is committed to excellence in patient care and strongly believes that an empowered and engaged workforce is the best way to achieve that goal. Even though the healthcare system is widely recognized for excellence, Fred is uncomfortable simply resting on the status quo. He realizes that the competitive forces in the region and in health care and sweeping changes in how health care is provided and reimbursed threatens the status quo.

He meets with his senior executive team and tells them, "We can't sit still and wait for the future to happen. We must invent the future and write the script for how we will interact with the forces that can either make or break us as a healthcare system. If we are truthful with ourselves, none of us really thrive in a constantly changing environment, and we often long for stability. Unfortunately, we don't live in a stable environment. We are seeing major changes in healthcare reimbursement, challenges with serving the community as it changes ethnically and economically, threats from a union environment that demands more than our organization can offer, and a constantly deteriorating physical plant that needs replacement or refurbishment. We are compelled to accelerate new and creative thinking to proactively address some of these challenges."

He goes on to tell the team that he is not comfortable with slow, incremental changes, and he challenges them to consider ways that the organization's leaders can incentivize innovation from the point of service all the way to the top of the organization. He informs them that he recently attended a national meeting of presidents of healthcare systems and that innovation was the most discussed and hotly debated topic at the meeting. It seemed as if all of the healthcare leaders were feeling the need to reinvent their organizations to position them for the new accountable care act and the consequences of other national issues, such as the potential for terrorist acts in their communities, natural disasters, growth of diverse immigrant populations, and the impact of an aging population that experiences many chronic and acute illnesses.

Fred recommends that a comprehensive strategy be developed to create a culture of innovation and instill excitement about developing new and more economical ways to meet patient needs while still supporting the enhancement of professionalism among caregivers. Fred states that this is not a new budget-cutting initiative to meet the financial bottom line, but rather a willingness to invest in new, innovative ideas that can revolutionize how care is provided in primary care settings, hospital settings, and the home environment after discharge. He wants the executive team to consider how the organization's leaders can partner with physician groups, community leaders, the organization's nursing leaders, and clinical directors to instill and incentivize a culture of innovation.

Later, Fred meets with all of the CNOs from the system's hospitals and informs them of his new vision for a culture of innovation. He states that he believes that nursing is a key stakeholder in creating innovations at the bedside and that he is willing to support key innovations in their testing phase and in implementing the changes.

The CNOs discuss Fred's vision and the need for innovative thinking. They are convinced that advancing the nurses' knowledge and expertise in evidence-based practice will be an important step in creating a culture of excellence and innovation. The CNOs ask the respective leaders in research and professional development to develop a plan to advance evidence-based practice at all of the hospitals. They also discussed the notion of having an annual nursing innovation conference that would recognize nurses who have developed innovations in care, education, or leadership and disseminate that knowledge to the entire healthcare system. They discussed a plan to financially reward the top innovation, which would be chosen by the executive team with clinical nurse representation and evaluated on financial, outcomes, and alignment with the health-care system's mission, vision, values, and behavioral standards. They agree to ask Fred for an innovation development budget that would finance an evidence-based practice institute and an annual innovation conference with financial prizes of $2,500 for the first-place winner, $1,500 for the second-place winner, and $1,000 for the third-place winner.

The evidence-based practice institute would use an established framework for the project development and a mentor–mentee format. The mentors would be the CNSs for research nurses initially, but it is anticipated that in the future mentors could be past graduates of the evidence-based practice institute. The mentees would be recommended by their unit managers and given 8 hours of pay per month to attend the evidence-based practice institute didactic classes and 4 hours of paid time to work on their evidence-based innovation projects. The institute would be conducted once a year with an annual evidence-based conference to recognize the new graduates and to disseminate the find-ings from their projects. The cost of the institute would also include expenses to have a nationally known nursing leader as a keynote speaker and to display poster presentations of the various projects, with podium presentations from those that meet the criteria and have the greatest impact on unit changes and patient outcomes.

The CNOs also lead the design and development of the annual innovation conference, but they decide to make this annual conference interdisciplinary and invite physicians and other discipline representatives to help plan the annual conference. Using the evidence-based practice institute as a model, they plan for a nationally recognized health-care leader to be a keynote speaker on the topic of innovation and then for the rest of the day to be filled with presentations from the healthcare system's employees and physicians who developed innovations to improve the workplace environment, patient outcomes, or workflow processes.

The CNOs are excited to present their proposals and prospective budgets to Fred and the senior executive team for consideration. They had one other proposal that they felt would advance the culture of innovation, and they realized that they would need Fred's help to initiate plan. The CNOs recommended that the healthcare system partner with major businesses in the region to expose leaders of all disciplines in the system to the re-search and development process and to engage business leaders in advancing innovations in health care. Several major healthcare vendors had corporate offices and production plans in the region, and they would be perfect partners to design, build, and finance in-novations in the physical plant, medical equipment, information technology systems, and workforce planning and resource procurement. Fred and the senior executive team are really interested in the three proposals and particularly like the notion of partnering with regional businesses to advance innovations in the healthcare setting. They also embrace the idea of advancing the knowledge and expertise of clinical nurses in evidence-based practice and the healthcare system's leaders in the R&D process in regional businesses. The annual innovation conference that was planned to be interdisciplinary is also well received, and the senior executive team commit themselves to support these initiatives and to allocate funding to ensure their success.

Questions

1. How do you think the three initiatives will facilitate the development of a culture of innovation in the healthcare system?
2. What types of incentives do you think would be necessary to encourage and facilitate innovation among clinical nurses or other clinical leaders in the healthcare setting?
3. How effective do you think the initiative to expose the system's leaders in the research and development of regional businesses will be in developing a culture of innovation?
4. What effect will advance nurses' knowledge and competence in evidence-based practice on innovations at the clinical level?
5. What purpose do the annual conferences for the evidence-based practice institute and the innovation conference serve in promoting a culture of innovation?

References

Alberto, P., & Colacino, P. (2008). Motivation strategies for knowledge workers: Evidences and challenges. *Journal of Technology Management & Innovation, 3*(3), 12–16.

Anderson, J., & Willson, P. (2008). Clinical decision support systems in nursing: Synthesis of the science for evidence-based practice. *Computers, Informatics, Nursing, 26*(3), 151–158.

Argyris, C. (1999). *On organizational learning.* New York, NY: Blackwell.

Ashley, J. A. (1976). *Hospitals, paternalism, and the role of the nurse.* New York, NY: Teachers College Press.

Baer, E. D. (2001). *Enduring issues in American nursing.* New York, NY: Springer.

Bahuth, M., Blum, K., & Simone, S. (Eds.). (2013). *Hospital-based practice: A guide for nurse practitioners and perspectives.* Chicago, IL: Springer.

Basole, R., & Rouse, W. (2008). Complexity of service value networks: Conceptualization and empirical investigation. *IBM Systems Journal, 47*(1), 53–70.

Busch, M., & Hostetter, C. (2009). Examining organizational learning for application and human service organizations. *Administration and Social Work, 33*(3), 297–318.

Carey, D. C., & Von Weichs, M.-C. (2003). *How to run a company: Lessons from top leaders of the CEO Academy* (1st ed.). New York, NY: Crown Business.

Cassey, M. (2007). Keeping up with existing and emerging technologies. *Nursing Economics, 25*(2), 121–125.

Colbert, A., & Witt, L. (2009). The role of goal-focused leadership in enabling the expression of consciousness. *Journal of Applied Psychology, 94*(3), 790–796.

Colley, J. L. (2005). *What is corporate governance?* New York, NY: McGraw-Hill.

Coyne, K., Clifford, P., & Dye, R. (2007). Breakthrough thinking from inside the box. *Harvard Business Review, 85*(12), 26–34.

Day, C. (2008). Engaging organizational support for the Magnet journey. *Nursing Management, 39*(12), 44–48.

Dickinson, H., & Mannion, R. (2012). *The reform of health care: Shaping, adapting and resisting policy developments.* New York, NY: Palgrave Macmillan.

Erwin, D. (2009). Changing organizational performance: Examining the change process. *Hospital Topics, 87*(3), 28–40.

Estrin, J. (2009). *Closing the innovation gap: Reigniting the spark of creativity in a global economy*. New York, NY: McGraw-Hill.

Fine, M. (2009). Women leaders discursive constructions of leadership. *Women's Studies in Communication*, *32*(2), 180–202.

Gkorezis, P., & Petridou, E. (2008). Employees psychological empowerment via intrinsic and extrinsic rewards. *Academy of Health Care Management Journal, 4*(1).

Goodman, J. (2009). Strategic customer service. *Business Book Review Library, 26*(26), 1–9.

Haffeld, J. (2012). Facilitative governance: Transforming global health through complexity theory. *Global Public Health, 7*(5), 452–464. doi:10.1080/17441692.2011.649486

Hall, B. (1993). Time to nurse: Musings of an aging nurse radical. *Nursing Outlook, 41*(6), 250–252.

Hertzberg, F. (1991). *Hertzberg on motivation*. New York, NY: Penton Media.

Heskett, J. L. (2012). *The culture cycle: How to shape the unseen force that transforms performance*. Upper Saddle River, NJ: FT Press.

Hickey, M., & Kritek, P. B. (2012). *Change leadership in nursing: How change occurs in a complex hospital system*. New York, NY: Springer.

Hildreth, P. M., & Kimble, C. (2004). *Knowledge networks: Innovation through communities of practice*. Hershey, PA: Idea Group.

Humphrey, W. (2008). *Managing for innovation: Leading technical people*. New York, NY: Prentice Hall.

Kalisch, B. (2008). Transforming of nursing organization: A case study. *Journal of Nursing Administration, 38*(2), 76–83.

King, A. E., Conrad, M., & Ahmed, R. A. (2013). Improving collaboration among medical, nursing and respiratory therapy students through interprofessional simulation. *Journal of Interprofessional Care, 27*(3), 269–271. doi:10.3109/13561820.2012.730076

Kuratko, D. F., Goldsby, M. G., & Hornsby, J. S. (2012). *Innovation acceleration: Transforming organizational thinking* (1st ed.). Boston, MA: Pearson.

Leong, J., & Anderson, C. (2012). Fostering innovation through cultural change. *Library Management, 33*(8/9), 490–497.

Lynch, M., & Verner, E. (2013). Building a clinical leadership community to drive improvement: A multi-case educational study to inform 21st century clinical commissioning, professional capability and patient care. *Education for Primary Care, 24*(1), 22–28.

Malloch, K. (2010). Creating the organizational context for innovation. In T. Porter-O'Grady & K. Malloch (Eds.), *Innovation leadership: Creating the landscape of healthcare*. Sudbury, MA: Jones and Bartlett.

Marshall, J. (2009). Jeff Immelt and the new GE way: Innovation, transformation and winning in the 21st century. *Financial Executive, 25*(5), 13.

Mazur, D. J. (2003). *The new medical conversation: Media, patients, doctors, and the ethics of scientific communication*. Lanham, MD: Rowman & Littlefield.

McCarthy, J. A. (2011). *Beyond genius, innovation and luck: The "rocket science" of building high-performance corporations* (1st ed.). Los Altos, CA: 4th Edition Publishing.

Moore, D. A. (2005). *Conflicts of interest: Challenges and solutions in business, law, medicine, and public policy*. New York, NY: Cambridge University Press.

Nadler, D., Behan, B., & Nadler, M. B. (2006). *Building better boards: A blueprint for effective governance* (1st ed.). San Francisco, CA: Jossey-Bass.

Nelson, M. (2009). A cloud, the crowd, and public policy. *Issues in Science & Technology, 25*(4), 71–76.

Nohra, N., Groysbery, B., & Lee, L. (2008). Employee motivation: A powerful new model. *Harvard Business Review, 86*(7–8), 78–84.

Perel, M. (2005). You can innovate in hard times. *Research Technology Management, 48*(4), 14–24.

Pink, D. (2009). *Drive.* New York, NY: Riverhead Books.

Porter-O'Grady, T. (1990). *The reorganization of nursing practice: Creating the corporate venture.* Rockville, MD: Aspen.

Porter-O'Grady, T. (2007). *Implementing shared governance.* Atlanta, GA: Tim Porter-O'Grady Associates.

Porter-O'Grady, T. (2009a). *Interdisciplinary shared governance.* Sudbury, MA: Jones and Bartlett.

Porter-O'Grady, T. (2009b). *Interdisciplinary shared governance* (2nd ed.). Sudbury, MA: Jones and Bartlett.

Porter-O'Grady, T. (2013). Building the practice community. In M. Bahuth, K. Blum, & S. Simone (Eds.), *Transitioning into hospital-based practice: A guide for nurse practitioners and administrators* (pp. 181–204). Chicago, IL: Springer.

Porter-O'Grady, T., & Malloch, K. (2010a). *Innovation leadership: Creating the landscape of health care.* Sudbury, MA: Jones and Bartlett.

Porter-O'Grady, T., & Malloch, K. (2010b). *Quantum leadership: A resource for healthcare innovation.* Sudbury, MA: Jones and Bartlett.

Rapport, M., McWilliam, R., & Smith, B. (2004). Practices across disciplines and early intervention: The research base. *Infants & Young Children, 17*(1), 32–44.

Rounds, K. E., McGrath, B. B., & Walsh, E. (2013). Perspectives on provider behaviors: A qualitative study of sexual and gender minorities regarding quality of care. *Contemporary Nurse.* doi:10.5172/conu.2013.2440

Salge, O., & Vera, A. (2009). Hospital innovativeness and organizational performance: Evidence from English public acute care. *Health Care Management Review, 34*(1), 54–67.

Schultz, S., Abercrombie, S., Crownover, B., Hoekzema, G., Krug, N., Maxwell, L., . . . Tuggy, M. (2013). Accountable care organizations: An opportunity for synergy. *Annals of Family Medicine, 11*(3), 283–284. doi:10.1370/afm.1530

Viney, M., & Rivers, N. (2007). Front-line managers lead and innovative improvement model. *Nursing Management, 38*(6), 10–14.

Walker, S. (2012). *Employee engagement and communication research measurement, strategy, and action.* Philadelphia, PA: Kogan Page.

Walumbwa, F., Lawler, J., Aviolo, B., Wang, P., & Kan, S. (2005). Transformational leadership and work-related attitudes: And the moderating effects of collective and self-efficacy across cultures. *Journal of Leadership & Organizational Studies, 11*(3), 2–16.

Webb, N. J. (2011). *The innovation playbook: A revolution in business excellence.* Hoboken, NJ: Wiley.

Weberg, D. (2012). Complexity leadership: A healthcare imperative. *Nursing Forum, 47*(4), 268–277. doi:10.1111/j.1744-6198.2012.00276.x

Yang, A., & Shan, Y. (2008). *Intelligent complex adaptive systems.* Chicago, IL: IGI.

Suggested Readings

Cristiansen, C., Johnson, C., & Horn, M. (2008). *Disrupting class: How disruptive innovation will change the way the world learns.* New York, NY: McGraw-Hill.

Metcalf, M. (2012). *Innovation leadership: Workbook for emerging managers and leaders.* Chicago, IL: Integral.

Ness, R. (2012). *Innovation generation.* New York, NY: Oxford University Press.

Skarzynski, P., & Gibson, R. (2008). *Innovation to the core.* Boston, MA: Harvard Business School Press.

Quiz Questions

Select the best answer for each of the following questions.

1. Which of the following best defines disruptive technologies?
    a. Normal changes that alter the way things work
    b. Radical changes that result from normal evolution
    c. Significant shifts that alter how we think, act, and behave
    d. The results of changing how an existing product or service looks and works

2. How have medical subsidiarity and subordinateness directly affected the nursing profession?
    a. By creating a lack of interdisciplinary collaboration, linkage, and interaction
    b. Through creating practice boundaries limiting nursing scope of practice
    c. By creating political and legislative limitations to clinical practice opportunities for nurses
    d. All of the above
    e. None of the above

3. How does focus on functionalism and process-oriented work affect innovation?
    a. By eliminating a broader focus on purpose and outcome, resulting in more responsiveness to innovation-based solutions
    b. By encouraging practical foundations for innovation
    c. By connecting innovation to real work issues
    d. By keeping people's imaginations focused on innovation as a part of their work

4. Equity is essential to innovation for which of the following reasons?
    a. Everyone does equal work in the organization.
    b. Equity reflects the value placed on an individual and his or her work.
    c. It is important to acknowledge that not everyone's work has equal value.
    d. Knowing what work contributes to innovation and what work does not is important.

5. Professions are different from employee in which one important way?
    a. They make more money.
    b. They are more important to the work of the organization.
    c. Professions are directed by their social mandate for the people they serve.
    d. Professionals are not obligated to the organizations with which they relate.

6. How can worker motivation best be described?
    a. Increasing monetary rewards to get better work performance
    b. Identifying the internal values that direct and satisfy individuals in their work
    c. Encouraging, directing, and reinforcing workers to be more productive
    d. Making workers feel better about their work so that they will do more of it

7. Why is innovation always driven from the point of service?
    a. That is where investment, engagement, and ownership of the outcomes of work are directly located.
    b. People do more work there, and that is where the money is made.
    c. People are more creative and innovative when they're in the front lines.
    d. It is always easier to get people to do new things close to the places where they do the work.

8. Why is partnership among the board, executives, and managers critical to innovation?

　　a. The staff are required to do what the board and managers determine.

　　b. Executives and managers must always do what the board directs.

　　c. Managers are solely accountable for making sure the organization works.

　　d. Each group has a specific role to play in the innovation process to make it successful.

9. Why is the most important leader in the innovation process the first-line manager?

　　a. He or she knows more about what is really going on in the organization.

　　b. This manager's proximity to the point of service exemplifies the strongest partnership with the staff closest to the place where innovation becomes action.

　　c. This manager does what he or she is told and translates that best to get the staff "on board."

　　d. This manager can make the most sense of the change and translate it in a way staff can best understand.

10. Which of the following characteristics demonstrates that an organization is innovative?

　　a. It is willing to always change and be ready for the next change.

　　b. It constantly creates new products and ways of doing work.

　　c. The collaboration and integration of all of its members demonstrate their commitment to their organization's vitality and sustenance in the presence of constant change.

　　d. The staff ensures that their organization can survive, constantly change, and produce new products and ways of working.

CHAPTER FIVE

Innovation Leadership

Man's mind stretched to a new idea never returns to its original dimensions.
—*Oliver Wendell Holmes*

Chapter Objectives

At the completion of this chapter, the reader will be able to

- Compare and contrast the work of innovation with the work of routine operations.
- Identify the rationale for innovation in healthcare organizations.
- Define key concepts and terms associated with innovation.
- Describe multiple strategies to advance the integration of innovation into the work of healthcare organizations.
- Evaluate multiple metrics for the measurement of innovations.

Traditionally, the emphasis in healthcare organizations has been on stability and goal achievement. Experimentation with patient care processes was discouraged to avoid additional expenses and to ensure that safe and effective patient care was administered. Leaders tended to delay process modifications until significant research documented evidence for new processes or the current process failed abruptly.

This approach is typical even when current processes are known to be only marginally successful in providing safe and effective patient care. Maintaining the status quo where cost and outcome are known is preferred to taking risks in which the costs and outcomes are not clearly known. More than 20 years ago, Wheatley challenged leaders to think differently about leadership. She challenged us to search for new ways of understanding leadership, and the integration of innovation more clearly into our leadership paradigm might be finally recognizing Wheatley's challenge (Stuke, 2013; Wheatley, 1992). To be sure, our current approach is understandable but shortsighted. Adopting a leadership mind-set that actively supports both innovation and effective operations is important for organizations to grow, sustain new practices, and excel in the future healthcare marketplace.

In today's healthcare environment, leaders and managers need a wide and varied range of competencies to manage not only the operations of the organization, but also the work of continually adapting to new evidence, new technology, and new processes. The work of

173

adapting to new approaches requires knowledge specific to creativity and innovation. This chapter presents the concept of innovation leadership, the rationale for innovation, leadership expectations, organizational structures and strategies to advance and integrate innovation, and metrics to measure innovation. The twenty-first-century leader must develop these skills to lead in a world in which innovations are the lifeblood of the organization (Kiechel, 2012).

The seemingly contradictory nature of healthcare leadership, which requires both sound business practices to create real value for the organization and a designing eye on the future, is a challenge that has become more intense with the advent of the Internet. Leaders have always been concerned about adopting new work processes, just not with the intensity and frequency they are currently exhibiting. This balancing of initiatives presents the greatest challenge to contemporary leaders: Focusing on the work that is known is much less stressful than working to modify and eliminate the known work in favor of the unknown and untested. The risk-adverse mind-set of traditional organizations too often leads to continually reworking ineffective established processes—much like the metaphorical rearranging of the deck chairs on the *Titanic*!

> ## Key Point
>
> A blockbuster innovation is not a guarantee of success, just an opportunity.
>
> DAVILA, TONY; EPSTEIN, MARC; SHELTON, ROBERT, MAKING INNOVATION WORK: HOW TO MANAGE IT, MEASURE IT, AND PROFIT FROM IT, 1st Edition, (c) 2006. Adapted by permission of Pearson Education, Inc., Upper Saddle River, NJ.

The believed lower level of risk associated with traditional operations encourages leaders to focus on this work at the expense of designing the future. Innovation leadership makes it possible for the leader to address this challenge and to balance the work of sustaining current operations that result in profitability; simultaneously, the leader can work to re-create the future as new developments emerge in the healthcare world. In fact, innovation leadership allows the leader to develop and present the new processes. Superior innovation, according to Davila and colleagues (2006), provides an organization with the opportunities to grow faster, better, and smarter than its competitors—and to ultimately influence the direction of its industry.

Innovation is more than just creating new technology; it is about the continual adaptation to the changing environment and available resources that includes creating new business models and strategies for the organization to survive and thrive into the future. Innovation leadership is about balancing the need for value/profit and the creation of new and improved approaches to health care. Innumerable references and resources are now available on topics of innovation (**Exhibit 5-1**). It is interesting to note that some researchers are challenging organizations to focus less on the traditional organization chart and more on how decisions are being made. An infrastructure that supports rapid, evidence-driven, and effective outcomes may be more localized in the job descriptions than in the organizational chart (Blenko, Mankins, & Rogers, 2010).

This chapter provides a new perspective and overview of innovation leadership as an essential competency of the quantum leader, the leader who approaches the work of health care from a systems perspective, continually recognizing the importance of sustainability, growth, and renewal for survival. The reader is encouraged to delve further into the rich and extensive writings on innovation.

Exhibit 5-1   Selected Innovation References for Healthcare Leaders

Burns, L. R. (Ed.). (2005). *The business of healthcare innovation.* Cambridge, MA: Cambridge University Press.

Christensen, C. M., Anthony, S. D., & Roth, E. A. (2004). *Seeing what's next: Using the theories of innovation to predict industry change.* Boston, MA: Harvard Business School Press.

Christensen, C. M., Grossman, J., & Hwang, J. (2009). *The innovator's prescription: A disruptive solution for health care.* New York, NY: McGraw-Hill.

Davila, T., Epstein, M. J., & Shelton, R. (2006). *Making innovation work: How to manage it, measure it and profit from it.* Upper Saddle River, NJ: Wharton School.

Fagerberg, J., Mowrey, D. C., & Nelson, R. (2005). *The Oxford handbook of innovation.* New York, NY: University Press.

Gottfredson, M., & Aspinall, K. (2005). Innovation vs. complexity: What is too much of a good thing? *Harvard Business Review, 83*(10), 63–71.

Hesselbein, F., Goldsmith, M., & Somerville, I. (Eds.). (2001). *Leading for innovation and organizing for results.* San Francisco, CA: Jossey-Bass.

Kelly, T. (2005). *The ten faces of innovation.* New York, NY: Doubleday.

Pauly, M. V. (2005). Competition and new technology. *Health Affairs, 24*(6), 1523–1535.

Porter-O'Grady, T., & Malloch, K. (2010). *Innovation leadership: Creating the landscape of health care.* Sudbury, MA: Jones and Bartlett.

Rogers, E. M. (1995). *Diffusion of innovations* (5th ed.). New York, NY: The Free Press.

Schumpeter, J. (1943). *Capitalism, socialism, and democracy.* New York, NY: Harper.

VonHippel, E. (2005). *Democratizing innovation.* Cambridge, MA: MIT Press.

Rationale for Healthcare Innovation

The rationale for innovation in health care is multifaceted but is primarily driven by the explosion of information on the Internet. Fragmented services, ineffective processes, patient safety concerns, and consumer expectations all have contributed to the need for change in the system. The transformation to a knowledge-based digital world, which includes the Internet, demands that leaders move faster, get optimized, and go global—all sooner rather than later. Contemporary leaders recognize that organizations cannot grow through cost reduction and reengineering alone. Neither can they survive when there is continual chaos and changing processes at the expense of providing value-based service. Organizations of the twenty-first century must be focused and flexible structures that meet the new demands of the technology age in a way that supports the introduction, testing, and integration of new ideas. Asking individuals to think outside the box is insufficient for integrated innovation; principles, behaviors, and metrics for success are

175

needed to support innovative thinking. Most important, new leadership mind-sets are needed for leaders to manage these seemingly contradictory expectations of stability and uncertainty.

Group Discussion

Is there any process, product, or technology that should not be changed or viewed as an opportunity for improvement? Is there any truth to the adage, "If it's not broken, don't fix it"? Identify examples of areas that are believed to be immune to change. If appropriate, describe strategies to gain support for evaluating opportunities for new and better approaches.

Healthcare innovation is not limited to creating an electronic medical record. It is about rethinking and re-creating healthcare methods of care delivery that include diagnostic approaches, communication methods with those involved in providing health care, documentation of services, and billing and payment services. Healthcare leaders are called to reinvent a healthcare system that was designed neither with safety in mind or to ensure organized and defined processes that support safety and minimize adverse patient outcomes. Innovations are needed to correct these inefficiencies. Interestingly, as leaders work to integrate the work of innovation into the organization, they are also challenged to identify those processes and treatments that lack evidence for efficacy and to eliminate them.

In the last 30 years, biotechnology has transformed the healthcare industry and has changed the way people are treated for disease. The convergence of biotechnology, information technology, and nanotechnology has transformed the way in which health care is provided. More than 300 biologics—drugs that target specific diseases—are now available (Kimley, 2006). It is now possible to improve treatment because biologics target specific diseases, turning many fatal diseases into chronic conditions. These innovations, although unequivocally beneficial for health, are not always welcomed and easily integrated into the existing healthcare system, which was designed for different products, services, and roles. Other areas that are also changing include patient care delivery processes, technology for diagnostics, patient record keeping, information integration, and the overall business model for health care.

Healthcare consumers are demanding care that does not require complex invasive processes and long recovery times. Providers of health care expect computerization, Internet access, and increasingly interconnected applications that integrate best practices and alerts to identify patient risk situations. Healthcare leaders and policymakers continue to expect more streamlined processes and expeditious communication of costs and transactions within the system.

Herzlinger (2006) identified three general categories that need improvement: methods of patient care delivery to consumers, selection and integration of technology, and the business models that support the entire healthcare system. **Exhibit 5-2** lists examples of areas for healthcare improvement within these three categories.

Exhibit 5-2   Healthcare Challenges

Patient Care Delivery
- Less invasive
- Less painful
- More convenient
- Less costly
- Increased consumer control

Technology
- Pharmaceuticals
- Diagnostic methods

- Patient record keeping
- Interconnected/integrated information

Business Models
- Less fragmentation of processes, providers, payers, settings, vendors, suppliers
- Increased vertical and horizontal integration

Group Discussion

Often, innovation is confused with creativity or performance improvement. In a small group, compare and contrast the definitions and expectations of each of these three concepts. Consider also the advantages and disadvantages of each. Is there a difference in sustainability for each concept? How is each of these supported and funded in your organization? Based on your discussion, what recommendations would you make to advance innovation in your organization?

Definitions and Concepts

Innovation is not a magical, fog-laden concept. Because the concept of innovation is used and defined in many ways that can be confusing or misleading, clarification can assist leaders. Getting to common ground on what innovation is and what it is not serves to minimize confusion and chaos.

Definitions and descriptions of innovation are as follows:

- Innovation is a historic and irreversible change in the way of doing things—creative destruction (Schumpeter, 1943).
- Innovation can be understood as a process of learning and knowledge creation through which new problems are defined and new knowledge is developed to solve them (Fagerberg, Mowrey, & Nelson, 2005).
- The power to redefine the industry; the effort to create purposeful focused change in an enterprise's economic or social potential (Drucker, 1985).
- Anything that creates new resources, processes, or values or improves a company's existing resources, processes, or values (Christensen, Roth, & Anthony, 2004, p. 293).
- The first, practical, concrete implementation of an idea done in a way that brings broad-based extrinsic recognition to an individual or organization (Plsek, 1997).
- The implementation of new or altered products, services, processes, systems, organizational structures, or business models as a means of improving one or more domains of healthcare quality (AHRQ Innovation Exchange, n.d.).

- Something new or different (*Webster's New Collegiate Dictionary*, 2001).
- The conversion of knowledge and ideas into a benefit, which may be for commercial use or for the public good; the benefit may be new or improved products, processes, or services (Erlendsson, 2005).

Related concepts are as follows:

- *Brainstorming:* A group technique of solving problems, generating ideas, and stimulating creative thinking by unrestrained, spontaneous participation in discussion (*Webster's New Collegiate Dictionary*, 2001).
- *Change:* To make different in form; to transform or modify (*Webster's New Collegiate Dictionary*, 2001).
- *Creative:* Having the quality or power to cause something new to come into being; imaginative (*Webster's New Collegiate Dictionary*, 2001).
- *Creative idea:* An original, novel thought.
- *Creative thinking:* Thinking in a new direction, away from or beyond current mental patterns toward some new pattern (Plsek, 1997).
- *Directed creativity:* Creativity on demand. Directed creativity involves using specific techniques that allow individuals to perceive things freshly, break free of the current mental models, make novel associations among concepts stored in memory, and use judgment to develop rather than reject new ideas. It is the purposeful production of creative ideas in a topic area, followed up by deliberate effort to implement some of those ideas (Plsek, 1997).
- *Disruptive innovation:* An innovation that cannot be used by customers in mainstream markets. It defines a new performance trajectory by introducing new dimensions of performance compared to existing innovations. Disruptive innovations either create new markets by bringing new features to nonconsumers or offer more convenience or lower prices to customers at the low end of an existing market (Christenson et al., 2004, p. 293).
- *Entrepreneur:* A person who organizes and manages an enterprise, especially a business with considerable initiative and risk (*Webster's New Collegiate Dictionary*, 2001).
- *Intrapreneur:* An employee of an organization allowed to exercise some independent entrepreneurial initiative (*Webster's New Collegiate Dictionary*, 2001).
- *Invention:* A new process, machine, improvement that is recognized as the product of some unique intuition or genius (*Webster's New Collegiate Dictionary*, 2001).
- *Process improvement:* The activity of elevating the performance of a series of actions, especially that of a business process with regard to its goal (Lock, 2007).
- *Research:* The investigation or experimentation aimed at discovery and interpretation of facts, revision of accepted theories or laws in light of new facts (*Webster's New Collegiate Dictionary*, 2001).

Innovation and the Quantum Leader

The role of the quantum leader is to create an infrastructure that integrates innovation into the overall work of the organization. Innovation leadership is about creating conditions, securing resources, and providing rewards for innovative work (Malloch, 2010). The desired culture supportive of innovation is one in which employees are encouraged and valued for both challenging existing work processes and providing services that ensure organizational viability. It is important to note that advancing one's culture to embrace innovation can be paradoxical—it takes time to shift a culture to support innovation with changing values, norms, and assumptions *and* the marketplace is demanding speedy changes (Miller & Wedell-Wedellsborg, 2013). Innovation leadership requires continually transforming and remaking structures and processes of the current system to integrate new processes and technology so that systems do indeed perform more effectively (Weberg, 2012).

The system complexity that accompanies healthcare innovation is a source of the accelerated uncertain expectations. Of significant concern for the contemporary leader is how to determine and manage the uncertain expectations associated with innovation, the speed at which change occurs, and the anticipated outcomes of new knowledge, technology, and process interactions with as little negative impact on the organization as possible.

By its very nature, there is no evidence for innovations in the making, only expectations. This reality does not deter most leaders from continuing to expect assurances and metrics for success. Risk taking is not viewed as a classic leadership behavior, and it is not traditionally welcomed and encouraged. Instead, risk taking is viewed negatively. It increases the organization's exposure to unforeseen hazards and to the loss of net income. Playing it safe and being a hardworking employee leads the organization nowhere because the intent is to sustain the past, to continue the practices that have been deemed to work yesterday.

Taking the initiative to advance innovation rather than clinging to the same old routine is now the work of the contemporary leader. This requires that leaders expose themselves to failure, avoid mediocrity, and embrace opportunities rather than retreat from them. The role of the leader is to inspire creativity and hard work and to challenge the past as the means to a better future. The work of inspiration requires not just inspirational phrases but inspirational behavior. Risk-disposed leaders motivate others by showing what can be done, not merely by sermonizing about opportunities. They also exhibit candor and vulnerability, identify value in marginally successful efforts, and allow others to take risks and experience success and failure.

Innovation Leadership Is Not . . .

Often, when an individual assumes the responsibility to manage the implementation of a technology product, the perception is that this work is innovation leadership. Innovation leadership is not project management. Innovation leadership is about who the leader is and how the world of work is approached. Project management is about the dissemination of processes using a top-down approach. Traditionally, the work of project management is done by a manager who is following and guiding the implementation of a clearly defined plan. However, as the healthcare industry works to better integrate innovation and operations, an innovation leader can also be a project manager for selected projects. This approach increases cross-fertilization of innovation and operations, and at the same time, it provides real-time opportunities for the innovation leader to correct course or modify the project plan to ensure optimal results.

Strategies to Integrate and Advance Innovation

The following considerations are suggested for leaders interested in advancing the work of innovation in the culture of the organization:

- Integrating mission, vision, and values within an innovation paradigm
- Assessing community and team needs
- Evaluating organizational structure
- Supporting organizational processes
- Measuring results

Integrating Mission, Vision, Values, and Innovation

The first consideration, to advance innovation, is a clear statement within the mission, vision, and values. It is important to formally define the organization's commitment to innovation as an integral part of the work of the organization. The mission incorporates the desire to provide a service or product that is continually viable and able to meet defined goals. The vision statement continues the expression of the desired service and the level of achievement necessary to achieve the mission. The values selected are those that support behaviors necessary to achieve the mission of value and innovation. **Exhibit 5-3** is an example of innovation-based mission, vision, and values statements.

Assessing Community Innovation

The second consideration is the identification of the needs of the community for innovation within the confines of the mission, vision, and values. Each organization is challenged to identify the unmet needs of the organization and its customers, the obstacles to excellent patient care, and the bottlenecks for efficient throughput as considerations when integrating the work of innovation with operations. Each of these three areas, according to Anthony, Eyring, and Gibson (2006), can assist the organization in creating a focus for innovation and avoiding the temptation to work on a great idea that is not consistent with the organization's needs.

Assessing Team Innovation Skills

In addition to knowing community and organizational innovation needs, it is also important to know the innovation skills of team members in the organization. Knowledge of comfort levels with different innovation skills can assist leaders in the reinforcement of existing skills

---

Exhibit 5-3   Innovation-Based Mission, Vision, and Values

Mission: To provide excellent patient care that provides value and makes a difference in people's lives.

Vision: To be the market leader of quality, service, and cost-effectiveness in health care.

Values: Participation, multiple intelligences, creativity, risk taking, respect for chaos, vulnerability leadership, evidence-based processes, and measurement.

---

and the development of new skills. The essence of innovation should be integrated throughout educational offerings. The opportunities to explore mental models associated with skill updates can be especially helpful.

Evaluating Organizational Structure

As previously stated, it is not enough to hold a one-day retreat and ask others to think outside the box. Structure and support are needed to fully embrace and realize the work of innovation. Interestingly, some believe that structure and process are the natural foes of creativity. Leaders often treat innovation as if it were magical, not subject to guidance or nurturing, much less planning. According to Samuel Palmisano, former president and CEO of IBM, that is not true. Rather, there are times, places, and conditions under which innovation does indeed flourish. Innovation and creativity require some restraint. Creativity with a vision, rules about how to get there, and deadlines support rather than hinder new ideas.

Valuing Natural Tensions

As one considers innovation structure, it is important to recognize the natural tensions and competing priorities that exist in a complex organization. There is a natural tension between being creative and delivering value from being creative. Leaders are very experienced in exploiting existing and known processes and less experienced in exploiting new opportunities for growth. Both the lack of time and the intense pressures within the existing work contribute to the limited attention and effort given to innovation. O'Reilly

> ### Key Point
>
> Certain types of individuals, physical facilities, authority designations, decision-making expectations, and systems to document and measure results are essential elements of an organizational infrastructure. An organization's infrastructure is a reflection of the mission, vision, and values. Innovation leadership is about embedding support for innovative thinking in the mission, vision, and values and from there throughout teams in the organization. Organizational structures are continually evaluated and reshaped to better match the work to be done. Roles are added, modified, or eliminated to improve performance and outcomes. Each change is accompanied by anticipated but unknown outcomes.

Group Discussion

To increase comfort with innovation thinking, begin small. One example is relooking at the impact and value of continuing education programs. Begin with challenging the assumptions and value of the 1–5 Likert scale for program evaluations. Instead of the ratings scale, would it be more helpful to ask participants if they could have obtained this information in a different manner? How will participants change their practice? When will they change their practice? How will the quality of patient care be affected?

181

and Tushman (2004) challenged organizations to become ambidextrous organizations, or those that emphasize balance between creativity and value capture so that the company generates successful new ideas and gets the maximum return on investment. Balancing these two seemingly disparate processes requires leaders to think differently and to continually develop the skills of middle managers to balance these same processes.

The tension between stability and innovation is especially notable in the area of patient safety. Serious efforts are in place to support high-reliability processes in which there is consistency and redundancy to ensure safe outcomes. Standardization is the goal. What is also known is that despite standardization many patient care processes do not result in safe outcomes. Patients are injured from falls, medication errors, wrong-site surgical procedures, and malfunctioning equipment. Processes to test, innovate, validate, and ensure safety can be achieved through the lens of innovation leadership, organizational resources, and a strong commitment to excellence and continual course correction.

There are two basic models for organizational structuring to support innovation. The first approach is to develop leaders and managers who have the ability both to be rigorously dedicated to value and to support the work of innovation. With this option, the balancing of goals and priorities is much more complex than the balancing required for two distinct groups.

The second approach is to develop two distinct but collaborative groups in the organizational structure: one group focusing on current business value, and the other group focusing on potential business. This approach deliberately secludes new ideas and intellectual property until the organization determines they are appropriate to release. With the two distinct groups, role confusion is also minimized. Interestingly, whereas this model is effective in the short term, separate innovation efforts and structures are at risk in times of economic stress.

Regardless of the approach taken by an organization, the leadership team must support operations that are multifocal in nature. The difference between the two options is in the amount of emphasis on each and the time required to support each approach. The skill to operate multifocally is necessary to effectively sustain business while exploring the future and minimizing organizational chaos. Choosing an approach is directly related to the levels of innovation anticipated by the organization and the available skill sets of employees. The integrated approach requires higher levels of leadership skills to plan, collaborate, negotiate, and synthesize when compared with distinct structures for current business and potential business. Seldom does an organization choose an all-or-nothing model. Rather, a combination of focused and integrated approaches is selected.

The anticipated expectations for innovations in the future should be considered in creating the structure. Levels of innovation range from minimal innovations to entire system innovations. Lower levels of innovations are described as incremental or partial and do not completely disrupt the work of an organization. Incremental innovations are introduced using project management methods and change management principles into existing systems to achieve diffusion of the innovation into the core of the organization.

Disruptive innovation, a concept identified by Christensen and colleagues (2004), is a unique approach to introducing innovation. The innovation focuses on disruption to the competitive landscape rather than incremental, semiradical, and very radical innovations that affect both technology and the business model. A healthcare example of disruptive innovation occurs when a large system builds a new healthcare facility that is designed to transform the healthcare experience. New technology, state-of-the-art technology, computerized patient records, and evidence-based architecture meld to create the backdrop for a culture revolution. Every work process and worker role is examined and remodeled to fit with the innovative healthcare facility. Not surprisingly, the work of design and construction is only the beginning. Identifying, role modeling, and sustaining new practices are the work of change management, negotiation, and teamwork.

Innovation Label Versus Innovation Role

Another consideration is the use of the innovation label. The label *innovation* can have both positive and negative effects on the intended goals of the organization. Some believe that using the innovation title should be avoided because it further separates the work of innovation from the traditional work of creating value and profit for the organization. Labeling a new team, department, or individual with the innovation label separates business from design. The designers or innovators are frequently perceived as better or different from those in routine operations. In contrast, when senior leaders are able to value and function in both the business and the design worlds, the innovation label recognizes that innovation work is different, is funded differently, and is an important segment of the organization in addition to operations. The goal is to select a title that is consistent with the mission, vision, and values; does not induce hostility or divisiveness among coworkers; and invites as many as possible into the processes of innovation (**Exhibit 5-4**).

Supporting Innovation Processes

Walking the talk of the innovation mission, vision, and values requires specific behaviors that reflect the value of innovation for the organization. There are several considerations to support innovation. It is clear that although the traditional culture is one that supports stability and patient safety, this rationale cannot be used to avoid innovations. Leaders need to be aware of the culture but not blame the culture for failure to advance. These processes can assist leaders in transforming the current healthcare culture from a

Exhibit 5-4   Innovative Leader Titles

- Chief Marketing Officer
- Director of Design and Brand Experience
- Chief Innovation Officer
- Champion of Innovation
- Chief of Design
- Director of Global Innovation
- Director of Strategic Marketing
- Innovation Champion
- Vice President, Enthusiast Services
- Vice President, Strategic Leadership and Competency Creation
- Chief Technology Officer

risk-averse model to one that balances both value creation for net income in the present and designing for the future. Support, measurement, and continual modifications are necessary to ensure the ultimate integration and value production. If this does not occur, the innovation dies a slow, sometimes painful, and sad death.

Interestingly, some organizations find that coming up with a great idea is the easy part; the more difficult work is selecting the right ideas and implementing them. There is no template or road map for innovation sustainability. What are available to leaders are the guiding principles of change management and conflict utilization, along with previous experiences in the integration of new processes and technology. Process activities that continually link innovation to the organizational mission through appropriate metrics and rewards reaffirm the commitment of leaders. Given the complex and multifaceted nature of innovation, no two innovation integration situations are identical.

Integrating innovation behaviors into the organization does not require a revolution inside of an organization. According to Davila and colleagues (2006), what innovation does require is thoughtful construction of solid management processes and an organization that can get things done. Employees want to be involved, valued, and know their work is meaningful (Goffee & Jones, 2013). Innovation should be routine rather than random, central rather than marginal, and exciting rather scary. Similar efforts to integrate quality assurance and performance improvement into the basic structure of the organization have occurred in health care and can be examined to assist in the integration of innovation work. Innovation leadership is about integrating two seemingly disparate worlds of business and design, and about integrating the need for patient safety and stability with the need to test innovations designed to improve patient safety and quality.

Democratizing Innovation

Another consideration of integrating innovation is to democratize innovation in the work of the organization. Hippel (2005) proposed this concept in an effort to demystify innovation and to develop the skills of all individuals to respect and value innovation as a core value and process of the organization. Democratizing innovation is considered a twenty-first-century strategy for success. It is not unlike the efforts of national quality or patient safety initiatives; the work is no longer isolated to a specific department but rather is a core competency for all employees. The diffusion of innovations process described by Rogers (1995) relies on the accountability of leaders to internally and personally adopt innovations before the critical mass diffusion processes across the organization can occur. Leaders are encouraged to identify those individuals who are innovators and early adopters (Rogers, 1995) of change and to support the development of new expectations and metrics for changing work. Greater numbers of colleagues dedicated to innovation create a critical mass of energy and effort dedicated to thriving in uncertainty—uncertainty that is channeled into the productive work of confronting, monitoring, and modeling innovative behaviors whenever possible.

Expect Evidence-Based Processes

Another consideration is work based on evidence. Evidence-based practice and innovation may seem contradictory on the surface. Practice based on evidence seeks consistency and standardization, whereas innovation is about creating new and different processes and products. There is an inherent relationship between evidence and innovation, one that is both dynamic and, at the same time, rigorous and structured. Indeed, both innovation and evidence are essential to each other because innovation frees evidence to alter the trajectory of our practice and evidence disciplines innovation to affirm the veracity of practice (Malloch & Porter-O'Grady, 2013). **Figure 5-1**, the cybernetic interface of evidence and innovation (Malloch & Porter-O'Grady, 2013), is a diagram reflecting the dynamic nature of innovation and evidence. Information is always in process, either as evidence at some level or as an innovation needed to close identified gaps in research, practice expertise, and/or clinical values.

Significant work has occurred in developing a commitment to providing patient care services based on evidence from research, the clinician's expertise and patient's values, and other recognized sources of knowledge (e.g., ethical knowing, sociopolitical knowing, and aesthetic ways of knowing) (Sanares & Hilliker, 2009). The relationship between evidence-based practice and innovation is apparent when there is a gap between research

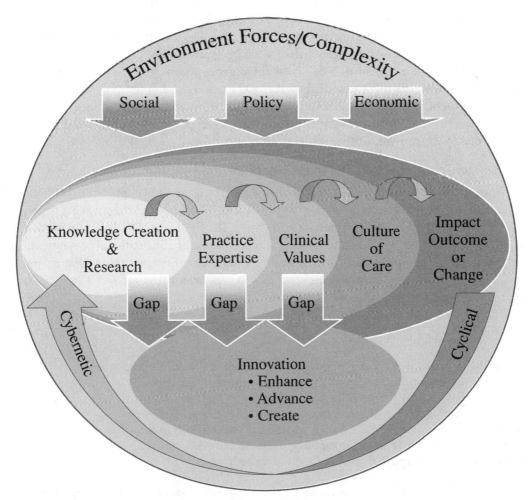

Figure 5-1 The Cybernetic Interface of Evidence and Innovation

evidence and patient values. The recommendations from valid randomized clinical trials are seldom appropriate for every patient; rather, these recommendations are generalizable to patient clinical conditions. Implanted defibrillators, insulin pumps, and transdermal medications are specific to patient clinical conditions. When a patient has difficulty functioning effectively with these recommended treatments, there is a need for exploration of other ideas and issues to discover innovative solutions.

Valuing Multiple Intelligences

Successful innovations result from a unique combination of ideas, perceptions, beliefs, and skills. The innovation leader creates conditions for the expression and valuing of many intelligences and wide diversity as sources of new ideas. In addition to the traditional valuing of linguistic and mathematical intelligence, additional intelligences are supported and encouraged.

Intelligence theorist Gardner (1993) posited that most theories of intelligence, singular and multiple, assume that intelligence is simply a biological entity or potential and exists in the brain distinct from context. Gardner's theory of multiple intelligences is helpful for innovation leaders. The seven intelligences identified by Gardner recognize other spheres of knowledge and intelligence that could be supportive of creative thinking and the work of innovation (**Exhibit 5-5**). These intelligences each describe ways of knowing the world and how different individuals perceive the world. Each individual's perspective is rich with perceptions, ideas, and potential ideas to transform current realities. Additional intelligences from other authors contribute further to recognizing the wide and varied perceptions from individuals that leaders can access.

Provide Time for Reflection and Idea Generation

The work of the leader is to continually challenge the status quo to encourage new ideas and better ways to provide health care. Most work processes have limited effectiveness times; new technology renders them ineffective and costly. The challenge is to determine which processes are the most obsolete and in need of replacement or elimination. Idea generation requires time and an open mind. Brainstorming, mind mapping, identifying what-ifs, model building, and future state mapping are strategies to support idea generation. Plsek (1997) described directed creativity as one of the essential strategies to assist individuals in bringing

---

Exhibit 5-5   Seven Intelligences

1. *Linguistic:* The capacity to use language to express ideas and understand others
2. *Logical/mathematical:* The capacity to analyze problems logically
3. *Spatial:* The capacity to recognize and use patterns of pictures and spaces in one's mind
4. *Musical:* The capacity to think in music, to hear and recognize patterns
5. *Bodily/kinesthetic:* The capacity to use all or parts of one's body to solve a problem
6. *Intrapersonal:* Having an understanding of oneself and one's limitations
7. *Interpersonal:* The capacity to understand other people

Source: From Frames of Mind: The Theory of Multiple Intelligences by Howard Gardner, Copyright (c) 1983 by Howard Gardner. Reprinted by permission of Basic Books, a member of The Perseus Books Group.

forth their creative skills and knowledge. Innovation laboratories also serve to intensely focus efforts on product idea generation from concept to reality. Leadership innovation laboratories are less obvious and are traditionally integrated into executive leadership programs in which leaders are continually asked to integrate new knowledge, challenge assumptions, and redesign leadership processes. Leadership of the twenty-first century now demands new processes and outcomes. The twenty-first-century leader works to find the appropriate amount of time and frequency in which idea generation can occur.

Recognize the Value of the Anomaly

Not everyone is ready and willing to explore and consider new ideas. Resistors to innovation or process modification can be hostile and totally unwilling unless there is an overwhelmingly compelling reason to change. The greatest obstacle to innovation is people and their comfort with existing and known processes. Although is it unrealistic to expect all individuals to embrace innovation at the moment of introduction, the opportunity to recognize and value the anomaly is present. Innovation leaders necessarily work to neutralize the organizational resistance that kills off good ideas because they are different from the norm and work to transform the resistance into a meaningful phase of the innovation process.

> ### Key Point
>
> Be cautious that creative zeal does not crowd out the reality of organizational effectiveness and survival.

New ideas are anomalous to the norm and require individuals to behave differently. The anomaly, a deviation from the common order, can be considered a potential vehicle to a better future or an aberrant event that will be ignored and soon become extinct. Anomalies present both challenges that are inherent in the nature of the change process and opportunities to design and mold future systems. Innovations, in the purest form, represent anomalies to the individuals presented with the new idea or process. Some will embrace the novelty, whereas most will respond along the innovation adoption continuum described by Rogers (1995). When faced with an innovation, five characteristic behaviors are present in individuals: innovator, early adopter, early majority, late majority, and laggards. Rogers (1995) described the innovators as venturesome, educated, needing multiple sources of information, and having greater comfort with risk taking. The early adopters are social leaders, popular, and well educated. The early majority are more contemplative and have many social contacts. The late majority are typically skeptical, more traditional, and in lower socioeconomic groups. The laggards get information about innovations from friends and neighbors and worry about costs.

Providing information about the innovation is a crucial first strategy to persuading others of its value, to supporting a decision to put the innovation to use, and finally to accepting it. Resistance to anomalies is not uncommon. The digital world could be considered an anomaly as the move from paper to electronic documentation emerged. Virtual healthcare services, in which there is no physical contact between the patient and the provider, are another. Once the anomaly gains acceptance and is believed to be the preferred way to do work, the leader begins the adoption process, using sound change management strategies to integrate the anomaly into the emerging paradigm.

Develop Capacity for Rational Risk Taking

Another consideration is proactive support for risk taking. Decision-making styles of leaders vary widely from very decisive to more contemplative. The risk of failure is ever present for all leaders and manifests in a variety of ways. Regardless, the risk of failure must not be paralyzing and counterproductive to organizational success. Rational risk taking is a skill to be learned and practiced within existing organizational structures.

Shifting the notion of risk taking as negative and costly to one of essential work in a complex and rapidly changing organization requires major organizational change in mission, role expectations, rewards and recognition, and measurement of outcomes. Traditional organizations view errors and negative outcomes as costly to the organization from both a quality and a financial perspective. Innovation leaders integrate the work of unsuccessful occurrences into the design work of the organization. These occurrences are viewed as opportunities for discussion and evaluation of the existing system structure and processes.

Rational risk taking is designed to enhance the organization, to support innovative processes, and to avoid obvious negative outcomes. Examples include advancing the organization and skill development. Adding new programs, expanding services, selecting equipment and technology, and selecting priorities are rational and minimize risk when choices are made on the basis of core values, respect for others, the safety of individuals, strategic goals of the organization, and available resources. Another example is developing the skills of employees. Gaining new knowledge and skills is considered a rational risk when those skills are needed to improve job performance or to develop abilities for anticipated opportunities. Examples include developing computer application, public speaking, sports, creative arts, and personal protection skills.

Risk taking is considered irrational in several situations. The first situation is when there is a history of failure and oppression. If the last attempt did not work and there is little interest, the risk should be questioned. It is important to recognize that something might not have been successful previously and could be successful in the future under the right conditions. Continuing to push an idea or product with new energy, new rationale, and new value is irrational. The second situation is poor judgment. Walking in traffic is an example where the risk of injury to oneself and to others is present and probable. This action is irrational and similar to the leader who continues to hire employees in the midst of a financial crisis. The organization incurs additional financial obligations and the positions of new employees will most likely be eliminated. The third irrational risk is in situations where there are unrealistic expectations or very little potential for success.

Group Discussion

The iPhone and GPS have contributed to the revolution of communication across the globe. As these tools gain increasing acceptance, their utility seems obvious and irrefutable. Reflect on these innovations and identify at least five obstacles that were offered to resist them. Consider the resistance from funders, policymakers, competitors, potential users, family members, and retailers.

Attempting to implement one more program when the staff is already overwhelmed and frustrated is not rational.

Form Uncommon Partnerships

Another consideration to advance innovation is the creation of partnerships that include individuals from diverse backgrounds and disciplines. Innovation requires teamwork and strategic partnerships that are in-person, verbal, and virtual online relationships. Networks of stakeholders are the building blocks for innovation. Strategic partnerships serve to allow organizations to create value that no single individual or organization could create alone. According to Adner (2006), innovation ecosystems bring both new opportunities and new risks. These new partnerships include risks specific to creating an initiative, ongoing coordination of activities, and adoption strategies to ensure the initiative is fully integrated into the system.

Multiple levels of collaboration and teamwork are needed to support innovation. Internal stakeholders, those who touch the innovation in any way, and others external to the process should be considered for brainstorming and idea generation. Often, those external to the process who could provide new insights are not easily identified. Many successful innovation leaders deliberately invite colleagues with differing viewpoints and points of reference to form a more complete approach. Examples of colleagues external to the process include stakeholders responsible for the location of services, payments, ownership and oversight of the processes, profit status, patient advocacy, technology development, legal accountability, policymaking, and quality measurement.

Measuring the Results: Innovation Metrics and Evaluation Strategies

New metrics are needed when innovations are introduced. In most cases, multiple interrelated metrics are required to adequately reflect the value of the innovation. Measurement

Group Discussion

Innovations in Communication: Blogs, Social Networking, and Podcasting

Blogs, social networking, and podcasting are recent modes of electronic communication. The organization is looking for ideas on how to improve patient throughput in the emergency department. How could each of these modes of communication, or a combination of the modes, be used to obtain ideas and provide new strategies to improve throughput? Consider who should be involved and create a problem statement and measures for success.

Blog: A weblog, usually shortened to blog, is an online publication with regular posts.

Social networking: Internet-based programs used to make connections with others.

Podcasting: A method of distributing multimedia files across the Internet. A podcaster creates content for an audience that wants to listen when they want, where they want, and how they want.

Exhibit 5-6   Guidelines for Selection of Innovation Metrics

1. Select metrics to assess innovation progress and costs in advance. Incremental benchmarks are especially important to track and trend progress. Different sets of funding, testing, and performance criteria for incremental, experimental, and potentially disruptive innovations are needed.
2. Aim to identify early successes. Major initiatives often require significant time to realize the full benefits. Interim achievements are necessary to demonstrate progress and the likelihood of achieving the full potential of the innovation.
3. Get data to back up your gut. Successful innovators begin with the "gut feeling" and must move quickly to develop the quantifiable supporting data.

---

of an innovation, both qualitative and quantitative, is essential and fundamental to the work of the organization. What is different about measuring innovations is that initially only historical and anticipated metrics can be selected to examine. The innovation leader selects a group of metrics knowing that they must be routinely evaluated for comprehensiveness and sensitivity and updated as needed as new and unexpected changes occur with an innovation (**Exhibit 5-6**).

Numerous organizational metrics specific to broad operations, human resources, supplies, technology, and patient outcomes are available. Often, single metrics are selected to evaluate effectiveness to simplify the measurement process. The disadvantage to single-metric evaluation is the loss of information specific to interim achievements that may ultimately affect the selected single metric. For example, selecting hours per patient day as the single metric to evaluate an innovative model for patient assessment would not consider the quality and completeness of the assessment data. Incomplete data could result in an extended length of stay and patient complications.

When different metrics or different groups of metrics are selected for analysis, additional uncertainty is introduced and the number of potential conclusions increases. The work of the leader is to identify the metrics that reflect the true value of the work.

> **Key Point**
>
> Innovation never occurs in isolation or by a single individual—it requires a team of dedicated individuals passionately committed to making a difference.

The greatest difficulty is to identify and measure what really matters—which metrics are the critical variables that indicate value, service, and cost outcomes accurately and comprehensively. Multiple related metrics are required to explain the causality of relationships; seldom does one variable explain one outcome. By its very essence, the complex and dynamic nature of health care renders it resistant to simple linear cause-and-effect metrics. For example, no one intervention is accountable for the resolution of a patient's pneumonia; diet, fluids, medications, and activity all contribute to the resolution of the chest congestion. Similarly, the hours per patient day metric cannot be simply linked and traced to the activities of a single unit leader; the competence of staff, level of illness of patients, number of interventions required, and availability of equipment and supplies all affect the level of hours per patient day used. With each modification of work, the outcome expectations change. New

Exhibit 5-7 Personal Calendar: Evolving Expectations and Metrics

Innovation	Expectation (Intent)	Metric
Handwritten calendar	Summary of information	Appropriate space allocation for entries
Computerized calendar	Automated, editable, accessible by multiple individuals, able to archive and retrieve information	Real-time availability, accessible to selected individuals to facilitate scheduling; decreased time in calendar management
Interconnected Internet-accessed calendar	Wireless, Internet access	Accessibility from multiple devices and multiple locations

mind-sets, new approaches, and new resources also evolve as expectations change. Consider the evolution of two processes: creating and managing one's personal calendar and the documenting process. It is important to note that as the innovation evolves and becomes more defined, expectations evolve reflecting the intent of the innovation. This evolution of expectations is an integral part of the process of adopting innovations (**Exhibit 5-7**).

Not all innovations require new metrics. Some changes in healthcare work result in new expectations for greater involvement of individuals or higher performance targets while the specific metric remains the same. For example, changing from nurse-administered pain medication to patient-controlled analgesia pumps does not change the expectation for pain control; rather, the intent of the change is to improve the level of achievement or performance of the specific metric. Patient satisfaction with pain control and comfort should be better with the patient-controlled analgesia than with nurse-administered pain interventions (**Exhibit 5-8**). Discussed elsewhere in this text are the challenges and nature of innovation valuing.

Course Corrections

Expectations for success are not realized for a variety of reasons. The wise leader works to minimize the time spent ruminating about the unsuccessful events and focuses on developing new solutions and course corrections to achieve the desired outcomes. Change often fails if the culture is not supportive or if leaders are not qualified to lead innovation. The lack of urgency, poor communication, or lack of teamwork are common obstacles

Exhibit 5-8 Barriers to Effective Innovation Measurement

1. The business model is flawed, resulting in selection of the wrong levers of value creation.
2. Subjective measures of effectiveness are excluded.
3. Available information technology for data mining and analysis are not used.
4. Information technology replaces analysis and judgment.
5. The right question is not asked about what is being measured.

Source: DAVILA, TONY; EPSTEIN, MARC; SHELTON, ROBERT, MAKING INNOVATION WORK: HOW TO MANAGE IT, MEASURE IT, AND PROFIT FROM IT, 1st Edition, (c) 2006. Adapted by permission of Pearson Education, Inc., Upper Saddle River, NJ.

(Ponti, 2011). According to Rogers (1995), rejection of an innovation may occur any time along the adoption process, which includes awareness of the innovation, interest, evaluation, trial, and then adoption. Discontinuance is a rejection that occurs after adoption of the innovation. Further, there are two types of discontinuance:

1. Disenchantment discontinuance, which is a decision to reject an idea as a result of dissatisfaction with its performance
2. Replacement discontinuance, which is a decision to reject an idea to adopt a better idea

Given the inevitability of rejection or discontinuance of a new work process, the emphasis, first, needs to be on making course corrections with evidence and rationales and, second, on realizing the information and lessons that can be learned from the experience. Before implementing course corrections or new strategies, the team must once again be sure that the values of the work continue to be congruent with the organization, and then the team can challenge the assumptions of the work processes that went awry and clarify expectations that new processes have a high degree of potential for success.

Conclusion

For innovation leadership, processes that require and improve performance on the basis of defined innovation as the way of doing business are essential. An assessment of current ways of doing business, identifying the unwritten rules about how work is accomplished and how these processes enable or inhibit innovation, begins the transformation to a balanced value-innovation culture.

Case Study 5-1

Innovative Strategies to Prevent Hospital Readmissions

Mission Medical Center is a 700-bed hospital in an urban city in the Southwest. Mission is part of a vertically integrated healthcare system with a number of physician medical groups, ambulatory care settings and surgical centers, a psychiatric hospital, and orthopaedic specialty hospital, and a children's specialty hospital. All of the hospitals are within a 50-mile radius of one another. At Mission Medical Center, the nursing division is organized under a chief nursing officer (CNO) who is also the designated chief operating officer (COO) for the medical center.

John has 25 years of experience in nursing leadership, and for the past 10 years he has been the CNO for Mission Medical Center. Six nursing directors report to John and provide supervision and direction to Medical-Surgical Services, Surgical Services, Maternal-Newborn Services, Rehabilitation Services, Intensive and Emergency Services, and Professional Support Services. John meets with the directors once a week for a Nursing Operations Council that focuses on the operational aspects of providing and coordinating patient care with other professional disciplines. Once a month, John meets with the directors and the clinical nurse specialists (CNSs) for Nursing Executive Council. The purpose of the Nursing Executive Council is to promote the professionalism of nursing, advance strategies and initiatives to improve patient care outcomes, promote research and evidence-based practice, and ensure a healthy work environment that attracts and retains nurses. Mission Medical has been designated as a Magnet organization and is currently working toward redesignation, which is scheduled in approximately 2 years.

As an organization, Mission Medical is very forward thinking and is considered to be one of the top hospitals in the state. One of the reasons that Mission has earned its reputation is because of its recruitment of top medical specialists, attractive new patient bed tower, the latest of capital equipment for patient care and surgical services, and a strong financial foundation. Whereas Mission Medical has strategically sought to advance its market penetration into competitor territory, it has also been thoughtfully conservative not to overbuild beyond its financial capacity. The strategy to emphasize excellence in patient care services, excellence in the work environment, and excellence in medical staff has attracted a constantly growing market share of insurers wishing to contract with Mission Medical and individuals in the community who have elected to purchase medical care through the Mission Medical Plan.

At one of the Nursing Executive Council meetings, a discussion ensues about changes that may need to occur as a result of the new Affordable Care Act. John and the directors realize that reimbursement will be strongly tied to patient outcomes, readmissions to the hospital within 30 days, and other operational metrics. Although the nursing-sensitive indicators, Hospital Consumer Assessment of Healthcare Providers and Systems (HCAHPS) scores, and satisfaction levels of patients, physicians, and nurses are extremely high, the directors realize that they must somehow motivate nurses to identify new ways of providing patient care that will minimize redundancies and maximize workflow. They also realize that they must ensure that every patient is ready to be discharged and able to care for him- or herself at home to prevent readmissions within 30 days of discharge. The directors and clinical nurse specialists discuss a number of ideas. John encourages the open discussion and listens to each of the ideas with interest. While he quietly listens to the input from the nursing leaders, he considers the various organizational structures and processes that might need to change to support some of the ideas. He realizes that he must also encourage the nurse leaders to consider how they will measure the effect of the changes that they would like to implement, but he doesn't want to discourage the open dialogue and freethinking during the initial stages of the discussion.

One of the major points of discussion is about the prevention of readmissions within 30 days of discharge. Because of the major financial impact that this issue has on the hospital's bottom line, John and the nurse leaders are keenly interested in any innovative thinking as to how to prevent these occurrences. After several hours of open dialogue, John asks the CNSs and the nursing directors to divide into three teams and challenges them to work together in their teams to identify strategy around preventing readmissions. To incentivize the groups, John states that the team with the best idea will be rewarded with a prize for their respective areas. He also tells them that their ideas must include not only the intervention, but also methods of measuring the effect of the intervention on reducing readmission rates. He suggests that the directors work with the chief financial officer (CFO) to develop a return on investment (ROI) on their respective ideas. The group agrees that they will reconvene in 1 month for each group to present their ideas.

Three groups return a month later with posters to illustrate their respective plans, formal PowerPoint presentations, and supporting evidence to substantiate their innovative thinking. Group 1 recommends developing a role in each unit for a discharge resource nurse, who would not be counted in the daily staffing, but who would be responsible for reviewing each patient's status for discharge. The discharge resource nurse would coordinate patients' needs with social services, the discharge planner, the physician, and the patients' family to ensure that all of the resources that the patient needs after discharge would be readily available upon arrival home. In addition the discharge resource nurse would assess patients' understanding of their illness each day and their knowledge of their medications, required therapies, and appointments with their primary providers. A significant part of the discharge resource nurse's role would include patient and family education and assessment of the patient's readiness for discharge. Group 1 suggests that they would measure success by reducing the number of readmissions per quarter from the existing baseline. They estimate that the cost savings from potential losses in reimbursement without the intervention would more than pay for the expense of the new discharge resource nurse position.

Group 2 proposes a very similar intervention; however, they based their proposal on evidence that demonstrated the effectiveness of a patient-centered approach to care in improving patients' knowledge and ability to care for themselves prior to and after discharge. Group 2 proposes defining "patient-centered care" to be patient empowerment, engagement, and activation in their care. The new definition of patient-centered care would reflect nursing's involvement in educating the patient and empowering patients with knowledge to be completely engaged in decisions related to their care, and thereby activating patients' own resources to care for themselves at home. Group 2 presents the notion that every nurse believes that he or she provides patient-centered care without fully understanding the concept or realizing the nurse's role and responsibility in ensuring patients' involvement in their own care. The CNSs in Group 2 propose an educational platform for nurses to promote the new definition of patient-centered care and provide standardized educational plans for high-risk conditions that have been correlated with readmissions in the past. The CNSs propose that they would measure the effectiveness of their plan by having patients and/or their families complete a Readiness for Discharge Assessment tool that they had reviewed in the literature and to measure the patients' knowledge and abilities to follow up with their proposed treatment plan during hospitalization and after discharge.

Group 3 recommends a collaborative, interprofessional approach using team rounding with the patient each morning to ensure that the patient and family are knowledgeable about the plan of care. In addition to the team rounding, Group 3 suggests changing the unit structure to include a clinical nurse leader (CNL) who would be assigned to approximately 12 patients with a team of primary care nurses. The CNL would coordinate all of the patients' care among the various disciplines and ensure that patients were being instructed and engaged in their care. In addition the CNL would coordinate with the discharge planner, social services, and other specific disciplines to meet with the patient each day of his or her hospitalization in preparation for discharge. Group 3 also proposes adding a responsibility to the primary nurse's role to call each of the discharge patients

1 week after discharge to ensure that they are adequately cared for and following up with medications, therapies, and provider appointments. Group 3's proposal includes the addition of several new positions. They present several studies where the role of the CNL saved money in other organizations and improved patient satisfaction, physician satisfaction, and nurse satisfaction rates and patient outcomes.

John invites the CFO, the CEO, and a guest consultant to hear each of the proposals and to provide feedback to each of the teams. It is a time of great excitement because of the competitive nature of the presentations, but also friendly engagement in discussions about the merits of each of the proposals. It is suggested that the best intervention would be a combination of all three proposals with the development of the CNL who would act as a patient care coordinator and a resource nurse to support the direct care providers. In addition it is suggested that the discharge nurse coordinators assume a greater role in assessing the patients' readiness for discharge and that the CNS group and nurse educators assume a greater role in assessing the patients' level of knowledge and ability to care for themselves and to follow up with the proposed treatment plan while in the hospital or after discharge. It is decided that a previously published instrument, Readiness for Discharge Assessment Tool, would be used with all patients to assess their level of empowerment through education, engagement in decision making and planning, and activation of their own skills for self-care. It is also decided that the Readiness for Discharge Assessment Tool would be used again in a follow-up phone call by a discharge liaison nurse (new role) who would contact each of the discharged patients for the unit on day 2, day 5, and then weekly for a month after discharge. In addition the group decides to develop a "Call A Nurse" hotline to facilitate decision making among discharged patients relative to their questions about their health status, follow-up instructions, or care questions.

The CFO offers to work with the directors to estimate the expense of the new positions and the return on the investment for minimizing the number of readmissions each quarter. All of the participants realize the risks involved in adding new full-time equivalents (FTEs), but also realize the potential loss of revenue that would result from readmissions within 30 days of discharge. The CEO and CFO are particularly impressed with the evidence shared from other hospitals that had implemented the CNL role and subsequently reported positive outcomes from having nurses with Master's degrees coordinating the care, discharge, and after-hospitalization experience of a small group of assigned patients. This idea coupled with the other support roles seems to be the best innovation to address the problem of loss of revenue related to readmissions within 30 days of discharge.

Questions

1. What are your thoughts about John's approach to using friendly competition among the three groups to motivate them to think creatively about solving the problem?
2. Of the three possible proposals, which proposal do you think has the greatest merit in reducing readmissions?

3. Because the three groups were charged with designing an innovative solution to the problem, how do you think that the morphing of their proposals into a fourth solution affected the nurse leaders' motivation to think creatively in the future?

4. What would you add to the final solution to ensure its success in decreasing the readmission rate for Mission?

5. What barriers, if any, do you think that the nursing leaders will encounter when implementing the final proposal to reduce readmission rates?

6. What stakeholders do you think should be involved in developing implementation and measurement strategies in the adoption of this new innovation?

Case Study 5-2

Using Innovative Strategies to Correct Unit Problems

There seems to be a serious problem among the nursing staff on the acute care unit at West Memorial Hospital. The unit manager has just received the employee opinion survey results for the past year and is shocked to find that the questions related to "respect among employees" and "open communication among employees" were scored in the 25th percentile. The nursing satisfaction scores on the NDNQI survey are also extremely low in comparison to other nursing units at West Memorial Hospital. The unit manager realizes that something needs to be done to improve the scores, but most important to improve the morale of the nursing staff and their satisfaction with the work environment. The unit manager shares the results with the clinical nurse specialist (CNS) and enlists his help in determining the root of the problem. The two decide to talk with some of the informal leaders among the nursing staff to ask their perceptions of why nurses would rate their satisfaction level and their respect and communication among their colleagues so low on the two surveys.

While talking with several other nurses, it becomes readily apparent that they are not willing to talk or share their feelings with the unit manager or the CNS, and in fact it seems as if some of the nurses are actually fearful of talking at all about the situation. One or two of the more courageous nurses who are interviewed share that they are fearful of reprisal from some of their colleagues. They share that several of the nursing colleagues on both the day and night shifts would refuse to talk with them or help them when they tried to approach them about improving communication among the nurses. The unit manager and the CNS are quite concerned about the situation but are uncertain how to approach correcting the problem.

Not long after the survey results are available, there are two reportable patient falls. When the nurses who were involved in the care of the patients are interviewed, they indicate that in one case the nurse did not ask for assistance from any of the other nurses to get the patient out of bed for the first time because there had been recent occasions when some nurses were openly hostile when asked to assist in patient care. In the second patient fall, the nurse involved indicates that she had asked for assistance from her colleagues, but they had openly refused to help her. Therefore, she tried to ambulate the patient on her own and was unable to prevent the patient from falling. These two incidents confirm in the minds of the unit manager and the CNS that something needs to be done quickly to correct the attitudes and behaviors of the nursing staff on the unit. Patient safety was at risk, and nursing morale was at the lowest it had ever been.

Although the unit manager tries to discuss the situation in staff meetings and asks the staff to be more collegial with one another, it seems that this message falls on deaf ears. It is quite obvious that the nursing staff are unwilling or fearful to speak to anyone about the specifics of the situation. It is also obvious that there were informal leaders among the nursing staff who may have instigated the bullying behavior toward some of the less experienced and younger nurses.

The unit manager invites a human resources representative, a counselor from the employee assistance program, the CNS, and a member of the Lean/Six Sigma team to a meeting to discuss the situation and to identify possible interventions to address the problem. The group decides to call themselves the "Innovation Team" and decides to use an innovative approach to solving the problem because the traditional method for a quick resolution had failed. After discussion among the Innovation Team, it is decided that a more detailed assessment needs to be done to determine the actual issues among the staff. Because talking with the nursing staff was not effective because of the fear factor, the employee assistance program counselor suggests having a series of education and discussion sessions regarding the importance of a healthy work environment, collegiality, and open communication among the nursing staff for their own well-being and for patient safety. She volunteers to develop a content outline that could be presented to the group at their next meeting. She also offers to have more time available for individual counseling should any of the nurses elect to participate. The CNS offers to do a literature search to find a survey or instrument that could measure nursing attitudes more specifically so that a definitive action might be taken. The Six Sigma representative reviews the problem using an A3 diagram to mind map all possible scenarios that could be causing the problem and also a fishbone diagram identifying the desired outcome and all of the potential barriers that were preventing the desired outcome in the current situation. The group realizes the severity of the problem and the potential for other patient issues; therefore, they place the actions in the high-priority category for implementation.

The CNS discovers several survey tools to measure collegiality, communication, trust, and respect among nurses and prepares a formal institutional review board (IRB) proposal to measure these attitudes and behaviors before and after the educational series. The series would be presented by the employee assistance program (EAP) counselor to raise the staff awareness and knowledge about the benefits of a healthy work environment and the risks of a negative, hostile, and uncooperative work environment to their own health and to the safety of their patients. It is decided that after a few of the educational sessions, the Six Sigma representative would engage the staff in conversations using the mind-mapping technique and fishbone diagrams to openly discuss some of the issues that the staff were obviously feeling. It is felt that this step cannot be taken until more trust is developed among the staff, which is expected after the educational series is presented.

After IRB approval of the proposal, the CNS posts flyers on the unit and announces in the staff meetings that a survey would be available for the staff related to developing a healthy work environment. He also announces that a series of educational classes would be presented by the EAP counselor on developing a healthy work environment and that he hopes that as many staff as possible would participate by completing the survey and attending the classes.

It seems that the nursing staff feels safe in recording their perceptions of the communication, respect, and cooperation on the survey instruments when they were not at all expressive of their feelings in individual meetings or group settings. After the presurvey is completed, the CNS tabulates the results and shares the findings with the nursing staff in the staff meetings. It seems as if the staff are shocked at the level of discontent that is revealed in the survey results. Perhaps these findings motivate the staff to attend the educational sessions offered by the EAP counselor, which focus on crucial conversations, crucial confrontations, collaboration, respect in the workplace, and attributes of a healthy work environment. It is stated in the classes that every employee has a right to feel safe in the work environment; supported by their unit manager and colleagues; respected for their individuality, knowledge, and skills; and accepted as a valued team member. Each class also includes time for discussion; however, in the initial classes most of the participants are absolutely silent. As they receive more content, many of the staff begin to participate by sharing their personal feelings and hopes that a healthy work environment could be achieved. By the end of the educational sessions, it is apparent that the staff are engaged not only in the class content, but also in a newly found commitment to improve the unit culture. Informal leaders with negative attitudes suddenly lose their power base and followers as many of the staff begin to demonstrate behaviors that they are more willing to place their affiliation with the group who wants to make a more positive work environment.

After the classes end, the EPA counselor keeps her promise and offers 1 hour of individual counseling to any employee who wishes to meet with her. Many of the staff accept that offer and meet with the counselor. The Six Sigma representative also meets with some of the more positive staff members, and they begin to identify specific causes of some of the issues and identify possible behavioral changes that could create positive changes.

Several months later the CNS readministers the postsurvey, and the findings reveal significant improvement in the staff's perception of open communication, respect among coworkers, nurse satisfaction, and perceptions of cooperation in patient care. Needless to say, the Innovation Team is excited about the findings and develops a strategy for sharing these findings with the staff. Tables and graphs of the improvements are prepared, and the findings are shared in a special staff meeting on both day and night shifts. The EAP counselor is on hand to facilitate discussion among the staff who also seem excited about the results. Many of the staff comment that the changes on the unit are palpable and that coming to work is a much more pleasant experience. It seems that the staff are engaged in resolving the issues and committed to making the work environment more pleasant.

The unit manager and the CNS are excited about the positive changes that they could see on the unit for themselves and that are reported to them by individual nurses who comment on how appreciative they are that steps were taken to change the work environment. The unit manager and the CNS decide to write an article about how their unit's culture changed once the staff realized how the problem was affecting them personally as well as negatively affecting their patients. Increasing the staff's awareness about the potential for a healthy work environment and the behaviors that would be required of them to create such an environment made a significant difference in their overall perceptions of the relationships with their colleagues. The Innovation Team also prepares an abstract for presentation at a national nursing conference on Innovations in Nursing Practice and is selected to share their process of problem identification, problem solutions, and measuring the outcomes of the innovative interventions.

Questions

1. What are your perceptions of the methods used by the unit manager and the CNS to resolve the unhealthy work environment on the unit?
2. What might have been some of the barriers that could have been anticipated by the Innovation Team in resolving the negative work environment?
3. What are the factors that might affect the adoption or rejection of the innovation that was used to improve the work environment?
4. How did the Innovation Team engage the staff in resolution of the poor unit morale?
5. What might you do as an innovation leader to ensure that this change was sustained over time?

References

Adner, R. (2006). Match your innovation strategy to your innovation ecosystem. *Harvard Business Review, 83*(4), 98–116.

AHRQ Innovation Exchange. (n.d.). Home page. Retrieved from http://www.innovations.ahrq.gov/

Anthony, S. D., Eyring, M., & Gibson, L. (2006). Mapping your innovation strategy. *Harvard Business Review, 83*(5), 104–113.

Blenko, M. W., Mankins, M. C., & Rogers, P. (2010). The decision-driven organization. *Harvard Business Review, 87*(6), 54–61.

Christensen, C. M., Grossman, J., & Hwang, J. (2009). *The innovator's prescription: A disruptive solution for health care.* New York, NY: McGraw-Hill.

Davila, T., Epstein, M. J., & Shelton, R. (2006). *Making innovation work: How to manage it, measure it, and profit from it.* Upper Saddle River, NJ: Wharton School.

Drucker, P. F. (1985). *Innovation and entrepreneurship.* New York, NY: Harper & Row.

Erlendsson, J. (2005). Innovation. Retrieved from http://www.hi.is/~joner/eaps/innodd.htm

Fagerberg, J., Mowrey, D. C., & Nelson, R. (2005). *The Oxford handbook of innovation.* New York, NY: Oxford University Press.

Gardner, H. (1993). *Frames of mind: The theory of multiple intelligences.* New York, NY: Basic Books.

Goffee, R., & Jones, G. (2013). Creating the best workplace on earth. *Harvard Business Review, 90*(5), 99–106.

Herzlinger, R. E. (2006). Why innovation in health care is so hard. *Harvard Business Review, 83*(5), 58–66.

Hippel, E. V. (2005). *Democratizing innovation*. Cambridge, MA: MIT.

Kiechel, W. (2012). The management century. *Harvard Business Review, 89*(11), 63–75.

Kimley, A. W. (2006). Biotechnology leads the way. *Harvard Business Review, 83*(5), 51–54.

Lock, D. (2007). Project management (9th ed.). London, England: Gower Publishing, Ltd.

Malloch, K. (2010). Innovation leadership: New perspectives for new work. *Nursing Clinics of North America, 45*(1), 1–9.

Malloch, K., & Porter-O'Grady, T. (2013). Innovation and evidence: A partnership in advancing practice and care. In B. M. Melnyk & E. Fineout-Overholt (Eds.), *Evidence based practice in nursing and healthcare: A guide to best practice*. Philadelphia, PA: Lippincott Williams & Wilkins.

Miller, P., & Wedell-Wedellsborg, T. (2013). The case for stealth innovation. *Harvard Business Review, 91*(3), 91–97.

O'Reilly, C. A. III, & Tushman, M. L. (2004). The ambidextrous organization. *Harvard Business Review, 82*(4), 74–81.

Plsek, P. (1997). *Creativity, innovation, and quality*. Roswell, GA: Quality Press.

Ponti, M. D. (2011). Why change fails. *Nurse Leader, 9*(4), 41–43.

Rogers, E. M. (1995). *Diffusion of innovations* (4th ed.). New York, NY: The Free Press.

Sanares, D., & Hilliker, D. (2009). A framework for nursing clinical inquiry: Pathway toward evidence-based nursing practice. In K. Malloch & T. Porter-O'Grady (Eds.), *Introduction to evidence-based practice in nursing and health care*. Sudbury, MA: Jones and Bartlett.

Schumpeter, J. (1943). *Capitalism, socialism, and democracy*. New York, NY: Harper.

Stuke, K. B. (2013). Understanding leadership through leadership understandings. *Journal of Leadership Studies, 7*(2), 55–61.

Weberg, D. (2012). Complexity leadership: A healthcare imperative. *Nursing Forum, 47*(4), 268–277.

Webster's New Collegiate Dictionary. (2001). New York, NY: Random House.

Wheatley, M. J. S. (1992). *Leadership and the new science: Learning about organization from an orderly universe*. San Francisco, CA: Berrett-Koehler.

Suggested Readings

Christensen, C. M., Roth, E. A., & Anthony, S. D. (2004). *Seeing what's next: Using theories of innovation to predict industry change*. Boston, MA: Harvard Business School.

Kellerman, B. (2006). When should a leader apologize and when not? *Harvard Business Review, 83*(4), 73–81.

Lindegaard, S. (2013). Innovation culture: The big elephant in the room. Retrieved from http://www.innocentive.com/innovation-culture-big-elephant-room

Middlebrooks, T. (2013). Introduction: New perspectives of leadership. *Journal of Leadership Studies, 7*(2), 32–34.

Mockler, R., & Dologite, D. (2006, May). Creating the digital hospital. *Healthcare Informatics, 47*, 50.

Rayport, J. F., & Jaworski, B. J. (2004). Best face forward. *Harvard Business Review, 82*(11), 47–58.

Schoemaker, P. J. H., & Gunther, R. E. (2006). The wisdom of deliberate mistakes. *Harvard Business Review, 83*(6), 109–115.

Quiz Questions

Select the best answer for each of the following questions.

1. Which of the following best describes innovation?

    a. Out-of-the-box thinking

    b. Something new or different

    c. A process that requires a laboratory for brainstorming, modeling, and testing

    d. A new product that is successful in the first month of introduction to the marketplace

2. Which of the following characteristics demonstrates the optimal organizational structure for innovation?

    a. It includes the traditional work of operations.

    b. It includes both departments of innovation and operational departments.

    c. It is complex and often confusing.

    d. It considers the innovation work to be done and the available skills of leaders.

3. What is the primary purpose of a department of innovation?

    a. To support creativity as an integral part of the organization's mission

    b. To isolate creative scientists and leaders dedicated to innovation

    c. To create an entity that is easier to develop a budget and goals specific to innovation

    d. All of the above

4. How can disruptive innovation be described?

    a. Work that does not support required healthcare services

    b. Work that requires new thinking by all customers

    c. An innovation that cannot be used by customers in mainstream markets

    d. Work that has been terminated because of poor outcomes

5. When is rational risk taking appropriate?

    a. New skills are being developed.

    b. There is adequate insurance coverage.

    c. No obvious changes are anticipated.

    d. Team members support the risk.

6. Which of the following best describes opportunities for innovation?

    a. They are limited to organizations focused on technology.

    b. They can be found in all walks of life.

    c. They are present in healthcare delivery systems, technology, and business models.

    d. They are difficult to identify and integrate in healthcare systems.

7. Which of the following best describes intrepreneurship?

    a. Creation of a personal business using company funds

    b. The organization and management of an enterprise or business with considerable initiative and risk

    c. An innovation laboratory

    d. When an employee of an organization is allowed to exercise some independent entrepreneurial initiative

8. Metrics for measuring innovation should include which of the following?

a. Cost of technology and personnel

b. One metric at a time to determine specific impact on the organization

c. Goals that can be identified once the innovation is in place and functioning adequately

d. Multiple variables that are believed to reflect the intended goals of the innovation

9. Which of the following describes course correction for organizations committed to integrated innovation?

a. It is an effective strategy to support risk taking and open discussion of the realities of innovations.

b. It reflects poor planning.

c. It is a strategy to cover up negative outcomes.

d. It is common for all innovations.

10. Resistance to innovation is a result of which of the following?

a. Personal discomfort and lack of experience with new ideas

b. Lack of understanding of the goals of the innovation

c. Excellent performance in one's current role

d. All of the above

CHAPTER SIX

Leadership and Normative Conflict: Managing the Diversity of a Multifocal Workplace

Cooperation is the thorough conviction that nobody can get there unless everybody gets there.

—*Virginia Burden*

The Process of Intuition by Virginia Burden Tower, Theosophical Publishing House, Wheaton, Illinois, 1987. Reprinted by permission.

Chapter Objectives

At the completion of this chapter, the reader will be able to

- Recognize the key principles of conflict resolution in dealing with a wide variety of conflict-based issues.
- Apply conflict management principles and processes in the everyday exercise of the leadership role.
- Distinguish between normal conflict management and the management of differences.
- Formulate personal insights regarding how to apply conflict management skill sets as part of the leadership role.
- Distinguish between identity- and interest-based conflict and describe the best approach to dealing with each type.

Conflict is central to all human interaction. Conflict simply codifies the deep and abiding understanding of the fundamental diversity of the human experience. Managing conflict is the vehicle through which we negotiate our differences and work to find passage to common ground. As a metaphor for difference, normative conflict represents the foundational aspect of human interaction and communication. The challenge presented by conflict is that it is often rife with pain and violence. However, that it frequently has those features is evidence of our inability to see conflict as normal and to develop mechanisms for managing it well (Kriesberg, 2003; Levinger, 2013; Werner, 2012). Because it is so much a part of the human experience, we would do better to learn the dynamics of conflict and incorporate its management into our human skill set. This chapter treats

203

> **Key Point**
>
> Conflict is normal. The challenge is to know what it is when it happens and what to do about it when it is recognized for what it is.

conflict as normal and offers a range of techniques and methodologies for managing it in such a way as to ultimately achieve purposeful action and improved relationships. The emphasis is on developing skills for facilitating the use of conflict as a tool for promoting good interaction and advancing relationships. The chapter also outlines the difference between interest- and identity-based conflicts and describes the processes used to address each.

Conflict is normal. It is present in every human relationship. It is a sign of the Creator's commitment to diversity and in fact represents diversity in action. It is the dynamic content of diversity. The management of human conflict is essentially diversity being both valued and negotiated as we facilitate effective relationships in the human community.

Conflict should never be avoided or suppressed. Instead, it should be embraced as a fundamental part of every human interaction. Conflict is the most frequently occurring dynamic in human relationships. And yet it is the most misunderstood and misused element in the whole arena of communication and interaction.

Embracing conflict is easier said than done, of course. A particular instance of conflict can involve a significant emotional overlay that adds stress to the interaction. This emotional component takes the conflict to a level of intensity that is uncomfortable and potentially destructive. At higher levels of intensity, the process of being in opposition becomes its own end, and the purpose and product of the conflict disappear in the dust raised by living in opposition. The emotional component creates so much unpredictable and untenable content that most people simply back away from the conflict, unable to figure out how to deal with it or cope with its pain.

In making conflict normative, the leader creates a frame for conflict that turns it from an event to a process. The more conflict is looked at as a normal occurrence, one that reflects the usual vagaries of human interaction, the more likely it can be handled appropriately. This notion of normative conflict is a relatively recent understanding of the role conflict plays in organizational dynamics. Good leaders recognize that the tensions associated with normative human conflict simply represent the usual and ordinary differences that exist between people at all levels of the human community. Conflict itself is never a problem. However, *unresolved* conflict continues on a growth trajectory that becomes increasingly problematic to the extent that it is ignored or unaddressed. The wise leader, therefore, never ignores conflict; in fact, he or she searches for it in the human community and, always finding it, addresses it in an appropriate and timely fashion.

The good leader recognizes that conflict cannot be avoided. In fact, this leader does everything not to avoid conflict. What the leader does is create an environment that provides a safe space for identifying and expressing conflicts. The leader recognizes that conflict management is the one fundamental obligation that he or she has in the leadership role. Knowing that conflict cannot be ignored, the good leader embraces it. The best way to deal with conflict is through the leader creating an environment that makes it comfortable and safe to engage conflict and a culture where conflict is accepted as part the interaction of the human community. More important, the leader recognizes that opening interactions to the noise, ambiguity, and challenge of expressing differences creates a safe milieu for the expression of those differences, even though it can often be especially demanding for the leader to manage.

Good leaders are responsible for creating a positive context for the work of others. Leaders are continually attempting to provide a framework for work that is positive, encouraging, and growth oriented. A good part of creating this context is building the kinds of relationships that evidence a high level of partnership, openness, and trust. When managing conflict is considered a regular part of the manager's responsibilities, confronting it directly becomes a part of effectively expressing the manager's role. The manager must begin to recognize that fear of confrontation is a significant impediment to resolving interpersonal and relationship-based conflicts.

The best time to address conflict is early in its expression. Seeing a conflict situation emerge is a forewarning that it is likely to blossom. The manager needs to know that conflict does not go away of its own volition. Because it is normal for almost all human interactions, when left unaddressed, conflict simply changes its form and emerges somewhere else in a kind of "wolf in sheep's clothing." The longer conflict simmers, the more difficult it is to resolve. Conflict is never a static process that just sits there, failing to gather energy. It is common for unresolved conflict to grow in intensity as it lies just below the surface, collecting energy and building toward a cataclysmic eruption. Unresolved conflict always intensifies. The good leader has an intuitive sense of the potential for conflict. This person knows that every interaction is rife with the seeds for conflict. Human differences drive its continual unfolding. If not recognized early, the conflict continues to gather potential and to grow in possibility until its more volatile expression becomes likely. The leader must do two things in the presence of the potential for conflict: Address it early and address it appropriately.

Leaders need to recognize that early engagement of conflict means recognizing it soon enough to address it without noise and/or overwhelming personal emotion. In the earliest moments of an interpersonal conflict, the beginning signs of the impending conflict are always present. An attitude of disrespect, an unkind word from one person to another, an offhand remark, or an inappropriate phrase can be early signs of the gathering storm of a conflict. The leader lets no remark or behavior that represents anger, misunderstanding, or personal apprehension go unaddressed. Each of these emotions is an indicator of an underlying set of concerns that begs to be addressed. Interrupting the course of a conflict in these early stages gets the real issues out in the open and raises the chance that addressing them will allay further opportunity for the conflict to accelerate.

In the earliest stages of conflict, the leader is constantly looking for people creating positions and taking sides. Indeed, in the earliest stages, the conflict-driven individual creates boundaries and limits to a view or position as a way of emphasizing the differences. This person often becomes exclusionary or exclusive to perceptions or notions that represent his or her chosen position. Ownership and expression of the position and extreme defense of it create the initial conditions and circumstances upon which further conflict can build.

Fear and avoidance of conflict are main causes of the problems that can arise when a conflict occurs. Another problem is ignorance and lack of use of the legitimate processes of conflict management. When a person becomes embroiled in a conflict, many feelings rush to the surface and begin to be expressed in one form or another, until eventually the person is dealing with feelings rather than the conflict that generated them. As a result, the original reason for the conflict can get lost in the interaction and may even be forgotten, replaced by another reason. In this scenario, ending the conflict amicably does not resolve the underlying problem, which has the potential to bring about another skirmish. The cycle can continue indefinitely, building layer upon layer over the underlying problem and making it ever harder to discern and resolve.

Growth and Transformation

All conflict provides a dynamic opportunity for growth and transformation, and leaders should treat conflict as simply another tool of good leadership. Peter Drucker (Edersheim & Drucker, 2007) has often said that 90% of leadership is addressing human behavior issues. A good proportion of this 90% involves addressing issues that have some form of conflict at their base.

The secret of good conflict management is simple, but the process is not. The secret is to get the parties in conflict to discern the root issues and mutually agree on actions to be taken. Actually building an effective process to accomplish this goal, however, is a complex task.

> **Point to Ponder**
>
> About 90% of the average leader's responsibilities involve dealing with human behavior and human interaction. Given that this is true, why do leaders spend so little time learning how to resolve the issues that arise out of human dynamics?

Conflict management takes into account that people differ in a whole range of ways and that factors as broad as culture, race, gender, social status, and income group and as specific as personal beliefs, family position, mental health, intelligence, and emotional maturity all can influence the onset and process of a particular conflict (**Exhibit 6-1**). It also takes into account that typically the parties to a conflict are unequal in some way, that one party may have a substantial advantage over the other (e.g., the lion's share of power). If a satisfactory outcome is to be obtained, the conflict management process must create equity at the table. It must utilize a mechanism that closely reflects the character and content of the conflict and moves it toward a mutually agreed-upon resolution. This mechanism must take into account the sources and contextual components of the conflict, as well as the content elements. It must also address the power equation so that any unevenness can be accommodated and the process can unfold in a balanced and fair way.

Much of the structural inequity alludes to individual and collective issues generated out of personal insecurity and inequality. In health care, there is an overwhelming and almost suffocating lack of scholarship and dialogue around issues of gender, power, and role inequity. Although frequently alluded to, formal structures and processes specifically directed to resolving conflicts related to inequity are few. The historical masculine and medical caste structure of the health system represents a serious relational disequilibrium and generates a set of values related to power, importance, significance, and value that subordinates roles and creates structural barriers to equity. As value-driven healthcare

Exhibit 6-1   Sources of Conflict

Environmental Sources	**Individual Sources**
• Culture	• Ego
• Nationality	• Personality
• Religion	• Identity
• Class	• Intimate relationships
• Economics	• Beliefs
• Politics	• Perceptions
• Society	• Perspectives
• Resources	• Education
• Race	• Position and role

reforms unfold with increasing intensity over the next decade, issues of collateral relationships, interaction, value, and mutual contribution will come to the fore and require formal processes that help construct more effective and collateral relationships among the disciplines.

Nurses have a unique set of concerns regarding conflicts and their resolution. In some ways, the history of nursing parallels the history of the women's movement, including the subordination and powerlessness experienced by both women and nurses (most of whom have been women). Recently, the education of nurses and other health professionals has gone far toward creating intellectual and role equity, but long-standing medical practices and legal constraints on the scope of practice for various health professionals make these professionals, including nurses, uncertain of the agendas of physicians and administrators and skeptical of the processes that have been used to resolve conflicts among the professions. In the view of many nurses, the relationship they have had with physicians and administrators has historically been one-sided and biased against them, and their sense of being ignored or even silenced has not created a good foundation for building equitable relationships and resolving conflicts, to say the least. Even as nursing practice has expanded to meet critical needs for advanced practice, pejorative enumerations and

Group Discussion

It has been said that health care is both risk adverse and conflict adverse. Discuss this claim. First, consider whether it is indeed true that health professionals avoid conflict to an unusually high degree. To reach a conclusion, it may be helpful to look at the following questions: Does the structure of healthcare services create unusually clear lines of demarcation between people? Is the hierarchical nature of healthcare services a promoter or preventer of conflict? Are there fewer or more personality issues in healthcare settings than in other settings? How does the physician's role and position affect the incidence of conflict?

identification of the role by other disciplines as "midlevel practitioners" or "physician-extenders" and the like characterize these practitioners in subordinating and comparatively subservient roles to those of the historically predominant superior role of physicians. Even though the competencies and skill sets of these practitioners bring a unique set of talents to the continuum of care, there remains a regulatory and structural need to ensure these roles are bounded and subservient rather than collateral, partnered, and equity-based.

As a result, out of frustration, nurses are sometimes inclined to engage in passive-aggressive, hostile, uncooperative, or avoidance behavior, even if the consequences are damaging to themselves. One explanation is that they have not always been able to avail themselves of the maturity that comes with development, dialogue, conflict resolution processes, and any aggregated measure of success. Another explanation may be that the practice and service delivery models in use generally do not require nurses to interact at a high level outside of their own discipline or with other disciplines. Most nursing work is designed to be performed by interdependent nurses or nursing teams assigned to defined groups of patients acting inside of the nursing community. Nurses primarily speak with each other regarding the specifics of nursing practice and the processes and values of nursing-driven decisions and actions. This type of work involves little interdisciplinary interface and sharing and keeps nurses from the vital multilateral interactions that would develop their broader relational skills. The conflicts among nurses and between nurses and other health professionals fall into the category of identity-based conflicts, and their ultimate resolution requires, among other things, reconstructing the relationship between nursing and the other professions.

Leaders, to do their job well, must acquire basic conflict management skills. Most lack these skills or have failed to master them, and as a result in many organizations a whole range of conflicts festers and grows. The avoidance of conflict is one of the singularly greatest sources of human relationship and interactional problems in the workplace. The possession of well-honed conflict management skills has become even more important because of the increasingly interdisciplinary nature of the workplace and because questioning or attempting to change these historically uneven relationships can easily raise the potential for conflict.

Avoiding Unnecessary Conflict

Because conflict is an essential component of human interaction, trying to create conditions in which conflict is completely absent is a pointless exercise. There is generally a prevailing sense that conflict is negative. Nothing could be further from the truth. Conflict is simply the indication of the presence of differences. Ignoring essential differences provides solid ground for encouraging unnecessary conflict. It is not a good use of the leader's skill or time trying to prevent inevitable conflict. Leaders instead should devote themselves to managing conflict, which also includes preventing unnecessary conflict. Some of the conditions that help prevent unnecessary conflict are described in the following sections.

An Environment of Open Communication

It goes without saying that creating a climate of openness and trust is an excellent way to facilitate work and relationships. However, some leaders believe that tightly controlling work creates the fewest problems and that a "tight ship is the best run ship." This is not true for the normal activities of work. Leaders must realize that the relationship between the members of the work team is the most critical factor influencing the extent to which any conflict situation becomes a way of life. A sense that there is nothing that cannot be dealt with, that there are no "undiscussables," is essential to avoiding unnecessary conflicts.

The leader of an organization has enormous influence over the organization's culture. The leader's personal style of relating to and communicating with others sets the tone for the workplace, and it does not take long for others in the organization to discern what is acceptable to the leader and what is not. The leader's behavior toward staff and his or her responses to the stressors and challenges of the work create the model of acceptable conduct and act as the framework for which topics can be approached and which behaviors are appropriate.

> **Key Point**
>
> An environment that abounds with "undiscussables" is an environment that breeds mistrust and unnecessary conflict.

Groups become very skilled at seeing and noting the permissible and the political. Group members know what they must "work around" to get things done. What cannot be dealt with openly and directly is addressed secretively and behind closed doors. It is when open communication is absent that the infrastructure of conflict begins to take form and processes leading to irresolvable differences begin to emerge.

Congruence Between Organizational and Professional Work Goals

A good way to prevent conflict is to ensure that the goals of individual workers and the goals of the organization support each other. It is commonly understood that complementary goals prevent conflict and competitive goals generate conflict. The history of work in America is rife with instances where organizational goals and processes were at odds with the goals and expectations of those doing the work and where inherent conflict sprang up as a result.

When there is goal congruence, people are more open, cooperative, engaged, and supportive and less angry and frustrated. When everyone is clear about expectations and processes and there is a supporting structure that contributes to the meeting of expectations, less conflict is generated.

Of course, congruence between goals is not always possible. Therefore, people must be given the opportunity to disclose what the differences are and how they are affected by these differences. If the reasons for the differences and the character of the differences can be made clear, people find them easier to accommodate or

> **Key Point**
>
> Facilitators must understand that the conflicts they attempt to resolve never belong to them. A conflict is owned by those who experience it, and transferring the locus of control is not good for the parties or the process.

accept. In addition, they find them easier to accommodate or accept if they understand that all issues and situations are transitional (subject to inevitable change) and all relationships operate within the context of the constantly shifting human and relational journey (**Figure 6-1** through **Figure 6-5**).

Managing Conflict Productively

Leaders should devote more resources to the task of recognizing sources of conflict soon enough to handle disputes in the right way at the right time than they should devote to avoiding conflict. Following are some rules for handling conflict appropriately and productively.

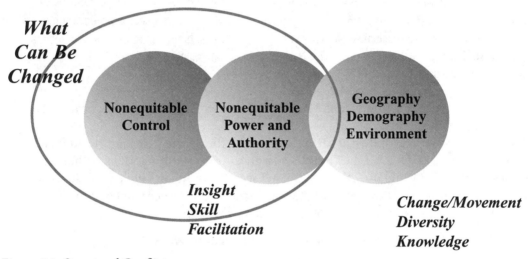

Figure 6-1 Structural Conflicts

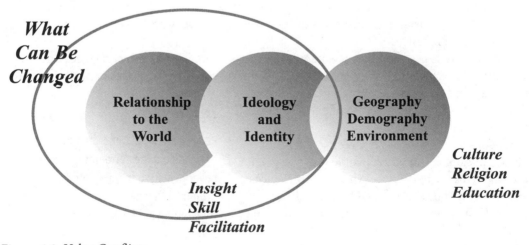

Figure 6-2 Value Conflicts

210

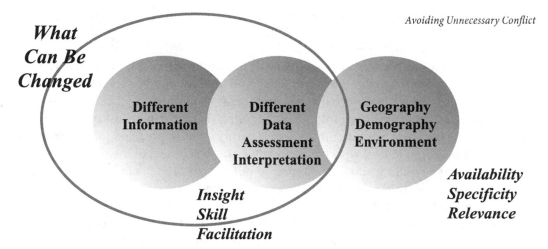

Figure 6-3 Information Conflicts

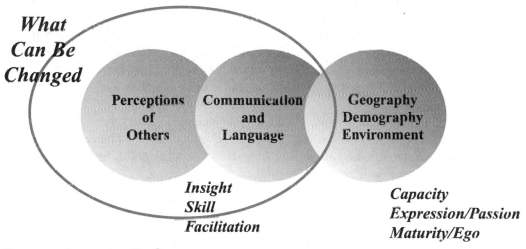

Figure 6-4 Interaction Conflicts

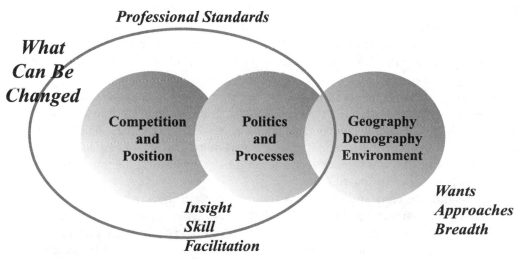

Figure 6-5 Interest Conflicts

Time and place can play a role in diffusing or inflaming a conflict. For example, if a conflict arises in public, the wise leader acts to remove the parties to a private place where the issues can be dealt with directly and freely. In many cases, a conflict first reveals itself at a critical or stressful moment, fooling the participants into believing that the situation is the source of the conflict rather than simply an occasion for its expression. In such a case, trying to deal with the conflict within the context of the situation will likely escalate the conflict, and so it is better to put the participants into a different environment or deal with the conflict at a later time when everyone can focus the dialogue on the issues, not the event.

Remember, conflict is primarily about behavior, not about people (although see the section titled "Identity-Based Conflict," which follows). In dealing with a conflict, the leader needs to be clued in to the behavioral patterns and concerns and their impact on the parties' relationship because the ultimate goal is to sustain their effective relationship. The leader is looking for accommodation and the ability to develop a working relationship that evidences the values and commitment necessary to do the work and sustain it. In addition, the goal is to fix the problem, not to affix blame. No conflict is unilaterally driven—there is always enough fault to go around (thus, faultfinding is a waste of time). Wasting time and resources on trying to affix blame invariably delays long-term resolution of the conflict.

The resolution of a conflict depends on the achievement of some level of agreement about the parties' behaviors or responses. Further, the agreement must be clearly articulated and must be understood by all parties. In addition, at some point the parties must formally/publicly define their common ground in a joint meeting.

If a conflict is to be resolved, the parties must have a sense of ownership over their own feelings and the resolution agenda. The leader must ensure that the parties own their feelings and do not cast them onto the shoulders of others and that they do not interpret what others mean without confirming that their interpretation is correct. The use of "I" approaches is critical to the dialogue. By making certain that each party's insights, feelings, and views are expressed from the party's own perspective and in his or her own language, the leader keeps both parties away from "us versus them" and "you" statements. The leader also can help maintain the focus and flow of the dialogue by making certain it stays within the limits of self-directed communication and personal ownership of the dialogue.

A flip chart or other visual tool can be used to get the conflict elements out in front of the parties in a two-dimensional way. The use of visual tools can overcome some of the obstacles likely to be raised by poorly chosen language and place the ideas of all the parties before their eyes in a way that automatically creates equity. It also can help balance the dialogue and move the issues closer to real resolution by expanding the foundation of understanding between the parties.

Vagueness must be constantly fought. Although a certain amount of ambiguity is unavoidable as people sort out their issues, continuing vagueness obscures the issues and stops the dialogue. The leader must work to facilitate clarity around every issue of concern. By naming names, identifying events, describing situations, and illustrating behaviors, the leader seeks to get down to basics. The goal is to ensure that the real issues and processes are laid out on the table in clear enough terms that all the players can see them plainly.

Each party is looking for something, and unless this something is obtained or willingly given up for something else, the conflict will not end. First, each party must articulate what he or she wants and what the other parties want in a way that all can understand and agree to. Second, each party must leave the conflict with a sense that he or she obtained something valuable, and each must feel good about what the other party got as well. In other words, the parties must view the resolution as equitable. This does not mean that what everyone gets is equal. It means instead that the resolution dispensed to each party is enough to satisfy that party, regardless of how important what was given or obtained may be to any of the other parties.

This advice on how to manage conflict is not all inclusive. For instance, leaders must take into account both situational and cultural factors when trying to facilitate the resolution of a conflict. The flexibility necessary to incorporate these factors is part of the conflict management skill set.

Team-Based Conflict Issues

Working together to provide healthcare services can be intense and difficult and can easily lead to conflict. To reduce the chance of unnecessary conflict, leaders must pay attention to relationship issues and create and keep an open and honest context for the work. Still, even in the best circumstances the behaviors and characteristics of people can lead to conflict (Behfar, Peterson, Mannix, & Trochim, 2008; Payne, 2010).

Different personalities deal with conflict in different ways. Some folks are naturally generators of conflict, whereas others are skilled avoiders of it. Most of us fall somewhere in between these two extremes. Because different interests and personalities are present in the workplace, there is always opportunity for conflict to emerge.

The leader of a healthcare organization should always be on the lookout for the potential for conflict. Because conflict eventually arises in any human environment, its potential is always present, at least to some degree. Further, if a conflict can be detected in its very early stages, it can be addressed soon enough to keep it from becoming critical and requiring extensive intervention. In general, the amount of effort needed to resolve a conflict is directly related to how early in the conflict's development the issues are dealt with.

Leaders must be aware of the main factors that lead to team-based conflict. Some of these are as follows. If team members believe they are on the receiving end of unfair or inequitable treatment, they will descend Maslow's hierarchy of

> ### Point to Ponder
>
> The team, not the individual, is the basic unit of work. The individual must always be seen in the context of his or her relationship with others. Because work is the aggregation of the efforts of many people, for work to result in sustainable outcomes these efforts must be coordinated and integrated. The task of any team leader is to synthesize the efforts of the team members and take advantage of the resulting synergy to achieve the team's goal efficiently and effectively.

needs. Conflict and acting out inevitably occur unless everyone is given an equal opportunity to provide input and have an impact. Another source of inequity is the tendency of people to use each other or the team for their own agendas or advancement. All team members must try to be just and fair in their dealings with each other to ensure the playing field is level and even and everyone is treated impartially.

Everyone does not need to know everything, but there must not be a lack of essential information, especially the information people need to do their work and to function and relate efficiently. In addition, team members must have a common understanding of the information and be able to see it within the correct context. It is common for people to believe they have the information they need but to discover upon further investigation that each has a different understanding of it, and so the team leader must make sure that everyone shares a common understanding. At the end of an interaction, session, or meeting, it is always wise for the leader to poll the group regarding their level of mutual understanding of what has been deliberated and decided on prior to anyone undertaking action. Also, team members need to share their knowledge, insights, and experience in a way that can influence the team and what it does. Expressing what they know and believe is critical to their own sense of value and place on the team and is likewise critical to the viability of the team.

Game playing always leads to conflict. The team leader must therefore be certain that the members are singing off the same song sheet. The rules that govern the team's activities should be clarified to and by the team members at the outset and often along the way. The members also need to be reminded that they will be held accountable for respecting the rules. Although any team must be able to accommodate different personalities, the interaction of team members must keep within certain boundaries. Processes that impede good interaction and communication between members ultimately lead to conflict.

Not acknowledging everyone's unique contribution can be a source of trouble. Every person approaches his or her work differently, has a different array of talents and skills, and has a different background and set of experiences. The team leader must not only recognize the differences between team members but must use them to advance the work of the team. For instance, some members are more reflective, and others are more active. The leader usually does not need to prompt the more active members to make themselves heard—they are usually the first to initiate dialogue or action—but the leader may have to ask the more reflective members for their views. Because the reflective members often have excellent insights and thoughtful opinions, they also must be involved in the team process to ensure the team's work is fully effective. Thus, the leader must recognize that the presence of personality and role differences can actually enhance the team's effectiveness and that getting the full range of contributions from members avoids conflict because no one feels unjustly neglected.

Behavior based on hidden agendas is a prevalent source of team conflict and is extremely difficult to address. Almost every team has members who are not "on board" because they are pursuing their own agendas. They attempt to realize their goals by manipulating others and preventing others from attaining their objectives. They tend to see the world solely from their own position and treat others simply as a means of advancing their own interests. Whether they keep the team from growing or move the team in the direction of their choosing, they damage the integrity of the team and its sense of purpose. The team leader must try to detect these patterns of behavior early in the team process and correct them before they do serious harm. If members are allowed to pursue their own agendas with impunity or for a long period of time, they reduce the team's effectiveness and eventually cause the team to descend into a state of chaos and conflict.

Lack of mutual appreciation among team members impairs team integrity. An old Zulu adage says, "I can only be me through your eyes." Who people are and the gifts that they bring are sacred and important. All team members should believe they have value and are there because they have a unique contribution to make. They should know what it is they offer and be acknowledged for it by the other members. Each member should be aware of the character and role of any other member and understand how to advance and honor his or her own role. By clearly articulating the gifts that everyone brings to the table and the value of those gifts, the team leader keeps all the team members mindful of everyone's importance and thus diminishes the potential for conflict and breakdown.

> **Key Point**
>
> Power is a sensitive issue in health care. For example, the word *power* is rarely used by health professionals, as if they do not really believe it operates in their relationships with each other. Of course, it always does. It is vital that the issues of power and authority be open for discussion because they are critical elements in the interaction of team members at every level of the system.

Power issues are a common source of conflict. How power is dispersed and used has a great influence on the occurrence and intensity of conflict within a team. In particular, conflict inevitably occurs if the expression of power is not seen as competent or balanced, or if the location of power is not seen as appropriate. A team operates like a community, and the team leader has the responsibility to maintain a sense of community among the members. The leader is always looking for breaks and potential problems in the relationship between members as a way of anticipating conflict and dealing with it before it develops into a major crisis requiring substantial time and resources (Zedeck, 2011).

Getting ahead of the conflicts that emerge is the best possible method for diffusing them and mitigating their consequences. The team leader should set up the team's structure and processes to make conflict a normal part of the interaction and relationship among members. The leader should not ignore conflict but instead implement strategies to expose the essential differences between members early enough to resolve the inevitable episodes of conflict as quickly as possible. By valuing and validating differences among team members and accommodating them, the leader reduces the number of conflicts and at the same time decreases the chance that any of them will become crippling.

Identity-Based Conflict

Conflicts generally fall into two categories: interest-based conflicts and identity-based conflicts. Interest-based conflicts arise from circumstances or interactions and often can be resolved quickly. Identity-based conflicts go much deeper and last longer. Rothman

(1997), in laying some foundations, suggested that identity-based conflicts are rooted in threats to people's need for dignity, recognition, safety, control, purpose, and efficacy. For these conflicts to be adequately addressed, their origin and their meaning to the opposed parties must be adequately appreciated. In general, identity-based conflicts have the following characteristics:

- Reflect the parties' culture and beliefs
- Involve questions of identity and sense of self
- Arise out of the parties' commitment to their values
- Are of long duration
- Are the most difficult conflicts to resolve
- Can be passed on from one generation to next

Sources of identity-based conflicts include the following:

- Values
- Religion
- Language
- Heritage
- Culture
- Family
- Community
- Country

Each person has a unique background and set of life experiences and brings a personal and a cultural framework to any dialogue or deliberation with others. Further, because everyone is a unique individual, relationships and interactions exhibit a dynamic pattern and identity-based conflicts are possible. The differences between people create life's mosaic—its fabric. The richness of human experience is driven by the broad diversity that is characteristic of human life and that forms the foundation for human interaction. It is no surprise that for conflict resolution activities to be successful, they must be based on an understanding of the ingrained differences between the parties and must encompass a respect for and appreciation of these differences.

Group Discussion

Look around the room at the other occupants and write down as many differences as you can in a few minutes. After listing all the differences on a flip chart, discuss how each might lead to a conflict. Also discuss how the resulting conflicts might affect relationships, interactions, and the work environment. Then, identify how the different types of conflict are related to each other and consider the possibility that together they could result in an irresolvable state of conflict. Finally, discuss how the conflicts identified could escalate and describe the impact such escalation could have on patient care.

Conflict is a normal part of all human affairs, from marriage to politics. Recognizing this fact encourages us not to ignore conflict, downplay it, or leave it unaddressed. The best strategy is to accept that conflict is inevitable and to acquire the skills and methods for safely and effectively dealing with it, including paying attention to what it means and the positive direction it is trying to move us toward.

Identity-based conflicts are very difficult to either define or resolve. Because they are rooted in historical, psychological, cultural, and experiential factors, their boundaries and content are hard to determine. Because they are deeply embedded in personal sentiments, the contending parties are less willing to compromise. Therefore, they demand a deep and creative engagement.

Protracted religious, ethnic, tribal, regional, and national conflicts are the best examples of the persistence of identity-based conflicts. Long-term, persisting "enemy images" create a permanent "other" that influences notions of equality, equity, value, and identity. Enemy images that are believed to be valid and that are stereotypic are embedded in a group's set of beliefs, hypotheses, or theories about another group. Over time these images become normative and set up intransigent images that reinforce the stereotype and hostility toward it. Group consensus around the beliefs and stereotypes reinforces acceptable enemy characterizations and socially entrenched opposition behaviors as normative parts of the sentiments toward the "enemy group." These behaviors, in fact, become a way of life such that not having them would be inconceivable. Because the idea exists over a sufficiently long time, the "enemy other" often becomes inherently inequitable, less than, innately subordinate, often subject to the grossest maligning, objectification, and the worst levels of inhuman violence. Such hostility reinforces hostility, generates more intensive hostility, and sustains hostility over generations. Like all conflicts, the longer it remains unresolved, the more entrenched it becomes and the more difficult it is to resolve.

Giving the Parties a Voice

When confronted with an identity-based conflict between two or more parties, a "third-party" leader must facilitate the resolution of the conflict. Acting as facilitator, the leader's first job is to give the parties a voice and listen to their essential insights and their perceptions of the conflict. They must be allowed to express where they are located in the conflict and what their feelings are about the conflict. Note that their perceptions do not have to be correct, right or wrong, because the main goal is to simply lay out what each party has experienced from inside the experience. The stated perceptions of each party constitute a personal expression of his or her experience of the conflict and of course are bound to be different from the stated perceptions of the other party. In some cases, the parties' perceptions are so different that an objective third person may wonder if each is describing the same situation, condition, or scenario.

> ### Key Point
>
> Difference is a cause of conflict and, as a prerequisite of dialogue, part of the solution to conflict. In fact, both difference and dialogue are necessary for good and sustainable human interaction.

Point to Ponder

Although conflict is normal, unresolved conflict is dysfunctional. Further, a particular conflict will remain unresolved if it remains unnamed or undiscussed.

Getting the parties to give expression to their perceptions of the conflict is an essential first step in understanding and resolving the conflict. The way the perceptions are formulated should reflect the feelings and sentiments of those who have the perceptions. This stage, when the parties give voice to their sentiments and perceptions, is not the time for structured clarification and process. The facilitator needs to allow the expression of perceptions to be natural and unconstrained. The result is sometimes uncomfortable because the emotion can be intense and raw. Yet intensity of feeling indicates to the parties how critical the process is and just what the stakes are.

These perceptions are accompanied by sentiments and emotions that are largely not grounded in sound facts or occurrences. Historical perceptions of a wrong or fault have often been embellished by story and mythology over the long term to the extent that it becomes difficult to separate the myth from the real, fiction from fact. As has often been done in emerging nations where ethnic groups have played enemy roles for generations, grievances have been acknowledged and accepted as true by all stakeholders, recognized as undeniable, and simply acknowledged as a part of history. Such processes are always followed by significant national or ethnic symbols of forgiveness and separation so that a new foundation or demarcation can be laid, upon which a fresh and emergent pattern of social compatibility can be structured between former divergent ("enemies") groups, representing a level of mutuality and agreement about the future that all parties can agree to.

For there to be movement toward resolution and/or acceptance, the facilitator must make sure that all the issues and all facets of the issues believed by the parties to be critical are laid out in detail, including issues related to dignity, recognition, value, and meaning. There is nothing more threatening to the process of resolution than for a party to believe that his or her story was not told, the story has not been fully heard, or the origin of the conflict has not been fully appreciated and, as a result, that the process is skewed and therefore flawed.

Identity-based conflicts are rooted in the parties' need to protect their value and identity (**Exhibit 6-2**). They believe there is a threat to who they are—a threat to the

Exhibit 6-2   Identity Characteristics

- Needs
- Self-image
- Insight
- Knowledge
- Skills

- Balance
- Clarity
- Investment
- Breadth
- Ownership

very foundation of their being—and they often
respond by going on the attack. For example,
conflicts between nurses and physicians over
practice are rooted in their notions of who they
are as professionals and their sense that their
value and even survival are threatened by the
other professional group. Physicians believe
that nurses jeopardize their independence as
practitioners and their economic well-being,
and nurses believe that physicians obstruct
their ability to practice, grow, thrive, and
contribute. In fact, each group views the other
group as a major threat to its own interests,
predisposing members of both groups to let
their negative perceptions of the conflict inform
every interaction they have on issues of practice
and service.

> **Key Point**
>
> Identity-based conflicts take longer
> to resolve than do interest-based
> conflicts. They arise out of people's
> identity—who people are as opposed
> to what they do—and often have
> substantial historical content. In an
> identity-based conflict, to reach a
> resolution the two parties must come
> to appreciate each other's value and
> respect each other's uniqueness—a
> very challenging task given the
> passionate attachment of each party
> to his or her own identity.

Interest-based conflicts, if left unresolved
long enough, can and often do become identity-based conflicts, but the latter, no matter what their origin, require strategies different from those used to resolve conflicts that are simply interest based. For instance, legalistic and negotiation-oriented strategies tend to alienate the parties to an identity-based conflict. These strategies limit the amount and types of dialogue that occur, preventing the parties from establishing the kind of relationship they need to deal with the issues affecting them. Using resolution strategies aimed at getting to an early agreement can poison the conversation and keep the parties from finding common ground and some points of mutual value and shared identity. People are not willing to compromise those things that they believe are fundamental to their own identity and survival. For them some issues simply are not subject to negotiation.

Time and Patience

In trying to resolve an identity-based conflict, it is a mistake to begin by pushing the parties to compromise, often the strategy of choice for interest-based conflicts. Another mistake is to try to get the parties to separate their feelings from the so-called facts of the conflict because their feelings, especially their sense of identity, are at the root of the conflict. Using a strategy that threatens their identity makes the parties more suspicious of each other and of the conflict resolution process.

The resolution of identity-based conflicts takes a great deal of time, especially the first stages of the process. However, these stages are the most crucial and warrant the extra time and patience. Naming and certifying issues, feelings, and positions clearly at the outset establish a firm foundation on which to construct a process that moves effectively to a successful outcome.

In a traditional negotiation process, the parties try, through compromise, to arrive at a place where they can essentially split the difference. This process works best when the issues are clear, the goals are well defined, and the parties are reasonably clear on what the common ground looks like. Unfortunately, the underlying issues in an identity-based conflict are blurred, and the parties feel especially vulnerable because the stakes are seen as so consequential. The parties therefore are hesitant to compromise early in the process, and moving too quickly toward a resolution could threaten the process itself and prevent the parties from dealing with the underlying issues, in which case these issues would ultimately give rise to another episode of discord.

Building Trust

Much of the early work in the resolution process is directed toward getting the parties to change the way they think about each other and agree on a process and method for interacting. The parties are essentially suspicious of each other. Their suspicion is itself a great source of conflict, and getting to a place where the rules of engagement are clear and can be used as the vehicle for dialogue increases the probability that the parties can work out their differences.

In an interest-based conflict, the root issues are not always put on the table, and the negotiation strategies are typically as important as the issues. In contrast, in an identity-based conflict, posturing and positioning are generally ineffective because the parties need to disclose their powerfully held sentiments and beliefs—those things that reveal who they are and what they do. To build a proper foundation for resolving the conflict, they must fully understand these sentiments and beliefs—their own and those of the other party—and identify whatever common ground exists.

> **Point to Ponder**
>
> Conflicts love to hide in ambiguity. If a conflict remains unclear or undefined, it also remains elusive and hard to eradicate. The parties, only able to deal with the symptoms, almost certainly will allow the conflict to have an impact on all their joint activities, leading to negativity and uncertainty far beyond the boundaries of the conflict itself.

Because of the high stakes involved in an identity-based conflict, the facilitator should move the parties toward negotiations slowly, after a trusting foundation has been established. Often, using informal familiar and familial interaction and relationship development humanizes the participants, makes them real to each other, gives them an opportunity to witness common frames of references related to children, family, and community. These informal opportunities at relationship help again humanize those who had lost their humanity through enemy metaphors of prejudice, objectification, humiliation, and subordination. In the initial stages of dialogue, the facilitator should encourage the parties to set practical goals, such as arriving at a common view of the conflict and agreeing to a description of the issues in a common language. By achieving these goals, the parties are more inclined to accept that resolution of the conflict is a real possibility and can feel comfortable with the resolution process. In short, the parties must develop a sense of relationship with each other before moving further along toward resolution.

The facilitator must realize that building a trusting atmosphere and getting the parties to recognize they each have a substantial stake in resolving the conflict are both essential steps.

By showing the parties their relationship to the larger context, the facilitator helps them see where their common values lie and what might be a resolution equitable to everyone.

The facilitator is likely to find that one or both parties exhibit a currently prevailing pattern of behavior characterized by deviousness, secretiveness, manipulation, and a sense of "us against the world." This pattern provokes a response of unilateral defensiveness that is hard to break through. To fight against it, the facilitator must try to nurture cooperative inquiry, establish credibility, and engage in relationship building. A good part of the resolution process must be devoted to creating a common identity around the issues in a way that allows all the parties to believe they are mutually contributing to a justifiable end of the conflict.

The parties must arrive at a place where they can honestly say what they value and believe. Getting them to this place may not be easy because the parties may have strong emotional blocks that prevent them from articulating their real issues. Sometimes the parties believe they are articulating the issues by stating how they feel, but in doing this they are focusing on the results of the issues, not on the issues themselves. The facilitator must get them to focus on what caused these feelings—the conflicts that lie at the heart of their emotions.

The long-term work involves helping the parties reconceptualize the conflict, perceive their relationship in a new way, change the language they use to describe the conflict, and even change the nature of the conflict altogether. The conflict may be rooted in a lack of clarity, and one or both parties may say things that are inconsistent with what they do. They both need to achieve a good understanding of their own motives and desires before attempting to move toward an end to the conflict. Otherwise, each will be unable to hear the other and understand where the other is coming from.

Finding Differences

As mentioned earlier, each person is a unique blend of differences, and their differences from each other are what make people exciting and intriguing to each other. We celebrate our differences and honor diversity in culture and personality. Yet differences can become an impediment to understanding and relationship, and given enough time any human

Group Discussion

In any organization, unresolved conflict eventually creates a culture of conflict, increasing the incidence of conflict at every level (LeBaron, 2003). After identifying personally experienced unresolved conflicts in the workplace, discuss the impact that each conflict had on relationships in the workgroup. In talking about this issue, consider the following questions: What kinds of factions formed? Did the one conflict lead to others? Did the group leader take any action to ensure that the conflict would be resolved? That it would not be resolved? What was the long-term impact of the unresolved conflict? Was the conflict ever resolved? How?

relationship will give rise to some level of conflict. When it does, those in the relationship must understand that it is not the conflict that is problematic but its nonresolution.

To figure out just what caused a conflict, the parties to the conflict must frame the issue in a way that gives it focus. One method is for each party to ask, what do I want here? To answer this question, each must be clear on how he or she stands on the differences between the two parties. Framing their notion of the conflict or of their position in relationship to it gives the parties a foundation on which to take a position. To get there, they need to ask themselves some specific questions.

Do the parties remember the period before the conflict existed? Looking at the before and after can help the parties give the conflict a time and a frame of reference, allowing them to identify its elements in a way that makes it real. Furthermore, the parties, in reviewing the period before the conflict, give the facilitator an opportunity to see how each perceives the beginning of the conflict and to detect any differences in their perceptions.

What antagonisms emerged? What did they look like? How did they feel? Here, the focus is on perceptions of the moment of conflict. The issues of resentment, behavior change, and cultural and personality differences get expressed in the unique language of each party. Both parties begin to express their special insights about the feelings and animosities that emerged and grew as a result of their differences, and the individual flavor of the conflict starts to become clear. The parties now get a chance to express not only how they felt but why and what it meant to them at the time, allowing the circumstances to be reflected through the lens of personal experience. This process disciplines their insight and forces them to focus on the conditions and circumstances that give form to their sense of the conflict.

Who is to blame and what is he or she to be blamed for? Answering this question is a good way to get to the dynamics of the conflict. In almost every conflict, a strong element of blame lies at its heart. The parties need to get some idea of what the blame is, where it resides, and what form it takes. Not only is it important to uncover the blame, the facilitator must push each party to describe the content of the blame it points at the other party and explain why it is justified. The explanation is likely to make reference to stress, pain, or anguish experienced by the party doing the blaming and indicates how the other party was responsible for it.

These questions get at the fundamental antagonisms causing the conflict. The parties' perceptions and feelings need to be articulated at the beginning of the resolution process for two reasons. First, both parties must see and say where they are in relation to their notion of the conflict. Second, the facilitator must get some sense of where the parties are at the start of the resolution process. The agenda for building the process and achieving reconciliation is constructed at the very beginning of the process. By getting the parties to delineate the differences in their perceptions and positions, the facilitator gains information about the work yet to be undertaken.

To get this information, it is best to talk with each party independently. The facilitator should keep the meetings informal and focused on gathering information and helping the parties get ready for their work within the process. These meetings also offer a good opportunity to discuss the rules of engagement that will be used when all the parties are at the table. Note, however, that the rules of engagement must be finally deliberated and agreed to when both parties are present.

Who Wants What?

People in conflict generally know what it is they believe they want. When individuals or groups are at the point of conflict, they generally have reached the stage of holding black-and-white positions—positions that are mutually exclusive and sit at some distance from each other.

To bring the positions closer, the facilitator must be steeped in the resolution process and look for every opportunity to foster congruence, strengthen trust, and improve the interface between the parties as their relationship begins to grow. As noted previously, the parties to an identity-based conflict must establish a relationship and not simply obtain a resolution of their issues. The facilitator helps them do this by knowing them as well as possible and being familiar enough with their issues and positions so as not to miss opportunities for bridging differences and constructing common ground because such opportunities rarely are presented twice. The facilitator's knowledge is his or her main tool for advancing the process and moving the relationship through the tough times.

ARIA Conflict Engagement Theory

In his seminal work on identity-based conflicts, Rothman (1997, 2013) suggests a format for the resolution process. The stages of the format, which he calls ARIA Conflict Engagement Theory, are antagonism, resonance, invention, and action. They are outlined in the following subsections.

Antagonism

In this first stage the facilitator pushes the parties to express their antagonism, which, besides helping the facilitator move the process along, helps the parties lay out their raw emotions in plain view and, in so doing, diffuses them, thereby reducing the temperature of the conflict. Given the proper context, this initial expression of antagonism also provides extra motivation to do something about the conflict and the negative feelings that it generates—to end the pain and discord and move to a better place, where there is more peace and stability and opportunity.

In addition, it can reveal to the parties their own limitations and constraints. They are able to see how their own intensity of emotion polarizes their views and positions. Although unlikely at this point to be able to make substantial changes, they can at least get a picture of what their positions look like and how strongly they hold their views, possibly opening a window to understanding. Indeed, expressing their antagonism and hearing it reflected back in the language of the facilitator may surprise them and finally make them realize just how fixed, strident, or polarized they have become. After all, the flames of antagonism are fanned by a wide range of emotions that, regardless of their legitimacy, are strongly felt and often just as strongly expressed.

> **Key Point**
>
> Parties to a conflict must be allowed to express their feelings, even their passionate feelings. If not expressed, these feelings become intensified and move deeply inward, poisoning every interaction and preventing a resolution from being achieved. Therefore, facilitators must create a safe space for the parties to get their feelings out.

Point to Ponder

Blame keeps the parties from owning their part of the conflict—from naming their own issues and identifying them as causes of the conflict—and thus keeps them from achieving a resolution. In pointing a finger, each party focuses exclusively on the other party's actions, whereas each should instead attempt to see clearly and admit to his or her role in the conflict dynamic.

In a typical conflict, one or both parties blame the other side to strengthen their own position, at least in their own eyes. Blame serves to escalate the conflict and give it a justification. It creates an "us and them" position, locates the enemy, and defines the terms of opposition. It puts the other party at fault and provides a reason to be angry at and in conflict with the other party. The natural tendency to place blame is best exemplified by the common childhood claim, "He hit me first."

Blame helps the parties avoid focusing on their part in the conflict. By concentrating on why it is the other party's fault, each party evades having to reflect on the role he or she has played. The parties never have to consider how they might have acted differently, experience the pain of admitting their own contribution to the conflict, or engage in the work of reaching a resolution. Indeed, blame suggests that a resolution to the conflict is not possible.

Blame helps keep the conflict external—safe and free of personal content. It puts the responsibility for resolving the conflict in the other party's court and suggests that if the other party would make certain changes or act differently, the issues and the conflict would simply disappear.

Blame never has any real inherent or intrinsic value. The facilitator's best strategy is to pursue naming the feelings of each party and their intensities. Even when restating accusations of blame, the facilitator does not spend time in the blame. Discussing the blame that has been leveled merely helps the facilitator figure out (1) where the parties are in relation to each other and to the issues at the root of the conflict and (2) how to move the parties toward reconciliation.

Blame also generalizes feelings and perceptions and keeps the parties from being specific and reaching clarity. The facilitator's role is to get the parties into and through the blame and on to focus on the particulars and delineate their own positions.

Group Discussion

Greg Shue, manager of a hospital department, was angry with the head of critical care. She had beaten him out of a part of the budget he needed to make programmatic changes in his own department. He occasionally referred to her in derogatory terms and seemed unable to get past his anger, which was beginning to have a serious effect on the relationship between Greg and the other department head and on the entire organization. You are the conflict mediator in this case. How would you begin the conflict resolution process? What would you do to get Greg to own his anger? What would you do to induce Greg to move beyond his feelings and begin dealing with the real issues?

Posturing and positioning commonly act as intensifiers of conflict. They support the culture of justification and rights and lead to rationalizations of the polarization that typically occur in a conflict. The parties give reasons for the polarization and construct a whole logic to support it. In other words, they "circle the wagons" and make the war their cause, rather than the issue at the root of the war. They then devote more time and energy to conducting the war than they ever did in pursuing the underlying issue.

At this stage, the conflict has taken on a life of its own. Nothing the other party does with regard to the issue is right or appropriate. Further, because each party is acting out of his or her own identity, the other party not only does the wrong thing but becomes wrong. The next step is to describe the other party as bad and to conclude that he or she must be opposed. If the one party did not oppose the bad party, the former would be bad too, and in the same way. This would be untenable. Thus, each side builds the polarization between the parties and raises the intensity of the conflict.

Also, as the characterization of each party by the other grows increasingly negative, the less necessary each believes it is to resolve the conflict. Who would want to resolve a conflict if it meant giving up a justifiable fight against what is bad, perhaps even evil? In the mind of each party, what needs to happen is for the other party to stop being bad. If that occurred, the conflict would automatically end.

The facilitator must realize that each party has a selective memory. Each vividly remembers events that led to the conflict and for which blame could be laid on the other party. On the other hand, each tends to forget contributing events for which he or she was responsible, not to mention their own dishonorable motives.

When the negatives run high, each party's desire to resolve the underlying issue wanes. Their energy is instead devoted to building a culture of opposition and to placing themselves in the right. They act to strengthen their position and get it validated by prospective allies. Correspondingly little energy is devoted to pursuing strategies that might lead to a resolution of the conflict.

As time goes on, each party becomes increasingly critical and disapproving of the behaviors, practices, and even culture of the other party. Words and actions become opportunities for the one party to challenge, skewer, or demean the other and further validate continuation of the conflict.

Projection is commonly used by parties in a conflict to strengthen their positions. Projection involves attributing to others problematic behaviors we engage in or embarrassing characteristics we possess. It is universally understood as a defense mechanism for avoiding responsibility for such behaviors and characteristics. In a conflict, one party, in addition to viewing the other party as fundamentally different, might project, for example, unacceptable motives onto the other party and thus avoid confronting the fact that these are his or her own motives.

If this occurs, the facilitator's goal of getting the parties to see what they share in common becomes even harder. Each party resists admitting that the other could in any way be similar because doing so might involve acknowledging parallel objectionable behaviors. Though daunting, the facilitator's task at the outset is to achieve as much clarity about the antagonism as possible, and his or her initial activities largely are spent on getting the parties past this part of the conflict so that they can pursue resolution strategies.

Group Discussion

The parties to a conflict each possess values and beliefs. If the conflict is identity based, their ownership of their values and beliefs and their sense of who they are unavoidably have an impact on their interaction with each other. Assume you are assigned the job of facilitating the end of an identity-based conflict between two people. How do you break through the identity issues to get the parties to talk with each other? What should you explore and settle with the parties separately before you bring them together? Break the discussion group into two and give each sub-group the role of acting as one party in an identity-based conflict (a conflict arising out of a difference in nationality, ethnicity, religion, or politics). List the elements of conflict as they come up during the ensuing dialogue.

Resonance

Resonance is the process of moving away from antagonism and toward the identification of common ground. Through *reflexive reframing* the parties begin to articulate their values and concerns and seek commonalities on which to build dialogue.

In the preceding phase, the focus of each party is on the behavior of the other. Each party's view is outward and other oriented. Reflexive reframing refocuses the gaze of the parties back to themselves so that they can clarify who they are and what they want before trying to fashion a resolution.

An identity-based conflict is likely to involve intangible and subjective issues. The facilitator might have a hard time believing the two parties are talking about the same concerns. In point of fact, they may not be. The two parties are likely to have different cultural and experiential backgrounds, have different perceptions of the conflict, and use different language to express their perceptions. The notion of objective truth is irrelevant because each party cannot help seeing the conflict through his or her own eyes and treating his or her own perceptions as true.

However, by expressing their deepest feelings and values, the two parties start to fashion a common frame of reference. Each begins to sense that the other shares certain sentiments and each develops a fuller picture of the other. By going deeper into their own experiences, the parties build the foundation for future dialogue. They discover that their initial views and positions—those expressed during the first stage—are inadequate and cannot be supported. The personal and "why" questions they ask help turn the conversation into a vehicle for learning about each other's different perspectives and values.

Reflexes come in two varieties, the automatic reflex to external stimuli and the reflective response based on study and assessment. The latter type is characteristic of good conflict management. It requires the ability to step back and look at issues and concerns from a far enough distance to see the whole landscape related to the conflict. The goal of the facilitator is to get the parties to take the necessary step back. Ideally, they would see each other's pictures of the conflict, understand the circumstances and variables placing them in the conflict, and understand how all of that stands in relationship to everything else. Ultimately, the facilitator wants to create a double-loop experience for the parties. Once each has articulated his or her experience and completed the circle of experience, the two parties would link their experiences in a way that exposes their similarities and intersections. Common elements and frames of reference begin to emerge as a result, and the relatedness of the elements become clear to the parties and form a foundation for further dialogue.

The two parties also need to see clearly that both have the same fears, uncertainties, meanings, and values and to recognize that they could find themselves saying the same things. When one party says, "I am concerned," "I am afraid," or "I am angry," the other should be able to admit honestly that he or she could easily utter the same statement. Furthermore, through the "I" form of the expression, the individual ownership of thoughts and feelings ultimately becomes mutual. It is precisely because of the deep ownership each has of his or her own insights and feelings that mutuality can begin to emerge without causing the threats of challenge, accusation, or alienation. It is hard to reject in another what you just affirmed in yourself.

Identity-based conflicts can exhibit elements of reaction. Each party's sense of self may actually be formed in opposition to the other party's sense of self. The parties' discernment of who they are not can sometimes be as important as their definition of who they are. For instance, they might see themselves as not having characteristics that they attribute to the other party, possibly just because they perceive the other party as having them. They are likely to view themselves not just as possessing different interests, but as *being* fundamentally different. Religious, cultural, ethnic, national, and sexual differences often serve as the basis of identity-based conflicts. After all, there is nothing any of us can do about our gender, nationality, ethnicity, or religion, and so these are seen as defining us and differentiating us from the "other."

In health care, discipline, role, function, and license can similarly act to divide people in fundamental ways and create a priori positions that are hard and sometimes impossible to get around. For example, "I am the doctor; the buck stops with me" or "I am the nurse; I manage the processes of care" or "I am the caregiver; I do the work of health care." Each of these statements is partially true, but by holding to them the parties can become polarized and entrenched. Moving them from their positions is a challenging task, but it can be done by persuading them that no role is the most special, important, critical, powerful, or viable and that no person can do what needs to be done if the other parties fail to meet their responsibilities. The fact is that "I am because you are." That is, we are all interdependent, and indeed the clearer I am as to how I stand in relation to you, the clearer I am as to who I am and who I can become. It is essential that the parties understand the interdependence of their roles so that they can reach a sustainable resolution of their differences.

Key Point

Fear keeps people from disclosing how they really feel and focusing on resolving the issues at the root of a conflict. Therefore, early in the conflict resolution process, the facilitator must give the parties a strong sense of safety so that they can confront their anxieties and talk openly and honestly.

227

The parties to an identity-based conflict are faced with a fundamental choice: They can continue to maintain an isolated identity against the world, or they can search for and uncover their common roots and frames of reference and find their mutuality. To get them to do the latter, the facilitator should help them move

- From blaming to articulating their sense of self
- From antagonism toward the other to identification with the other
- From the attribution of negatives to understanding
- From projection to ownership
- From anger to acceptance
- From fear to a sense of safety

As the parties move through these initial stages of the conflict resolution process, they clarify the conflict, obtain ownership of the process, and explain to each other what is most present in themselves, thereby deepening their self-understanding and establishing a foundation for the later stages.

Invention

During this stage, the parties begin to see some payoff for the work they have done. The focus is on inventing solutions that can take the parties to a place where they can live in peace and engagement. In short, they begin the work of resolution.

Their main task is to look at solutions through a larger lens or use a greater frame of reference—in other words, to think outside the box. They should try to develop new ways of looking at the conflict and come up with new solutions. As noted, in identity-based conflicts negotiating a compromise is fraught with difficulty because the parties would view compromising as giving up something of who they are, not simply something they have, and would thus find it unacceptable.

Instead of seeking compromise, the facilitator must challenge the parties to apply a broader framework and see the situation in a new way. They both have a stake in the outcome and stand to gain from a solution. They must therefore reconceptualize the conflict, which is the purpose of the invention process. This process is about developing whole new ways of seeing the issues and working through them. It demands a focus on the practical and the real, and by going through the process, the parties should be able to develop a different vision of their concerns and a different image of each other. In particular, they should recognize that they are interdependent and need each other and that the resolution of the conflict requires everyone to get on board.

The first step is to develop and agree on statements of objectives. These are derived from statements of the issues. They help the parties see and say what they want to get from the process, especially as relates to their fundamental needs for safety, security, value, dignity, and so on. They also inform the more detailed discourse the parties will engage in regarding the steps and processes intended to move the parties to where they would like to be.

> **Point to Ponder**
>
> In trying to resolve an identity-based conflict, the facilitator should help the parties differentiate themselves and develop a clearer sense of who they are and what they bring to the table.

This step includes components that allow the parties to educate each other on what they need and to explain their reasons why. The education expands on what has already been shared but with a new focus on safety, security, values, and so on. Because the issues at the root of the conflict are identity issues, the parties must try to explain how what they are asking for advances or protects their identity.

Working out the details is critical. Watching negotiations, uninformed observers often believe that the haggling that occurs over the smallest detail is disingenuous and foolish. In an identity-based conflict, each detail has implications for the identities of the parties after the resolution, and thus each one counts.

Note that there is a significant difference between interests and needs. Interests generally play a central role in resource- or interest-based conflicts but a subsidiary role in identity-based conflicts, where needs are primary. Consequently, in an identity-based conflict, the most critical task is to get parties to express their needs and then to reach an understanding of their interests based on their needs. For example, as they see it, the nurses in a healthcare organization need to give care to patients unconstrained by financial considerations. On the other hand, the managers, as they see it, need to ensure the financial health of the organization. Both needs—the nurses' need to give good care and managers' need to ensure financial viability—relate to a common interest, ensuring the existence of enough financial resources to render good service to the public. If the two groups understand that because of their needs they share an interest, they are more likely to reach a resolution of their conflict.

Of course, achieving a resolution does not mean that the parties get everything they desire. At best, they can negotiate a method for meeting their needs—a method that may involve working together, such as one of those described next.

Sometimes differentiating between the parties more clearly, that is, accentuating and enumerating their differences, can lead to a more suitable resolution for each. Although their needs may differ, clarifying them and seeking alternative ways to satisfy them through common action can help move the parties to a new place. For example, imagine a respiratory therapy union is seeking greater recognition for its members and a stronger role for its leaders, whereas the management wants a reduction in complaints and

Group Discussion

Nina Conners really did not want to settle the issues she had with Frank Kliener. They had been feuding for 3 years. Both she and Frank used their conflict as a way of getting more for their own departments and keeping their staff energized and competitive. However, the organization has been paying the price, and its goals are sometimes held hostage to the war between the two departments. Discuss how a mediator would begin to resolve this conflict. What are the apparent issues? What might be the real issue? How would the mediator structure the resolution process? As part of the exercise, create a resolution plan that contains steps for addressing the issues and resolving the conflict.

grievances instituted by the union. Both groups agree to apply a different method of problem solving, one in which the union leadership plays a more direct role. The result is less use of the grievance procedure. Here, the different needs of the two groups provide a basis for resolving their conflict creatively.

A second technique involves expanding the playing field so that the parties can each get more of the resources they need. For example, nurses may request more staffing, and management may want to save more money. The two groups may agree that if the nurses meet set productivity targets, management will use part of the savings to hire more nurses. By consenting to work together to expand the organization's resources, they each help meet their own needs and those of the other party. The result is a win–win resolution of their conflict. To reach a mutually beneficial resolution, the parties usually have to identify joint activities that move them past the issues that prevented them from ending their conflict in the past.

If the parties find that their needs are seemingly irreconcilable, the solution may lie in offering compensation for not meeting a certain need by bestowing something different of equal value. If one party is asking for money that the other party cannot afford to give, it may agree to accept something it views as equally valuable, such as more vacation time. The two parties must engage in clear and creative dialogue to ensure that the substitute is truly viewed and explicitly accepted as equivalent; otherwise, the issue of just compensation will likely arise later and cause problems and further conflict.

The leader-facilitator must look for signs of enough movement and energy to take the parties to the next step—or provide the necessary energy. There is nothing like a small success now and again for maintaining the momentum. Once successes begin to occur, they serve to spur the process and move it in ways that nothing else could. The process, energized by the successes already achieved, begins to change the dynamic, the emotions, and the relationship of the two parties without any further intervention. Through good timing and careful pushing, the facilitator can get the parties to work on the more difficult issues in the midst of good momentum, increasing the chance that they will be finally settled.

The inventing stage is when the parties' interaction changes from being oppositional to being collaborative. It is an essential stage on the journey to a resolution, and the techniques of differentiation, expansion, compensation, and momentum all have the potential of increasing the probability that the parties will achieve an end to the conflict.

> ## Key Point
>
> Conflict resolution is a process with its own timing and techniques. It requires training and experience. Leaders should develop the necessary skills and practice using them until they are adept at bringing parties in conflict step by step through the process to a sustainable settlement of their differences.

Action

The final stage is devoted to crafting a plan of action. There is nothing more disheartening than to get through the touchy issues and concerns, establish a strong commitment to pursue possible solutions, build an effective relationship, and then have the process fall apart because an action plan either could not be constructed or was not detailed enough to guide the parties to a final resolution.

As the process progresses toward action, the parties need to reaffirm where they have come from and where they believe they are in relation to their own needs and their interaction with each other. The mutual understanding that results serves as the ground for the subsequent focus on action. In the action phase, the new questions are what to do, who is to do it, why is it being done, and how to do it.

The first step is to set the agenda for action. What are the priorities of the agreements reached? Where do the parties start? What are the items that must be translated into substantive work, enabling the agreed way of relating and behaving to be realized? These questions serve as the basis for the next level of critical dialogue. Here again patience and attention to detail are required from both parties and from the leader-facilitator.

Setting the agenda includes deciding the priority of actions, their timing, their criticalness, and what other actions must be done in preparation. It also includes reaching an agreement on who is to be accountable for the actions.

New kinds of structures and institutions may have to be constructed as vehicles for implementing the actions. If built early on, they provide a framework for implementing the actions and evaluating their progress. They also help ensure that the issues important to the parties are addressed as expected and that any problems or concerns that arise are defined precisely (Moore, 2003; Ramsbotham, Woodhouse, & Miall, 2011).

Once problems are defined, they need to be solved, which means building problem-solving mechanisms into the implementation process. Unaddressed problems have the potential to negatively affect the relationship between the parties and eliminate the progress made to date.

The parties need to clarify immediate and long-term goals and priorities based on the critical elements identified during the reflexive reframing process (which occurs in the second stage of ARIA). They also need to ensure that the principal, pivotal, and relational items are handled first during the implementation.

The facilitator must try not to upset the delicate balance achieved between the parties. The facilitator's tasks include

> **Point to Ponder**
>
> A conflict resolution facilitator must keep the parties centered by reminding them what is at stake and which issues need to be addressed. The facilitator must also remind the parties of the expectations agreed to so that these can be reaffirmed or altered as the process moves forward.

determining the specific needs each party wants to satisfy as a result of the implementation process and devising an evaluation schedule so that progress can be assessed at critical points. Evaluating the process regularly keeps the parties on board and ensures the process remains in line with their expectations.

Equally critical is the assignment of accountability for specific outcomes. Who does what should be a practical rather than a political issue, yet at this stage politics often take precedence in a way they never should, typically because the skills, talents, and roles of the participants have not been discussed in advance of the assignment. These must be ascertained before the point of assigning accountability if political machinations are to be kept at a minimum.

Content (goals) must always be placed before process (methods). Once the parties set their goals, however, they need to choose methods for achieving them. In thinking about methods, they need to anticipate potential impediments and select those methods that are most likely to succeed.

The parties should keep in mind that each is going to judge the other by his or her actions because these actions are the visible evidence of that party's commitment to the agreement. They represent what the one party has done on the other's behalf. The parties' actions therefore require as much attention as any of the other components of the resolution process.

The leader-facilitator must always keep the parties focused on what is at stake and how important it is. The parties must have the sense that they are a part of a meaningful effort that is larger than their own contributions and that will lead them to a better place.

In any conflict resolution process, no matter whether the conflict is interest or identity based, the leader-facilitator must establish his or her neutrality at the outset. If that cannot be done, the leader-facilitator may consider relinquishing his or her role. A facilitator who is seen as too close to the issue or unable to act in a neutral manner is more of a hindrance than a help.

The facilitator must be as committed to the process as to the parties. He or she has an important position of trust and is responsible for moving the dynamic in critical ways. If not careful and skillful, the leader-facilitator will cease to be credible to the parties and will lose their confidence, thereby crippling the process and ensuring that further problems will arise.

The facilitator must make it clear at the outset that he or she is working for the whole, not one side or the other, regardless of how he or she got there. Further, the parties must agree to the notion that the facilitator is neutral or the process simply will not progress. If one side or other is paying for the facilitator's services or the facilitator holds a specific role in the organization, accommodation may have to be made at the outset of the process to ensure that the parties trust and support the leader-facilitator equally.

Although identity-based conflicts are the most difficult of all conflicts to deal with, they can be resolved using the processes and mechanisms outlined here. Many of them are allowed to continue because leaders have no idea that these tools even exist and mistakenly try to use approaches suitable only for interest-based conflicts.

In the current world of health care, the potential for conflict is greater than ever. The various disciplines and workgroups are being forced to revise their relationships and their boundaries—or even establish them for the first time. Team-based and continuum-driven approaches to service place a great emphasis on who people are rather than simply what they do (Caspers & Pickard, 2013; Cooperrider, Whitney, & Stavros, 2008). Thus, a vital part of the leadership role in the new age of health care involves working through the differences between professionals and building mutuality as a basis for preventing unnecessary conflict and resolving unavoidable conflict when it arises.

Interest-Based Conflict

Interest-based conflicts are situations that present the potential to affect or compromise the impartiality of a person or an issue because of the likelihood of a conflict between an individual's self-interest and professional interest or public interest. In legal terms one representation of interest-based conflicts is a situation where an individual party's responsibility to a second party limits the first party's ability to discharge its responsibility to a third party because of interest conflicts. In negotiating interest-based conflicts, the substantive assumption is that parties in conflict are much more amenable to reach mutually satisfying decisions when their respective interests are honored and met in a way that suggests mutual advantage or satisfaction.

Most interest-based conflicts involve questions related to the distribution of interest among the disputants, often related to money, property, personal benefit, or obligations. With these sources of conflict, questions relate more to a symbolic "pie" and just how equitable the pieces of that pie can be distributed among the stakeholders that have some investment or interest in all or parts of the pie. Interest-based negotiation depends much more strongly on win–win processes, and many of the elements of interest-based dialogue and negotiation are directed to achieving that kind of outcome.

Types of Interest-Based Conflicts

Like any other human dynamic, conflict has content, particular elements, and specific processes. Kinds of conflict generally fall into relationship-based, value-based, structural-based, data-based, and related interest-based categories. Each one has its own characteristics and elements that mark it as unique. The leader becomes skilled at identifying the kinds and characteristics of conflict being dealt with and the responses that best address them.

Because the leader is always looking for specific conflicts, it is wise to become skilled in identifying the particular characteristics of conflict that most often appear within the culture of the service or department. Each setting is unique with regard to the makeup of the staff and the stressors on them and the work that they do. The good leader makes a conflict-potential assessment as a part of delineating which strategies are going to be most helpful in dealing with conflict. In this assessment, the leader attempts to get a handle on those specific potentials for conflict that will most often be a concern in the ordinary management of the service.

The leader looks at the makeup of the staff, the demographics (both cultural and age related), the breadth of the work, and the skill level of the staff. Embedded within these factors is the potential for specific kinds of conflict that may recur. In this manner, the leader makes the potential for conflict a normal and usual part of her or his organizational and resource planning. This leader knows that the greater the awareness of the circumstances and characteristics of conflict, the earlier it can be addressed appropriately.

Relationship-Based Conflicts

In any work environment, there are a number of personalities and situations whose vagaries create conditions that can lead to conflict. Differences between people always provide a source for a variety of relationship-driven crises or conflicts. Differences in personality create problems in interaction and communication and often lead to misunderstandings.

These differences can frequently lead to specific altercations reflecting emotional involvement and personal animosity. Left unaddressed, these differences can escalate and create real polarization between the involved parties and those who relate to them. Relationship conflict is the most frequently experienced conflict in most organizations. Communication irregularities emerge and miscommunication becomes common. Negative behavior becomes repetitive and, if not resolved, becomes a way to sabotage and offend the opposing party, which can affect the work, workers, and those they serve.

The good leader recognizes the potential for this conflict early in the process. Usually, unkind words, snide comments, asides, negative comments to others, and avoiding behaviors are the early signs that a relational conflict is present. Because the leader always expects some level of conflict to exist, she or he is able to see these signs and begin to take action right away.

The leader first must get at the originating source of the conflict. Confronting both parties separately with regard to the behaviors expressed is the critical path to getting at the root problem underlying the behaviors. Beginning the questioning with an open-ended approach is best. The leader might say one of the following:

I'm noticing that . . .
Can you tell me . . .
I'm wondering if I'm seeing . . .
Help me see if I'm perceiving this right . . .

At this stage, the leader is just trying to get a level of understanding about the existence of a problem and the basic perceptions of what the problem might be through the words of each party. Through this process, the leader is simply validating whether a problem exists and the underlying nature of the concern. The leader is also ascertaining the degree of perceptive agreement that exists between the parties regarding their issues. The leader initially responds to emotions and feelings. It is impossible to get at the problem without first going through the emotional content of each party's issues. In relationship conflict, the parties are reacting to their own feelings and impressions of what has happened to them and how they are feeling about it, rather than to the real issue that may be the causative factor.

If the leader tries to get to the causative issues too soon, the parties may block and refuse to move there because they have not had an appropriate opportunity to work through the emotional content related to the issue. Sometimes the leader might need to carefully move individuals through their feelings by validating and supporting the person while clarifying the underlying issues along the way. The leader attempts to get the individual to a more reality-oriented place from which some rational work might be done as the individual moves through the conflict. At some point, the parties must be in the same place to move the conflict closer to resolution. The leader attempts to prepare each to understand where both individuals are in relation to feelings and content. The leader, acting as a neutral, seeks to have each party express his or her feelings with a language that accurately expresses feelings without further polarization, energizing a new level of emotional intensity.

As the process moves toward engagement, the leader seeks to focus on expression and rules of engagement as well as to remind each party of the expectations regarding communication and conflict management in the service or the department. Having created an appropriate milieu for conflict management, the leader wants to ensure that the parties are aware of the expectations and need to resolve issues that impede the ability of the staff to communicate and deal with differences. The leader identifies the conflict resolution process as one of the mechanisms that exemplifies the components of communication within which the unit operates. It is only at this point that the leader begins to bring the parties together to a dialogue and to work through their differences.

Values-Based Conflicts

Perhaps one of the most difficult classes of conflict to resolve is one that represents differences in values. Conflicts of these types are often categorized within the context of identity-based conflicts discussed earlier in this chapter. Every person brings different experiences and beliefs to the expression of their human journey. Cultural, social, religious, moral, and personal values are all part of what defines an individual. In a multicultural society such as that reflected in the American experience, cultural and personal differences are a common experience. Yet with the richness of these differences comes the inevitable conflicts that arise when individual values come in conflict with the values of others. The leader creates a culture of acceptance and openness to differences and to the vagaries of response they reflect. In anticipation of the potential for conflict, the leader sees to it that cultural and value awareness is inculcated into the educational and developmental activities of the service. Everyone should be expected to participate in activities that teach them about the value and practice of acceptance and about the negative behaviors that are unacceptable between and among different ethnic, cultural, national, and religious groups.

Like identity-based conflict, values-based conflict is very difficult to resolve late in the cycle of conflict management; it is wise to confront it at the earliest possible moment. A breach in the code of conduct or expectations of behavior should be addressed as soon as it happens. The absolute unacceptability of such patterns of behavior should be clear to everyone at the outset. Refusal to conform one's personal behavior to these rules of good relationship should be grounds for the strongest disciplinary action. Ethnic discrimination has no room for dialogue or debate. Any discrimination based on color or disparaging remarks that reflect on ethnic origins have no legitimacy. In a world of many colors and ethnic backgrounds reflecting the broadest array of human beings, any conflict based on this has no room for negotiation and misunderstanding. In the human experience, there are some a priori considerations that operate beyond question. Race and ethnicity are two of them. The only room for conflict in this arena is where a misunderstanding or misrepresentation of one's remarks or behavior has occurred and needs clarification and restating between the parties. Cultural or language difficulties or misrepresentations can create a perception that simply may not have been intended. The process of continuous cultural and values education for staff should keep such misunderstandings to a minimum.

Religious and values differences can create significant problems. A number of problems can arise from religious differences related to beliefs, practices, and accommodation. Special considerations to religious and values practices can create negative feelings in others who do not hold the same beliefs. Resentment and feelings of preference can emerge, creating conflict. Here again, being clear in advance about what the expectations are regarding the presence of staff with different practices and the impact of those on the staff relationship is a critical obligation of the leader. Adjustments required in the schedule and even assignments and role adjustments need to be clear to all staff members with attention paid to how equity is maintained between and among staff members. Achieving equity between and among staff members with different religious or values needs is challenging for the leader and the staff. Dialogue and negotiation regarding these adjustments must be delineated up front with the staff. This approach keeps the issue before the staff, makes it a part of their ongoing work experience, and creates an expectation that such accommodations are always a part of the work environment.

When accommodations to the expression of particular religious practices are especially difficult for staff to accept or verge on creating resentment, the leader must reanimate dialogue around the differences in light of reinvigorating acceptance. The leader and staff can find creative ways of addressing the related issues and resolving the conflicts these issues generate. If the leader has been successful in the aggressive creation of an environment of acceptance and openness, the expectation is that such problems can be dealt with and ultimately resolved.

In cases where there is intractable religious-based conflict, it is often wise for the leader to expand the dialogue and include experts from outside the service to guide the discussion and advance resolution. It is often helpful to involve pastoral assistance from representatives from the religious traditions at issue and have them help the participants find some common ground and define areas of resolution or accommodation. The leader always acts as a resource purveyor when conflicts require an alternative mechanism for resolution.

In values-based conflicts, it is also helpful for the leader to expand the dialogue to values that can be shared by all participants. Those values that operate in the broader human context and reflect common human needs and interests can help refocus the issue to one that engages human experience, regardless of value tradition or expression. Attempting to find common areas of value (such as family, home, nation, loyalty, sentiment, children) can change the emotional and relational content of the conflict and create a common frame of reference for its resolution that might not have originally been anticipated.

Finally, it is important for the leader to know that it is sometimes necessary to allow people to agree to disagree. Values are sacred to the individual who holds them; they can't easily be surrendered to others. The leader may have to get the parties to determine how they will live with their differences and make the necessary accommodations to those differences as a part of their relationship. Respect is critical to effectiveness of this process. If each can respect the position of the other, common ground can be found and progress can be made with regard to the quality of the work relationship.

Structure-Driven Conflicts

Structure-driven conflicts recognize inequities inherent in the system or structure of work. These can be classified as inadequate or unfair policies, processes, rules, behaviors, and practices, as well as contextual and organizational factors that inhibit cooperative relationships.

The leader recognizes that no workplace is free of structural and operational challenges to the capacity to do work and to build relationships in the system. Differences in pay grades, benefits policies, reward systems, and job and role status all contribute to perceptions of structural inequity. Even if there is a rational basis for these practices, the inherent inequity needs to be addressed as a possible source of unresolved conflict.

The leader recognizes that there must be openness with regard to people's specific concerns about any particular structural inequity. The leader acknowledges its presence and clearly enumerates the logic behind the apparent inequity. Understanding the value of implementing a particular advantage by one group in relationship to others is a valuable first step. In those places where the inequity established is sufficiently egregious, mechanisms and efforts at self-correction must address the structural element. Where such inequities can be changed or struck down in the organization, they should be, as soon as possible, with a solution that can actually be implemented.

There is a perceived inequity and imbalance at the professional level in a number of organizations. These perceived imbalances generally indicate that one profession or work group is preferred or treated favorably compared with another profession or work group. This perceived inequity often creates much internal conflict in the organization that may not always be directly expressed. Hidden conflict operates as an organizational subtext or frequently lies just below the surface. In this specific set of circumstances, the leader must recognize the foundations of the perceived inequity early and clearly. If it is status inequity evidenced by differentiation of role or reward, the justifications and support for these differentiations must be clear enough to make sense to the group that feels disadvantaged. Although these inequities cannot always be changed, they can be understood. The role of the leader is to generate such understanding.

Where there are more challenges in justifying the inequity and it does not appear to be legitimate or functional, the leader must support individuals in undertaking a process in which the inequity can be actively addressed and pursued further. In such circumstances, advocacy for a particular approach or solution, communication with the appropriate leadership individuals, or structural or organizational approaches to finding solutions must be determined by the stakeholders in the conflict. Without the leader advocating for a specific process for problem resolution, the structural problem will continue to frustrate and challenge the effectiveness and integrity of the work group.

Additional structural challenges that can generate conflict relate to the environmental or the architectural construct within which work unfolds. In many clinical organizations, the structures of the organizations impede the effectiveness of the work. Where the structures can be altered, they should be. Where the architectural and structural elements of work cannot be altered or adjusted, those affected by the structural impediments can explore mechanisms and methods for accommodation or modification. In addition, continuing leadership attention and focus must be centered on addressing the structural barrier in a way that ultimately removes it. This emphasis indicates that the leader is committed to supporting the clinical work. The leader also represents in this activity an understanding that these issues are part of her or his role in continuously challenging those structural elements that do not support the clinical work of the organization. Whether the architectural modifications or structural adjustments can be undertaken is not as important as the commitment of the leader to continuous support of the staff by challenging organizational leadership to modify structural impediments and evidence of this commitment to the clinical work of the organization.

Data-Based Conflicts

Conflicts related to data are generally driven by either limited access to information or lack of information. Information is critical to the effectiveness of organizations in today's clinical workplace. Without appropriate information in a useful configuration, clinical work cannot be successfully undertaken. In fact, the complex of information necessary to do the work now makes the work completely information dependent. This information is critical to the ability of any of the disciplines to fulfill their obligations in rendering clinical service throughout the healthcare system. Furthermore, business, clinical, support, and material information must interface to create a sufficient data foundation upon which effective clinical choices can be made. Information now must be seamless with the work and reflect a portability and mobility that links the provider in real time with data essential to work quality and effectiveness. The growing intensity of the generation and interface of information creates some of the most difficult and intractable contemporary problems and conflicts.

Information is resource intensive. As a result, there is wide variability related to the distribution and quality of hardware and software across the healthcare system. Emphasis has historically been placed on building a business infrastructure and information system, and much business sophistication has emerged as a result. In the growing accountable care environment, clinical information infrastructures are just now being expanded, perfected, and linked to business and clinical infrastructure in ways that can have an impact on resource use and clinical decision making. However, information priorities, mechanisms for generating information, tools for using data, distribution of resources in building information infrastructures, and the quality and kind of information generated all have an impact on organizational effectiveness and integrity. Therein lies the source for the emergence of conflict. Each of these issues can generate its own internally fixed sources of conflict from access, availability, accuracy, quality, efficacy, and utility of information.

The leader must recognize that a fit is necessary between resource allocation and information usefulness. Because there are intersecting groups, all requiring various components of the information complex, some level of agreement must be achieved as to what information is necessary, important, and vital to clinical decision making. Organization-established priorities and clinically useful data processes and information must be interfaced in a way that is wise and reflects service utility. In addition, the leader must ensure that there are structural and process formats within which these priorities and elements should reflect the useful and common set of criteria to which all stakeholders have contributed.

The leader's role is to reduce the structural opportunities for conflict by ensuring that appropriate processes and interfacing regarding information collection, management, and generation have been delineated and structured in the organization. The leader makes sure that the right stakeholders are present so that deliberations include those whom decisions will affect. When issues have been overlooked or forgotten, the leader, recognizing that the process is fluid, brings the stakeholders together again to deliberate and reassess, with the intent of establishing a process that works successfully. Where there are challengers to the skill set and ability of the stakeholders, the leader ensures that appropriate experts and expertise are available to guide the team to correctly delineate needs and resolutions for information management solutions. Through this complex of activities and systems approaches to handling the information infrastructure, the leader creates an ongoing mechanism that embeds conflict resolution in the information system utilization process.

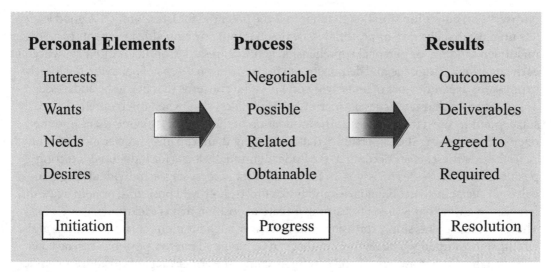

Figure 6-6 The Interest-Based Conflict Resolution Process

In each of the arenas of interest-based conflicts are specific and unique activities related to resolving conflict. Although this chapter certainly introduces some of the steps leaders can take to address conflict, it isn't comprehensive. The leader must recognize that conflict management is a significant skill set and obtain as much development and education as necessary to build conflict management skills. Facility in conflict management comes with discipline, practice, and time. The leader, recognizing how important conflict management is to successful group interchange and group dynamics, therefore commits considerable time and energy to understanding and developing those skills.

In dealing with all interest-based conflicts, a leader acts essentially as a mediator, a neutral third party who helps the parties resolve their issues and bring closure to the conflict. There is much more negotiation and give-and-take than in the resolution process for identity-based conflict. Offers are made and countered as the parties try to work out an agreement consistent with their interests.

The mediator typically undertakes two kinds of intervention: contingent and non-contingent. The noncontingent interventions focus on the processes necessary to any mediation. The contingent interventions are implemented in response to specific circumstances arising from the process itself. Problems, emotions, issues, and other contingencies can individually or collectively have an impact on the mediation process (**Figure 6-6**), and the mediator occasionally has to respond by adjusting the process accordingly.

Isolating Interest-Based Conflicts

As with all conflicts, as we have emphasized in this chapter, leaders must recognize that early engagement of a conflict is important in interest-based conflicts. Here, the leader recognizes as early as possible the need to address the "noise" related to an emerging conflict between parties. From the earliest stirrings of conflict between persons, signs of the impending conflict are present. If the leader is aware, she or he notices an attitude of disrespect, unkind words from one person to another, offhand remarks, an inappropriate phrase, or an emerging situation that has in it the potential for later conflict. A good leader lets no remark, behavior, or potential issue that has in it any embedded elements of anger, misunderstanding, or personal apprehension go unaddressed. Conflict is often evidenced in early emotional language and demonstrated in particular patterns of behavior. Such early expressions are indicators of underlying or emerging concerns that beg to be addressed. These are early characteristics of interest-based conflicts that, when interrupted in an early stage, point to substantive issues at the foundation of the conflict, moving them into the open and increasing the opportunity that addressing them can allay acceleration of conflict.

In these earliest stages of conflict, the leader continually looks for individuals creating positions or taking sides on issues. In fact, in the very earliest stages, individuals begin to drive conflict, construct boundaries and limits for strongly held positions, or demarcate differences in a way that represents a strong unilateral position that is exclusionary or exclusive. The individual ownership, expression, and defense of such positions create conditions and circumstances upon which further conflict can be built and interest positions can be taken.

Through constant awareness and careful listening, the leader prepares to address conflict at the earliest possible moment using appropriate tools. It is vital for the leader to identify the key elements of the impending conflict situation as quickly as possible. What most often appears are signposts to real issues that are deeply buried and of which the emerging conflict is symbolic. The ability of the leader to dig deeper to find the source of the conflict is critical for problem solving (double-loop problem solving). Often, the conflict-laden language represents feelings, not circumstances. These feelings generally mask the true roots of the conflict.

In interest-based conflict resolution, the leader's role is to enumerate feelings and sentiments, allowing them a language and expression, with the intent of finding the underlying issues that are driving the conflict expression. There are often triggers, remarks that serve to indicate the intensity of feeling and perception, the leader will need to sort through and get past to enumerate the conflict. Often the leader hears feelings and response triggers similar to the following:

"She always does this to me."
"He is forever dumping this on me."
"She never stops criticizing me."
"He always makes me so angry."
"What she says or does just wants to make me scream."
"He is mean to me all the time."

These comments are filled with reactive emotional content. These sentiments represent feelings of powerful emotions representing a sense of impotence and helplessness. Sometimes these feelings are even accompanied by related behaviors; at times they are merely feelings. Either way, these feelings are powerful indicators of an impending and a potentially irresolvable conflict if they are not addressed.

Of course, not all conflict can be addressed by the leader on the spot. Good conflict resolution may require that the conflict temporarily goes into the leader's "parking lot" of responses until it can be more reasonably and fully addressed. Even so, when the leader hears comments from an aggressor in the conflict or from the offended individual, it is important that an immediate response be offered while noting the potential for longer-term follow-up action. Short, yet key, immediate responses from the leader to the individual are advisable. Some sample responses are the following:

> "I'm concerned about what I'm hearing; I'll need to talk with you about it after we finish this task (work, procedure, meeting, etc.)."
>
> "I hear what you're saying, and I think we need to talk about it after we're done here."
>
> "I'm very unclear about what you are saying, and I think we need to talk about it right after we're done here."
>
> To the offended person the leader might respond:
>
> "I need to know more; let's talk when we're done here."
>
> "I'm concerned about how you're feeling right now. Let's talk when this task (meeting, procedure, work, etc.) is finished."

Note that the leader addresses the fact that there is an issue but postpones focusing on the issue to a more appropriate time. Also, note that the leader does not address all parties to the conflict immediately. The leader needs to establish clarity around individual perceptions and reactions to the conflict before purposeful collective resolution activities begin. At the outset simply getting notions, perceptions, and facts related to individual responses to the conflict is a critical element in the initial data-gathering process that informs the later resolution processes.

Perhaps the most important aspect of straightening out the underpinnings of conflict is found in gathering all pieces of the information related to the conflict. The good conflict leader pays attention to what is being said and what is being felt. Getting to the facts of the conflict requires travel through an emotional landscape, dealing with perceptions and feelings first because these lead ultimately to a deeper understanding of the situation, clear contextual framework for the conflict, and opportunities for the parties to be fully heard and to express sentiments early in the process. What happens most often is that the leader seeks to resolve the conflict too early in the process, hoping that by doing so the leader can short-circuit the conflict and its emotional content in that way keeps it from escalating. However, the opposite occurs. In moving too quickly the leader fails to address strongly felt personal sentiments, emotions, feelings that, left unaddressed, cloud and slow the movement to meaningfully addressing the facts of the conflict.

Ten Steps to Resolving an Interest-Based Conflict

The resolution of an interest-based conflict typically includes 10 steps (**Figure 6-7**). Each step requires a different amount of time and a different approach. By keeping track of each step of the process, the mediator can discipline the parties and keep the process moving steadily in the right direction.

Establishing the Initial Relationship

The mediator's first task is to establish credibility with the parties and introduce them to the process. A conflict resolution process has components and rules that the parties must understand and agree to if the process is to result in a resolution.

Developing Strategies to Guide the Process

Discussing approaches and processes, as well as the rules of engagement, with the parties up front is a good way to strengthen the relationship between all the participants.

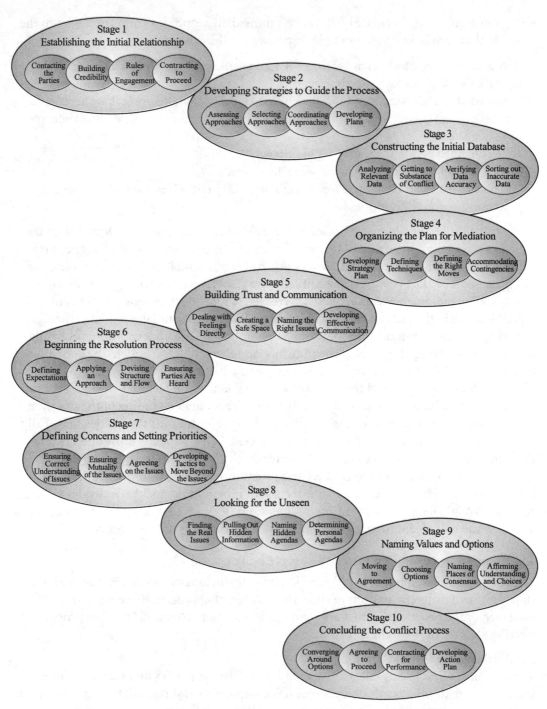

Figure 6-7 The 10 Stages of the Conflict Resolution Process

In addition, it helps the parties learn about the process and select those activities they determine will best assist them in moving effectively toward resolution.

Constructing the Initial Database

The mediator needs to become familiar with the parties and the issues as soon as possible. Thus, early in the process the mediator should ask the parties about their histories and experiences and for their insights to build a foundation for establishing priorities and deciding on an approach. Verifying the accuracy of the collected information and the central issues of concern is part of the data-gathering process. After the gathering stage, the participants should spend time reflecting on the content of the conflict and its implications for the resolution approach and process. Here again, they get to know each other better. In particular, the mediator obtains a view of the personal processes and behaviors of the parties within the context of the mediation process and can adjust the approach accordingly.

Organizing the Plan for Mediation

In this stage, the mediator considers the approach and structures to use for the mediation. The goal is to develop a plan of approach that fits the situation and the parties, accounting for the contingent factors discernible thus far. The mediator designs the noncontingent structures, considers process elements that could move the parties closer to agreement, and constructs a framework for guiding the process. The plan is simply contingent and is not cast in stone. The participants need to be flexible and adjust the process in response to the inevitable emergence of new information and unexpected factors.

Building Trust and Communication

It is essential to build trust between the parties and to strengthen the parties' trust in the mediator. The challenge is obvious: The parties have entered the mediation process precisely because they are in conflict and have negative feelings toward each other. The mediator's job is to get the parties at least to trust the process enough to get from it what it has to offer. Through exploring the emotional component of their perceptions of each other and of the process, the participants can lay a firm foundation for the subsequent work they will do.

Beginning the Resolution Process

The first stages of the conflict resolution process set up the parties for everything that is to follow. The mediator clearly lays out rules of engagement at the beginning, ensuring that the parties understand what to expect and how to proceed. These rules include guidelines for meeting together and for expressing feelings. The mediator also clarifies the areas of focus and the mechanisms used to proceed and apprises the parties of the opportunities they have to be heard, have their issues considered, and be included in deliberations. Familiarizing everyone with the structure of the process is essential because that increases the participants' flexibility. Flexibility is especially important for the mediator because he or she must respond appropriately to what emerges along the way and take advantage of any opportunity to bring the parties to agreement.

Defining Concerns and Setting Priorities

Here, doing one's homework pays off. The mediator, having come to understand the beginning issues, gives the parties an opportunity to explain their individual perceptions and how they formed their related expectations. The mediator also gets agreement from the parties on their understanding of the issues. The participants discuss the substantive points and positions until they are clear to everyone, work out the flow of events, and express their expectations of the methods for dealing with the issues.

Looking for Hidden Information, Agendas, and Interests
The mediator constantly focuses on what the real issues are and on finding clues that could direct the parties toward sustainable solutions. During this stage, many issues, concerns, and problems are likely to emerge, and the mediator must be on the lookout for opportunities to get the parties to work them out. The seeds of solution are to be found in the parties' dialogue. The parties are engaged in a great amount of detailed work, sometimes together and sometimes apart or one on one with the mediator.

Finding Potential Solutions and Determining Their Value to the Parties
As the parties move closer to an agreement, the mediator concentrates on getting them to understand where they appear to be in accord. The mediator's main task is to help the parties work out and state in detail any points of agreement between them, assess the applicability of potential solutions to the issues, determine their acceptability, and do whatever else is necessary to bring closure to the issues. As part of this process, the participants figure out the expected benefits and costs of meeting the obligations of the solutions.

Formalizing the Agreement
Once all the issues in the dispute have been dealt with and the parties understand what they have agreed to and find it acceptable, the mediator and the parties fashion an official agreement that is both clear and acceptable to the parties. Depending on the breadth and complexity of the agreement, different levels of documentation may be necessary. The parties must make certain they all have the same understanding of what they have agreed to. In this final stage, the mediator prepares the documentation that formalizes the agreement and forms the foundation for carrying out the solutions. The parties, once they are satisfied there is a mechanism for implementing the agreement, formally accept it.

Keeping the Process on Track
The conflict resolution process summarized here is of course influenced by the issues, behaviors, personalities, and circumstances of the parties to the conflict. Some of these are unanticipated and move the process in directions not initially imagined by the mediator. However, the mediator, by paying attention to the dynamics of dialogue and remaining flexible, can guide the process in a way that ultimately gets the parties to an agreement and/or an end to the conflict.

The mediator uses many techniques to get the parties unstuck and moving toward a workable consensus. Taking the parties aside and working

> **Key Point**
>
> Mediating any dispute involves helping the parties remain "unstuck," often a time-consuming task. It is all too easy for the parties to retreat to known territory, pushing for their own advantages and sustaining the polarization that has occurred. The best strategy is to stay focused on the larger picture and on the mutual benefits to be gained from a resolution.

with them individually (commonly called caucusing) helps each deal with the issues in a way that is impossible when they are all in the same room. Getting more information, expanding the options, introducing new considerations, moving horizontally on the issues, pressing the parties to consider other factors, and expanding the parties' perceptions, among other strategies, are all tools in the mediator's tool box.

The mediator attempts to move the parties toward a negotiated settlement by means of a joint problem-solving process in which the parties work out the solutions themselves. The mediator is not invested in any particular outcome. The parties must be satisfied. They own the issues and the solutions. The mediator simply provides them with tools and a structure within which the resolution can be more assuredly achieved. The mediator stays neutral, not favoring either party and moving both toward a state of mutual satisfaction.

The mediator is also constantly aware of the need to maintain a balance of power between the parties. In any dispute, issues of power are embedded in the process, and each party is tempted to pursue his or her own advantage to the exclusion of the other party's interests. Aware that jockeying over power occurs, the mediator does everything possible to make sure that the balance of power remains constant so that no party is disadvantaged as a result of the process. The mediator must not become an advocate for one party and must not act in a way that creates a perception of favoritism. The best strategy for dealing with issues of power is to be as public as possible about maintaining a balance, making it clear to the parties that this is a necessary feature of mediation.

Conflicts come in all shapes and sizes and levels of complexity, but in any conflict the mediator's role is to guide the process of problem solving and solution seeking for people who have been unable to get through this process by themselves. Although the details of the mediator's role are subject to debate, the mediator must recognize that the issues and their solutions belong to the parties. The mediator can bring his or her insights and skills, as well as sophisticated techniques and new concepts, to the process, yet the parties essentially own it. Whatever solutions are obtained are chosen by the parties and implemented by them. This is not to deny that sometimes the parties might want the mediator to control more of the process or take over responsibilities that properly belong to them, either because they view the responsibilities as too difficult or see the mediator as better placed to handle them.

The mediator must keep in mind that the process lends itself to tricks and stratagems that can slyly or inexplicably change the character or context of the interaction between the parties with such subtlety that it happens unnoticed. To avoid such shifts from occurring, the mediator needs to remain constantly focused on the process and its dynamics, evaluating its viability and efficacy and working to ensure that it is unfolding as it should.

People and Behavior

In conflict situations, stress levels are high and not everyone is at his or her best. Further, because of the history of conflict and people's general attitude toward it, people in conflict are not disposed to engage in relationship building and problem resolving.

Parties to a conflict generally take the position that someone must win and someone must lose. The role of the mediator is to see that this outcome does not occur. It should be clear that only a mutually satisfying solution is likely to end the conflict permanently.

In the effort to "win," either party might try one or more tactics to unbalance the situation. The mediator needs to be on the lookout for these tactics and counter them through good techniques and a good process. In addition, the mediator needs to be aware of other factors that often influence the outcome of a conflict resolution process, such as those discussed next.

Communication Technique

The mediator must always be listening. And not just listening but listening actively, which means continually restating points in a way that is understandable to all the parties and that gets the issues out in the open. Almost any conflict is rife with emotional energy, and the mediator must manage and diffuse as much of it as possible through being clear and understandable and by translating every nuance and every embedded message into an explicit assertion. The parties are more likely to come to an agreement if they fully comprehend all the issues and each other's positions.

Meeting Setting and Schedule

The meeting place should be comfortable and not favor any particular party. The room should exhibit balance, the table should be round instead of rectangular, the seating arrangement should be comfortable and informal, and the lighting should be conducive to dialogue and therefore not bright or irritating. It is important to schedule the meetings at a time of the day when the parties are alert and invested instead of tired and worn out. By being sensitive to the possible influence of the environment on the resolution process, the mediator can ensure that the meeting place is pleasing and congenial and supports the process rather than works against it.

Demeanor

Mediators come from all kinds of backgrounds and have all kinds of personalities. Personality is always a consideration in mediation, and there must be a good fit between the mediator and the parties. If there is not a good fit, the mediator will have difficulty moving the process forward, possibly to such an extent that the process comes to a dead halt. The mediator must exhibit confidence and competence and present him- or herself as someone the parties can depend on in the times of challenge. The mediator is responsible for the process and its culture and dynamics, and by showing a proper demeanor and gaining the respect of the parties, the mediator can do much to create a suitable culture and stimulate movement toward resolution. When the fit between the mediator and the participants is not aligned, mediators must recuse themselves from the mediation process and make room for a neutral mediator who can create a better fit and help facilitate moving the resolution process to success. Mediators should not be offended by their lack of congruence. In many aspects of the human interaction, relationships do not always work as anticipated. Recognizing this and moving on are often the critical moments in accessing successful problem solving.

Information Exchange

During a conflict resolution process, lots of information is laid out. The mediator must facilitate the transmission of correct information. The more accurate the information exchanged between the parties, the more likely the process will move along smoothly. There is always a danger of having more information than is necessary for good decision making. Having lots of information is not the same as having the right information. The mediator tries to ensure that the parties have the information they need and can differentiate between desired data and needed data (needed data are data they can use to fashion an agreement).

Use of Experts

The mediator tries to provide the parties with access to whatever will help them resolve their conflict. Because no mediator can be an expert in all the elements and processes associated with every kind of conflict, others may need to be involved in the process. There are no rules limiting access to what or who is needed to resolve issues. Planning for and scheduling the use of experts or other resources and determining the focus of their use are among the critical responsibilities of the mediator.

Conclusion

Resolving conflicts is a fundamental part of managing human relationships. All relationships have the potential for conflict embedded deep within them, especially in our increasingly diverse healthcare system, where professionals with widely different backgrounds and roles are required to work together. As they sort through their unique contributions, they face many opportunities for conflict and are almost guaranteed to fall into disputes and disagreements (Posthuma, 2012; Tojo & Dilpreet, 2007). Healthcare leaders are responsible for supervising the relationships between the disciplines, and as the roles of the disciplines change and their relationships become more complex, the leaders have the critical task of helping all who work in the health field to respond to the changes and build stronger more positive relationships.

The kind of intense interdisciplinary interaction characteristic of continuum-based teams is new to health care. Historically, there were only a very few types of professionals, and each type performed a wide variety of tasks. With the advances in technology that have occurred, more types of professionals exist, but the activities of each type are more narrowly focused. As a consequence, more people will be negotiating the clinical practice landscape, and, to complicate matters, these people will have more divergent roles and views. Working through their differences to find common ground will be essential to creating a more aligned and integrated healthcare system. Leaders have an important role to play in bringing this kind of system into existence by assisting others in solving problems and resolving conflicts.

Dealing with conflict is a normal part of the leadership role as it currently exists, and therefore leaders must understand the basic elements and learn the essential skills of conflict management. The implications for the role will only accelerate in the emerging and growing interdisciplinary work environment. Finding common ground among the disciplines and achieving true relational equity will imply the management and resolutions of many heretofore unaddressed relational and interactional conflicts. Like any skill, conflict management leadership requires continuous development. Leaders must recognize this and persevere in their learning efforts. The payoff is that these skills serve any leader well in dealing with the increasingly complex set of relationships in the delivery of health services. To the extent that a leader develops the necessary skills and takes on the role of conflict resolution facilitator, he or she will strengthen the relationships between health professionals and, most importantly, increase the effectiveness of health care.

Case Study 6-1

Managing an Unhealthy Work Environment

Isabella is new to the management role and has been the nurse manager of the Mother Infant Care (MIC) unit for 6 months. She recently graduated with her master's of science degree with an emphasis on leadership in micro healthcare systems. She was excited to be chosen from a candidate pool of five more experienced nurses, and she was eager to apply what she had learned in graduate school in shaping the culture of the MIC unit. After getting to know the staff and the assistant nurse managers, Isabella made some changes to put structure and processes in place that would facilitate staff involvement in decisions related to patient care and their practice of nursing. She encouraged the assistant managers to change from developing the staff schedule to allowing self-scheduling based on a few rules and principles that the staff had part in developing. It was decided that the more senior staff would have first choice in their schedule, followed by the part-time, and finally the per diem staff. Requests for time off were to be submitted to the assistant managers prior to the new schedule being posted so that the unit would be staffed appropriately.

All seemed to be going fairly well with the self-scheduling system for the first 4 months, but with the holiday season approaching, Isabella was receiving feedback that some of the staff were extremely unhappy with the system. There had been some arguments among staff in the nursing lounge, and Isabella was informed that one of the staff members left work in tears. Apparently, some of the more senior staff were being unreasonable with the less tenured full-time staff and refused to cover personal requests. The assistant managers informed Isabella that a powerful clique had formed with a few senior staff who were bullying some of the new nurses and refusing to assist them in patient care activities or to answer any of their questions. It seemed as if the situation was becoming quite unsettling, and two of the newly hired nurses had put in a request to be transferred to another unit.

When Isabella interviewed the nurses who had resigned or were transferring to another unit, she was surprised to hear their stories of verbal abuse, the "silent treatment" with no communication, or refusal to cover for them during required break times. She was also told that several of the more senior nurses refused to assist in turning patients and often withheld information that was important to patient care. Although Isabella was not able to convince the nurses to stay on the unit, she realized that the culture of the unit had to be changed.

Isabella called all of the assistant managers together and told them that they needed to work as a team to change the culture on the unit. She listened to their perspectives on what was happening and quickly identified that some of the assistant managers may have contributed to the problem because they had refused to become involved in managing the situation on their shift. It seemed to Isabella that the assistant managers may have been afraid of some of the staff members and, therefore, weren't comfortable confronting them about their inappropriate behaviors in the workplace. The small group of senior staff seemed to have control over staff members as well as the assistant managers. Some ethnic clashes also contributed to the problem.

Isabella decided to meet with the human resources specialist for her area and her director to apprise them of the situation and to ask for assistance in developing a strategy to resolve the conflicts. After discussing the situation and identifying potential options for resolution, they decided that the problem needed to be discussed openly at staff meetings and that performance and clarification of expectations would be discussed with offending staff individually and all staff collectively. A series of short presentations by a clinical psychologist on workplace bullying was planned with follow-up discussions with the staff.

New group norms for professional behavior and consequences for unprofessional conduct were presented and discussed with the staff. Each staff member was asked to sign an agreement outlining his or her knowledge of and acceptance of the new behavioral standards. This process allowed Isabella to meet with each staff member with the individual's assistant manager to reinforce the importance of acceptable behaviors in the workplace. Isabella and the human resources specialist helped the assistant managers give disciplinary warnings to the more offending staff members, and Isabella reiterated her expectation to these staff members that, if they could not accept the new behavior standards or demonstrate the necessary changes, she would assist them in "making other career choices."

Finally, Isabella announced a zero tolerance policy for workplace bullying and unprofessional conduct. She told the staff that "everyone had a right to feel safe, respected, and valued when at work. How we feel at work affects our ability to provide the best possible care to our patients." She told the staff that each of them could expect to be treated fairly and that she wanted them to feel safe in expressing their feelings in a professional and positive manner. She listened to their views on how to improve the self-scheduling process to ensure fairness for all. Isabella also arranged for every staff member to attend educational sessions that included discussions on cultural, gender, and age diversity in the workplace. Every staff meeting included open discussion on progress that was being made on each shift toward resolving the conflicts and creating a healthier work environment for all of the staff. She encouraged the staff to meet with her if they had any concerns about conflicts on the unit, and she made frequent rounds to speak with individuals and to make her presence visible among the staff.

Isabella also worked with her assistant managers to increase their leadership competencies in facing conflict and developing strategies to resolve the conflict rather than choosing to ignore the situation. She reminded them of their responsibility as leaders to face the conflicts early before they became unmanageable. She discussed the need for improved teamwork among the assistant managers to ensure support for one another during these times of crisis. She reassured them that she would be available to each of them to support them through any difficult situation, and that she would secure any resources needed to create a healthy work environment for them and for the staff.

Questions

1. What were some of the sources and possible causes of the conflict that emerged on the unit?
2. What were some of the signs that the conflict had escalated to an unacceptable level?
3. What leadership roles did Isabella assume in managing the conflict process?
4. How did the assistant managers' actions affect the level of conflict and the resolution of the conflict?
5. If you were Isabella, how would you have handled the conflict and mediated the situation?

Case Study 6-2

He Said, She Said, and No One Is Listening!

It started out a good day, and Mike reviewed the long list of items that he needed to accomplish that day. He had planned to meet with his managers to discuss the operational budget goals for the department and to initiate discussion about needed capital equipment that had to be projected for the upcoming year. Mike was the director of Medical Surgical Services and had six direct reports who were nurse managers over the Oncology unit, General Medical unit, Postoperative Surgical unit, Bariatric unit, Orthopaedics, and an Observational unit. In addition to the six nurse managers, the medical director for Internal Medicine and the medical director for Surgical Services also reported to Mike. The management team was an eclectic group with very different levels of education and experience, which made for lively discussions in their team meetings.

Each nurse manager brought a list of capital needs to the meeting. It quickly became apparent that there was more need than there was allocated budget because Mike's service line was only one of four for the entire hospital. As the nurse managers began to present their proposed capital needs, the group dynamics began to change from friendly to conflicting and competitive. The Orthopaedics department had the longest capital need list with the biggest dollar amount. As the other managers began to defend their list of needs, the nurse manager of the Orthopaedics department mentioned that his service line also contributed the greatest amount of revenue as compared to the other departments. He used that fact as a rationale for why his department should receive a larger piece of the allocated budget. The other nurse managers argued fiercely about their contribution to the hospital's bottom line and the value that their department brought to the organization. When the discussions became heated, Mike suggested that they take a recess as a "cooling off period." They agreed to meet again the next day to finalize the capital budget plan.

The next day the nurse managers came prepared to defend their units' needs, and they had formed a coalition against the nurse manager of Orthopaedics. They had met outside of the meeting and agreed that they might have more power in the discussion if they presented their needs collectively as contrasted to individually.

The nurse manager of Orthopaedics also had a strategy. He had met with the chief of the Orthopaedics service line and the medical director of Surgical Services. He asked them to join him in the meeting and indicate how important it was for Orthopaedics to receive the requested capital budget items. He also presented information about the threat to the hospital's market share if the Orthopaedics department did not keep up with state-of-the-art equipment.

Not long after the meeting started, it was clear to Mike that the cooling-off period had not worked, but rather had served as an opportunity to strengthen the conflict. As each of the nurse managers stated their case and rationale for their requests, tempers began to flare, and accusations were made on both sides. Mike realized that further discussion was not going to be helpful in resolving the conflict. Although the capital budget for his department was due in 2 days, Mike decided to stop the meeting once again. He informed the group that he would meet with two representatives from the coalition group and two representatives from the Orthopaedics group. Although the others were not happy about this plan, they were also not happy with the group's inability to negotiate a fair and equitable capital budget plan within the overall allocated amount.

The next day Mike met with the four representatives in a quiet, subdued setting that he felt would facilitate the mediation process and create a favorable environment for open dialogue, negotiation, and resolution. His opening remarks addressed the need for the four representatives to make decisions for the entire team that would be appropriate within the budget limitations. Mike had reviewed in his head the steps of the negotiation process and reminded himself not to take sides or contribute to the discussion until both sides were able to find common ground and begin to develop some realistic solutions.

Mike led them through a meeting norming process with the participants agreeing to "rules" for the meeting. They agreed that they would (1) respect the person speaking, and only one person would speak at a time without interruption; (2) focus on the common good in contrast to their individual units' needs; (3) create a list of the top 10 priorities for the entire department, and then negotiate the list down to the allocated budget amount; and (4) vote on items until consensus was reached. Needless to say it wasn't easy in the beginning, and Mike had to continually remind them that there was a finite amount of money that could be allocated and that they needed to make decisions for the whole based on the allocated budget amounts. With this constant reminder and norming process, the four began to work together using the strategic plan for the department as a foundation for their decision making. They also developed rationale for each of their decisions that could be presented to the whole group. It took a full 2 days of meetings to finally have a proposed budget that could be presented to the rest of the group.

Mike called the entire group together and informed them of the decision-making process that led to the proposed budget. Two of the representatives prepared a presentation for the entire group and provided handouts of the proposed budget with rationale for each item suggested. As it turned out, Orthopaedics did receive a greater allocation than the other units, but there was clear justification using the strategic goals for the department as a foundation. Not everyone in the group was happy with the proposed budget, but they did agree that the rationale was sound. After discussion, the group finally decided to adopt the new proposed capital budget and to develop proposals for the hospital's foundation to fund some of the other items that they felt were important to their units.

Mike submitted his final capital budget on time, but he recognized that there was still some discontent among some managers within the group. He realized that he couldn't please everyone, but the method that he used to resolve the open conflict resulted in a budget that was supportive of the department's strategic initiatives even though some capital items were not approved, as some had hoped.

Questions

1. Identify the potential causes for the conflict among the managers.
2. If you were in Mike's position, what might you have done differently to manage and resolve the conflict?
3. What are your thoughts about why the splintering among the group occurred when they began to form a coalition and bring other team members into the process?
4. How did Mike help or hinder the negotiation process?
5. Although the capital budget has been submitted, what work does Mike need to focus on to improve the group dynamics?
6. Describe the power imbalances that existed within the group and discuss how these imbalances affected the group dynamics.
7. How were the 10 steps to conflict resolution used in developing the final solution to the capital budget plan?

References

Behfar, K., Peterson, R., Mannix, E., & Trochim, W. (2008). The critical role of conflict resolution in teams: Up close look at the links between conflict type, conflict management strategies, and team outcomes. *Journal of Applied Psychology, 93*(2), 170–188.

Caspers, B. A., & Pickard, B. (2013). Value-based resource management: A model for best value nursing care. *Nursing Administration Quarterly, 37*(2), 95–104.

Cooperrider, D., Whitney, D., & Stavros, J. (2008). *The appreciative inquiry handbook: For leaders of change.* San Francisco, CA: Barrett-Koehler.

Edersheim, E. H., & Drucker, P. F. (2007). *The definitive Drucker.* New York, NY: McGraw-Hill.

Kriesberg, L. (2003). *Constructive conflicts: From escalation to resolution* (2nd ed.). Lanham, MD: Rowman & Littlefield.

LeBaron, M. (2003). *Bridging cultural conflicts: A new approach for a changing world* (1st ed.). San Francisco, CA: Jossey-Bass.

Levinger, M. (2013). *Conflict analysis: Understanding causes, unlocking solutions.* New York, NY: Institute of Piece Press.

Moore, C. W. (2003). *The mediation process: Practical strategies for resolving conflict* (3rd ed.). San Francisco, CA: Jossey-Bass.

Payne, D. (2010). Harnessing conflict. *Library Leadership & Management, 24*(1), 6–11.

Posthuma, R. (2012). *Conflict management and emotions International Journal of Conflict Management: Volume 23, Issue 1* (pp. 1 online resource (110 p.)). Retrieved from http://proxy.library.oregonstate.edu/login?url=http://OSU.eblib.com/patron/FullRecord.aspx?p=896031

Ramsbotham, O., Woodhouse, T., & Miall, H. (2011). *Contemporary conflict resolution.* Cambridge, UK: Polity Press.

Rothman, J. (1997). *Resolving identity-based conflict.* San Francisco, CA: Jossey-Bass.

Rothman, J. (2013). ARIA conflict engagement theory. Retrieved from http://www.colorado.edu/conflict/peace/example/roth7516.htm

Tojo, J., & Dilpreet, C. (2007). *Appreciative inquiry and knowledge management.* Northampton, UK: Edward Elgar.

Werner, E. K. (2012). Peacemaking: From practice the theory. *Library Journal, 137*(5), 132–133.

Zedeck, S. (2011). *APA handbook of industrial and organizational psychology* (1st ed.). Washington, DC: American Psychological Association.

Suggested Readings

Busch, M., & Hostetter, C. (2009). Examining organizational learning for application and human service organizations. *Administration and Social Work, 33*(3), 297–318.

Cahn, D., & Abigail, R. (2013). *Managing conflict through communication.* London, England: Pearson.

Cheung, F., & Tang, C. (2009). The influence of emotional intelligence and affectivity on emotional labor strategies that work. *Journal of Individual Differences, 30*(2), 75–86.

Deutch, M., Coleman, P., & Marcus, E. (2006). *The hundbook of conflict resolution: Theory and practice.* San Francisco, CA: Jossey-Bass.

Fine, M. (2009). Women leaders discursive constructions of leadership. *Women's Studies in Communication, 32*(2), 180–202.

Late, J., & McCurdy, D. (2008). *Conformity and conflict: Readings in cultural anthropology.* Chicago, IL: Allyn & Bacon.

Malloch, K., & Porter-O'Grady, T. (2009). *The quantum leader: Applications for the new world of work.* Sudbury, MA: Jones and Bartlett.

Nye, J. (2008). *Understanding international conflicts: An introduction to theory and history.* London, England: Longman.

Quiz Questions

Select the best answer for each of the following questions.

1. Conflict in everyday relationships is _____.
   a. To be avoided
   b. Unacceptable
   c. Normal
   d. Destructive

2. Conflict resolution facilitators must recognize the value of _____.
   a. Uniformity
   b. Diversity
   c. Anxiety
   d. Humanity

3. When is conflict destructive?
   a. When it is not resolved.
   b. When it is accompanied by anger.
   c. When it is secretive.
   d. When it becomes physical.

4. The perceived imbalance of power can lead to conflict. To mitigate its potential for mischief, how should power be handled?

   a. It should be viewed as a necessary evil.
   b. It should be placed in the hands of managers.
   c. It should be placed in the hands of staff.
   d. It should be distributed equitably across the organization.

5. What do two parties in conflict generally know?

   a. Each other's position
   b. Why they are angry
   c. What they want
   d. What they dislike

6. Which of the following is an accurate description of interest-based conflict or identity-based conflict?

   a. Interest-based conflict concerns how the parties view themselves.
   b. Identity-based conflict concerns how the parties view themselves.
   c. Identity-based conflict involves tangible issues.
   d. Interest-based conflict is harder to resolve.

7. What is the primary role of a conflict resolution facilitator?

   a. To bring the conflict to an end
   b. To establish a good resolution process
   c. To keep the parties moving through the process
   d. To help both parties get what they want

8. What must a conflict resolution facilitator never do?

   a. Take sides
   b. Stop the process
   c. Get angry
   d. Interject personal insights

9. To reach a successful completion of the 10-step conflict resolution process, what does the mediator ensure happens?

   a. The interaction between the parties is friendly and their dialogue is courteous.
   b. The parties use effective techniques for communicating and exchanging information.
   c. The parties always meet with the mediator together, never one on one.
   d. The parties receive all the information the mediator is able to acquire.

10. The attribution by each party of negative motives and qualities to the other party usually indicates what about the parties?

    a. They hold fluid positions.
    b. They have an accurate understanding of each other's positions.
    c. They do not fully understand the issues at the root of the conflict.
    d. They want to avoid dealing with the real issues.

CHAPTER SEVEN

Leading Constant Movement: Managing Crisis and Change

For the past 33 years I have looked into the mirror every morning and asked myself: "If today were the last day of my life, would I want to do what I am about to do today?" And if the answer were "no" for too many days in a row, I know I need to change something.

—*Steve Jobs*

Chapter Objectives

www

At the completion of this chapter, the reader will be able to

- Define crisis and expand on the essential elements of crisis within a leadership context.
- Enumerate the complexity of systems and the role crisis plays in moving them to change.
- Explain the role of crisis in the change process and identify the characteristics of crisis in the process of change.
- Understand and apply the concepts of predictive and adaptive capacity in the role of the leader.
- Use a systems model for crisis management as a way of systematically confronting and addressing crisis as a normative part of the change process.

This is a time of great transformation for healthcare systems. The increasing digitalization of health service and its related data, major initiatives related to national health reform, and the growing technical transformation of therapeutics and service delivery all converge to create the perfect storm of chaos and complexity throughout the health system. Leaders increasingly understand the vagaries of complexity and chaos and the implications of unplanned events in their leadership. In fact, the unexpected has become the norm. Increasingly, unplanned events are part of the way of doing business and natural occurrences in the cycle of human experience. All the planning in the world and all the anticipation that accompanies it cannot change the fact that contingencies are now a constant and response to them is a fundamental part of the leadership experience.

Crises have always been with us. Since the dawn of time, natural and human events have combined to create conditions and circumstances that have raised the intensity of human life and even threatened its very existence. From natural disasters and environmental shifts to human-made war, conflict, and social and cultural change, crises have accompanied human beings on the human journey. Only in the last couple of decades have we begun to study crisis and to sort through its characteristics, elements, and all aspects that operate to affect the "critical" human experience. Through studying crisis and understanding its vagaries and variables, humans can anticipate, perhaps even predict, crises in a way to help us better manage the impact on our social and individual experiences (Kanel, 2006; Lerbinger, 2012).

Normative Crisis

Crises are not always stimulated by cataclysmic events. Sometimes, crisis can be stimulated by simple occurrences. An accidental moment of invention, turning down the wrong street, a casual conversation with another individual, and the choice of where to spend one's vacation all represent simple decisions and actions that might result in significant and important challenges and shifts in events and experiences. These kinds of critical events and unanticipated situations can be the end product of a convergence of forces unknown at a given time, yet operating inexorably to create an impact or cause a result that was fully unanticipated.

> ### Point to Ponder
>
> Crisis is a fundamental component of the human journey; it will always accompany all change.

Although unplanned events are normal parts of human existence, people do not like crises and significant change events. Individuals demonstrate most discomfort when normal patterns of human experience are interrupted with a radical or immediate shift in reality or conditions. This apparent contradiction between the normality of unplanned events and people's unwillingness to accommodate them creates the foundations for much of the conflict and anxiety related to confronting and addressing normative crisis. If crisis could be seen as a routine and fundamental element of everyone's personal experience and life process, perhaps more attention would be paid to developing adaptation, anticipation, and coping mechanisms to help people accommodate and deal with the crises that inevitably occur in their lives.

Early Warning

Crises very rarely occur without some level of early warning (Penuel, Statler, & Hagen, 2013; Noble, 2011). The critical factor in early engagement of crisis is the development and presence of tools and mechanisms that enable leadership to become aware of the potential for crisis in advance of crises actually occurring. The first step of any early warning system is the leaders' understanding and acceptance that the occurrence of crisis is a normative part of the human experience and crises are to be anticipated rather than surprises. This understanding of the inevitability and normative circumstances related to the potential of the onset of a crisis best conditions organizational leadership to create a programmatic and systematic approach to confronting crisis. In short, a systematic framework—a model—needs to be incorporated into the operational and structural characteristics of the organization as a way of ensuring that well-planned mechanisms for addressing the onset of a crisis event are in place long before crisis actually arises.

Hospitals and health systems are very good at anticipating clinical crises as well as community and natural disasters. Their capacity for disaster planning is unparalleled. However, these crises tend to be the least common occurrences affecting the viability and stability of the hospital or health system. Usually, other major significant crises place the hospital or health system at greater risk than do natural or clinical disasters. Crises related to readiness for health reform, finance, management, market, competition, environment, and operations create more significant risks for the organization than do natural or clinical disasters.

Much of the reason for the impact of this kind of risk is the lack of systems that predict and anticipate changes in current conditions and challenges threatening the status quo (Lodge & Wegrich, 2012). For all leaders, the ability to develop the skills requires a deep understanding of social and organizational complexity and the processes associated with facilitating human dynamics within the context of complex systems. The ability to comprehend the action of complexity and the human response to immediate and dramatic change is an important leadership skill that is required as a basic foundation for the expression of leadership competencies related to the management of crisis. Complexity theory and science have provided leaders with major new insights regarding predictive and adaptive capacity and the need to incorporate particular dynamics and applications into the ordinary and usual management practices of organizations (Weberg, 2012).

The ability to understand both the complexities of and applications essential to a positive response to crisis demands an understanding of the cybernetic nature of all action and human experience. Leaders must recognize the cyclical nature of all action, including human action, and the inevitability and eventuality of major and dramatic shifts in both experience and reality. Because of this inevitability, all human organizations must reflect a strong capacity for adaptation and change. Because change is the only constant in the universe, structuring organizations to be continuously adaptive and mobile is a critical requisite for long-term viability. The need for an organization to continue to thrive calls for its leadership to be ever vigilant with regard to the continuous and unrelenting risks embedded in change dynamics operating both internally and externally and having both negative and positive implications for the organization's health and life (Dickinson & Mannion, 2012).

The Leader's Perception of Crisis

Contemporary leaders must recognize the importance of adaptive and predictive skills related to managing crises. The contemporary leader must understand that crisis management is as important a part of the process of

> **Key Point**
>
> If the leader is unable to accommodate the critical variables embedded in the crisis of change, followers will be no more successful in confronting the demand to change.

management as the normative operational considerations of day-to-day function. At the same time, crisis is not always appropriate in the work environment. The leader must be able to separate crisis management as a functional activity from crisis leadership as a strategic imperative. Leaders who continually manage within a crisis mode create the conditions and circumstances that ultimately blind people to the legitimate and normative crises that confront their lives and work from time to time. At this level of intensity, crisis management both prevents people from dealing effectively with the crisis and creates a set of circumstances that makes them uniquely unprepared to adequately address a legitimate crisis.

Often, leaders who manage in a crisis mode like the intense feeling of the "high" that comes from living at an accelerated level of energy. For these people, everything has a serious potential for implications beyond what normally can be expected in a given situation. Raising this level of crisis and applying it to routine and ritual functions and activities ultimately causes people to burn out and become immune to responding appropriately to situations that might be potentially significant or dangerous. This kind of leadership is neither effective nor valuable; in fact, it is destructive. Wise leaders recognize the value of conflict and crisis, understand its appropriate context, and prepare for it without living it.

Understanding Crisis

Crisis comes in all forms, from natural disasters to human-caused crises such as war, national disasters, and economic meltdowns. In human organizations, the more complex the system, the more likely the onset of crisis. Human development has resulted in a burgeoning of technologies and systems that create increasingly more complex infrastructures. The more complex the infrastructure, the more interdependent the elements that make it up become and the more likely it is subject to the vagaries of external and internal forces causing the crisis. Technologies themselves increase the intensity through magnification of processes, elements, and experiences in ways that advance the human experience and the opportunity for a wide variety of human expressions. Technologies may be identified in the instruments of creativity and in the products of human ingenuity. From medicines to new products, from ideas to new insights regarding the technology itself, the impact of human ingenuity is increasingly vital to everyday human activity (Estrin, 2009; Goldstein, Hazy, & Lichtenstein, 2010).

> **Point to Ponder**
>
> Technology is accompanied by crisis. Destructive technologies always radically change our lives.

Technology further refines the human experience. In the presence of technology, the quality of human life is advanced and improved such that illnesses can be healed, diseases prevented, discomfort alleviated, and enjoyment and comfort in the human experience advanced. Technology becomes the means for fulfilling every human desire and expectation. Through the use of technology, the human experience can be expanded, deepened, and broadened. A part of the impact of technology, however, is the complexity that it brings to human experience.

Complexity and Technology

Human beings have lived in organizations of every level of complexity. We depend on the well-being and functioning of complex human systems in small and large aggregates of human interaction and relationship. Organizational and relational issues are highest on the priority list of human interest and exploration. As the human culture has grown in diversity, breath, and complexity, it has become increasingly complex and challenging to both understand and manage (Curlee & Gordon, 2011; Zimmerman, Lindberg, & Plsek, 1998).

Human beings shape the form of their organization through cultural, social, political, and relational interactions. The impact of each of these has led to highly complex and successful societies emerging from the earliest experiences of human history. From Greek societies and Chinese culture, to the Roman Empire, to the development of European and Asian powers, to the emergence of North American cultures and the political and social influence of the West, social and political aggregations of human organizations have continually made an impact on the human experience and the dynamics of change.

Our world has become more complex and diverse. In this diversity, it has also become more prone to the conflicts that difference creates. The crises that result from these conflicts usually demonstrate problems with the regulation of human organizations, the ability to control function and interaction, and the inability or unwillingness of various cultural organizations and groupings to deal effectively and peacefully with others.

Group Discussion

Identify a recent global or national social shift like health reform or a national tragedy and the unknown and unanticipated elements of the event. List the ways in which people were unprepared and identify how being unprepared contributed to the crisis. What elements of the crisis drove people into chaos and uncertainty? What role did the lack of technology play in exacerbating the crisis? How do human beings behave in the absolute absence of technology? What role does technology play in anticipating and managing crisis? In this scenario, is technology a means or an end?

Conflict in the Human Community

Many crises can be traced to problems within and between the organizational infrastructures of human communities (Deutch, Coleman, & Marcus, 2006; Diller, 2011). As a result of these inadequacies, various pathologies emerge out of the conflicts, representing inadequacies in groups and between groups to deal with the issues that negatively affect other groups. Various systems technologies have been developed within societies, organizations, and large groupings. These approaches deal with the complex interactions of variables that affect the quality of the human experience. From the development of economics, sociology, politics, psychodynamics, engineering and architecture, and other innovative and creative technologies, social groups find ways to optimize their collective and individual experiences and to create opportunities to advance their organizational infrastructure even at the risk of challenging current organizational configurations. Entire fields of science have been developed within the context of emerging complexities of human societies and organizations for researchers to find ways to solve the problems associated with large, complex human communities. Out of these sciences have emerged intellectual, theoretical, and practical processes directed to managing and creating ways to advance the social experience; ensure that societies live in harmony, peace, and comfort; and reduce the potential for war.

In the past two decades, scientific endeavors have led to a deeper understanding of the complexity of systems and the elements of complexity as applied to human dynamics and human organization (Dekker, 2011; Hazy, Goldstein, & Lichtenstein, 2007). This examination attempts to move past assumptions and serendipitous models of human process into understanding more complex systems and creating an increasingly adaptive and broad-based field of inquiry with regard to systems and human organizations. A variety of systems theory and cybernetics has emerged that recognizes the unfolding of a growing language for complex human organizations. A wide breadth of variables affect human relationships and the ability of societies and organizations to work and thrive in increasingly complex circumstances. Out of these systems approaches, a new synergistic understanding of human systems and organizations and the processes of human dynamics, interaction, innovation, and complexity has emerged, recognizing a complexity of processes and utilizing the insights and skills of a wide variety of disciplines.

> **Key Point**
>
> Complexity sciences now form the foundation for thinking about existence, organization, and human functioning.

Understanding complexity in systems requires understanding the integration, coordination, and facilitation of complex human groups. Understanding complexity in organizations enables leaders the ability to control the variables affecting human interaction, decision making, innovation, technology, and direction. These skills have become critical to the sustenance and advancing of both societies and organizations. Complexity science requires an effective conceptual foundation for successful social systems management. This brings to mind the need to manage the dynamic cybernetic capacity of human experience that lies embedded within this complexity, with all the related organizational and human challenges that implies. The cybernetics of organizational human life (cycles of unrelenting change) and the application of complexity science related to explicating it and communicating complexity become a management skill of translating understanding of human dynamics and social enterprise. The leader's capacity to do this helps to better articulate human interaction, autonomy, behavior and values, and significance in the application of work and issues related to advancing the human experience and achieving self-actualization.

Complexity and Organizations

Human organizations, especially those organized for work, are exemplars of both a broad and a narrow aggregation of human activity. However, to thrive and grow cybernetic and life-generating intelligent organizations require a systematic integration of a number of forces.

Human organizations must adapt to changing circumstances. Adaptation is a critical factor in an organization's ability

to continue to thrive and succeed. Adaptation is a fundamental predictor of continuing existence and requires a clear conceptualization of the elements and processes necessary to ensure thriving. Thriving means building a goodness of fit in the intersection between an organization's external and internal relationships and circumstances in the broader world. As the world continues to shift as a result of improving conditions, changing technology, or environmental transformation, organizations must reflect those changes within the context of their own operations. Nothing remains constant. Organizations must expect that the ever-transitioning environment will be challenging, perhaps even threatening, because the transforming social conditions and circumstances affect what the organization does and its place in the world.

Effectively managing change means leaders create an internally and externally adaptive environment that has the capacity to anticipate, even predict, the impact of changes, internal and external, that affect its ability to continue to function. The management of change is a constant rather than an exception and is a critical leadership skill in complex systems. Because change is ever present and continuously affects the organization, leaders must recognize in their own roles an adaptive capacity that helps the organization and its people shift and adjust practices, processes, and behaviors in the face of a shifting demand for them.

Adaptive Capacity and Change

Several factors need to be addressed for an organization to adapt to its changing realities. First, of course, senior management needs to be fully invested and committed to the change dynamic (Leban, 2007; Shaw, 2011). This level of leadership requires that the strategic frame for the organization incorporates change as a normative part of the operating decision-making infrastructure. Strong executive leadership requires that a strategic focus and a well-planned process related to contingent and disruptive conditions be incorporated into the normative planning activities of the organization. Senior leadership's commitment, skill, investment, and ability to organize and plan systematically around the potential for crisis are strong indicators of effectiveness in the face of constant change.

Key Point

Adaptive capacity is the ability to identify the key responses necessary to thrive in a change situation and to build new and related responses.

Second, there must be organizational commitment both in the design of the infrastructure of the organization related to its work and in the processes associated with undertaking work. Change never occurs when expected. Although predictive processes in the organization can look for the signals and triggers that indicate imminent change, these shifts often cannot be anticipated at a particular or given time in the organization's history. However, through the incorporation of a broad-based organizational construct for crisis, change, and contingency and an organized response to the possibility of a change event, the potential for crisis can be incorporated into the ongoing expectations of all in the workplace. In this way, successful organizations can demonstrate clear and specific goals for all the issues at every level of the organization that are affected by the potential change event.

The third factor is the need to understand the elements of the change process and a coherent organized response to the dynamics of change. Change is neither difficult to understand nor difficult to incorporate into the operating realities of an organization. Addiction to historical rituals and routines, often present in clinical environments, can impede or block adaptation to change. Leaders must articulate the vagaries and characteristics of change, incorporate that understanding into the work processes of all workers, and show by their own behaviors a willingness to adapt and change to the new realities brought on by critical events. In addition, the communication system in the organization must adapt and adjust to the various emerging demands that arise at any given moment. Communications systems require a multifocal, multichannel approach to information generation and the management of communication around specific change events. The communication of particular signals indicates an impending shift in the way of doing business and links those signals to the trigger events initiating the organizational action stage. This operates in response to the external and internal signals that anticipate a need for a change in a way of doing business. Also, the communication channels must not impede patient service and clinical activities in a way that interrupts the viability and effectiveness of the services. Although change may occur in a number of different forms, from payment changes to environmental and contextual changes and even clinical and technological changes, the patient experience should never be threatened or undermined as the organization responds to the demand for change.

The many challenges of health reform create both context and content to which most of the tool sets identified in this chapter are applicable. Significant whole-systems reconceptualization, redesign, and recalibration are the fundamental work of change agents across the health system. Moving from a volume-driven to a value-based approach to delivering service and paying for it calls for fundamentally rethinking at the environmental, systems, tactical, operational, and point-of-service arenas of increasingly complex health systems. As health service and system regional mergers and integration accelerate along the current trajectory to improved accountable care and broad-based population service models, the structural and contextual framework identified in this chapter is increasingly relevant and critical to ensuring full-scale system-wide approaches are well led and sustainable. Failing to adequately and thoroughly address the demands of each stage of change, component of response, and network action limits the development of an adequately supporting infrastructure and the sustainable processes that advance health system viability and success.

The Human Resources Focus

Good human resources management systems are critical to the organization's ability to adjust and adapt personal behaviors and work processes to critical change events. Human resources focus on the value and processes associated with normative change. These responses should be included in the ongoing education and development of all workers. This means incorporating the understanding of change elements and the management of change into every level of educational development within the organization. Clinical education, as well as organizational and management leadership education, should incorporate the elements, characteristics, and stages of crisis. Increasingly of concern is the alignment between clinical resource demand and the disposition of adequate human resources that meets the numbers, kind, and quality necessary for specific population and service demands in the emerging accountable care environment. The complex relationship between these factors must be considered if related problems are to be appropriately resolved. For example, addressing the need for better-educated nurses prepared in advanced practice for the growing primary care infrastructure of health reform is impossible without addressing the aging and diminishing numbers of competent faculty necessary to prepare them.

Effective human resources models should include cybernetics and change management as fundamental parts of the role expectations of leaders and the professional staff. Many organizations suffer in the face of inevitable change because their human resources have not been educated in the processes and activities of complexity and change management and the impact of inevitable change on clinical and service processes and response. In an era of service innovation, evidence-based practice, and accountable care, it becomes even more important to incorporate adaptive skills into the professional skill set of every clinical leader in the organization.

Group Discussion

Identify a particularly rancorous change process in your organization (health reform provides many such opportunities). Discuss and then list the particular elements that made this specific change event difficult. Also include in your discussion the personal and emotional reactions that occurred in the center of the change event. What were the particular elements of this change that created problems? What were people's attitudes toward the need for this change? How were people prepared and incorporated in determining the need for this change? How was engagement of the stakeholders in this change incorporated into determining how best to respond to it? How would you do it differently, if it were to be done correctly?

A crisis critical planning process should be incorporated into the operating activities of the leadership of the organization. All healthcare facilities have disaster plans and plans for specific critical events. These focus on the occurrence of particular crises that are environment or disaster related. Disaster, however, no longer is the only driver of crisis. Broad-based immediate social, political, and economic shifts create their own level of crisis, shortening response time and intensifying the degree of risk related to effective immediate, incremental, and sustainable responses.

Response planning should also encompass those normative strategic and alignment changes that affect the ability of an organization to continue its work. Because of the growing digital infrastructure and its ability to compress data, time, and response, traditional Industrial Age response mechanisms are no longer sufficient. Often, the introduction of a new technology or new regulations regarding payment policy or patient safety can create as much impact as a critical environmental event or community disaster. Recognizing that ongoing operational and planning activities should relate as much to normative change as to exceptional change is a vital leadership capacity for the twenty-first century. Incorporating these elements of the organization's critical planning processes and the activities associated with adapting to environmental and contextual changes ensures that the organization remains constantly vigilant as it reviews signals and trigger events that may lead to a change in the conditions and circumstances within which clinical practitioners work. Leaders must always be aware of the need for and the processes associated with deliberation of the critical action steps to organizational, contextual, and strategic shifts affecting the viability of the organization. These effects are as significant to the organization's success as any environmental or disaster-related critical event.

Adaptive Capacity in Human Organizations

Traditionally, organizational activity and learning have been considered continuous and dynamic processes that reflect inclusion of the organization's adjustments and adaptations to internal and external individual and collective contingencies that affect individuals' ability to learn and adapt. Resulting from this process are practices and routines that reflect the normal life and activity of the organization in response to strategic, market, and process demands. Each individual, when joined with the collective effort, contributes to these organizational values and routines in a way that reflects consistent and viable performance, reliability, and the achievement of expectations and outcomes. In this way, the organization maintains a continuum of rituals and routines that, when uninterrupted, comprises the usual and ordinary processes of work and contributes to achieving desirable outcomes.

At the same time, people and organizations live in a larger context. The dynamics of internal and external vagaries and variability have a direct impact on the life and activities of individuals and organizations. The influence of these random factors frequently create a level of organizational and individual uncertainty and ensure an embedded ambiguity. This condition, called noise, creates a level of personal and organizational interference with the continuum of normative work and the sustenance of the rituals and routines associated with it. The organization's availability and adaptability to these vagaries give form to its general adaptive capacity. The ability of an organization to accommodate these uncontrolled factors, making adjustments in work processes and individual behavior,

> **Point to Ponder**
>
> Organizations are dynamic living organisms. They operate less like a machine and more like an organism. Leaders must now see them as ever-changing dynamics with no permanent form.

reflects the level of flexibility and fluidity built into the organization's work processes that ensure its continuance.

Still, uncontrollable variances create instability in the mind of the worker and the processes of the workplace. Often, learning processes and programs in most workplaces employ process learning and apply it in a way that assumes a normative continuum of activities and stable, uninterrupted work processes. Rarely are the influence and force of constant, uninterrupted change embedded in the processes of organizational and individual learning. In many ways, it is assumed that these interruptive patterns of behavior are nonnormative and exceptional and are therefore not to be included in the usual processes of learning. Yet every worker is reminded that "change is constant" and that they must be willing to accommodate it. What often fails to be communicated is the notion that "change is the norm" and that stability, ritual, routine, and process activities are, themselves, nonnormative. Contemporary and adaptive organizations recognize this reality and must now begin to incorporate into their operating framework the continuous and unrelenting demands of continuous external and internal adaptation.

Organizational learning theory was based on a mechanistic notion of organizational life. Contemporary organizational learning approaches shift away from that foundation and now reflect the belief that organizations are not so much like machines but more like organisms. This biodynamic approach indicates that organizations and individuals can learn and adapt to external change and stressors through behaviorally oriented cognitive and adaptive processes. Adaptive approaches in human organizations enable the organization to adapt through learning processes that incorporate those realities.

> **Point to Ponder**
>
> Leaders frame adaptation by looking carefully for the intersections and interaction between seemingly unrelated systems and processes and dynamically managing these connections.

Chaos, Complexity, and Crisis

Contemporary chaos and complexity theory characterizes complex human systems and organizations as spontaneous and self-organizing (Mitchell, 2009). This approach recognizes behavior as nonlinear, understanding that small changes and shifts in behavior can have significantly large implications. Complexity theory goes beyond simply defining the impact of randomness and universal disorder. Furthermore, the theory recognizes that order can be found deeply within the seemingly random complexities. In addition, chaos theory reflects the constant contest between stability and chaos where the activities of creativity unfold. Chaos approaches attempt to understand the impact of change on systems; complexity theory attempts to understand how organizations and environments adapt to changing circumstances over time (Yang, Cao, & Lu, 2012).

The interaction between seemingly unrelated systems and processes creates the frame for adaptation. The notion of emergent order is consistent with adaptation. In complexity theory, emergence suggests that a fundamental and inherent order exists within an apparent disorderly and chaotic condition. Adaptation contains within it a certain

> ### Point to Ponder
>
> The potential for crisis is constantly present. Understanding this concept of potential is critical to the exercise of good leadership. The wise leader is always living in this potential.

amount of spontaneity and self-order that result from awareness of the connections and intersections to which the organization reacts or responds. Imbedded in the adaptation process are all the necessary elements: goodness of fit, feedback loops, and organizationally responsive strategies.

This borderland on the edge of chaos at the intersections between systems represents the conflict between stability and chaos. It is here that innovation, adaptation, creativity, and flexibility thrive at once. In essence, these elements create a dance of interaction, the confluence of which results in the conditions, circumstances, and forces that require human and organizational response and adaptation. In this place creativity and learning, adjustment and adaptation, flexibility and fluidity combine to encourage new patterns of behavior, action, and organizational response. However, this set of circumstances also creates the conditions for crisis.

Crises are embedded in the juncture between contemporary and normative organizational activities and occur at the critical moment when the external and internal forces converge to force a change in the organization's circumstances (Crandall, Parnell, & Spillan, 2009; Weberg, 2012). Crisis is often not easily anticipated, yet can always be expected. For the leader, anticipating crisis is a state of mind; responding to its inevitability is an organizational construct. The potential for crisis is consistently present regardless of the stability apparent within any current state. By understanding this potential, the leader can see that through the constant movement across time, the opportunity for the impact of change is ever present. One of the most significant leadership skills is the leader's ability to recognize the constant potential of crisis and identify the signs of convergence of factors and forces leading to a paradigm shift for the organization and its people.

Strategic Crisis Management

The key to thriving in the context of crisis conditions is a strategic ability to anticipate, identify, and respond. Organizational leadership should focus on developing the resources, both financial and human, that create a frame of reference to ensure that the organization adapts to crisis, and does not simply react to it. Because there will always be unanticipated surprises that can negatively affect the organization, the more strategic tools, supporting infrastructure, and planned approaches available to the leader, the better likelihood of sound response and recovery. Whenever models exist, they must be dynamic and represent the organization's continuous effort to anticipate and identify those internal and external factors affecting the work of the organization. This process must be inculcated into the operating structure of the organization and become a part of the life and work expectations at every level of the organization. The ability to read signals and to anticipate challenge can be generated at any place in the organization where the indicators and signs of impending impact can be diagnosed. From the front lines to the executive office, points of intersection within the system, between systems, or with externally generated variables can be anticipated and responded to regardless of position or role.

Leadership must enroll practicing professionals and managers by structuring and framing work activities so that workers can quickly assess and respond to crisis influence and impact. Furthermore, the cybernetic process, which is any action in a system that generates a change in its larger environment and cycles back to further "trigger" a system's change of whatever dynamic mechanism is built must make it possible—indeed desirable—for workers at all levels of the organization to own the obligation of identifying and responding to shifting realities that affect their ability to address the purposes of the organization and undertake their own work. A systematic and organized response to building the infrastructure that makes such fluidity and flexibility the frame for doing business and undertaking action is a critical variable that results in either negative impact or positive response.

The model for addressing critical variants needs to contain several elements. First, it must address team activities and relationships in the course of doing business and the activities of the organization in everyday rituals and routines. Every member in the organization must be aware of his or her connection to the strategy, mission, and purposes of the organization and how individual and collective work contribute. All the work elements of the model must tie the individual and collective action of the work team to fulfilling the goals of the organization. The work must also meet the needs of the various constituencies and customers, ultimately resulting in advancing the health of individuals and the community. In contemporary, value-driven care, evidence of the impact of such a model is witnessed in the seamlessness of service connections, supply chain supports, the clinical continuum, and the continuous highest level of healthy functioning of patients, populations, and communities.

Second, the model must assist the organization and its players, and every point in the system, in anticipating and predicting the impact of external and internal forces and how their convergence affects the work of the organization. Local and global influences affect the organization's viability and responsiveness to changes in its contextual circumstances. These often can be identified at the clinical sites as changes in practice, technology, therapeutics, or clinical evidence. Identification of the signals, such as health reform legislation and policy formation, that indicate a convergence of forces and triggers of change that will impact the organization should occur wherever they can be first anticipated. This demonstrates the need to inculcate the value at every level of the organization of the role of all players in sharing the identification, prediction, and adaptation of the organization to realities that affect its continuing viability.

Third, crisis planning must not simply be isolated to particular dramatic and critical events, as often associated with disaster planning. The model should encompass the inherent but less clearly visible crises embedded in contextual and external social, political, and economic changes, which are not so easy to respond to because of the organization's focus on current-stage work. Crisis planning should include the construction of an organizational frame within which predictive and anticipatory transformations and changes can be incorporated in the ordinary course of doing business. Developing these planning components for the normative trajectory of transformative crisis helps to normalize the notion of critical change and inculcates into the lives and activities of workers in every part of the organization the processes associated with predictive and adaptive capacity.

Group Discussion

Organized and systematic response is necessary to building a good infrastructure that supports constant change. Particular elements of this infrastructure are necessary for it to be effective, such as addressing team activities and relationships. What are some of the other elements that are necessary in creating an effective adaptive model (think of the necessary adjustments and changes embedded in responding to the demands of health reform)? What would you do to incorporate this model into your way of doing work? How would it affect the expression of leadership? And what would be the role of workers in making the model work effectively?

Dynamic Cybernetic Team Model (DCTM)

Teams are the fundamental unit of work in the contemporary workplace. If an organization is to fully engage the full range of activities to respond to both process and critical events and seek to be successful, it will do it through teams. Therefore, any model that focuses on predictive and adaptive organizational response to external and internal variances requires full engagement of teams. As previously identified, the ability to isolate environmental signals and triggers that indicate organizational impact may occur anywhere in the organization. Effective and adaptive organizations access insight and response from wherever in the system the indicators of change or crisis first appear.

Most important to the organization is the formalization and construction of rational and sequential approaches to team action (**Figure 7-1**). These responses should be tied to such action and to the purpose, mission, and goals of organization. This operationalizes the work of teams, such that team processes are strongly linked with all the major system characteristics and processes that can make the team ready and available to do its part in anticipating, predicting, and responding to critical indicators.

The team's participation in engaging the challenges to organizations cannot occur effectively unless a frame or discipline is available to give form to the team's work. This framework must be structured enough to provide direction and context, yet fluid enough to respond nimbly to whatever vagaries and variances might confront the organization. Critical to this format is evidence of synthesis of the various flow components of the team's action and the systems framework that gives form to the team's work.

Synthesizing External and Internal Factors

Creating a predictive awareness of the potential of critical events to affect the work of the team requires the team to maintain a broad focus on issues that influence its actions. One

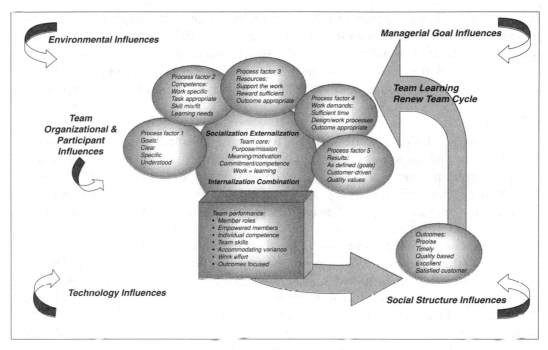

Figure 7-1 Dynamic Cybernetic Team Adaptation Model

of the most significant problems with clinical teams is their disciplinary isolation, hyper-focus on the issues of the day, and lack of awareness of the influences and circumstances affecting team viability occurring outside the immediate locus of the team's action. Environmental and contextual changes in health policy, finances, market, clinical and service characteristics, technology, social structure, priorities, and organizational goals all have a direct impact on the viability and vitality of the team's work. However, team member efforts are often diluted by the team's focus on function and action. There is a belief that the quality of a team's activity is sufficient to ensure its effectiveness, when, instead, external realities have a greater impact on the team's viability than its own actions do.

From a broad view, it is frightening to note how often teams are surprised by shifts in the prevailing reality that affect their ability to succeed in their work. Most teams have a complete lack of awareness of contextual, business, social, and relational changes that affect their work. Even more concerning is leaders' lack of insight regarding how important this level of contextual awareness is to successful action and interaction of team members with the system and with those they serve. Whatever model is created to

Point to Ponder

The team is the centerpiece of all work. It is important that the team be involved in the change process from first identification of the need for change to final implementation of the processes of change.

systematically address team operation and its predictive and adaptive capacity to anticipate and respond to crisis, it must be formalized and become a fundamental part of the discipline in the expression of the role of the leader. This model must be fluid enough to alter priority and practices, yet sufficiently structured to ensure the necessary continuum of actions that attempt to focus the work on reaching goals and achieving outcomes.

Strategic Core

Any systematic activity associated with the team's work must reflect how closely aligned the activity is with the strategic priorities of the organization. In this arena most healthcare organizations reflect the greatest dissonance. Clinical teams often see their focus unilaterally as how well they serve particular patient needs. What they often do not recognize is a broader strategic obligation to which they must contribute. This broader obligation operates at a level of complexity that requires teams at every level of the organization to frame their activities within the context of contribution to the strategic, financial, operational, and service goals of the organization. Simply providing adequate work performance to meet individual patient needs may actually be an impediment to advancing the strategic priorities of the health organization. Failing to make a difference in the health of the community, lack of evidence of the relationship between clinical activity and positive patient outcomes, and a level of resource use intensity that outstrips the financial viability of the organization are examples of how the team's unilateral focus on patient-related activities and functions actually limits or impedes its ability to adequately address the strategic imperative to create a healthy community.

Leaders can demonstrate focus on critical factors by encouraging team members to align patient-related activities with strategic priorities in the conscious application of team thinking and team members' work. Continuous awareness of the alignment of purpose, mission, and professionals' motivation and competence enables leaders and staff to focus on the constant need for goodness of fit between the organization's strategic core and the functional priorities and actions of its clinical providers. Partnership between each team member's personal effort as aggregated in the team's work and the strategic priorities of the organization represents the continuous, seamless thread of collective commitment to ensuring the organization's vitality.

> ### Key Point
>
> Once a strategy has been redefined, the leader must always inform the team and engage it with regard to how the change will affect the way the team does its work.

A part of the flexibility of strategic direction is the fluidity and adaptability of that strategy when external and internal (externalization/ internalization) forces and factors create a need to reconceptualize and reconfigure direction and goals. The tremendous external obligation to create more strongly aligned models of accountable care and the partnerships that sustain it is just one such example. Once a strategy has been redefined to reflect the changing parameters influencing the team's work, the leader must inform the team and inculcate the new factors on the template of the team's mental model and work processes to incorporate changing expectations into team action (socialization/internalization/combination) (**Figure 7-2**). Addressing adaptive processes

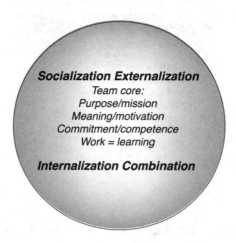

Figure 7-2 Strategy Core

is a critical component of the leader's role. Leaders at all levels of the organization are required to contribute to the fluidity and flexibility of the organization's strategy in responding to the continuously changing circumstances that affect the system priorities and the team's work (Edmonds & Meyer, 2013; Parker, 2003).

Team Performance

Essential to a team's capacity to respond to change and critical events is its basic internal, structural, social, and relational integrity. For a team to function well, it must be clear about the goodness of fit among team members in terms of relationship, competence, and work capacity. The degree of integration, efficacy of interaction, and intersection among team members is critical to smooth and effective functioning of the team. Leaders who do not spend sufficient time constructing effective teams pay a price for this failure at the time of a team's encounter with crisis or conflict.

Teams are themselves small systems, reflecting the same level of complexity as other levels of systemness do. Effectiveness with regard to work styles, communication, and clinical skills and an individual's ability to think critically, express competently, work well with others, accommodate differences, and approach work activities with a high level of flexibility are all requisites for successful team membership (**Figure 7-3**). Failing to balance these essential elements in team construction challenges the leader as the team members attempt to work together. Although learning to develop these capacities is possible for each member of the team, a basic facility with these skill sets must be present at the outset if effective team synthesis is to be ensured.

To ensure long-term team effectiveness, it is important for the leader never to settle for less than a good level of synthesis between and among team members. The leader must establish corollaries with regard to basic clinical competence, conceptual skills, social skills, personal attributes, and the balance of skills between and among team members because these are priorities that influence team effectiveness. The wise leader creates a competency grid related to the clinical, social, personal, and collective parameters

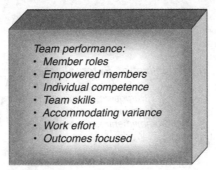

Figure 7-3 Team Performance

necessary to create a frame for defining an effective team within the specific clinical and service characteristics of the department. This "setting the table" for subsequent team interaction and action is perhaps one of the most critical elements of effective team construction.

Once the individual characteristics of team members are combined to create the team's "personality," it is important for the leader to focus on making clear the performance and work expectations that define the functional elements of the team's activities. Here, the leader establishes the link between performance and strategy such that the work efforts of team members are tightly aligned with the purpose and goals of the organization as represented in the focus and activities of the specific clinical service. Here, the leader begins to match the characteristics of the team with the performance expectations and activities represented in the team's work. In an evidence-based approach to structuring team effectiveness, the leader makes sure that team members are aware of expectations, goals, and the specific outcomes to which good performance must ultimately lead.

Once the basic elements of team construction have been configured appropriately, the leader must determine the team's adaptability to changing circumstances and address how vagaries embedded in their work life can be addressed appropriately through team action. Although it is important for teams to work effectively and to undertake their day-to-day routines with care and consideration, the forces of change are always working inexorably on the periphery of organizational life. Weighted by a growing content, the forces of change operate sometimes directly and other times discursively to create a shift in conditions and circumstances that affect the viability and sustenance of work. Sometimes this can be predicted and anticipated; more often, it cannot.

However clearly change can be anticipated, group adaptation and adjustments to the realities and impact of a given change must be part of the work construct of the team. Here, the leader must ensure that appropriate education and development of team members in their role of identifying and adapting to change events are part of the ongoing expectation for team effectiveness. To make sure that the team responds appropriately to critical events, the leader must ensure that team members expect these events to be normative and to appear in ways that directly affect the ability of the team to undertake its work processes. Ultimately, the team must demonstrate its ability to incorporate the demand for adaptation and change into team routines and rituals and, indeed, approach these changes as a normatively interruptive reality.

This critical and adaptive capacity must be present in all levels of team effort in the organization. From the board and executive team focusing on strategy and goal development throughout the organization to include administrative and financial support teams, organizational and clinical support, and clinical services, each makes a contribution to synthesizing and incorporating the demand for change into the collective and individual work processes that result in sustainable outcomes and the ability of the organization to thrive.

Team Outcomes

Teams have no purpose or meaning if purpose and meaning are not driving their work. Contemporary focus on outcomes ties the notion of strategic imperative and work process to the achievement of goals and sustaining work outcomes (**Figure 7-4**). This focus on outcome requires the team to have clearly delineated deliverables against which its performance can be measured. However, all too often in the clinical environment, the clinical team's work becomes an end in itself such that the process becomes the outcome where clearly articulated deliverables are never really expressed. In an evidence-driven and value-grounded world, this circumstance is not acceptable. As digitization of clinical practice and communication, accountable care, and value-based health practices increasingly become the norm, the expectation for the team is that some evidence of impact, of a difference being made, must be incorporated into the performance expectations of team members, just as it is the expectation of the organization.

Value-based practice requires that the team's work activity is viewed from the perspective of the difference it makes, the impact it has, and the health it produces, rather than simply from the view of the quality of the work processes. Teams might work well and with a high degree of commitment and precision and still not make a difference or achieve specific health objectives. This has been the Achilles' heel of most clinical teams in the past. Incremental and unilateral patient impact has historically remained

> **Key Point**
>
> A leader must always make the team aware of the realities affecting advanced planning, which demonstrates commitment to the normative construct and dynamic of change. In this case, adaption is even more important than anticipation.

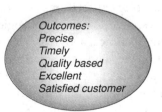

Figure 7-4 Team Outcomes

unconnected or unlinked to other like patient efforts such that an aggregate body of knowledge regarding specific and definitive clinical activities related to defined clinical outcomes has yet to be achieved. The potential for clinical standardization has created the fear that somehow a "cookbook" approach to clinical practice might emerge, robbing it of responsiveness and spontaneity and creating a clinical format that may be disconnected and unfeeling. This fear of standardization has kept clinical professions from developing a broad-based standard of clinical performance that can be effectively compared and contrasted and out of which would emerge clear notions of what worked best and what did not (value-driven, evidence-based practice). Now with the ability to aggregate information across a broad frame, the possibility of creating such foundations for practice is real and increases demand on the clinical team to align its work with a broader body of knowledge.

Standardization can now be seen as simply a mechanism for establishing the "floor" of practice, the norms of clinical decision making and action understood by every practitioner and forming the platform upon which any improvement or advancement occurs. Value-based efforts at finding points of excellence at the "ceiling" of practice demand increasing levels of clinical and service customization made possible by increasingly sophisticated levels of digital utility and applicability. In this dynamic, neither standardization nor customization remains a static notion. When they are continuously informed by increasingly discrete and sophisticated data, clinical practices simply reflect appropriate and timely reactions. On this dynamic trajectory, practice changes are the normative response to evidence that both informs and provides the impetus for continuous practice change.

User Expectations

With the emerging digital tools, teams can now be more objective and definitive with regard to clinical action. They can measure performance against an aggregated database to determine effectiveness and efficacy. Teams must think within this practice framework. As part of evaluating and delineating the most effective clinical processes likely to achieve defined expectations and outcomes, they must adapt strategies that integrate their unilateral action with the action of other similar teams. In generic terminology, outcome value must also include customer (patient) satisfaction, but only if that satisfaction is based on clearly enumerated, legitimate user (patient) expectations. Team members now must ensure providers and patients (users) have a clearly understood set of expectations with regard to what is legitimate to achieve under the circumstances.

In achieving sustainable outcomes, one of the performance expectations of team members is reeducation of the user, shifting expectations and roles as the parameters and conditions of service change in response to new technologies, therapeutics, and interventions. The constant enhancement of clinical activities over increasingly shorter periods of time requires that user reeducation be a constant activity of the clinical team in relationship to those they serve. Also, outcome expectation includes more clearly defining the performance roles of users (consumers or patients) in managing that part of the clinical journey for which they are primarily accountable. As healing increasingly occurs in settings other than the clinical institution, user accountability in undertaking activities and roles related to the individual's healing process is now a fundamental work expectation of the clinical team. Indeed, this is one of the centerpieces of value-driven health reform.

Notions of excellence and value with regard to outcomes must also include how clearly specific clinical and performance outcomes have fulfilled the overall strategic purpose and goals of the organization. The clinical team must always maintain a two-pronged focus on outcomes. First, it must meet the individual clinical needs of

> **Point to Ponder**
>
> Excellence in performance is no longer optional. Therefore, teams must focus on value and outcomes, not just processes. What the patient receives—not just what the provider gives—is important. For providers, there must be strong goodness of fit between process and outcome to achieve and sustain value.

the population it serves as those are defined from the perspective of the user (patient). Second, the overall organizational goals, which include community impact, overall health status, reduction in process risks, and any other specific clinical performance goals, must also be included in the performance expectations of team members. Making the connection between individual consumer impact and aggregated organizational effectiveness becomes the frame for delineating outcome value at the point of service and within the context of the work of all teams, regardless of where they are located in the system.

Here again, crisis and critical events are constantly lurking at the boundaries of the organization's intersection with the larger community and the team's intersection with the organization and consumers (patients). Inherent in all team action is the team's continuing awareness of and preparedness for environmental, financial, technological, social, and market changes that dynamically intersect with current operations and occasionally converge to create a demand for change in strategy, operations, and clinical practice. At best, in the course of doing business teams can adjust to predicted and anticipated changes with sufficient time and resources. However, just as likely, other critical events, disasters, and unanticipated and unplanned events will require teams to change behaviors and practices immediately, demonstrating their inherent flexibility and fluidity as well as the applicability of their crisis planning model.

The Partnership Team Process Factors

The best methodology available for confronting crisis events is an infrastructure that builds on the normality of good process. Building a good process infrastructure creates a frame for response to any particular work activities and, further, provides a construct within which critical events can be addressed through good form, format, and structure.

Process factors break down the framework for work activities into a series of steps that relate specifically to the work itself and the staged activities that represent particular points of reference in relationship to the work (**Figure 7-5**). In addition, process factors tie each stage of the work process to the goals and purposes that give direction and meaning to individual work. Process factors structure the work activities so that they best relate to the goals and objectives to which those work activities are directed. In the midst of a crisis or critical event, dependence on the stability that comes from process factors provides a solid frame of reference. What often happens in the midst of critical process is the loss of the routine and

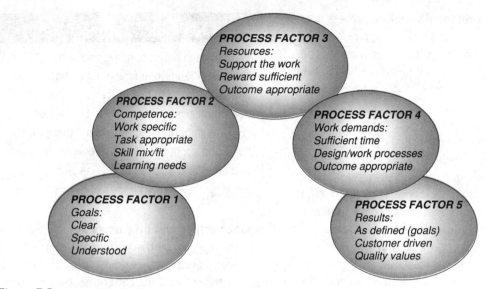

Figure 7-5 Process Factors

ritual embedded in process factors. Through this loss, organizations become chaotic and directionless and fail to incorporate the critical process into a ritualized series of activities that can ensure all issues affected by the crisis are addressed appropriately.

Process factors can be broken down into five types: goals, competence, resources, work demands, and results. There is a sixth factor that follows the successful flow of the five process factors, and that factor is the outcome, evaluation. This factor is separate from the other process factors because evaluation depends on their successful implementation and action related to them. The elements that identify and explicate outcomes are clearly enumerated in the first five process factors.

Process Factor 1: Goals

In moments of crisis or in the midst of critical events, organizations lose their bearing, their sense of directedness, and as a result become reactive and focused on the short term. They can be "eaten up" by the immediate issue or situation, often at the expense of other important factors. The purpose of goals is certainly clear during the normal processes of the organization in the absence of critical events (**Figure 7-6**). However, critical events do not change the need for goals; if anything, they advance them. An important and appropriate role of leadership during a critical event is refocusing the organization on its goals and

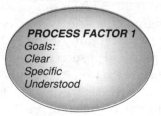

Figure 7-6 Process Factor 1: Goals

276

purposes so that, in responding to the critical event, the organization does not wander away from its key purposes and directional priorities. Goals serve as a point of demarcation even in the most critical change event, such that when a change occurs, a clear delineation of the impact of the change can be better made when compared to the originating goal.

Leaders help the organization in crisis by bringing leader and staff attention to the fundamental purposes and values of the organization as it confronts its crisis and attempts to continue to thrive. This notion of thriving is important in the midst of crisis. Often, during crises organizations move to survival mode. Although some of the immediate actions may focus on precise and definitive responses to the crisis, the organization should not forget its fundamental drive to achieve its goals and fulfill its purpose in a way that both acknowledges and accepts the impact of a change on originating goal content. Failing to do so maintains a crisis format for the organization and keeps it from returning to a focus that represents its core values and goal priorities.

Goal clarity and specificity are the two most important elements of goal setting. Goals must be defined in such a way that the purpose and mission of the organization are made transparent to all members and can be clearly articulated by individuals and workgroups whose activity ostensibly fulfills the purposes of the organization. The ability to clearly enumerate particular goals and priorities helps the organization keep focus on the purposes of work and the long-term values to which even critical responses must ultimately be directed. Furthermore, it keeps workers grounded and promulgates the particular values that relate to the organization thriving and the activities necessary to ensure that happens.

> **Point to Ponder**
>
> Competence is not simply what people know. Competence is what people do with what they know and how well that makes a difference for others.

Process Factor 2: Competence

Ensuring competence at every level of the organization is never so important as during a critical period of events. Lapses in identifying and managing issues of competence become especially risky when critical events intervene. At these times, the organization needs to depend on the ability and skills of those who do its work (**Figure 7-7**). If the critical competence factors necessary to ensure effective work processes are missing, the price that is paid during a critical event is additionally burdensome to the organization. Assurance that every level of work operates at a specific level of competence becomes very important in positioning organizations to address the inevitable noise and crises that

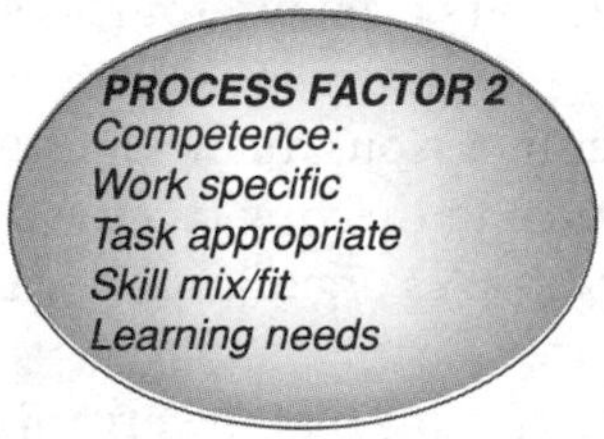

> **PROCESS FACTOR 2**
> Competence:
> Work specific
> Task appropriate
> Skill mix/fit
> Learning needs

Figure 7-7 Process Factor 2: Competence

come with unplanned occurrences. Individuals need to act independently and interdependently at a number of critical levels in the midst of a crisis event. This expectation, that the organization can count on the skills and talents of its workforce, is an important factor in the organization's preparedness and readiness for any crisis events.

Competence includes not only the skills, abilities, and capacity of performing job assignments, but also workers' ability to take focused action. The focus is on individual competence as well as on team response. Teams are the basic unit of all work. The ability of teams to respond appropriately and with efficiency to crisis depends on team members' ability to act in concert with each other, in direct response to the crisis as it affects the team's work, and in relationship with other teams with specified roles in responding to the critical event. This notion of the centrality of teams to work is especially critical in the development and refinement of models of accountable care where transdisciplinary partnerships, interactions, and relationships are central to obtaining high-level and sustainable clinical outcomes and advancing community health.

Competence in crisis also means the ability to adapt to additional challenges and activities necessary to ensure the organization's appropriate action in the face of crisis. Sometimes a crisis broadens role expectations beyond the usual and ordinary course of an individual's or a team's working over time. Critical events may change the mix of work expectations and demands, requiring workers to shift roles, performance, and expectations. Competence means the flexibility, fluidity, and adaptability necessary to meet the challenges and shifting demands that frequently arise in moments of crisis.

Incorporated in the notion of competence is the commitment of the organization, teams, and individuals to continuing education and development in preparation for or anticipation of inevitable crises or critical events. Continuing education and development of individuals and teams to respond to potential crises are important parts of the organization's development program. Although every kind of crisis cannot be anticipated, the demands of crisis are often generic and can be incorporated into the learning curriculum of employee development. Incorporating the elements of crisis, characteristics of crisis response, and individual and collective roles in reacting and adapting to crisis and addressing issues of flexibility and fluidity in the presence of crisis are all important learning elements that can advance the competence of leaders and teams in the face of inevitable critical events.

Process Factor 3: Resources
It is surprising how few organizations manage their fiscal distribution and operational budgets in a way that includes the anticipation of critical events and crisis situations. A certain amount of the organization's capital resources should be directed to addressing inevitable critical events. Often organizations that have failed to adequately create resource reserves find themselves in serious financial trouble too late in the crisis cycle to adequately respond and to return to thriving (**Figure 7-8**). In fact, this set of circumstances most often permanently cripples organizations in the face of crisis, ending in serious decline or corporate failure.

Appropriate resource allocation means that the organization has set aside sufficient financial, material, and human resources to respond immediately and effectively to crises

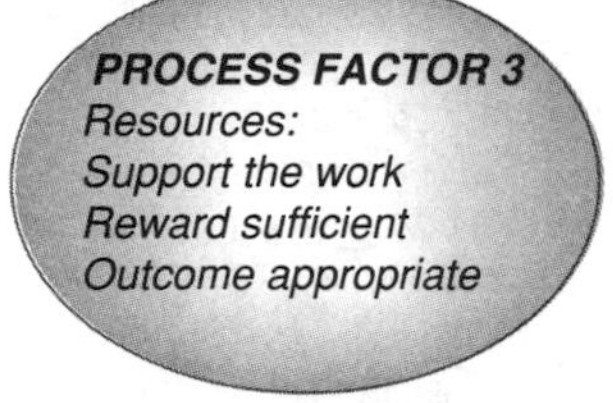

Figure 7-8 Process Factor 3: Resources

that affect the normative operations of the organization. The ability of the organization to adapt specific job functions, roles, and fiscal commitments to address crisis plays a major part in ensuring the organization can quickly recover from critical events and move forward into normal operations. Taking additional time and resources to adjust the normal flow of business to respond to the crisis, if not carefully managed, can be a formula for failure. Quickly responding to critical events and creating a goodness of fit between the response and the demand of the event indicate a good allocation of appropriate resources and an ability to adapt the focus of the organization to the issues immediately affecting it. This ability to reallocate and shift the distribution of capital and resources creates the level of flexibility and fluidity necessary to respond appropriately to crisis. Furthermore, flexibility reflects the organization's understanding that the social milieu for all organized human activity in the current digital social reality is to remain continuously portable and mobile in every endeavor. All levels of the organization should consider their individual and collective ability to shift focus and resource capacity to adequately address critical events without endangering the long-term viability and service provision of the organization.

One can imagine the secondary crisis created in an organization where staffing and financial resources are already tightly configured. The introduction of critical events often places additional demand on existing work infrastructure, making it virtually impossible for resources to meet the demands of the crisis and the routine and usual expectations for work (Alvesson & Willmott, 2012; Hamlin, Keep, & Ash, 2001). Not adequately accessing additional resources or adjusting the focus of existing resources in a timely fashion creates a double demand on staff, further burdening them with additional work, increasing levels of emotional stress, and decreasing their ability to focus and respond to immediate issues of concern. And yet it is common for just such secondary crisis events to occur in many organizations in the midst of crisis. The staff's inability to respond and the narrowly allocated resources with no financial flexibility create a serious constraint on the organization's ability to respond to crisis. This is a far more common set of circumstances than is often perceived. A critical leadership requisite is balancing long-term operational resource needs with the resources required for inevitable crisis occurrences.

Process Factor 4: Work Demands
The configuration of the elements of work and workload become important considerations in critical events. Most organizations operate as efficiently as they can, recognizing the need for appropriate productivity and maintaining a tight relationship between work

279

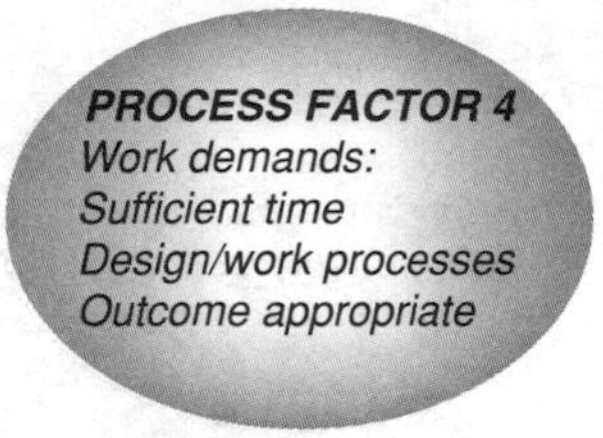

PROCESS FACTOR 4
Work demands:
Sufficient time
Design/work processes
Outcome appropriate

Figure 7-9   Process Factor 4: Work Demands

demands and workload. Although this is certainly an appropriate measure of performance in organizations under normal conditions, planning must include flexibility related to specific work objectives when crisis arises (**Figure 7-9**).

The design of work must include options related to responding to critical events and changes in the normal course and routine of work. In clinical organizations, different levels of census create shifting demands and require a flexible staffing and resource use plan. Insight into and need for staffing and resources during critical events are heightened. If a disaster or an unplanned event changes the normal routine, a different resource use plan that accelerates or shifts human resources allocation must be accessible. The crisis planning process should develop such a plan. Staffing and scheduling programs routinely need to be addressed in light of shifting demand and accelerating changes that affect work distribution and workload. Incorporating flexibility and fluidity into the human resources staffing plan increases the likelihood that the organization can adapt to particular crisis events.

Consider some of the challenges associated with health reform. An emphasis on late–stage, bed-based services is shifting quickly to a focus on earlier engagement of services along the continuum of care and new service configurations that reduce the dependency on bed-related services. Those persons staffing bed-related services are therefore poorly positioned to thrive. Quickly shifting human resources to new care models and retraining them for different roles are critical to hospitals' ability to accommodate changing care and service requirements and practices.

Many organizations build contingency staffing plans based on changing customer demand or productivity and workload issues. These contingency plans help the organization respond to shifting work demands that include a different service mix or accelerated product or service demand cycle. These flexibility plans also can serve an organization well in the midst of planned and unplanned events. Using this approach to variability in resource demand and staffing helps the organization adjust resources based on the nature of the crisis and the skills of and demands on the workers.

Continuing education and specific role development with regard to unplanned and critical events are important corollaries to the routine education and development of teams and workers. As in the process factor related to worker competence, it is important that the ability to act in a complex or crisis situation is also expected and incorporated into the role and routines of specific workers in the organization. Here again, many crises are unplanned, yet the nature of crisis often requires timely and effective response.

The talent and ability to anticipate and respond in crisis can be likened to volunteer fire departments and voluntary medical emergency units: The focus is on skill development of individuals whose primary work activity is focused in another arena. Using this dynamic in corporate crisis response helps prepare key workers to play specific roles in unplanned or critical events and ensures a heightened level of preparedness of the organization.

> **Point to Ponder**
>
> Almost all crises are unplanned for. Understanding that, leaders always make sure that there is a system for crises, an infrastructure that makes it possible to anticipate and to respond to unplanned-for crises.

Process Factor 5: Results/Impact

Results normally validate the achievements of goals to which the team and individual work has been directed. Clearly, the goodness of fit between the goals and the achieved results is an indicator of the level of success of the organization and its members. In critical situations, the notion of focus on results is as important as in the normative and routine operations of the organization. A significant difference between the two is that results orientation of normal work processes is long term and continuing, whereas the results orientation of critical events has a much shorter cycle of productivity and performance. Critical events lead to redefining and reconfiguring goals and results based on the immediate activities and actions that must be undertaken to return the organization to thrive status. Results in a critical situation must be defined early so that work processes can be focused specifically on achieving corrective short-term objectives in an efficient and effective manner (**Figure 7-10**).

Short-term goal orientation related to crises should still at some level be evaluated against the long-term operational goals of the organization. Critical intervention intends to return the organization to its normative level of operation. To do this, leaders must continually assess the critical goals directed to stabilizing and renewing the reorganization in the context of the longer term functional goals that supply the drive and purpose to the work of the organization. Matching critical goals helps create a process that fits with the return to normalization necessary to stabilize the organization and ensure its long-term viability. Leaders at every level of the organization must be aware of this need to address both the normative long-term goals and the short-term and immediate goals necessary to normalize activities of the organization.

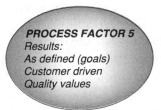

Figure 7-10   Process Factor 5: Results Focus

Impact on Outcomes

Focusing on the orientation to outcome during a critical event becomes important when considered from the perspective of the customer/user. Critical events have an impact on the will of the organization to serve its users and meet their needs. This orientation to user sensitivity is vital during crisis experiences. Users must be aware of the shift in emphasis, adjustment of resources, and impact on the service or product. The immediate inclusion of the user in consideration of crisis response helps reduce the impact of the crisis, the stress of responding to the crisis, and the negative impact on the user or plan needs. Often, when the focus of a crisis takes emphasis away from meeting the needs of the client or user and when the client or user can be incorporated into the dynamic of solutions seeking or problem solving, the stress and critical nature of the crisis can be significantly reduced. In addition, the client or user can participate in finding alternatives and changing his or her own demand in relationship to pressure on the organization during a critical time frame. Through partnership with the client or user, the organization in crisis can often better identify and address appropriate responses and solutions and return to long-term normative operations.

Group Discussion

In hospitals and service organizations, crisis has a special impact on patients and people. In planning for and building infrastructure for managing crisis, how does the leader incorporate the patient or the public in responding appropriately to the crisis? What roles do the patient (the user) and significant others play in responding to a clinical or an organizational crisis (such as that indicated by implementation of the various elements of health reform)? Should they be involved in constructing plans for a systematic response to crisis? How are they involved? What processes of communication are necessary in the system to make sure patients (users) are aware and informed of their participation?

Certainly, these process factors play a significant role in an organization's response to crisis. The more committed the organization is to systematically and effectively organizing around its specific process factors, the better the tool set the organization has to respond to unplanned events and crises. The discipline with which a company or clinical organization follows its process plan is an important factor in determining that organization's ability to respond well to a crisis. Although, clearly, subsequent processes and dynamics need to be in place to ensure appropriate response to a crisis, the foundations laid by an appropriate team-based process action plan incorporated into the clinical and operating framework is valuable for successfully responding to critical events. In addition, because this is a cybernetic process the impact and value of process factors in a normative work environment are continuous, dynamic, and cyclical in nature. The adaptation of these factors to a critical environment indicates the same level of dynamic, only on a shorter and more heightened cycle. The ability of the leader to apply process factors to the cycle of crisis intervention as a foundation for evaluating progress and successful intervention is an important indicator of effective crisis management.

Cybernetic and Interacting Environmental Scanning Process

The ability of an organization to respond well to crisis directly relates to the organization's ability to anticipate it. Anticipating and predicting crisis are important parts of the role of leadership throughout the organization. Leaders must recognize the fundamental obligation of leadership: ensuring the environmental influences that have an impact on the organization's ability to do its work have been considered and any change in them has been noted, especially with regard to a shift in the organization. The work of the organization is affected by a number of internal and external forces. These

> ### Key Point
>
> The model that is created for responding to crisis is cybernetic; that is, it includes processes that are continuous, dynamic, and cyclical in nature. This cybernetic system is what ensures that the processes are continuously fluid, flexible, and mobile.

forces continuously interact, and the leader, recognizing this level of interaction, realizes that a change in response may be indicated by a shift in conditions and circumstances.

Organizations are dynamic and living entities. As such, they must achieve a goodness of fit and interaction with the prevailing environment and the context within which they function (**Figure 7-11**). Because living organizations exist in a field of continuous and

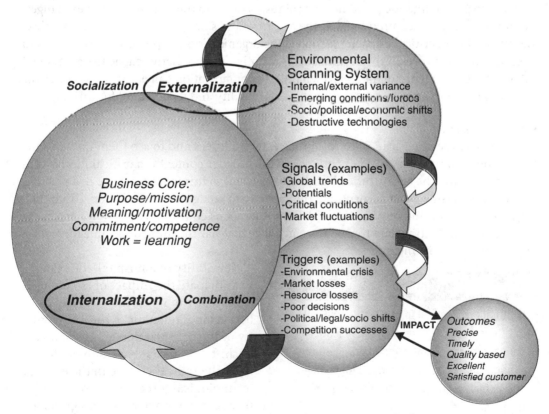

Figure 7-11 Cybernetic and Interacting Environmental Scanning Detail of DCTM

dynamic change, the circumstances and conditions within which an organization functions are constantly shifting and adjusting, frequently representing an ever-emerging set of factors that alter the organization's reality and change its operation and action.

Wherever the external environment of the organization comes in contact with the internal mechanisms of the organization, the urge and intersection for change occur. The leader, recognizing that these intersections are indicators of the potential for critical events or unplanned circumstances, constantly surveys the landscape for elements and contents of conditions or circumstances and the potential they have for shifting and adjusting organizational reality (Young & Hester, 2004).

Internalization and Externalization

Human organizations do not function in isolation. There is a convergence of interactions and intersections within which organizations operate in a continuously dynamic yet cybernetic environment. The external forces at work on organizations relate to social, political, economic, market, and human conditions and circumstances that constantly bombard the organization with different influences. For the most part, these forces can be anticipated and visualized early enough for the organization to respond appropriately. Occasionally, however, these forces converge in an unplanned or unanticipated way and create conditions that force the organization to respond immediately. For example, health reform can be planned for; an unanticipated number of respondents to the state insurance exchanges cannot be so easily accommodated. If the organization is not prepared for the eventuality and possibility of critical impact, reaction is the organization's response to the condition or circumstance. However, if the organization's adaptive and predictive capacities are refined sufficiently to deal with unanticipated change, the organization can actually use the change event as an opportunity to expand or extend its viability and its potential for thriving.

External Forces

The ability of the organization to recognize external forces and to see them in the context of the organization's lived experience in the broader context is a critical mechanism for guaranteeing the organization's ability to respond to immediate change in a positive fashion. Leadership must incorporate the capacity to recognize critical change into the organization scanning mechanisms. These mechanisms continuously scan for external forces and broadly translate those forces in a way that has meaning and value for the organization and its members.

Point to Ponder

External and internal forces lend equal weight to the process of change. The wise leader can incorporate both external and internal dynamics in assessing the need for change and in building a systematic and organized response to it.

The ability of a hospital, for example, to anticipate the impact of changing technology in its cardiac services can be a strong indicator of the adaptability of the organization and its ability to shift its internal environment to meet the radical change in the external technological forces. The movement from coronary artery bypass grafts to drug-eluding stents and/or emerging pharmacological responses is a classic example of the need for an organization to quickly shift its infrastructure, clinical dynamics, and payment processes to address an important new technology. In addition, a healthcare system's move to refining an electronic medical record documentation system is a radical shift in the mechanisms of information management and documentation such that skills, ability, systems, adaptation, and clinical process are all affected by the improvement. Anticipating the increasing demand at the policy and payment levels and with regard to utilization of resources and workload reorganization, the organization must adapt critically and appropriately to this shift in clinical process. Both are examples of external forces having a dramatic and direct impact on internal mechanisms, causing an organization to shift its resources and activities to respond to a new demand, not necessarily a part of its existing infrastructure.

Internal Forces

Internal forces, too, have a strong impact on an organization's ability to respond to changing circumstances and demands that affect its ability to thrive. Structural and operational forces work together to create a context for organizational activities. Unless internal forces are adequately configured to support the organization's ability to address changes and challenges that affect work goals, processes, and outcomes, the ability of the organization to thrive may be compromised. A traditionally satisfactory response to address prevailing or emerging demands may no longer be adequate and, as a result, can actually impede the organization's ability to engage and change.

Internal support structures, work processes, management systems, supply chain, and communication processes may work individually or collectively to create conditions that limit the organization's ability to address real-time issues and concerns. There is a real need for leaders to ensure a true goodness of fit between the internal work structures and processes so that when emerging demands, both external and internal, operate to create a change in the mechanisms of work, the organization can respond quickly and effectively (**Figure 7-12**). This notion of nimbleness is a critical element in the leader's

> **Point to Ponder**
>
> The internal environment must respond to crisis and change in a fluid and flexible manner because there is now no long-term recovery time between components of the change process.

understanding of contemporary work dynamics. There is not a significantly long period of time for adjustment and adaptation. Leaders must adapt and reframe work dynamics in a relatively short time and in a way that ensures appropriate linkage between work processes and changing demand (fluid and flexible). Examples of new medication administration systems, materials management supply chain systems, pharmacy distribution/control/monitoring systems, and an intranet communication infrastructure all represent the internal arena of work structures and processes. They must represent a commitment to reconfiguration and synthesis of changing technologies and processes in the internal work dynamics of the organization.

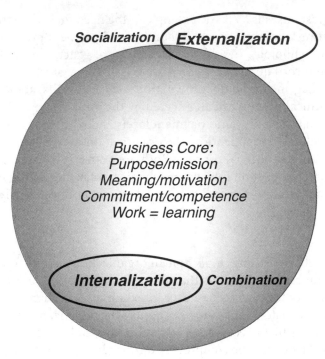

Figure 7-12 Externalization/Internalization

Ensuring a Strong Service Core

In hospitals and health systems, it is easy to see how leaders can be co-opted by business opportunity, fads, and new ventures in a way that causes them to lose sight of their core work (**Figure 7-13**). Exciting and innovative options can lead an organization down new paths. However, unless these options are disciplined by consistency with mission and purpose, they can also draw the life out of an organization. Leaders must understand that a change in any one part of the structure creates pressures and demands on other parts of the system, leading either to collective sustenance or to failure. To moderate this situation, new ventures and directions should be consistent with the vision, mission, and purposes of the organization.

When a mission reflects the vision and values of the organization, it must be inculcated into every person and activity in the organization. For workers, either clinical or support, the meaning and value of their work can become unilateral and nonaligned if it is not both

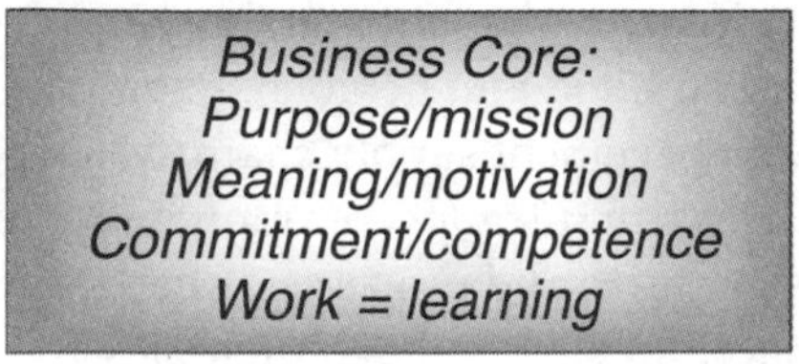

> Business Core:
> Purpose/mission
> Meaning/motivation
> Commitment/competence
> Work = learning

Figure 7-13 Business Core

286

informed and disciplined by purpose and clearly delineated work objectives. Successful organizations require that all stakeholders at any place in the organization be fully committed to living and working consistently with the mission and purposes of the organization. Affirming this ensures that the mission is inculcated in the fabric of the organization and that the work activities of every participant

> **Point to Ponder**
>
> Mission and purpose are fulfilled through an organization's work. Therefore, workers must understand the relationship between their own work efforts and the fulfillment of the mission and purpose of the organization through the commitment of their own effort.

create a core around which all strategic and operational activities can unfold. When this connection is not delineated for everyone in the system, employees often substitute sectional and unilateral purposes and goals and begin to fulfill their own purposes instead.

A strong focus on mission and purpose leads to ensuring that all workers in the system are motivated and committed to achieving positive organizational purposes and, it goes without saying, the success of the organization. Individuals are fully aware of how much their ability to thrive depends on organizational success. Building a membership community around this core of understanding and continually reinforcing it establish a firm and continuous foundation on which every work activity can build. In addition, leaders make sure that all activities related to knowledge generation, learning, experimentation, and innovation are evaluated against the mission and purpose. At every level of the organization, the direction, conversation, performance requisites, and work outcomes of all employees should reflect how every participant in the organization fulfills mission and purpose.

This requires leaders to translate the usually esoteric language of strategy and mission into a language that can be understood at the organization's points of service. Clinical practitioners, service providers, and support persons collectively need to be assured that their individual contributions are valued within the context of advancing the mission and purposes of the organization. The language of leadership must reflect the requisites of embracing the mission, identifying how individual work effort contributes to it, and ensuring that work outcomes advance the organization's mission and purpose. This series of activities, linkages, and integration, facilitated by the leader's commitment and effort, ensures the strong point of reference in the midst of intense change. In evaluating critical events or intense moments of change and unplanned crises or challenges, mission and purpose serve as the lens through which leaders can more accurately and appropriately determine specific response. The organization's place in the world is viewed through this lens, which creates both the frame and the discipline for leaders to evaluate crisis and select the most successful responses to it.

Crisis and Environmental Scanning

The wise leader is always aware of the constancy of change. This change comes in many forms and can emerge at almost any point in the life cycle of an organization. This constancy of change is the only true context and has a universal impact on all life processes. The skilled leader recognizes this dynamic is part of the constancy of work and relationship. The leader is ever vigilant to the conditions and circumstances, both internal and external, that indicate a significant organizational impact.

In times of great change, such as our current work environment, a talent for environmental scanning becomes vital (**Figure 7-14**). Mobility and the constant transformation of human work and communication systems create the conditions that call the leader to a broader and deeper understanding of the influences and circumstances affecting the organization and the work of its people. Through the development and refinement of strong environmental scanning skills, at every level of management meaningful change can be sorted from fad and superficiality, and appropriate shifts in strategy and work can be more clearly articulated. The effective leader, at every level of the organization, understands the internal work dynamics and relationships within the organization with a high level of proficiency. This leader knows the value and contribution the individual departments or units of the work system make to the whole organization. The reverse is also true: Capable department and unit leaders are aware of the impact of the larger system (both external and internal) on the ability of the individual department or unit to function and thrive. This awareness should raise the value of synthesis in the perception of all leaders and emphasize the need for consistency and integration in every level of system decision making and action.

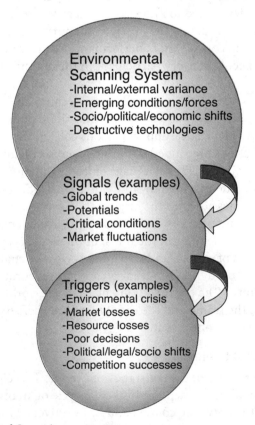

Figure 7-14 Environmental Scanning

Effective leaders assess information and resources that lead to understanding the convergence of dynamics that create the conditions that influence or affect current operations or work. The strategic decision to implement a high-portability electronic medical record system or paperless processes throughout the clinical organization is a strong indicator of a significant change in information management, documentation, technology, and work applications. Seeing the significance of these forces early in the strategic process provides

> **Key Point**
>
> Unit or departmental leaders see their role from the perspective of the whole system. They don't just lead departments or units, they lead the whole system from the perspective of the department or units where they are located.

a response framework for the leader that raises questions related to impact on work design, clinical roles, new learning, support systems, communication, and worker behavior. Once the strategic implications are fully understood, issues of timeline, planning, education, orientation, experimentation, and application can be better defined.

Systematizing this strategic environmental scanning process and formalizing it provide leadership at every level of the health system with both the tools and the processes necessary to anticipate and even predict essential change. Reinforcing in the leader the requisites to read broadly, to stay current with clinical and systems innovations, to remain invested and involved in strategic discussions, and to synthesize information from diverse sources is invaluable in developing effective environmental scanning skills. Leaders at every level of the organization must be free to honestly and openly recognize incongruence between current work conditions, circumstances, and processes and prevailing or emerging realities that challenge or threaten them. These variances create the context for new thinking and raise the challenge for developing innovative approaches. The leader recognizes that in response to these shifting realities, work processes never remain the same and must always shift to accommodate new technical or process realities. Here again, the leader creates this cultural frame, this context, if you will, within which worker attitude, behavior, responsiveness, and action can demonstrate a willingness and competence to respond in a timely fashion and to act appropriately.

Emerging conditions and forces often can be seen far ahead of their direct impact on organizations and people. Often, leaders suggest how they saw and recognized the coming change but never believed it would have the powerful impact it subsequently did. Anticipating constant change and incorporating it into the discussion related to strategy and response are strong indicators of organizational predictive competence. Also, using alignment strategies that create connections and linkages among emerging technical and work conditions and forces, social and political influences, dramatic economic shifts, and even destructive technologies is useful in determining the specificity and degree of the impact the future change may have on the organization and its people (Bridges, 2004; Hickey & Kritek, 2012).

Signals
Leaders are constantly alert for those major indicators or signals of impending change that are strongly predictive of an impact on the organization and its work (**Figure 7-15**). Changes in therapeutic modalities occur; for example, the movement from coronary

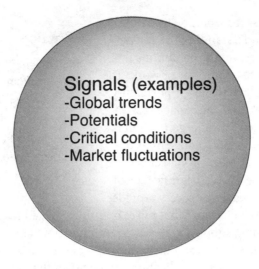

Figure 7-15 **Signals**

> **Point to Ponder**
>
> Leaders must help those they lead understand the impact of external trends and changes and how they alter the conception of the work, the way the work is done, and the activities of all workers related to undertaking change in their own way of doing work.

artery bypass grafts to pharmaco-therapeutics for cardiac support indicates a major shift in the clinical therapeutic modality for cardiac vein occlusion. This therapeutic shift creates intense conditional and process challenges, causing hospitals, diagnostic services, cardiac therapies, finance systems, and support systems to alter both their infrastructure and their work approaches. Because of the "noise" involved in such a dramatic shift, organizations often avoid the upfront conversations and interactions necessary to appropriately anticipate the significance of this therapeutic change and to directly confront the requisites of organizational and personal adjustment. The potential for conflict in neither having anticipated this significant shift nor having undertaken a planned strategic review of the signals ultimately creates reactive noise and increases the challenge of appropriate adaptation. Without adaptation, the conflict between cardiac surgeons and therapeutic cardiologists is accelerated, and marketing and payment schemes related to this therapeutic transformation, as well as service and operational adjustments, are severely challenged.

Leaders must regularly scan broad information sources and evidenced-based documentation related to health care or particular health services, identify the signals obtained from this activity, share them with key stakeholders, and undertake dialogue with regard to appropriate response. Leaders must now help their stakeholders assess global trends, clinical potentials, critical changes in environmental and work conditions, significant shifts in the market, and new technology if they are to ensure sufficiency in adaptation, prediction, and response.

Triggers

Recognizing significant events or indicators demonstrates the leader's ability to read signals and to draw inferences from them with regard to their potential impact on their organization and service. Eventually, however, all signals converge with external or internal conditions and circumstances to create critical moments. These critical moments serve as trigger events for organizations and people with regard to the dire, immediate, or direct impact of crisis, change, or transformation on the organization and its people (**Figure 7-16**). Still, at this level of intensity trigger events can be missed. When overlooked, they drive the organization into reactive strategies, away from proactive anticipation and response, causing a spiraling down of leadership and staff response toward reactive patterns of behavior; recidivism; poor decisions; market, business, and service losses; and negative human dynamics.

Organizational intelligence is best represented in the effectiveness and success of a system's ability to adapt in a cybernetic way to the vagaries of change that affect it. Sound environmental scanning processes help the organization anticipate strategic, operating, clinical, and technical potential for problems. Trigger events ultimately address any one or all of these in any given moment in time. These triggers can be anticipated if appropriately and properly identified through enumerating the signals that, upon convergence, create them. The ability of leaders at every level of the organization to identify signals and respond to trigger events precisely and quickly indicates the degree of adaptation really present in an organization.

Trigger events are the organization's last line of defense against an impending or inevitable shift or change. Triggers indicate that the change impact is "at the door" and now directly influences the strategy and work dynamics of the organization. Ignoring trigger events generally leads to a higher level of organizational crisis and ultimately extends to influencing the viability of the entire system. Developing in leaders effective

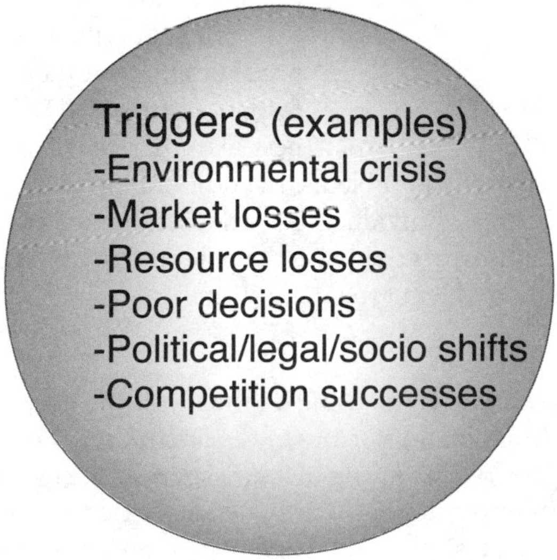

Triggers (examples)
-Environmental crisis
-Market losses
-Resource losses
-Poor decisions
-Political/legal/socio shifts
-Competition successes

Figure 7-16 Triggers

environmental scanning skills and formalizing methodologies in the organization for identifying signal indicators and processes and anticipating trigger events become requisites for systems adaptation and thriving.

Crisis Preparedness

Although environmental scanning is an essential skill, it is not, by itself, sufficient for addressing potential and inevitable crises or critical events. The organization's ability to predict and anticipate the potential for critical processes in today's world requires solid strategic planning. Any contemporary organization must now have an operating format or infrastructure that specifically incorporates into its management processes adaptive and predictive strategies and crisis preparedness.

Hospitals and health systems are excellent at developing a variety of community disaster plans. These plans have proven to be excellent templates for healthcare organization responses to crisis and disaster. However, few hospitals and health systems have crisis preparedness plans that are directed to helping them identify and respond to strategic, operational, and service crises and critical changes that directly affect the hospital or health system. In a time of fast-paced technological and therapeutic change, it is no longer optional for hospitals and health systems to anticipate and prepare for significant critical events that affect their very viability and sustenance. Crisis preparedness planning needs to confront the hospital's or health system's strategic, operating, human, and technical problem types that invariably result from the impact of a whole host of critical events.

> **Key Point**
>
> Crisis preparedness should be incorporated into the organization's strategic processes. Critical events should not be seen as external and not be planned for in advance. The ability to predict and adapt to inevitable crisis and build it into the infrastructure of strategy helps ensure the organization's ability to thrive.

Planning for critical events requires that the organizational leadership understand that each problem type must have specific planning processes that enumerate the organization's response to a crisis. Effective crisis preparedness planning needs to clearly identify specific response plans for each type of problems. In addition, the crisis preparedness plan needs to sufficiently address individual or particular threats: environmental, technical/mechanical, and human threats that have the potential to affect the clinical organization through one or all of its problem types.

Planning

A good crisis preparedness plan focusing on the life of the hospital or health system addresses particular functional priorities of the organization in each of its problem areas (**Figure 7-17**). Effective planning includes specific engagement and anticipation of leadership response in implementing designated activities in response to signal or trigger events. In crisis preparedness planning, a crisis plan group should be identified and each member should have specific tasks and responsibilities. Members of this group should

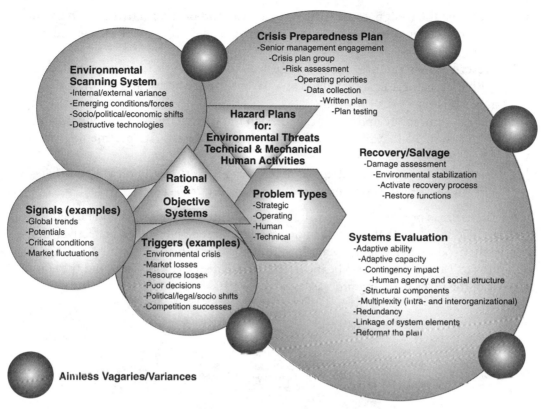

Figure 7-17 DCTM Details of Components for Assessing Adaptive Effectiveness

come from the various forums and levels of the organization representing the breadth of its service and support structures. This group ties crisis planning to the environmental scanning system and anticipates the potential for specific responses. This requires a well-refined mechanism of assessing risk potential and anticipating risk impact on the organization. Effective crisis planning identifies and defines particular risk-specific operating priorities that can potentially best respond to an impending crisis. The group clarifies these operating priorities and details responses from the involved departments, services, and people in the organization. The group can use environmental scanning processes and data from potential signals and likely trigger events to develop a database that informs particular critical response stages or steps.

The crisis preparedness plan should address the following issues:

1. Describe the various levels and activities associated with leadership engagement and the roles various leaders will play in response to specific categories of crisis
2. Form the crisis plan group, whose role is to coordinate the activities associated with crisis plan development and application
3. Identify and determine specific arenas of sensitivity or potential external and internal risk factors that may be associated with the cause of crisis

4. Describe the design, form, format, structure, and process activities associated with operating priorities at a time when trigger events impinge on the usual work cycles

5. Describe the structure, methodology, technology, and processes associated with data gathering and analysis as a part of the predictive and adaptive data mechanisms

6. Clearly enumerate and specifically design the written crisis preparedness plan and make it available to all the pertinent leaders and departments of the organization

7. Implement a regularly scheduled mechanism for testing the veracity and effectiveness of the crisis preparedness plan (**Figure 7-18**)

A written crisis preparedness plan should include all these elements and be detailed and clear enough such that it can be understood by all stakeholders and effectively implemented in response to a critical event. In addition, a mechanism for regular testing (6 months to 1 year) should also be included to evaluate the components and the effectiveness of the crisis planning process.

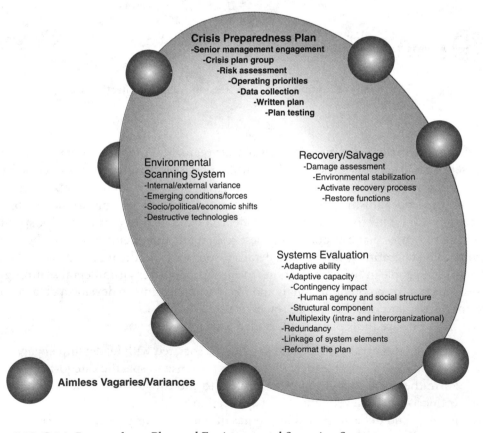

Figure 7-18 Crisis Preparedness Plan and Environmental Scanning System

Recovery/Salvage Stage

As a part of the cycle of crisis preparedness, hospitals and health systems must also recognize the need for quick and immediate response to prevailing factors that affect their clinical work and effectiveness. Crisis preparedness activities assume that, given sufficient time, normative crisis invariably occurs. Immediate crisis response activities and teams should be able to identify specific responses and activities necessary to address both short- and long-term issues in a way that configures the organization's response to a specific critical event (**Figure 7-19**). This intense focus on critical intervention requires attention on the part of involved leaders and staff. This frequently requires suspension of emphasis on normal activities to ensure a timely and correct adaptive response to the critical event.

In this recovery stage the effectiveness of the critical response enumerated by the crisis preparedness plan can best be demonstrated. Quick damage assessment and immediate corrective action processes enable the organization to establish a short-term investment in critical response, ensuring that the broader normative activities can be resumed as quickly as possible. Whether the critical event is a competing hospital's new cardiac accountable care program,

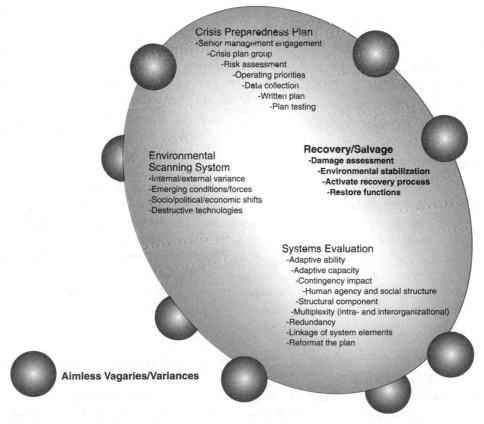

Figure 7-19 Recovery/Salvage and Environmental Scanning

which is drawing away an important population of patients, or the complete shutdown of an electronic medical record system, which requires immediate manual documentation, the crisis preparedness activities should focus on a response strategy in a short period of time. Through this dynamic, the specific recovery activities and the necessary reconceptualization or reconfiguration of specific responses should be facilitated. Leaders should recognize that temporary refocusing of resources and efforts may be required in the short term as a necessary part of redesigning and structuring an appropriate response to the crisis.

Adaptive Effectiveness

In any organizational disruption, whether technical, operational, or human, the strategic activities of the organization are directly affected. Any process associated with a hospital's or health system's ability to adapt must also be linked to its environmental scanning processes. In the three-part model provided in this chapter, the interface between multilateral health team effectiveness, environmental scanning, and critical response or crisis preparedness provides a dynamic and cybernetic approach of continuous adaptation and adjustment as an organization responds to the implications and vagaries of change in a highly transforming environment.

In an effort to mitigate strategic challenges and disruptions, the organization's adaptive capacity and response must address immediate needs in a timely fashion. The organization's response must stay one step ahead of the negative forces embedded in a change event. Strategic and operational responses need to be flexible enough to adapt to both the predictable and the unpredictable variances that accompany a significant change event (Bridges, 2002).

> **Key Point**
>
> The relationship among external forces, the leadership's ability to scan the environment, and the organization's preparedness for crisis is a strong indicator of whether an infrastructure for sustainability exists in the system.

The adaptive capacity of an organization must be exemplified in its ability to resume normative activities consistent with its mission and purposes as soon as possible. Executive leadership needs to be clear about the adjustments related to the interface between strategic, operational, and clinical services. Although a critical event may occur in any one of these arenas, ultimately each one is affected by the other. Leadership must recognize this interface of influencing forces and acknowledge that an issue arising out of one element (strategic, operational, or clinical) ultimately affects the others. Leadership synthesis and demonstration of an integrated response to a critical event are important indicators that the organization has successfully accommodated the crisis and can return to normal operations.

Systems Evaluation

No predictive and adaptive system or approach can succeed unless it is continually monitored, adjusted, and adapted to emerging conditions and circumstances. Such systems need continuous monitoring to ensure sufficient response capacity and a real goodness of fit between the organization's environmental scanning system (which includes its crisis preparedness plan) and the prevailing emerging external and internal realities, which are

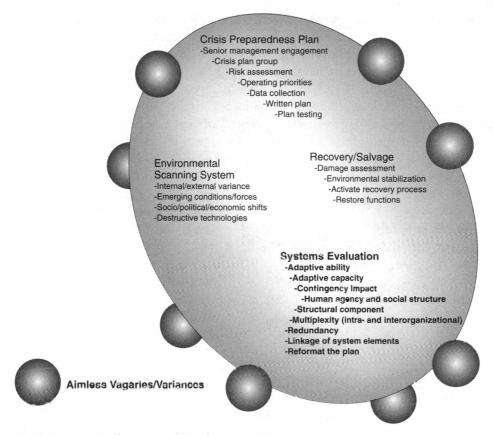

Crisis Preparedness Plan
-Senior management engagement
-Crisis plan group
-Risk assessment
-Operating priorities
-Data collection
-Written plan
-Plan testing

**Environmental
Scanning System**
-Internal/external variance
-Emerging conditions/forces
-Socio/political/economic shifts
-Destructive technologies

Recovery/Salvage
-Damage assessment
-Environmental stabilization
-Activate recovery process
-Restore functions

Systems Evaluation
-Adaptive ability
-Adaptive capacity
-Contingency Impact
-Human agency and social structure
-Structural component
-Multiplexity (intra- and interorganizational)
-Redundancy
-Linkage of system elements
-Reformat the plan

Aimless Vagaries/Variances

Figure 7-20 Systems Evaluation and Environmental Scanning

constantly in a state of flux and affect the organization's continuing viability. The content and character of any crisis represent the environmental conditions or circumstances that initiated it. As timing and technology work to create a different contextual framework, crisis planning and intervention processes must shift to reflect these changes. Close attention must be paid to the content of the crisis preparedness plan that addresses the external and internal contextual challenges that are constantly influencing the organization and its work.

A systems evaluation focuses on the application interface of each component in the process in the system's adaptation to real-time crisis (**Figure 7-20**). The interface between the cybernetic elements of team process, environmental scanning, and crisis preparedness is indicative of a whole systems approach to ensuring the effectiveness of the strategic operational and clinical activities of a hospital or health system. The ability of systems leaders to see a cybernetic process such as this as an integrated model and to demonstrate their own skills of synthesis and fluidity in its application is the strongest determinant of a successful model.

Appropriate systems evaluation should include the elements related to the organizational and human response to broad-based change and to critical events. Leadership must demonstrate that the system is effective in its ability, first, to anticipate and predict potential change and, second, to adequately respond in the presence of critical events and unplanned occurrences. Structuring this as a part of the organizational framework ensures that the system and its people can better anticipate, predict, and respond in the presence of a critical change and can consistently reproduce the necessary work and social processes to achieve operational normality within the context of a new change.

Accountability and authority in the implementation of a systematic approach to creating an operational infrastructure for environmental scanning and crisis planning demand a level of clarity across the organization. Individuals located at various points in the organizational structure must know they have access to and can communicate with key individuals, who can respond in a timely and appropriate way to broad signals and to external and internal triggers that suggest a need for an immediate response. At the same time, the system must have sufficient integrity to avoid a consciousness of crisis and to maintain as normal an operating milieu as possible.

> **Point to Ponder**
>
> Evaluation must always be included in the design of the system's response to crisis. Evaluation of the plan must represent as much patient impact and change as are part of the character and content of the crisis. Leaders must always use the insights they gain from evaluation of past appropriate responses to inform how they will manage future crises.

Good systems evaluation should include an assessment of successful approaches that represent the organization's adaptive ability and capacity to respond to the need for immediate change. The impact of the change on the organization's operating environment and the responsiveness of staff to that change give leaders some sense of the contingency impact of the immediate changes created in the organizational system. The ability of individuals and groups to respond and adapt quickly to the demand for a change in context or content of work is a strong indicator of the ability of the organization's social structures to quickly adjust to new ways of working and shifting outcome demands. Systems effectiveness is based on an evidence-driven frame and uses previous experiences, best practices, and innovative approaches to ensure the organization's response to changing environmental conditions or crisis is both consistent with the demand of the crisis and creates the foundation for sustainable normal operations.

Strong systems evaluation includes reviewing the impact of multiplexity (layers of change), of the diversity of interactions and relationships that operate between different elements of the organizational networks, and of redundancy. This review ensures that there is sufficient slack (open time) in the organizational system to anticipate, assess, plan, and adjust human response to a significant change or critical event. Making this time available is especially problematic in health systems and hospitals. The unrelenting focus on time-based productivity at every level of the organization has eliminated sufficient slack in the role of leaders and staff, virtually guaranteeing the organization's lack of preparedness with regard to immediate environmental, operational, and clinical crises.

Assessing the system's responsiveness to critical events requires the leader to synthesize all the components of the system and the structures of the organization. Understanding the nature of the flow of work processes, external and internal events, and the character of response strategies at the conceptual center of the system creates the proper frame for effective systems evaluation. The ability to see this linkage of multifocal team activity, environmental scanning and influence, and critical response provides the frame for ensuring systems competence and capability with regard to general adaptation.

The three major components of the cybernetic process—team-based synthesis, environmental scanning, and adaptive effectiveness (crisis planning)—each play their part in meeting the demands of the whole system approach to critical management in response to change. As in all systems approaches, each component must generalize to support the whole, and the whole must converge to ensure consistent and appropriate response to change, resulting in effective adaptation and successful outcomes. In a performance-based, evidence-driven, accountability-based, and outcomes-oriented health system driven by increasingly sophisticated clinical, service, and support technology, leaders must demonstrate systems skills, a capacity for innovation, and a high degree of adaptation. This is especially true as health systems work to adapt to the demands of health reform and value-driven models of service. Comparable effectiveness between health systems in their service, quality, and price commitment to those they serve will be a transparent witness to the degree of an organization's effectiveness. The future of health care depends on the ability of clinical systems to interface well and work together across the disciplines and the organization, to adjust to increasingly complex technology applications, to operate in a high-mobility accountable care arena, and to ensure that the health needs of individuals are met and the health of our communities is advanced.

Conclusion

Clearly, it is vital that health leaders understand the requirement to be prepared to confront the unexpected. In today's environment, with the complexity of changes that are occurring at a quantum rate, it is no longer optional for leaders to have the capacity to respond to immediate and dramatic change events. This ability to respond to the dynamics of crisis and critical change is not only an inherent leadership skill, it must now be inculcated within the very fabric of the organization and its operation. From the development of strategy through operational efficiency and effectiveness, leadership behavior, and work practices, every element of the system must reflect an ability to both predict and adapt to the drama of crisis and change (Porter-O'Grady, 2013). Developing a systematic and integrated approach that is evident at both the behavioral and operational levels of the system is the critical variable that ensures adaptation and the ability to thrive over the long term.

Case Study 7-1

Building a High-Performing Rapid Response Team

The chief nursing officer (CNO) at Pine Valley Medical Center has received a written proposal and business plan from the directors of the emergency department and medical surgical services for a new rapid response team (RRT). The two directors recently attended a national conference outlining the benefits of an RRT in improving patient outcomes and preventing cardiac arrest in unstable patients. Their proposal and business plan present a compelling case for the benefits of an RRT and outline the costs and benefits of the new program. The directors discussed how clinical nurses can perceive the deteriorating condition of a patient as a major crisis as they attempt to assess and intervene with the patient while also juggling the needs of other patients and their assignments. It was proposed that an RRT could provide a valuable service in assisting the less experienced nurses in assessing the status of patients and prevent untoward events from occurring from missed observations or interventions. The CNO and the other executives agreed to allow the two directors to develop and pilot the program for 6 months, and then evaluate the program for its success or to identify any changes that might be needed.

Frank, the director of the emergency department, and James, the director of medical surgical services, identified individuals they believed were important stakeholders for the development of an RRT and invited these individuals to the initial planning meeting. James reviewed the past year's data for cardiac arrest in the emergency department and throughout the hospital, patient transfers from medical surgical services to critical care, and other statistics. He shared evidence from the literature and speakers at the national conference who presented data demonstrating how an RRT improved patient outcomes by preventing deterioration of the patients' conditions. Another major benefit noted was the nurses' and medical staff's positive response to an RRT program because it was recognized as an important resource to improve patient outcomes.

James led the group through a process to identify the vision, mission, and purpose of an RRT for Pine Valley Medical Center. The group seemed to be very engaged in the process and quickly embraced the vision for the RRT. Although the group had interprofessional representatives, John and Frank invited the members to identify others who might add value to the planning process.

At the second meeting the group identified the critical attributes of a high-performing RRT, including (1) competence of the individual members, (2) team competence, (3) resources for staffing the RRT, (4) metrics to measure outcomes, (5) team roles for each interprofessional team partner, (6) group norms for reviewing performance of the team, and (7) patient scenario practice drills for the team. It was decided that several teams would be needed to cover the hospital 24/7. The initial planning group adopted the name of RRT Steering Committee and agreed that they would organize the initial teams and be the quality review team to review individual and team performance and recommend changes for continued improvement. The steering committee also identified a number of learning modules that would be beneficial to the new rapid response teams to enhance their understanding of team formation and development, interprofessional communication and collaboration, and assessment and monitoring results.

As the new rapid response teams developed over the next 6 months, an *esprit de corps* developed among the team members, who were considered as "the elite" and most competent nurses, physicians, pharmacists, and others who supported the effort. The individual teams practiced various patient scenarios, always looking for ways to improve their response and performance. They also held post-event reviews to critique themselves as a team and identify ways to improve their performance individually and as a team. At the end of 6 months, the CNO and other executives reviewed patient outcomes and staff and physician responses to the RRT, and the program was fully adopted with funding appropriated in the annual budget.

Questions

1. How does the Dynamic Cybernetic Team Model described in this chapter provide a framework for the organizing efforts of the RRT Steering Committee?
2. What might be some of the external and internal forces that could trigger recognition of the need to develop a rapid response team in a hospital?
3. Describe your perceptions of the process using the Dynamic Cybernetic Team Model that the steering committee put in place to identify their respective individual and team roles and practice these roles in various patient scenarios.
4. Describe how a rapid response team fits the description of a complex, adaptive, self-regulating system as described in this chapter.
5. How could you apply the Dynamic Cybernetic Team Model to other crisis teams?

Case Study 7-2

No One Could Have Prepared Me for This Experience

Sierra Mountain Hospital was well known for its stellar reputation for nursing and medical excellence, great leadership, and fantastic work environment. The new chief operating officer and her team had done wonders in totally transforming the organizational culture over the past 5 years and dramatically improving the patient, operational, and financial outcomes for the hospital. The executive team had recruited and hired top medical and surgical specialists and talented nursing leaders to create centers of excellence that were second to none for tertiary-level community hospitals. Sierra Mountain Hospital sat at the base of the Sierra National Forest and was surrounded by beautiful, well-established pine and Sequoia trees. The hospital had recently been recognized in the national press as one of the top 50 hospitals in the nation for excellence in patient outcomes and patient, physician, and employee satisfaction.

Sierra Mountain Hospital had the usual policies and procedures and annual competency reviews for various crisis situations, particularly disaster planning. The procedures outlined roles and responsibilities of the command post leaders and participants and sites for the safe location of patients for any type of disaster. Every employee in the organization was required to review the disaster policies and procedures annually and to demonstrate their knowledge and competence in carrying out their specific individual roles and team roles in case of a disaster.

In extreme weather conditions with winds recorded at 90 miles per hour, an electrical transformer was blown over and started a fire in dry timber conditions. With the high winds, the fire spread rapidly to the surrounding areas and embers were blown about as if they were laser darts. As the fire encroached on homes in the community, local fire brigades were dispatched to evacuate residents who were in the fire's expected path. Within hours the state National Guard and other fire brigades were en route to provide assistance in containing the rapidly spreading fire. Per protocol, the leadership of Sierra Mountain Hospital assumed their roles in the command post to assess resources needed, identify patients who could be discharged or immediately moved, identify patients who would need assistance, and determine the level of danger from the fire situation. The nurse director was in radio contact with the police and fire departments and was informed that she would be contacted should patient evacuation be necessary, but it was not expected.

As the command post leader began calling in staff, she realized that the expected number of staff from the callback might not meet expectations because many were actively involved in protecting their own homes and families. Some of the staff indicated that they would come in only if they could bring their young children and pets because they were afraid to leave them behind with other family members who were engaged in trying to protect their homes. The command post leader, knowing that she would need additional help to relieve staff who needed to return to their homes, told the callback staff that they could bring their children and animals to the hospital in this crisis situation. Immediately, the command post leader contacted the facility director and asked for a space to be designated for the care of young children and a space for animals. This situation was certainly one that no one had anticipated when practicing various disaster scenarios.

Within a few hours the nurse director called the police and fire captains for more information about the encroaching fire. It was obvious that they had become so involved in their work that they did not inform the nurse director that the fire was spreading rapidly and in the direction of Sierra Mountain Hospital. It's never an easy decision to make the call for evacuation of all patients, but the nurse director felt that it was in the best interest of the patients and her staff. Evacuation procedures were clearly outlined in the disaster protocol, so the nurse director implemented those procedures and called for the immediate removal of all mobile patients to a safe area in the community's high school on the other end of town. She asked the police department for assistance to use school buses to transport the more mobile patients. Higher acuity patients would be transferred by any available ambulance, and the nurse director mobilized all of her leaders to set up temporary critical care units in the school's gymnasium for the more critical patients who would be transferred with as much equipment and supplies as possible. She made calls to neighboring community hospitals to send ambulances and staff to help. The hospital had several trucks that were used to transport medical supplies and equipment, and these were mobilized to transport the sicker patients in their beds and with their equipment.

The next day authorities determined that it was safe for patients to be returned to Sierra Mountain Hospital, so the staff began the process of moving patients back. After the crisis was over, the nurse director, the command post leader, and others reviewed the situation and how the various unit and department disaster teams performed using the policies, procedures, and practiced roles. Although they were pleased that none of the patients were compromised in the process of protecting them and transferring them to a safe location, the team realized that there were several issues that needed to be addressed to prepare for future disasters. A list of potential changes was identified for implementation. The nurse director and other realized that staff who were called in were reluctant to leave their children and pets. Therefore, it was decided that the hospital would purchase a number of portable pet crates of various sizes and temporary fencing for the containment of animals on the grounds and in large storage areas. Cots and bedding would also be purchased for use when staff needed to bring their children to the hospital during disasters. The role of child caretakers was created and staff were identified for this purpose. Because of the knowledge gained from the review of the fire disaster, Sierra Mountain Hospital led efforts in the community to identify various safe locations for patients and storage areas for cots and other supplies should patients need to be evacuated again in the future.

Questions

1. Using the Dynamic Cybernetic Team Model as a framework, how would you assess Sierra Mountain Hospital's disaster preparedness?
2. From your own knowledge and experience, what other steps could the leadership of Sierra Mountain Hospital have taken to prepare for this or any other disaster?
3. Describe your perceptions of the review process after the disaster was over in planning for changes that would prepare them for future disaster response.
4. Describe how disaster response teams fit the description of a complex, adaptive, self-regulating system as described in this chapter.

References

Alvesson, M., & Willmott, H. (2012). *Making sense of management: A critical introduction.* Thousand Oaks, CA: Sage.

Bridges, W. (2002). *Way of transition.* New York, NY: Perseus.

Bridges, W. (2004). *Transitions: Making sense of life.* New York, NY: Perseus.

Crandall, W., Parnell, J., & Spillan, J. (2009). *Crisis management in the new strategy landscape.* Thousand Oaks, CA: Sage.

Curlee, W., & Gordon, R. L. (2011). *Complexity theory and project management.* Hoboken, NJ: Wiley.

Dekker, S. (2011). *Drift into failure: From hunting broken components to understanding complex systems.* Burlington, VT: Ashgate.

Deutch, M., Coleman, P., & Marcus, E. (2006). *The handbook of conflict resolution: Theory and practice.* San Francisco, CA: Jossey-Bass.

Dickinson, H., & Mannion, R. (2012). *The reform of health care: Shaping, adapting and resisting policy developments.* New York, NY: Palgrave Macmillan.

Diller, J. V. (2011). *Cultural diversity: A primer for the human services* (4th ed.). Belmont, CA: Thomson Brooks/Cole.

Edmonds, B., & Meyer, R. (2013). *Simulating social complexity.* New York, NY: Springer.

Estrin, J. (2009). *Closing the innovation gap: Reigniting the spark of creativity in a global economy.* New York, NY: McGraw-Hill.

Goldstein, J., Hazy, J. K., & Lichtenstein, B. B. (2010). *Complexity and the nexus of leadership: Leveraging nonlinear science to create ecologies of innovation* (1st ed.). New York, NY: Palgrave Macmillan.

Hamlin, B., Keep, J., & Ash, K. (2001). *Organizational change and development: A reflective guide for managers, trainers and developers.* New York, NY: Financial Times/Prentice Hall.

Hazy, J., Goldstein, J., & Lichtenstein, B. (2007). *Complex systems leadership theory: New perspectives from complexity science on social and organizational effectiveness.* New York, NY: Vintage Press.

Hickey, M., & Kritek, P. B. (2012). *Change leadership in nursing: How change occurs in a complex hospital system.* New York, NY: Springer.

Kanel, K. (2006). *A guide to crisis intervention.* London, England: Wadsworth.

Leban, B. (2007). *Managing organizational change.* New York, NY: Wiley.

Lerbinger, O. (2012). *The crisis manager: Facing disasters, conflicts, and failures* (2nd ed.). New York, NY: Routledge.

Lodge, M., & Wegrich, K. (2012). *Executive politics in times of crisis.* New York, NY: Palgrave Macmillan.

Mitchell, M. (2009). *Complexity: A guided tour.* New York, NY: Oxford University Press.

Noble, C. (2011). *Conflict management coaching.* Toronto, Canada: Cynergy.

Parker, G. M. (2003). *Cross-functional teams: Working with allies, enemies, and other strangers* (2nd ed.). San Francisco, CA: Jossey-Bass.

Penuel, K. B., Statler, M., & Hagen, R. (2013). *Encyclopedia of crisis management.* Thousand Oaks, CA: Sage.

Porter-O'Grady, T. (2013). A new context for service: Healthcare for the 21st century. *American Journal of Maternal Child Nursing,* 5–9.

Shaw, R. (2011). *Management essentials for doctors.* New York, NY: Cambridge University Press.

Weberg, D. (2012). Complexity leadership: A healthcare imperative. *Nursing Forum, 47*(4), 268–277. doi:10.1111/j.1744-6198.2012.00276.x

Yang, S., Cao, J., & Lu, J. (2012). A new protocol for finite-time consensus of detail-balanced multi-agent networks. *Chaos, 22*(4), 431–434. doi:10.1063/1.4768662

Young, H. D., & Hester, J. P. (2004). *Leadership under construction: Creating paths toward transformation.* Lanham, MD: Scarecrow Education.

Zimmerman, B., Lindberg, C., & Plsek, P. (1998). *Edgeware.* Irving, TX: VHA, Inc.

Suggested Readings

Barton, L. (2007). *Crisis leadership now: A real-world guide to preparing for threats, a disaster, sabotage, and scandal.* New York, NY: McGraw-Hill.

Berstein, J. (2011). *Manager's guide to crisis management.* New York, NY: McGraw-Hill.

Crandall, W., Parnell, J., & Spillan, J. (2009). *Crisis management in the new strategy landscape.* Thousand Oaks, CA: Sage.

Fink, S. (2013). *Crisis communications: The definitive guide to managing the message.* New York, NY: McGraw-Hill.

James, R. (2007). *Crisis intervention strategies.* Three Lakes, WI: Cole.

Malloch, K., & Porter-O'Grady, T. (2009). *The quantum leader: Applications for the new world of work.* Sudbury, MA: Jones and Bartlett.

Mitchell, M. (2009). *Complexity: A guided tour.* New York, NY: Oxford University Press.

Regester, M., & Larkin, J. (2008). *Risk issues and crisis management and public relations: A casebook of best practice.* London, England: Kogan Page.

Wankel, C. (2008). *21st century management: A reference handbook.* Los Angeles, CA: Sage.

Watkins, M. (2013). *The first 90 days: Proven strategies for getting up to speed faster and smarter.* Cambridge, MA: Harvard Business Review Press.

Quiz Questions

Select either true or false for each of the following questions.

1. True or False? All conflict is normative and a fundamental characteristic of human behavior.

2. True or False? All crises are stimulated by cataclysmic events.

3. True or False? Adaptive and predictive skills are now requisites for twenty-first-century leaders.

4. True or False? In truth, all crises can be prevented if the leader exercises sufficient proactive skills to avoid them.

5. True or False? Organizations shape human beings by directing their cultural, social, political, and relational interactions.

6. True or False? Most crises can be traced to problems within and between the organizational infrastructures of human communities.

7. True or False? The complexity of an organization really has no impact or influence on the number or intensity of potential crises.

8. True or False? Effectively managing change means leaders create an internally adaptive environment rather than simply dealing with crises as they arise.

9. True or False? Clinical education should incorporate the principles and processes associated with good conflict management, just as leadership education does.

10. True or False? A good crisis planning process should be developed by the senior leadership of the organization and directed to every other leadership individual in the system.

11. True or False? Crises are embedded everywhere in the organization, not just at the junctures or intersections between external and internal forces in the life of the organization.

12. True or False? Crisis management planning should incorporate all key stakeholders and have an impact on functions and activities at every level of the organization.

CHAPTER EIGHT

Living Leadership: Vulnerability, Risk Taking, and Stretching

Take comfort in the notion that we have never been in control!
—Anonymous

Evolved people respect differing views, understanding that life's meaning is to be found everywhere. They are open, always learning and growing. An evolved person knows that there is only one truth, but many different ways of seeing it.
—Lance Secretan
Reprinted by permission of Dr. Lance Secretan

Chapter Objectives

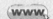

At the completion of this chapter, the reader will be able to

- Understand vulnerability as a positive leadership trait.
- Identify four essential relationship skills that support vulnerable leadership.
- Discuss the process of complexity communication.
- Evaluate open communication as a means of improving leadership expertise.
- Critique vulnerable leadership as a moral imperative.

I don't have all the answers; am I a failure? Traditional organizations hold leaders to standards of rationality, clarity, and foresight—yet most leaders cannot meet these standards because they are human and face an incredible amount of unpredictability and fallible analyses of data. To be able to prosper and thrive in the current millennium, the leader must shift from the somewhat comfortable position of control to one of great uncertainty and vulnerability. In reality, uncertainty and need for vulnerability have always existed for leaders. With the current explosion of information technology and availability of information, leading using command-and-control behaviors is no longer an option. To be sure, no leader is alone on this journey. Colleagues, patients, and the community are aware of the plethora of data, data sources, and lack of clear pathways.

Leaders of postmillennium quantum organizations must use resources effectively in an environment in which control and direction are uncertain. They must grow comfortable with the idea that uncertainty is the norm and that one cannot know everything there is to know. They must be willing to take risks, recognize that their colleagues come from a wide range of backgrounds and experiences, and realize that they will never obtain a complete picture, no matter how accomplished their communication with others. Finally, they must use new strategies based on vulnerability principles if they are to succeed in designing a healthcare system that works.

In the Industrial Age, leaders were expected to be in control. Whether chief executive officers or case managers, they were viewed as being in charge and in possession of the information that consumers and employees wanted and needed. According to the classical theories of management, good leaders knew everything and could do everything better than anyone else. They held all the information necessary for operating the organization and shared this information with employees only when appropriate.

Today things are much different. Information is currently available to the masses and in great quantities, minimizing any leader's potential for being in control of anything. Furthermore, all leaders have limitations and as they move through the chaos of the transition into the Information Age, they typically experience feelings of defenselessness, helplessness, and inadequacy. Leaders, to act with vigor in this time of great uncertainty, need to replace their old skills with new ones.

Leadership Fitness in the New Millennium

The leadership fitness profile is very different from the leadership role of the past, which was basically one of command and control. In the new millennium, leaders find themselves in an environment of great uncertainty, and to navigate in this environment they need to be comfortable with taking risks, being vulnerable, and stretching the boundaries of current thinking and current practices. They also need to coach employees to develop the same performance characteristics. Engaging the staff to work collectively to interpret the events of change in a way that makes sense of them is essential for success.

> **Point to Ponder**
>
> Becoming vulnerable is a growth process—a process without a roadmap—yet one that opens up endless opportunities.

Vulnerability, risk taking, and stretching are required for several reasons. First, the present is very different from the past, and the skills that will be needed in the coming age, the Information Age, are very different from those needed in the Industrial Age. Past practices of bureaucratic command and control cannot be assumed to be effective in a new environment in which the distribution of knowledge has been radically altered and the skills needed to manage the environment are undeveloped. The quantum leader, besides exemplifying the spirit of incompleteness, must shift from managing content to guiding process and outcome over and over again until order finally emerges.

Second, the leaders of the healthcare professions need to maintain a focus on creating a new framework for each profession, a framework that allows them to understand and manage the future rather than sustain the past. As part of this process, they need

Group Discussion

Compare the behaviors of classical management and those of vulnerability leadership. Examine the practices of coaching, facilitating teams, building relationships, and empowering others in each model.

to scrutinize the relationships between the professions, examine the specific services provided by each profession, and assess the value of these services in the marketplace. The services that add value will be retained, and those that do not will be eliminated.

Vulnerability

In the Industrial Age, vulnerability in a leader was seen as a weakness. Indeed, the word *vulnerability* tends to conjure the idea of susceptibility to physical or emotional injury or to corrupt influence. This type of vulnerability is very different from the type required of leaders in the Information Age. The essence of *vulnerability*, as the term is used in this book, is openness to others and to new ideas (**Exhibit 8-1**). It encompasses being able to

- Examine long-held beliefs and change one's mind without feelings of inadequacy
- Recognize personal limitations and strengths
- Work from a clearly defined personal identity

Vulnerable leaders know and show their limits, whether these pertain to knowledge or to abilities. Rather than work beyond their limits, they allow people with the right kind of aptitude to assume responsibility for particular tasks. According to their mind-set, their role is to create the conditions that allow employees to make their maximum contribution and simultaneously enjoy their work.

Leadership vulnerability is not about weakness or incompetence. Team members and colleagues do not want leaders to be weak, ailing, or whining. They look for strength and self-confidence, but the kind of self-confidence that permits someone to admit his or her limitations and not maintain a stance of immunity to anxiety, fatigue, or doubt. Leadership vulnerability is also about creating conditions that encourage safe and healthy dialogue as the way to do business.

Exhibit 8-1 Leadership Vulnerability

Facilitators	Barriers
• Openness to new ideas	• Aloofness, arrogance
• Recognition of personal limitations	• Strong ego
• Feelings of adequacy	• Fear of losing control
• Self-awareness of strengths and weaknesses	• Fear of discovery
• Absence of ego	• Believed immunity to anxiety, fatigue, illness, and overwork
• Trust in others	

In contrast, leaders who act out of a sense of invulnerability tend to be aloof, separate themselves from those they lead, and avoid making time for the meaningful discussion of complex issues. Their purpose in behaving in this manner is to keep control over situations and to abstain from dialogue that might lead to the revision of their chosen courses of action. Charisma, too, is suspect. There is a dark side of charisma that requires attention. Chamorro-Premuzic (2012), in *Harvard Business Review*, noted that the short-term effects of this type of leadership or charm serve to engage people; however, in the long term there are four significant downsides:

- Charisma dilutes judgment.
- Charisma is addictive.
- Charisma disguises psychopaths.
- Charisma fosters collective narcissism.

The traits and behaviors associated with invulnerability play a big role in protecting the leadership ego. Traditionally, leaders have feared not just losing control, but also being found out. They have worried that others would discover that they are not what they seem to be, that they do not have all the answers to all the questions. Quantum leadership, on the other hand, is about the absence of ego. Quantum leaders seek exposure of their limitations as a means of improving organizational performance. According to Torbert (2000), vulnerability is paradoxically powerful. When power is exercised by a leader who remains vulnerable or open to transformation, the result is voluntary transformation in others, rather than mere external conformity and compliance (or resistance). In addition, there is no point in fearing discovery or losing control because in reality no one is really in control.

> **Key Point**
>
> Quantum leadership is about the absence of ego, not its presence.

Relationships in a quantum organization are based on three principles:

1. Power is a pluralist, not an elitist, commodity.
2. Diversity of knowledge, individuals, social status, and so forth is essential.
3. Personal boundaries must be clearly defined.

These principles provide the framework for developing new and more effective relationships.

Power

The notion of power has both positive and negative connotations and often produces feelings of ambivalence. Further, because power is associated with the conflicting ideas of strength, influence, coercion, and dominance, it is difficult both to understand and to use. Yet as we move into the Information Age, leaders must comprehend the nature of power and make use of it in their relationships.

> **Point to Ponder**
>
> Knowledge really is power. Intellect is a gift, but learning is hard work.

First, quantum leaders consider the quantity of power to be infinite and thus conclude that sufficient power is generally available for all individuals to exert influence, mobilize resources, and meet their goals. They view power as located in each person, not centralized in an elite group, and they treat the legitimate exercise of power as a right that belongs to everyone. These beliefs are most clearly reflected in a complexity leadership model (Uhl-Bein & Marion, 2008).

In a traditional organization, power is concentrated at the top of the hierarchical pyramid, and work is compartmentalized and controlled from that central point. The organizational power structure always benefits some at the expense of others. If anything, revisions of the structure tend to enhance the power of those who have it. In other words, leaders seldom design themselves out of a position.

Group Discussion

Consider power from both an elitist perspective and a pluralist perspective. How is power perceived in your organization? In your department? Describe the power behaviors that occur in your organization as a whole and in your department. Identify at least two opportunities to shift power behaviors from elitist to pluralist.

In a quantum organization, the response to centralization is not decentralization but uncentralization. Uncentralization, unlike decentralization, does not attempt to preserve hierarchical workways by subdividing and parceling out the work while hanging on to central control through the use of more and more creative accounting systems. The new organizational structure is fluid and flexible, allowing easy rearrangement of work groups to meet point-of-service needs.

To be sure, there are still distinctions between organizations. In some the style of leadership is more informal and collegial, whereas in others recommendations mostly go up and orders mostly come down. The intent, however, is the same: to minimize bureaucratic control and the concentration of power and to maximize involvement while still getting the work done.

The point is not to create "nobody in charge" systems. Yet regardless of how the leadership power transition occurs, some leaders experience real or perceived threats to their power, and their instinct for self-preservation may override their concern for organizational goals.

In many cases, employees who have high expectations are quickly disillusioned by the leaders' perceived failure to meet their expectations. In fact, traditional employees discourage leaders from becoming vulnerable. This means that leaders not only must change their own mind-set, but also must create the conditions for employees to adapt to the new culture. As the necessary changes proceed, the resulting battles for survival are likely to cause organizational confusion and even chaos.

Authenticity Is the Key

Leadership is often described as transactional, transformation, or complexity (Gill, 2011). It is interesting to note that there is no single accepted definition or theory of leadership nor is there an agreed paradigm for the study and practice of leadership. According to Kurtsman (2010), there is no consensus on what leadership is, how leaders develop, or how to become a more efficient leader. Despite this lack of consensus, leaders must continually ensure that their efforts match the needs of the organization and provide value to the users. At times leaders unknowingly adopt one style of leadership in the hopes that it will serve the entire organization when in fact the chosen theory or model may address only one aspect of leadership. No one style, however, is absolute or appropriate for all situations. This plethora of leader styles can be daunting for the emerging leader. Formal monitoring programs provide guidance and recommendations to support role development. Yet conforming to the normative leadership style of the organization or the recent literature recommendation can spell disaster for the leader. According to George (2004), great world leaders all had very different leadership styles—George Washington, Winston Churchill, Margaret Thatcher, Mother Teresa, and John F. Kennedy all led in their own unique way.

In reality, the success of the leader is more closely linked to personal authenticity than to a particular leadership style. The leader's authenticity—not the leadership style—really matters. Attempting to emulate another's leadership style can be disastrous. New leaders may desire a model of shared leadership but must understand and live the basic values in their personal lives to make shared leadership a reality. A lack of congruence between personal and professional values creates a reality gap that is obvious to team members. This gap compromises leader authenticity because the leader talks the talk of shared leadership but is unable to fully live the values consistently.

The values of the authentic leader are shaped by personal beliefs and developed through study, reflection, and dialogue with others. These values create a moral compass for the leader and provide guidance in determining the right thing to do rather than blindly attempting to emulate the style of another leader.

A broad understanding of leadership styles serves merely as background information to understanding behavior options. Being one's own person is the key to developing an authentic leadership style that is consistent with one's personality and character. Ongoing development of the leader's personal leadership style continues as the leader encounters different situations and different people.

The authentic leader accepts personal faults as well as strengths and avoids attempting to win approval of others by covering up shortcomings and thus sacrificing authenticity to gain respect from others. There is no way a leader can do everything—be on top of the incoming mail, read the most recent literature, and be responsive to everything and everyone. Attempting to be such a leader is foolhardy. According to Lencioni (1998), vulnerability is essential for building trust and requires behaviors that reflect caring about others and their success. The authentic, vulnerable leader knows what he or she knows and what he or she does not know and is content with the limits of his or her capacity.

Integrity is closely linked to authenticity for the effective leader. In addition to personal authenticity, the vulnerable leader exhibits integrity, a characteristic that is not just the absence of lying but the presence of telling the whole truth, no matter how difficult it might be. Leadership integrity is the uncompromising adherence to moral and ethical principles. From authenticity and integrity, trusting relationships emerge.

The Cycle of Vulnerability

Learning to live and thrive in vulnerability is a lifelong journey. It is often a circuitous journey, reversing on itself and then moving forward. For the purposes of discussion, learning to live and thrive in vulnerability is presented as a cyclical process (**Exhibit 8-2** and **Figure 8-1**). The seven stages of this cycle are as follows:

1. Becoming vulnerable
2. Taking risks
3. Stretching one's capacity
4. Living the new reality
5. Evaluating the results
6. Cherishing the new knowledge gained
7. Begin the cycle again

Becoming Vulnerable

The first stage in the cycle involves recognizing the value of being vulnerable. You need only enroll in a computer class with a teenager to discover the value of vulnerability—the value of being open to receiving new ideas about how to use a computer. By admitting you are uncertain and not all-knowing, by being willing to put aside long-standing mental models, you open yourself to the possibility of incredible growth and rewards.

Frustration and fear typically fuel the search for certainty, a search that wastes significant time and effort. In any organization, situations and relationships are usually too complex to be predictable, and therefore a degree of uncertainty is unavoidable. If fear of the unknown is allowed to rule, the result is organizational inertia and continued reliance on past practices. Despite believing in the need for change or in the savings to be gained from a new technology, leaders place too much emphasis on the failure of past innovations and sit back and do nothing.

Employees, as well as leaders, long for certainty. Formerly, securing a position in an organization meant getting employment for a lifetime. This is no longer true. As organizations face more challenges than ever before, employees face more uncertainty, particularly about the security of their jobs. As a consequence, they experience additional stress as well as feelings of isolation. In struggling to find a new vision, they become frustrated and often panic. What they should do instead is learn to tolerate and respect the discomfort of their uncertainty and thereby unleash their creativity in the interests of organizational change.

Exhibit 8-2   The Seven Stages of the Cycle of Vulnerability

1. Become vulnerable and open to new ideas. Recognize and value uncertainty.
2. Choose to take risks that challenge the status quo.
3. Stretch organizational capacity by stimulating the latent potential of employees.
4. Live the new capacity.
5. Evaluate the outcomes.
6. Cherish the resulting new knowledge.
7. Begin the cycle again.

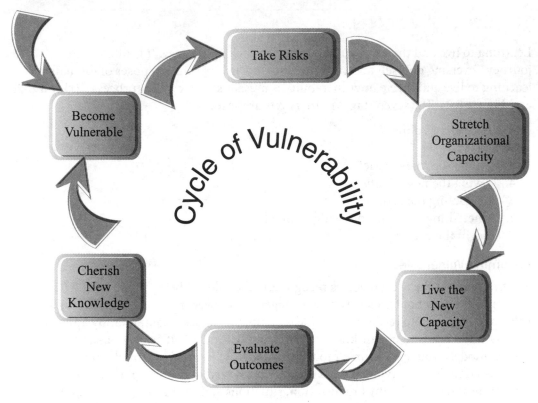

Figure 8-1 The Cycle of Vulnerability

Quantum leaders need to give up the quest for certainty and discover the benefits of admitting fallibility. One benefit is that leaders can expend their efforts in designing the future rather than becoming petrified by feelings of panic and loss of control. After all, leaders never have possessed a crystal ball capable of predicting the future. Leadership judgment is called judgment because certainty is missing. Besides judgment, what leaders can use is creativity. To do this, though, they need time for thinking, for designing the future. Unfortunately, many leaders deny they have any extra time. Most believe they are working at their highest level of productivity and are unable to fit in additional work, especially if it is merely inventive headwork.

The common occurrence of unpredictable challenges places significant demands on leader creativity and imagination. Striving to understand and mediate uncertainty is the most appropriate and logical approach for leaders, rather than working to eliminate variety and hope for stability. Working to achieve stability is irrational given the complex nature of healthcare work. According to Weick and Sutcliffe (2001), recognizing the complex nature of organizations, detecting incredibly weak warning signs, and taking strong decisive action when appropriate are the hallmarks of a high-reliability organization (HRO). HROs have gained credence for their ability to become highly reliable in minimizing errors and thereby increasing patient safety. In addition, HROs have achieved greater stakeholder motivation, time savings, and cost efficiency. These organizations demonstrate the ability to build effective practices and identify unexpected events early on and then respond to these unexpected events in ways that are adaptive rather than destructive. Leaders of HROs thrive in vulnerability, identify different approaches to issues, and take risks in addressing situations in nontraditional ways.

The reality is that their organizations suffer severely unless they make the time to engage in creative thinking. In some cases, new employees have the extra time and energy to explore possible innovations and reforms. More often, the necessary time can be found by examining current work from a value perspective and eliminating particular tasks that fail to add value (i.e., that fail to make a difference in patient care). The time formerly spent on these fruitless tasks can then be used to think creatively and work toward constructing a vision of the future.

Taking Risks

The second stage requires leaders to begin to take risks. Much like vulnerability, risk taking is not viewed as a classical leadership behavior and is rarely welcomed or encouraged. Instead, it is seen as increasing the organization's exposure to unforeseen hazards and to the loss of net income.

Classical leadership behavior encompasses strategic planning and the purposeful review of ideas. With the recent advances in information technology, these processes are becoming increasingly ineffective. New approaches, such as the "tinkering" described by Abrahamson (2000), a management professor at Columbia Business School, will become the norm.

Too often leaders are reluctant to express ideas for fear of retaliation or rejection. Past experiences and assumptions about the potential reactions of others render the health-care professional immobile and ineffective. Leaders must become open and honest in three key situations: sharing opinions and assessments during interview processes, communicating with the media, and providing feedback when negative events occur. Leaders must not only develop competence in these three areas, they must become experts and resources for those with whom they work.

Efforts by quantum leaders to reverse the practices of institutionally imposed powerlessness, which expects nurses not to assert themselves individually or collectively, will continue the journey to optimal authenticity. Overcoming this silence leads to increased personal authenticity and greater public awareness of the importance of the role of nurses and all other healthcare professionals. As greater personal and professional authenticity emerges, feelings of low self-esteem, powerlessness, and lack of collegial support can only decrease. Reversing the spiral of silence begins with regular discussions of situations within the three key situations that identify specific events in which silence negatively affects open and honest communication.

Tinkering, in fact, is a good way to learn how to take risks because it involves making small changes to reconfigure existing practices and business models rather than creating new ones. A little tinkering and a lot of expertise enable small groups of providers to make changes with big goals in mind and to evaluate the changes efficiently. In addition, the providers' skills are stretched with little risk to the organization. Support for

---

Exhibit 8-3   Risk Taking

- Encourages creativity
- Supports "tinkering"
- Requires continuous evaluation
- Allows for mistakes
- Requires vulnerability
- Requires resiliency
- Is avoided by leaders
- Is inconsistent with classical leadership behaviors

---

constant tinkering minimizes the chance that the organization will drift into inertia. Risk becomes the norm, change is internalized as essential for survival, and employees gain new experiences and develop new skills.

Embedded in tinkering processes is the expectation that leaders routinely challenge the status quo—indeed, seriously challenge it, which means not asking questions out of idle curiosity but looking carefully at current dogma and raising issues that open the door to substantial improvements. For quantum leaders, examining the work of their organizations is not a meaningless exercise but is intended to guarantee accountability and make certain that all work is value producing. Asking the unaskable questions about structure, principles, and customs requires an ease with vulnerability and an openness to and passion for new realities (**Exhibit 8-3**).

When leaders ask the unaskable, they are ostensibly inviting employees to mention the unmentionable, which the employees can perceive as very risky, especially when the leaders' body language says, "Do not raise difficult issues." Brusque or otherwise unwelcoming behavior must be replaced with genuine openness so that the employees feel safe and the inquiry into problems can be fruitful and lead to growth. Although decisions made under conditions of incomplete information sometimes fail to have a positive outcome, leaders must be willing to risk changing course if there are good reasons to do so. No one knows the future for certain, as shown by the

> **Key Point**
>
> Leadership judgment is called judgment because certainty is missing.

many mispredictions perpetrated by supposed experts. (Perhaps none is more famous than the implicit prediction regarding the future course of movies that was contained in the question asked by Warner Brothers in 1927: Who the heck wants to hear actors talk?)

Some risky decisions have paid off well. Consider the cash register, which was introduced in the late nineteenth century by Patterson as a help in cash management and as a means of double-checking the honesty of sales clerks. Patterson took an incredible risk in challenging the status quo, and indeed at first everybody resented the product. Owners, for example, refused to have this "thief catcher" in their stores. Patterson had to use great leadership skills to convince others to accept his idea and to motivate his sales force to sell the product. Today, of course, no store is without one.

The role of the leader is to inspire creativity and hard work and to challenge the past as prologue, recognizing that the past is past. The work of inspiration requires not just inspirational phrases but inspirational behavior. Risk-disposed leaders motivate others by showing what can be done, not merely by sermonizing about opportunities. They also need to exhibit candor and vulnerability, to identify value in marginally successful efforts, and to allow others to take risks and experience success and failure.

Group Discussion

Harlan Cleveland (1972) in *The Future Executive* notes that "planning cannot be done by a few leaders, or even by the brightest whiz-kids immured in a systems analysis unit or a planning staff. Real-life planning is the dynamic improvisation by the many on a general sense of direction. The sense of direction is announced by a few . . . but only after genuine consultation with those who will have to improvise on it." Do you agree with Cleveland? Review the current strategic planning processes in your organization and then challenge the status quo by modifying them. Consider and challenge such things as the length of the plan, percentages of employees involved, achievement of value for you as an individual employee. Is your work more meaningful as a result of strategic planning? What is the rationale for your recommendations? List the advantages and disadvantages of the suggested revisions.

Risk-disposed leaders develop a very high level of self-discipline that allows the processes of risk-taking to evolve. A strong sense of commitment can be more valuable than intelligence, education, luck, or talent. Leaders adept at taking risks neither surrender nor overreact to crises or marginally successful efforts; they regroup and return. They take stock of the situation, often pulling back temporarily (but not too long) while they plan the next steps. They realize that sometimes it is best to put aside personal feelings and let bygones be bygones. Finally, they focus on the present and the future, both of which offer perils and possibilities, rather than on the past, about which nothing can be done.

Resiliency is the key. Leaders must be resilient to manage the uncertainty and inherent risks that are features of the leadership role. They must act with confidence, purpose, and enthusiasm rather than hesitation and self-doubt. To manage risks through resiliency, they must apply determination and energy, inspiring those around them at the same time.

Rational Risks and Negative Fantasies

Negative fantasies often cause leaders to become paralyzed or reluctant to take risks. In reality there is little, if any, chance for such fantasies to be realized. Perhaps the most common negative fantasy in health care is the perception that one will be fired for taking risks and speaking up. Individuals often worry that speaking up will have a negative outcome on their reputation, their ability to communicate openly and honestly with others, and, ultimately, the security of their position. Leaders can minimize negative fantasies through discussion with colleagues and clarification of the issue and its importance. Further, leaders can examine the issue and determine whether indeed there is rational risk involved.

The four areas in which risk is considered rational are (1) advancing the organization, (2) developing skills, (3) mandatory reporting, and (4) whistle-blowing (Porter-O'Grady & Malloch, 2011). Each risk serves a different purpose:

1. *Advancing the organization:* Every organization strives not only to survive, but also to thrive in the best way possible. To ensure contemporary services, the leadership team evaluates numerous programs, systems, technology advances, and products. Leaders are routinely faced with choices about clinical programs, initiation and expansion of new services, hiring, firing, selecting equipment, and prioritizing which issues are addressed and which issues wait for attention. Choices that are rational and minimize risk are those choices that are made on the basis of core values, respect for others, the safety of individuals, strategic goals of the organization, and available resources.

2. *Developing skills:* All individuals need new skills to continue to exist in the ever-changing environment. Acquiring new knowledge and skills is considered a rational risk when those skills are needed to improve job performance or for other available opportunities. Considerations should be given to personal physical capability, resources, and family obligations to support rational risk taking. Examples include developing skills in computer programs, public speaking, sports, creative arts, and personal protection.

3. *Mandatory reporting:* Many state licensing agencies require licensees to report to the licensing board the unprofessional conduct of other licensees. Protecting the public from licensees who commit repeated errors, abuse alcohol or drug substances, and/or are incompetent to do the work often requires professionals to identify issues and take risks to speak up and address the situation. This action is not an option in many states and requires collegial support to meet this expectation. Examples include unprofessional conduct, repeated medication errors, boundary violations, and theft from patients. Mandatory reporting is a rational risk required by statute.

4. *Whistle-blowing:* Whistle-blowing is about righting a wrong—a wrong that is believed to be deceitful or that results in the mistreatment of others. To be sure, the need for whistle-blower protection arises when the culture of the organization does not support open communication, differing opinions, and rational risk taking. Individuals believe they have not been heard on an issue or believe the public interest is compromised and there is danger to the public or the environment. The intent of the federal whistle-blower act, also known as the False Claims Act, is to combat fraud and corruption and to protect those who exposed information from wrongful dismissal, allowing for reinstatement with seniority, double back pay, interest on back pay, compensation for discriminatory treatment, and reasonable legal fees. Although the whistle-blower legislation is present, this approach is considered a rational risk and involves personal and professional risk regardless of the outcome.

The influence of the workplace on ethical or principled practices is significant because it may render the leader vulnerable to conflicting peer opinion, loss of colleague approval, physician conflict, and patient dissatisfaction. More often than not, leaders risk changing their relationships and reputation in creating and sustaining an ethical climate. Many organizational cultures discourage employees from challenging or disagreeing with others and label such behaviors as negative and disruptive. A culture of trust and openness, in which employees are encouraged and expected to identify and confront ethical dilemmas as a team, often requires risk taking to make the best decisions and simultaneously value employees.

Employees who participate in decision making and have access to the information necessary to make informed decisions are empowered and contribute significantly to organizational performance. A culture that fosters and reinforces the value of risk-taking behaviors is an essential characteristic of a high-performing organization. The following questions should be considered to ensure ethical decisions are made:

Is the action under consideration legal?
Is the action consistent with organizational policies and guidelines? If not, should a policy be developed or modified?
Is the action consistent with organizational values?
Am I personally okay with the proposed action?
Would I be satisfied if someone took this action with me?
Would the most ethical person I know do the same thing?

Determining when to take a risk is seldom straightforward and linear. Learning to fly an airplane is steeped in risk but is also supported by extensive safety processes. In addition to one's personal comfort and competence with risk taking, the context in which the risk is taking place can be either supportive or not supportive. The same risk may be viewed and managed quite differently in different organizations, with some viewing it as positive and others viewing it as negative and disruptive. Leaders are encouraged to assess their perceptions of risk taking and risk takers and work to create a culture that is open, trusting, and supportive of new ideas.

Stretching One's Capacity

In the third stage of the vulnerability cycle, the leader of an organization works to stretch the organization's capacity. In doing this, the leader looks for new and untapped potential. Typically, this potential lies within the organization. For example, new and long-standing employees in continuing education programs represent two main sources of serviceable potential.

Despite the chaos and uncertainty in organizational operations, quantum leaders learn to mitigate and overcome their reluctance to implement new processes in the face of economic downturns and perceived dangers, including the threat of failure. This is not to say that the dangers are not real. Yet there are also serious dangers that arise when an organization fails to adapt to the changes in its environment or undergoes unmanaged change.

Risk taking serves to stretch the organization's capacity. Indeed, overcoming risks by making use of the potential of the members of the organization should become the new golden rule. Once everyone in the organization sees the emperor has no clothes, the best strategy is to put new ideas out into the open and begin to design new services and products once thought unattainable. By sharing the uncertainty, leaders can increase the level of trust in the organization and strengthen the social connections, thereby raising the levels of reciprocity, information flow, collective action, happiness, and wealth.

Kellner-Rogers (1999) stated that a complex web of relationships and creating meaning characterizes all living systems, including organizations, gangs, families, and political movements. This web is not describable using neat organizational charts or flow diagrams. Even more important, it cannot be used to predict outcomes. The relationships that make up a living system display an incredible capacity for engaging in sophisticated coordinated behaviors. These behaviors, however, are seldom the result of directive leadership, strategic plans, or engineered solutions but instead usually occur when the conditions that support risk taking and creative stretching are present. In short, they emerge to the degree that the members of the organization are open, vulnerable, and willing to take risks.

Capra (1982) described the emergence of coordinated behaviors using the analogy of chemical combination. Sugar is made up of three atoms: oxygen, hydrogen, and carbon. Where is the sweetness? The sweetness is in the relationship between the atoms. It is not a quality of any of them individually but emerges in the molecule as a whole. Likewise, when vulnerability, risk taking, and stretching enrich the communal capacity of an organization, out of the relationships of the members tend to emerge behaviors that produce positive results, although not always.

In fact, less than optimal results often lead to a new and better order, as shown by the following story. In a Midwestern village at the end of the nineteenth century, a common orchard was used by all of the villagers to feed their livestock. Over time the villagers, despite working diligently, went bankrupt and even faced starvation. What happened? Before the collapse, each villager had thought, "The more livestock I have, the better off

Group Discussion

As described in the text, at the end of the nineteenth century a common orchard was used to graze livestock by everyone in a small Midwestern village. Because the feed was free, everyone felt the temptation to add animals to their herd. Eventually, after a rapid increase in the total number of livestock, the grass became depleted, the trees died, the livestock starved, and the villagers went bankrupt. Obviously, new rules were needed. Who should create the new rules for use of the orchard? What strategies would you recommend to correct the situation and make the village prosperous again? How should the strategies be evaluated? What is the relevance of this case history to the role of leadership in the transition from the Industrial Age to the Information Age? Identify at least two scenarios in your organization that bear some resemblance to the case history and critique how the main issues were managed.

I will be. The feeding is free, so I will increase my herd as fast as I can." The number of livestock grazing in the orchard increased so rapidly, however, that the grass was soon depleted and the trees died. The livestock began to starve and the village faced destruction. The main problem was that the villagers all engaged in the same behavior without awareness of their interdependence and of the impact of their behavior on the village as a whole. It was by experiencing the dire outcome of their actions that the villagers were able to recognize their interdependence and to gain the power to reverse the course of events.

Living the New Reality

The fourth step is living the new reality. Living the new reality is about trial and error, about learning what works and what does not work. Once a new path has been identified, the leader, along with the team members, supports the unfolding of additional capacity (new work processes or services). Ideas become reality by being applied by the organization on a trial basis. For the organizational leader, living the new reality involves

- Allowing the new work processes (or services) to become integrated into the system
- Determining the fit between the processes and the stakeholders (patients, employees, and the entire organization)
- Accepting that unanticipated outcomes will occur, both positive and negative
- Coaching others to sustain the new knowledge
- Encouraging vulnerable behaviors
- Leading the way to a state of mutual trust

During this phase of the cycle, the leader and team might easily lose sight of the original purpose. The tendency is for them to become so anxious and pressured for success that they do not always examine the new processes carefully enough to determine the full range of their effects. The goal here is not to ensure the success of the new processes but to allow them to become integrated into the system to evaluate their goodness of fit (i.e., their advantages and disadvantages for the organization, the employees, and the patients).

The leader and the team must allow the new work processes to unfold, to live and breathe, rather than expecting perfection immediately. The leader and the team must carefully examine the processes from all perspectives, looking for opportunities for improvement. Timely evaluations become the norm. What the leader and the team should not do is implement the new processes as if they were permanent and fully refined, hoping that no rework is necessary and that no additional costs are incurred. Continual tinkering should be the norm.

Evaluating the Results

In the fifth stage, the results of implementing the new work processes or services are evaluated. Mechanistic principles of thought presuppose linear cause-and-effect relationships. Given the nature of healthcare organizations, such principles are inappropriate for evaluating work processes and must be replaced by nonlinear evaluation models for two reasons. First, the increasing complexity of work in the Information Age minimizes the number of simple cause-and-effect relationships. Second, living systems, especially systems that encompass human beings and their behavior, cannot be understood mechanistically.

Exhibit 8-4   Performance Measurement Matrix

	Quality Indicator	Productivity	Cost
Customer	Satisfaction	Service time/event	Unit cost of service/product
Employee	Satisfaction	Turnover	Cost of labor and benefits
Organization	Reputation	Net income margin	Administrative cost of overhead/all costs

Source: Malloch, K. 1999. The Performance Measurement Matrix: A framework to optimize decision making. Journal of Nursing Care Quality, 13, no. 3: 1–12, copyright 1999, Aspen Publishers, Inc. Reprinted by permission of Wolters Kluwer Health.

Because of the complexity of organizations, the assessment of processes and outcomes requires the use of multiple indicators and a nonlinear evaluation model such as the Performance Measurement Matrix. This model accommodates different data levels, data measures, and traditional performance measures while taking into account the limitations of cost-to-benefit analysis. It examines nine categories of data that represent quality, productivity, and cost measures (**Exhibit 8-4**).

The Performance Measurement Matrix provides a framework for assessing the impact of selected indicators on organizational performance and can help minimize the tendency to make a decision on the basis of one positive indicator. In some situations, for instance, it might show that a course of action, despite increasing the organization's net income in the short term, negatively affects all the other eight indicators, including customer and employee satisfaction and the organization's reputation, in both the short and long terms. The matrix also can be used to compare two or more options and their overall impact on the organization.

Whether the matrix is used or not, the goal of this stage of the vulnerability cycle is to

- Measure multiple process and outcome indicators
- Evaluate the quality, productivity, and cost of the new work processes
- Avoid simple, linear, cause-and-effect assumptions

When the risk results in a less-than-optimal outcome, the work becomes that of course correction and remediation. The new knowledge gained from the unsuccessful effort is critical to continuing success; this information serves to inform others of a course of

Group Discussion

Suppose your organization is exploring which of two possible employee retention programs to implement. One applies to all employees, whereas the other applies only to nurses, who have an especially low retention rate. The same amount of funding is available for each program. Select indicators for the nine dimensions of the Performance Measurement Matrix to evaluate each program, and then identify the potential positive and negative effects of each on the organization. Which program offers the greatest benefit to the organization? Explore other scenarios in which the Performance Measurement Matrix could be applied.

action that should not be repeated. Six actions are recommended when a negative outcome is identified:

1. Acknowledge that the outcome is less than expected.
2. Correct negative outcomes quickly; ensure personal safety.
3. Apologize quickly to those affected.
4. Review the goal and the selected process and identify areas of vulnerability. Be sure the work is still the right thing to do. Determine whether the goal is still appropriate.
5. Modify the process to avoid further negative outcomes.
6. Never be reluctant to abandon the goal and the process if safe and effective processes cannot be determined.

Cherishing the New Knowledge Gained

The goal of this step of the vulnerability cycle is to cherish and make use of the knowledge gained by going through the entire cycle. Each time a risk is taken, an outcome occurs—an outcome that may not have been anticipated. Consider the following two scenarios. In scenario A, an organization implemented a new work assignment process based on the recommendation of the staff employees. The project was more successful than anticipated. Not only were the original goals accomplished, but the professional behaviors of the employees improved and their job satisfaction levels increased (because of their involvement). In scenario B, the management team selected a reputable work management system without input from the employees. The employees did not support the system, and the costs for additional education and monitoring were much greater than anticipated. Employee satisfaction declined. Both projects were well thought out, and positive results were anticipated in both scenarios. In scenario A, the new process was retained. In scenario B, the project was discontinued or modified in step 5 (evaluation), and the knowledge that the style of implementation used was ineffective was retained and applied in future projects.

Group Discussion

The seven stages in the cycle of vulnerability present leaders with different levels of challenge. Consider two recent projects that were implemented in your organization, one believed to be a success and the other not. Using the cycle of vulnerability, determine for each project the stage at which the implementation processes were most successful and the stage at which interventions would have been especially helpful.

Beginning the Cycle Again

At the end of the vulnerability cycle, the challenge is to identify what was valuable and what was problematic and begin the process again with the next opportunity or challenge. Repeating positive efforts is as important as avoiding negative results. Although

Point to Ponder

Preparing an environment that will nourish creativity is, in itself, a creative activity. Spontaneity, dynamism, fun, humor, freedom from fear of failure, incentives, sympathetic values and culture, a soulspace, and celebration are just a few of the essential ingredients of a creative culture. Leaders who seek to liberate the soul through creativity must establish a sanctuary in which failure is not punished but valued as a learning experience.

—Lance Secretan

sometimes it is easy to see the value of implementing new processes or services, at other times it is difficult to discern anything more than that the implementation was not effective at this time and place. Nonetheless, leaders should always document both the positive and the negative results and try to view the implementation as a lesson in the value of vulnerability.

Coaching and mentoring employees in the development of vulnerable risk-taking behaviors are the logical next step. To guide employees toward these behaviors, a leader must first establish a culture of trust. The leader and employees must then discuss the value of risk taking and its potential impact on organizational productivity and morale. The coaching process—in which leader and employees learn together rather than alone—becomes transformative for everyone and for the organization as a whole. Guiding each other to become more vulnerable requires attention to both the content of the situation and the new relationships that emerge once the culture supports vulnerable behaviors.

Quantum leaders must develop patience to wait for the vulnerability cycle process to emerge, learn to trust in the value of fostering a vulnerability culture, and maintain their confidence in the inevitability of progress. Mutual trust evolves when the leader and employees experience the positive realities of the vulnerability cycle and when employees are valued for their efforts as well as the results of their efforts.

In addition, leaders serve as facilitators to guide employee and team member empowerment rather than as directors. Facilitating is not about judging behaviors and offering advice; rather, it is about recognizing new behaviors when they occur and inviting the employees to offer feedback on their performance and perceptions of success. It is also about maintaining composure and showing tolerance because vulnerable behaviors and risk taking are learned slowly, and employees who have yet to acquire the necessary skills may only partially finish new behaviors. Finally, it is about communicating well and developing and sustaining the kind of relationships that support new behaviors.

Group Discussion

Imagine you are a leader coaching employees in the acquisition of vulnerability behaviors. Develop a coaching outline that (1) describes the components of the vulnerability cycle, (2) provides examples of the relationships that emerge in a vulnerability culture, and (3) presents three strategies to sustain vulnerability behaviors.

New Relationships

Although much attention has been given to the differences between the Information Age and the Industrial Age, the fact is that successful leaders in all periods of history have valued information and knowledge. Being well informed with timely information has allowed leaders to facilitate the development of effective solutions to problems. Seldom do leaders rely on secondhand or outdated information. Instead, they develop networks of reliable sources to provide them with steady streams of current information. Indeed, their relationships with information sources in the organization and in the community take on ever greater significance as the availability of information increases.

Noted leadership expert Kouzes (2000) believes that, for leaders, social capital is as important as intellectual capital, if not more important. After all, leadership is about relationships. Who people know and what they can do for each other facilitates the work of the organization. This is not to say that brains or intellectual capital are not important, especially in the Information Age, but knowing is different from doing and does not necessarily translate into action. Making something happen requires having information and good relationships. Furthermore, with the opening of the floodgates of digital communication pathways, relationships are even more complex than before. Removing the traditional hierarchies of communication brings new obligations, such as the need to value diversity and personal privacy and to respect boundary setting and self-disclosure (**Figure 8-2**).

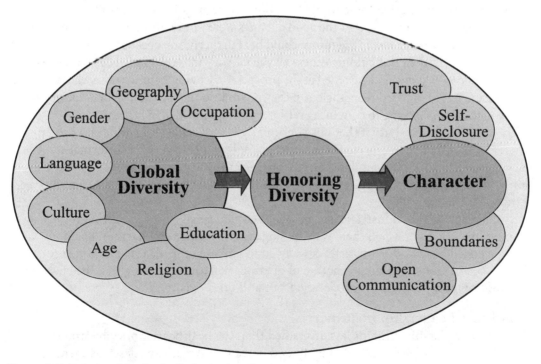

Figure 8-2 Relationships in the Information Age

Inclusivity: Valuing Diversity in a New Way

People differ in more than gender, race, and ethnic background. People grow up in different geographical locations, speak different languages, practice different religions, and belong to different generations. In addition, people think and act differently. Some think quickly, some slowly, some are analytic, others are creative, some are detail-oriented, some prefer the big picture, some want facts, some depend on intuition, some are outgoing, some are reserved—and the list goes on. Given these differences, it is a wonder that we can relate to each other at all. Yet the diverse reality of our universe requires that we maximize our efforts to form relationships, despite the prejudices that unfortunately form because of our differences.

Labeling individuals who differ from us and profiling their behaviors may make it easier for us to function at times, but labeling and profiling create irrational biases and often prevent people from forming meaningful relationships or fracture the relationships that do become established. Creating expectations of inclusivity rather than valuing diversity provides a positive approach to including the multiple attributes of our humanness. Thus, the benchmark for evaluating the breadth and depth of a team now focuses on openness and inclusivity rather than searching for documentation of the diversity of races, sexual orientation, and gender present in a team.

Perhaps the greatest obstacle to valuing inclusivity and developing new relationships is the common reluctance of individuals to accept change. Even when they are given a clear explanation of nonmechanistic processes, for example, and shown how these processes have led to success, many people continue to adhere to mechanistic and linear approaches and remain convinced that these would have brought about still better results. In short, these people resist admitting that the good old days were not really all that good, not even as good as today or as good as the future could be. Furthermore, because of their reluctance to change, the challenge of guiding others on the journey into the next age is monumental, and leaders can become disheartened at the prospect of leaving behind those who, for whatever reason, have cold feet. Nonetheless, if they are to lead the journey, leaders cannot afford to spend their time trying to convince everyone that the world is in fact changing.

The beauty of inclusivity it that it is continually emerging. Seeing differences as enhancements rather than as deterrents is increasingly important in the Information Age because attempts to filter out data can discourage creativity and obstruct an organization's creative potential. Keeping an open mind is necessary for gaining a richer, more complete understanding.

By contrast, in the Industrial Age creative thought was discouraged and consensus was encouraged. "Be a team member" was the slogan. The former emphasis on harmony and accord should be abandoned; instead, we need to embrace the idea that organizational success lies in transforming our notion of organization and accepting that the chaos of competition and the order of cooperation can and do coexist.

Healthcare Leadership Inclusivity

Healthcare leadership remains less diversified than the healthcare workforce and the overall population (Weber, 2000). Eighty-two percent of Americans describe themselves as white, 13% as black, 11% as Hispanic, 4% as Asian or Pacific Islander, and approximately

1% as American Indian, Eskimo, or Aleut. Healthcare organizations employ 11.5 million workers. Approximately 75% of the workers are white, 15% are black, 7% are Hispanic, and 3% are Asians or Native Americans. Of the 50,000 healthcare leaders, a remarkable 98% classify themselves as white. Given this lack of inclusivity of representative percentages of the population, opportunities certainly exist for including more (and more widely varied) perspectives in leadership decision making, not only for purposes of fairness but also to better serve ethnically diverse communities by delivering care that respects cultural traditions. Healthcare organizations have a responsibility to understand and meet the needs of their communities by developing partnerships with representatives from all local cultures.

Opportunities for Change

When things go wrong, what usually goes wrong are relationships, not physical objects or processes, and these go wrong because of poor communication. Unfortunately, as a society we have very little idea how to get along with one another. Wars rage around the globe, the divorce rate is higher than 50%, and violent crime is rampant. The legal profession has been dubbed "the undertakers of relationships."

Fortunately, healthcare leaders are realizing the importance of establishing and maintaining productive relationships. In particular, current healthcare reform expectations include effective partnerships with patients, partnerships that facilitate effective engagement that positively affects health. Furthermore, although the Internet is a valuable new communication tool, there are reasons to worry about its dehumanizing effects. For example, it allows people to inhabit a virtual world and spend less time relating directly to others. Although technology is necessary for leading an organization, it is not sufficient. Who one is in relationships with others may be just as important as what one does in the way of delivering technologically sophisticated care. Quality relationships are characterized by trust, the honoring of differences, clear personal boundaries, comfort with self-disclosure, and open communication—all of which confer a degree of vulnerability.

Privacy

The explosion of the Internet as a means of communication has made privacy into a hot political issue. Historically, privacy advocates have had difficulty building support for their position. Now, Internet users are becoming especially concerned about their privacy, largely because of the numerous available sources of information from social media sites and

> **Point to Ponder**
>
> Leaders have always been set on stage, in sight and view of the whole world. The Internet puts the leader under the microscope for all to see in the finest detail.

the well-known trails of e-commerce "cookie" crumbs that make it easy for companies to gather and sell customers' personal data to other companies. Recently, practices that inform consumers of their privacy rights and offer the option to opt out of further data sharing have become commonplace as well as cautions to social media users to filter their contributions to the widely accessed social media sites.

Furthermore, whether out of boredom or curiosity, we are spying on one another like never before. Tiny wireless cameras are used not just for espionage but to detect shoplifting in department stores, and a world of websites publish our dirty laundry and private thoughts. Although people in general need to be more open to ideas, to be more vulnerable, they also understandably want barriers around their private lives. For example, few people, if any, are willing to allow the rest of the world access to all of their personal, financial, and health information. Where the boundaries lie is unique to each person, and determining what to consider private and public in the Information Age requires careful reflection.

Unfortunately, it is not a simple process to identify what will be shared with whom and at what time. For one thing, individuals do not present appropriate component parts of themselves whenever these are desired. Instead, individuals are unified wholes. Mary Parker Follett, noted management expert, pointed out:

> It is unrealistic and wasteful to organize work on the basis that a person can be abstracted from the totality of their being and put into the exercise of one particular skill, taught to perform it to a certain standard, and expect continuous performance at that level—and nothing else. One cannot disconnect themselves, leaving most of themselves at the work-gate and take in just that bit relevant to their job. (Graham, 1995, p. 75).

The lack of clearly defined personal boundaries (personal firewalls) is a major cause of relationship problems. As privacy diminishes, the importance of personal boundaries increases. Personal boundaries are different for each individual, and creating effective boundaries requires a healthy sense of identity. Boundary violations often run rampant in organizations. Saying no is frowned on. Yet excessive overtime, for instance, violates employees' family boundaries. The best course of action is to respect assumed or articulated boundaries until permission is given to cross them.

Personal boundaries include physical, mental, and spiritual boundaries. In general, a person's physical boundaries extend beyond the person's skin to encompass a space surrounding his or her body. Hugging or standing too close is a violation for some and welcomed by others. A person's physical boundaries also pertain to his or her possessions, money, time, and energy. Touching personal belongings in someone's office may be viewed as acceptable or as a violation. Mental boundaries pertain to beliefs, emotions, and intuition. They are violated, for example, when people are told they do not have the right to feel and appropriately express their emotions. Spiritual boundaries pertain to people's self-esteem, their sense of identity, and their relationship with a higher power. Destructive criticizing, yelling, and uttering abusive words are violations of spiritual boundaries.

Group Discussion

Create a list of expectations regarding your physical boundaries, emotional boundaries, and spiritual boundaries. For example, would you consider your physical boundaries to be violated if someone stood very close while talking to you? Touched you on the arm? Ask a colleague to create a similar list and then share your expectations with each other.

Traditionally, boundaries and boundary violations in health care have been assessed from a patient–provider perspective. The point is that the patient is especially vulnerable by virtue of illness or injury and is dependent on the provider for help, whereas the provider has access to sensitive information about the patient and may uncover medical problems that the patient normally would share only with intimate friends. Given the imbalance of power, the provider has very clear responsibility to delineate and maintain appropriate boundaries.

The power imbalance between managers and employees creates similar expectations. In any relationship between a manager and an employee, both are responsible for delineating their personal boundaries, a task that is an essential step in creating an effective working relationship. Lack of boundaries blurs the purpose of the relationship, creating an ambiguous situation in which harm to either person may result. In addition, uncertainty is unnecessarily increased, to the detriment of the relationship and the entire organization. For far too long, command-and-control leaders have unwittingly violated the personal boundaries of employees without their consent—not with malicious intent but to ensure that the work of the organization was completed in a timely manner. The challenge for leaders today is to avoid dwelling on the rights and wrongs of past practices and instead to move forward and create the conditions in which personal boundaries are acknowledged and respected.

Self-Disclosure

No relationship can develop fully until the participants expose something of their deeper selves to each other. Revealing oneself to others—one's thoughts, feelings, and intentions—is about telling one's story. Self-disclosure leads to greater understanding, trust, compassion, and commonality—in short, to a better relationship.

The idea that self-disclosure is valuable is often difficult to embrace, especially in a business context, because it runs contrary to classical management theory. In traditional organizations, people who stand around talking about matters unrelated to work are seen as wasting time. The obsession with efficiency is an obstacle to appreciating the value of strengthening relationships through casual conversation.

Self-disclosure is based on trust, on having total confidence in the integrity, ability, and good character of the other person. In other words, the person making the personal disclosures must believe the other person reliably follows through on commitments, has the competence to carry out his or her responsibilities, is emotionally balanced, and consistently chooses the "right" action.

Relationship Skills

In establishing relationships with employees and helping them develop a vulnerable and open style of behaving on the job, leaders must not assume that the employees have well-honed relationship skills. In fact, many employees, like many leaders, have less-than-adequate skills. Relationship skills, unfortunately, are not necessarily learned by growing up in a family. Many adults, because of how they were raised, have developed patterns of behavior that obstruct learning and accountability (e.g., conflict avoidance and assuming a victim attitude). In addition, many have failed to acquire the skills needed to cope with change, deal with personality differences, and communicate effectively.

Rather than becoming Information Age aliens, quantum leaders learn when to spend time building relationships and when to focus on tasks. In a healthy organization, the distinction between performing tasks and building relationships becomes blurred. For one thing, the latter can be used to develop the relationship skills needed to incorporate vulnerability and open communication into the organization's work and grow its capacity. Developing these skills takes time as well as a strong commitment on the part of leaders. In addition, leaders can enhance the effectiveness of these skills by using the principles of complexity communication.

Complexity Communication

In sharp contrast to traditional hierarchical organizational structures, the new organizational structures are virtually flat, with a minimum of midlevel layers between executive management and staff. Using information networks, organizational staff in different divisions communicate and collaborate with each other in a moment's time. Multidirectional communication is the norm rather than the exception.

In many organizations the entire focus is on sending information, which is only one-third of the communicative interaction. The assumption is that the receiver understands what the sender intended. This assumption is often wrong, and the full exchange should include the sending of information by one person, its reception by one or more people, and, finally, a confirmation of their understanding.

Complexity communication is presented as an integrated process for improving the effectiveness of communication (**Figure 8-3**). It requires sensitivity to the myriad interrelationships and interdependencies that are characteristic of a quantum organization. It is based on three behaviors: critical listening, critical questioning, and critical thinking. The term *critical* here should not be taken as having a negative connotation; it is intended to have roughly the same meaning as *analytical*. This process is continually iterative and dynamic.

Critical Listening

In a conversation each listener has the responsibility to get the message, but often listeners are too busy thinking about what they want to say to listen carefully enough. People often understand only half of what is said to them. Being vulnerable requires expert listening skills—skills that many people obviously cannot claim.

The greatest challenge for listeners is to "still the mind," to stop the self-talk and mental rehearsing of what they intend to say when it is their turn. Stilling the mind is also about dismissing mental models, at least temporarily. Its consequences include allowing listeners enough time to formulate enduring and just solutions and minimizing the tendency to seek quick fixes.

> **Point to Ponder**
>
> Rest assured, no matter how bad it looks, I will not judge you until I have heard your side. Once a leader puts expedience above fairness, his reputation and integrity crumble away like something rotten.
>
> —Elizabeth I

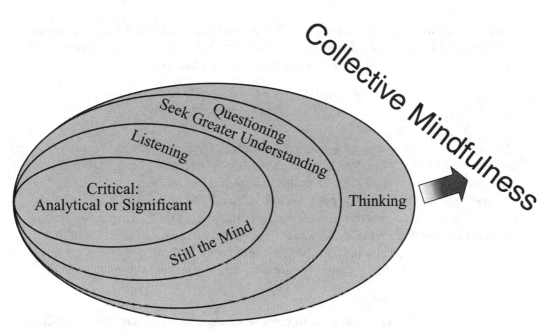

Figure 8-3 Complexity Communication Leads to Collective Mindfulness

Our deeply held internal images of how the world works have a powerful impact on how we listen and react to information. Putting aside our perceptions of power, money, gender, culture, physical appearance, and so on is simply impossible. Nevertheless, leaders who listen with an open mind and create the conditions for employees to do the same see better outcomes from their decision making.

Another challenge is to deal with information overload. Some individuals want to tell everything they know or at least provide more information than the listener needs, which puts a strain on the listener. The listener must then listen even more carefully to discriminate between what is worth retaining and what is not. Managing information is not an easy task, but it is essential for effective and efficient communication.

Critical Questioning

Lawyers are schooled never to ask a question that they do not already know the answer to. Vulnerable leadership requires the opposite. The purpose of critical questioning, or asking for significant information, is to check individual perceptions of an issue or situation and render it more manageable. Leaders in the Information Age need to ask new types of questions, including questions about progress, value, and satisfaction. Asking for clarification is also a good way to minimize misinterpretation.

The wise leader never leaves a meeting without going through a checkout procedure. This procedure involves asking the participants questions such as the following: How do you think the meeting went? Did we accomplish what you thought should be accomplished? What was accomplished?

Asking questions about the value of work done ensures that all of the work planned or completed will in fact make a difference. Examples include these: What difference will this work make? To whom will it make a difference? At what cost?

Group Discussion

Staffing is the largest expense for most healthcare organizations. One reason is that the uncertainty of patient care needs requires a healthcare organization to have sufficient staff on hand to cover upward swings in care delivery, including emergency situations. Use the principles of vulnerability and complexity communication to create an effective and efficient staffing system that incorporates staffing by ratios and/or patient acuity. Discuss the advantages and disadvantages of the system. How can you be sure that the right care provider is with the right patient at the right time? Is the highest quality care provided at the lowest cost?

Questions about the skills and roles of employees are also important. Do the skills of the employees match the needs of the marketplace? Is there a need to eliminate or add job duties? Are the organization and the community better off because of the services or products provided?

In asking questions like the preceding, leaders attempt to learn more about those being queried and their perspective on issues related to their work and the organization. In the fast-paced world of health care, leaders run the risk of overgeneralizing from past experiences, and asking lots of questions can help prevent this mistake in reasoning. Unfortunately, listening is not always easy for leaders.

One of the keys to critical questioning is to refrain from offering advice or commentary to the person being questioned. Most leaders are comfortable providing guidance to others, and they readily give advice. Critical questioning requires something more—the gift of an ear. Asking questions garners the questioner more information if the respondent is allowed to express pertinent opinions. Examples of questions leaders might ask are listed in **Exhibit 8-5**.

Exhibit 8-5   Examples of Critical Questions

- What is your understanding of this situation?
- Why is this important to you? To others? To the organization?
- Which issue do you think this situation is related to: technical, systems, or people related?
- What do you need to know to make a decision on this issue?
- What assumptions do you think others have made about this situation?
- Who else cares about this issue as much as you do?
- This sounds very rational. What do people believe about it?
- This sounds very emotional. What do people feel about it?
- What are the choices in the situation?
- What would you find helpful in this situation?

Receivers of information, or listeners, need a safe space to ask clarifying questions of the senders. In other words, the open exchange of information depends on the existence of a safe forum. If the sender of a message feels threatened by the receiver asking questions about the message, the resulting hostility can quickly end the questions and cause a breakdown in communication. If the receiver feels unsafe asking questions about the message, the resulting silence could easily be misinterpreted as agreement and understanding. When leaders misconstrue the absence of questions as acceptance and understanding of their messages, they commit a grave error.

For some leaders the challenge is different. Those who are steeped in the classical command-and-control leadership culture rarely ask questions to gain information. In their view, they are expected to be experts on all matters related to their role and are reluctant to ask for information for fear of exposure. Although their concern about looking less than competent is generally unfounded, they still are not able to listen very well or feel comfortable asking for advice from others. In the new age, their main challenge is to allow themselves to become more vulnerable and hence more open to input from others.

Critical Thinking

The ability to think critically has long been recognized as a necessary management skill. What is different in complexity communication is the sequence of events. The process begins with critical listening, followed by critical questioning, and then critical thinking. It does not make sense to engage in analysis before listening and asking questions to clarify content so that all vital data can be considered. Further, complexity communication is a team process, and it involves the participants assimilating information and then reaching a logical conclusion as a team, not individually.

Critical thinking encompasses the following components:

- Analyzing the use of language
- Explicating assumptions
- Formulating problems
- Weighing evidence
- Evaluating conclusions
- Discriminating between arguments
- Justifying claims
- Clarifying values

Critical thinking is helpful for seeking deeper meaning, validating perceptions, and setting priorities. The proper attitude for engaging in critical thinking is a mix of reflective skepticism and tolerance for ambiguity. Openness is essential for examining evidence. Too often people proclaim they are thinking critically when in fact they have prejudged the issues, and their discussion supports preconceived notions rather than exploring the range of available options. Managing the complexity communication process requires a more critical or analytical style of thought and communication.

For many leaders and employees, engaging in dialogue runs counter to the prevailing culture within their organizations—a culture that instead fosters internal competition and sets hierarchical limitations on who can contribute to the decision-making process.

These leaders and employees find it especially difficult to recognize and practice openness and self-disclosure, suspend judgment, and promote collaboration as ways of increasing collective intelligence. In complexity communication it is normal to view disagreement as an essential aspect of dialogue and to avoid suppressing differences merely for the sake of preserving the peace. Although intensely painful at times, learning the necessary skills and engaging in complexity communication dialogue have a value that can hardly be overstated.

Developing dialogue skills and communicating with others based on the belief that every person is of value but has a limited view represent an overwhelming challenge. In this type of communication, careful listening is integrated with questioning for clarification, and then messages are analyzed using critical thinking skills. Many leaders are quickly able to develop the three distinct skills of listening, questioning, and thinking but have difficulty with sequencing the application of the skills. Leaders commonly think or make a decision first (often before all the information is presented), request information and clarification second, and then listen as the final step—the fire–aim–ready approach. Despite the fast-paced work environment, which hinders contemplative communication practices, quantum leaders recognize the benefits of complexity communication and coach others to use the associated skills to mediate the internal competition and reinforce new and more effective behaviors.

Collective Mindfulness

Complexity communication skills are especially important in health care, where the potential for catastrophic outcomes, should employees fail to communicate, can be significant. Given the critical nature of the services they provide, healthcare organizations often develop what is known as the power of collective mindfulness, a phenomenon described by Weick and Sutcliffe (2001). Collective mindfulness is the capacity of groups and individuals to be keenly aware of significant details, notice errors in the making, and have the shared expertise and freedom to act on what they notice.

Consider the case of a patient who is experiencing cardiac arrest. A team of nurses, respiratory therapists, and physicians quickly assembles, prompted by a prearranged code call. Within minutes the patient's heart rate is stabilized, respiratory function is restored, and the team disperses. Those unfamiliar with emergency departments might believe the actions of the health professionals had been tightly scripted and well rehearsed. Rather, the professionals all knew their particular role, had experienced similar situations in the past, and had only to listen to what was happening, ask for additional necessary information, and think through and integrate past experiences with the current event to perform the rescue.

To be effective in potentially catastrophic situations, health professionals depend on their mastery of standardized routines and on complexity communication at its best. They listen intently and with full presence, question only for clarification, and intervene as a finely tuned unit.

Collective mindfulness is not limited to clinical situations. It is evident in many types of situations in which there are complex interpersonal relationships. Consider healthcare staffing. Healthcare leaders are continually challenged to deliver reliable services in the face of fluctuating conditions, such as shortages of qualified employees and reductions in reimbursement. Quantum leaders create a culture that allows employees to be flexible (but in orderly ways) and to focus energy and expertise where and when they are needed. They can then use the employees to assist in dealing with the difficulties that arise by creating strategies that address the appropriate issues.

Group Discussion

Select two teams, one composed of experienced employees and the other composed of newer employees. Consider an emergency situation in which a patient is experiencing chest pain. Compare the two teams with regard to their working relationships, communication skills, and ability to prioritize and make decisions. Create a plan to develop the skills of the less effective team.

Hidden within the spirit of collective mindfulness is the essence of vulnerability—being open, searching for new solutions, taking risks, trying new strategies, retaining what works, and discarding what does not work. What emerges is a delicate balance of processes that encourage continuous learning and improvement, while at the same time promoting order and reliable performance, a very powerful combination.

Strategies for Cultivating Leadership Vulnerability

In this section, two strategies for fostering vulnerable or open leadership are proposed: open communication and syndication. Both strategies have inherent risks and require leaders to stretch current thinking. Although many other strategies support open leadership, these two are designed to begin the process of changing mental models and moving to practices that fit with the work of the quantum organization.

Open Communication

Some leaders have confused dialogue with behind-the-scenes consensus building and decision making. Making decisions before all the information is considered leads to poor outcomes and decreases trust in the integrity of the decision-making process. Although according to the classical management model conducting business in informal settings such as the dining room and the golf course may have some merit, recent advances in information technology have brought both challenges and opportunities to the way business is conducted. In particular, by aiding in the removal of secrecy and increasing the ease of dialogue they support the open communication model.

The open communication model is based on the same principles as open meeting laws (**Exhibit 8-6**). The idea behind these laws, which have traditionally applied to meetings of public bodies, is that publicizing meetings and conducting them openly maximize public access to governmental processes. All 50 states have enacted some type of legislation to recognize the public statutory right to openness in government. The laws require

---

Exhibit 8-6   Basic Principles of Open Meeting Laws

1. A meeting is considered to be a gathering that can occur not only in person but also through technological devices.
2. All meetings of a public body shall be open meetings, and all persons so desiring shall be permitted to attend and listen to the deliberations and proceedings.
3. An "open call to the public" is permitted but not required. The purpose of an open call is to allow members of the public to address the public body on matters not listed on the agenda.
4. Executive sessions will be used to seek legal advice and review confidential records. No votes are taken in executive session.
5. Appropriate notice of each meeting will be given (usually not later than 24 hours before the meeting), and the agenda and meeting location will be posted.
6. For each meeting, there will be written minutes or a recording that will include an accurate description of all actions proposed, discussed, or taken and the names of members who propose each motion.
7. The minutes or a recording of any meeting, except an executive session, must be open to public inspection no later than 3 working days after the meeting.

Source: Data from http://www.sec.state.vt.us/municipal/pubs/openmeeting/

meetings of public bodies to be conducted openly and for notices and agendas for such meetings to be provided to the public. Open meetings expose the conduct of the business of government to the scrutiny of the public and prevent decision making in secret, thereby ensuring that appointed members of boards and commissions truly serve as representatives of the broader community and that the actions taken are in the best interests of the community.

The open communication model applies the principles of open meeting laws to organizations, based on the belief that the work of any organization belongs to all its members and that encouraging open communication enhances organizational effectiveness and capacity. The principles focus on the manner in which members communicate and make decisions, and their overall goal is to increase the fairness of decision-making processes and prevent them from being influenced by off-the-record communication between decision makers and others. The following seven principles, if followed, increase the incidence of open dialogue, improve trust among employees, and decrease bureaucratic processes:

1. The business of the organization shall be conducted during open meetings, which are defined as gatherings of people physically, telephonically, or electronically. This principle requires that issues brought before a committee are discussed in the presence of all members of the committee. It is not appropriate to discuss any topic without involving all the parties. Ex parte communication considers only one side of a situation and as such violates the first principle of open communication. E-mail communication, telephone conversations, and casual dialogue at social gatherings about committee meeting topics are not allowed. The intent is to eliminate selective collaboration and pre-voting on issues before the actual meeting. Decision making that is inclusive from the start results in decisions that, because everyone is highly invested in them, are more likely to succeed.

2. The date and time of each meeting, its location, and its agenda shall be posted. Publicizing this information allows unofficial but interested members to learn the issues to be covered in the meeting and to discuss them with other members ahead of time. It also helps eliminate the chance that decisions will be made in secret. In the meeting itself, only issues identified as being on the official agenda are discussed, which means that no surprise or unanticipated issues are dealt with. Although posting meeting information may be cumbersome at times, it minimizes the chances of reactive decision making.

3. Every meeting shall be open to all persons desiring to attend and listen to the deliberations and proceedings. The intent of this principle is to remove even the appearance of secrecy. It is based on the belief that the satisfaction felt by employees, along with their job performance, is highly correlated with their involvement in decision making that directly pertains to their work.

4. Every meeting shall include a "call to the attendees" to allow members of the organization or the community a defined allotment of time in which to address the official members on matters discussed. Although dialogue on the issues is restricted to official members of a committee, other attendees should be afforded an opportunity to react to what the official members say. Allotting a specified amount of time for comments keeps the meeting from running past its scheduled end. In addition, the official members are not required to respond but are requested to consider the additional information when making decisions.

5. Executive sessions shall be used for the purpose of seeking expert advice or reviewing information defined by law as confidential but not for the taking of votes. Some types of information, such as performance evaluations and salary and wage data, are protected. In executive sessions, issues involving confidential information are discussed, but no voting or decision making occurs.

6. Each meeting is documented by written minutes or a recording that includes an accurate description of all actions proposed, discussed, or taken and the names of the members who voted for each motion. Documenting the work of a committee fully prevents decision makers from hiding behind the cloak of the summative vote count. It also forces decision makers to own their opinions and makes them accountable to the membership at large. Minutes serve as an historical record of the decision-making process.

7. The written minutes or the recording of any meeting except an executive session must be open to inspection no later than 3 working days after the meeting. Ensuring that a record of discussion in the meeting is available to all interested parties in a timely manner again helps lift the shroud of secrecy.

Interestingly, the two most common violations of open meeting laws are discussion of agenda items without the full board or committee present (ex parte) and inappropriate use of the executive session. The same violations should be expected during implementation of the open communication model because collaboration and pre-voting on issues have been a traditional practice in organizations, as has the use of executive sessions for dealing with matters of organization-wide concern.

Syndication

The second strategy for cultivating leadership vulnerability is organizational syndication, which is basically a way of structuring business to tap latent potential. Based on the recognition that information is now widely available, syndication uses resources outside of an organization to benefit the organization.

Organizations, according to Dee Hock (1999), are extremely good at some things, are very good at many things, but are not good at everything. In fact, organizations are pathetic at some things. Although much organizational work is believed not to be amenable to syndication, significant work elements might be, especially those at which organizations are pathetic.

Syndication, which originated in the entertainment world, is now beginning to define the structure of e-business. It involves the sale of the same good to many customers, who then integrate it with other offerings and redistribute it, similar to the way television programs or news stories are managed.

Syndication is a radical new way of structuring business (**Table 8-1**). It requires leaders to rethink their strategies, to reshape their organizations, to change the way they interact with customers and partner with other entities, and to pioneer new models for collecting revenues and earning profits. Integrating syndication into an organization is similar to creating a "chaordic" organization, as defined by Dee Hock (1999). Hock is credited with devising a new concept of organizations based on the belief that chaos and order, competition and cooperation, can be harmoniously blended. He conceived of a global system for the electronic exchange of value, and the result was VISA International, which is owned by 22,000 member banks that compete with each other for 750 million customers and honor each other's transactions across borders and currencies.

Chaordic organizations present an unambiguous challenge to the traditions of independent organizations by bringing into existence an interconnected international reality once believed impossible. They also offer courage to those considering syndication for selected services or products. At the moment, the chaordic model is mainly a learning aid, however, and cannot be quickly imprinted on existing organizations.

TABLE 8-1   Business in the Syndicated World

	Traditional Business	Syndication
Structure of relationships	Linear supply and demand	Loose weblike networks
Corporate role	Fixed	Continually shifting
Value added	Dominated by physical distribution	Dominated by information manipulation
Strategic focus	Control scarce resources	Leverage abundance
Role of corporate capabilities	Sources of advantage	Products to sell
Role of outsourcing	Gain efficiency	Assemble virtual corporation

Source: Werbach, K. (2000, May–June). Syndication: The emerging model for business in the Internet era. *Harvard Business Review*, 90. Reprinted by permission. Copyright 2000 by the Harvard Business School Publishing Corporation, all rights reserved.

Group Discussion

A group of healthcare organizations has decided to apply the syndication model to its employee development program. Imagine you are on the team creating the product to be syndicated. Using the principles of syndication, your team has been assigned the work of content originators. Describe the content origination process and continue to model development with the creation of packaging and distribution plans for the education program. What are the advantages and disadvantages of syndication as a way of developing and implementing programs? Who would support or oppose the syndication model? What performance measures could be used to evaluate it?

Syndication is based on the realization that needed expertise is often found not inside an organization but beyond its boundaries. In a syndication network, the roles of originator of content, syndicator or packager of content for distribution, and distributor of content to customers are quite different from the traditional roles of content developer and distributor of content to employees.

In a syndication network, the content originator has greater responsibility and accountability than in traditional organizations. In some situations, leaders have established collaborative initiatives that can be moved to the syndication level. Health centers for indigents, school health education and treatment clinics, hospice centers, and training programs developed through cooperation between communities and financiers are candidates for syndication. Because of their need for standardization of services (to ensure quality), operational cost savings, and conservation of capital, each could be syndicated to create a greater network without substantial duplication of effort. The role of the originator is to assess and consolidate the work of many products into a single product desired community-wide.

The second key role, that of syndicator, encompasses packaging the content and managing the relationships between originators and distributors. The syndicator's goals include achieving consistency of products and services, uncovering user expectations, and supporting the established relationship between product users and the syndication processes. Time-limited agreements would support state-of-the-art products and services that provide appropriate quality at the lowest cost because failure to meet the standards would cause users to turn to other syndicators.

Finally, the distributor is responsible for delivering the goods from originators to users. As the virtual world develops, many more information services and education programs are likely to be distributed through the Internet.

It is no longer cost-effective for every organization to provide every service. Not only is it costly, but individual organizations lack the necessary concentration of expertise. The syndication model offers opportunities for current providers of services to generate revenue through a shared process as designated originators. Designated originators provide the content of their expertise to the product and become co-owners of the syndication model. If syndication became common in health care, those organizations with significant expertise could earn income as a result of contributing to the origination process, whereas those with limited expertise could have access to standardized state-of-the-art products for a reasonable cost.

Is There a Choice?

Are leaders obligated to develop a vulnerable leadership style? Do they need to replace closed leadership behavior with open leadership behavior? The obvious response is yes, there is no choice, the value of vulnerability is too conspicuous to deny. The move into the Information Age requires different skills and knowledge than those required in the Industrial Age.

However, some leaders may have difficulty making the transition. Some, for example, might support the concept of open leadership, but because of the perceived threat in admitting to a lack of answers or information, they might be resistant to living the new behaviors. They also might have great difficulty in creating a culture supportive of open leadership because their failure to walk the talk of vulnerability hurts employee morale and lowers the level of trust within the organization.

Thus, the best strategy for leaders right now is to critically assess their personal status and their ability to assimilate vulnerable behaviors and integrate them into their performance. Acquiring the skills needed to implement the open leadership model is a long-term process that requires understanding, commitment, and persistence. Ethically, developing open leadership skills is the right thing to do. In addition, as successful behaviors emerge, leaders will see some of the benefits to be gained from changing to a better model for the times.

Conclusion

Currently, it is nearly impossible for a single person to know more than 10% of what there is to know about a particular topic. This is most disconcerting to leaders who have worked and studied diligently to know as much as they can. Unfortunately for these leaders, it is even apparent to their colleagues that they do not have all the answers. In addition, they have no chance of catching up because information continues to accumulate too rapidly. The good news is that everyone is in the same situation; no one ever has all the answers.

Consequently, the new challenge for leaders is to become comfortable managing the information that is available—to become competent as information access finders and relationship makers. Furthermore, as this chapter points out, the best approach to leadership today is to understand that the high speed of change, among other factors, makes total control impossible, and to therefore accept that vulnerability and open communication are required. In addition, throughout the journey of learning to become openly vulnerable, leaders necessarily will become competent in managing uncertainty, encouraging risk, valuing diversity, and communicating with others based on principles of complexity and respect for privacy and personal boundaries. Increasing vulnerability increases leadership excellence, but no leader can achieve this desirable result without significant commitment and effort.

Case Study 8-1

Positioning for Positions

Everest Health System is located in the Midwest and is the largest healthcare system in the region, with three large acute care hospitals, a mental health hospital, two smaller community hospitals, and a rehabilitation hospital. In addition to the inpatient facilities, the corporate structure of Everest Health System owns a physician group with 10 outpatient clinics distributed over the large metropolitan area of nearly 3.2 million people. Everest also contracts with an independent group of physicians who are recognized as "Everest physicians" and share in negotiated group insurance rates for inpatient and outpatients services. In addition, Everest has an outpatient sports medicine and rehabilitation center, an outpatient MRI diagnostic center, two outpatient surgical centers, a cancer center, and a standalone infusion therapy center. The three large acute care hospitals are all Magnet designated, and two are recognized with the Planetree designation as well.

All of the chief executive officers (CEOs) of the inpatient and outpatient centers report to an executive vice president for patient care, and the chief operating officers (COOs) and chief nursing officers (CNOs) report to the CEOs at their respective facilities. Being a progressive healthcare system, the executive VP for patient care desires to develop an Institute for Nursing Excellence, an idea that also appeals to the executive for philanthropy because there is a potential donor who might be willing to fund the new institute. An outside consultant has been hired to facilitate the development of the new institute. It is decided that the membership of the newly formed institute will consist of the CNOs and the directors of research and development for each of the inpatient facilities who report to each of the CNOs.

During the first few months, the consultant facilitates the meetings. The group spends considerable time and process to identify what they consider to be the characteristics of an Institute for Nursing Excellence. Using this as a foundation, they developed a mission and vision statement and created a professional practice model that would serve as a conceptual model that could be used to articulate the purpose, mission, and vision of the institute internally and externally. After these foundational documents were developed, they decided to focus on meeting the recommendations of the Institute of Medicine's *Future of Nursing* report and look for opportunities to improve measures of nursing quality across the system. After 8 months of meetings, the CNOs met privately and decided to lead the meetings themselves and terminate the services of the consultant. One of the CNOs of the larger acute care hospitals volunteered to be the leader of the group.

Over the next year, the group worked on developing a strategic plan with measures for expected deliverables for quality, research, education, and nurse-sensitive indicators. The CNO leader also developed a job description for a director for the institute that was approved by the full membership. The position description was written to indicate that a doctorate in nursing was strongly preferred and that the applicant should have previous experience in a nursing leadership positions. There was considerable discussion about the title of the position, with several options considered such as director, vice president, and executive vice president.

Another area of consideration was the reporting structure for the new position. Several concerns were raised among the members, but these were not openly discussed in the meetings. Some of the CNOs were concerned that if the new position reported to the executive VP of patient services, the position might evolve into a chief nurse executive (CNE) position for the entire healthcare system and that they might be required to report to this person in the future instead of the hospital CEO. The CNOs indicated they don't want this new person to "interfere in the operations of their hospitals" and "tell them how to run their business." The directors of research and development also were concerned that they too might be required to report to this new centralized position; some of the directors prefer to report at the entity level rather than the system level. There was significant discussion about the new person reporting to the CNO in current institute leadership role because this structure would elevate that person above the other CNOs.

After several months of discussing the pros and cons of reporting structures, titles, and levels of authority for the new position, the job description was written to place the position one level below the CNOs with wording that the person would report to the entire CNO group. The position was viewed by the CNOs to be at an equal level of the directors of research and development. The position was then posted for recruitment.

A few applications were received, but they were reviewed first by the CNOs in their regular CNO meetings before they were shared with the entire institute membership. Applicants who seemed appropriate were interviewed by phone by the CNOs, and then vetted to the entire institute membership for a second phone interview or a face-to-face interview. It soon became apparent that most applicants with strong leadership experience were uneasy about a position that reported to a "group" instead of to one individual, and because most applicants had been CNOs or directors of nursing schools, they were not satisfied with the title "director" instead of "vice president." Months of debate ensued with no resolution to the reporting structure, title for the position, or selection of applicants willing to take such a position.

Because the new position remained unfilled for more than 18 months, the "interim director" position was rotated among the CNOs, but the directors of research and development were not considered in the rotation. With months of tenure in the interim director role, the lead CNO was in the spotlight for interviews and collateral materials developed to showcase the Institute for Nursing Excellence. This led to some of the CNOs voicing concern that the interim director CNO was "taking all the credit" personally for the institute's accomplishments without sharing the recognition and awards among all of the CNOs.

Over months of meetings, evidence of nursing excellence (publications, research, certifications, and newly earned degrees) were collected from each respective entity by one of the directors for research and development and published in a document highlighting nursing excellence at Everest Health System. The funding received from the major donor was used to provide nursing scholarships, and the group met to develop the application process, selection criteria, and the selection process. The money was distributed in scholarships for applicants bridging the associate degree to baccalaureate, the baccalaureate to master's, and the master's to doctorate. The institute membership seemed to work well together when given a specific task to accomplish.

The directors of research and development talked among themselves and voiced concerns that they felt that the institute had lost its vision and that the CNOs were controlling the work of the institute without recognizing the contributions or value that the directors brought to the institute. As issues were discussed at the institute meetings, any observer could see rolling of eyes and other nonverbal expressions of discontent among the members. Some members were meeting outside of the institute meeting to analyze what they believed was the "true agenda" of some of the CNOs. Some members expressed that they believed that decisions were made from a fear perspective: fear that hiring a real leader for the institute at the vice president or executive VP level might compromise the CNOs' power or disrupt the existing CNO reporting structure.

Communication among the group was guarded; positions on issues were calculated; and there was little transparency in expressing real feelings about important issues. When there was an application from and interview of a nationally known nursing leader for the position, the group began to speak of elevating the position to a VP level, but the reporting structure remained with the position reporting to the institute CNO leader. The applicant subsequently rescinded his application, and he stated that "he perceived that the group was not working well together and he was not willing to take a position at a director level that reports to a group as contrasted to an individual."

Questions

1. What is your perception of the forces that may be at play among the institute members?
2. What might you do as an institute member to facilitate a higher performance among the group?
3. What might be the risks, gains, and personal vulnerabilities in trying to redirect the group?
4. How might outcomes be different if there was more vulnerability and transparency among members?
5. What would be your vision of what could be done to create an exemplar Institute for Nursing Excellence?
6. If you were a CNO, using the six stages of the cycle of vulnerability, what might you do to try to facilitate change in the group dynamics?
7. How might collective mindfulness help the group to achieve the original vision for the institute?

Case Study 8-2

Taking the Next Step

Ashlee has worked at Midwest Medical Center for the last 10 years as the director of medical surgical services. She has really enjoyed this role and has led her team of nurses to accept many new changes to improve their scores in patient satisfaction and physician satisfaction. She has prided herself on advancing the skills and competencies of her direct reports (nurse managers) and has encouraged them to become certified in their nursing specialty areas. Ashlee also meets with the general staff at least once a month and provides information to them relative to the progress toward the nursing division's overall goals and other hospital information. She makes every attempt to meet with the staff of both days and nights and make certain that she has a presence with the staff during their unit meetings at least once a month.

Ashlee is well liked by her direct reports and all of the staff in general. Her managers have an opportunity to provide input into Ashlee's annual performance appraisal, and they frequently cite examples of how Ashlee has supported them and helped them to grow in their roles. On the annual employee opinion survey, the nursing staff of Ashlee's departments comment that she is visibly present on the unit and open to discussing issues of concern with them. Ashlee is very comfortable in her role and has a good working relationship with the other nursing directors and directors of other hospital ancillary departments and specialty areas. Ashlee has no desire to change her position or leave the organization, but she is constantly looking for ways to create new energy for herself in the workplace. Occasionally, the chief nursing officer (CNO) asks Ashlee to assume responsibility for other nonnursing departments as the interim director until a replacement director can be hired, or Ashlee is asked to assume the leadership of various project task forces for the organization. Ashlee has a great relationship with her CNO and looks to her as a mentor in her own career. The other directors indicate their appreciation for the chief nursing officer as well.

Ashlee is surprised one day in the Nurse Executive Council when the CNO announces that she will be leaving Midwest Medical Center in the next 30 days because she is relocating to another state with her husband, who has assumed a very prestigious position in one of the major universities there. The CNO announces that she has been selected as the chief operating officer (COO) of the Northwest University Medical Center, which is a huge promotion for her as well. The CNO announces that the Human Resources department will be placing advertisements in local and regional newspapers, in major nursing management journals, and on the organization's website for a replacement CNO. She also suggests that the directors consider applying for the position themselves because they are familiar with the organization and the strategic vision for the nursing division.

Ashlee leaves the Nursing Executive Council with mixed feelings—sadness at losing her personal mentor and conflicted with internal confusion as to whether she should apply for the position herself. She had never thought of herself as leaving her current position, and she begins to question her capabilities and skills for a CNO position. She is certain that at least one other director will apply for the position because he has often talked about wanting to be the CNO in an organization. For the next few days, it seems that Ashlee can think of nothing else but the CNO position. She tries to visualize herself in the role and consider all of the responsibilities that the role would entail. She knows that applying for the role would be a risk because she would be leaving a very comfortable position and moving into a position that would require new skills, new relationships with other healthcare executives, and a much broader scope of responsibilities.

She also feels the risk of applying for the position and not being selected. How would this look in the eyes of her colleagues? How would this look in the eyes of her staff, who have been as supportive of her as she has been of them? At times her mind is filled with the negatives of the role and all that could go wrong. She is aware that there is a constant threat of union organization because many of the other hospitals in the city are already under union contract. Midwest Medical Center is the only hospital that has not been organized. She is also painfully aware of the financial pressures that she would have to assume in the CNO role, and she has observed the current CNO struggling with budget cuts, managing negative budget variances, and advocating for the needs of the nursing department. Ashlee wonders if she has the skill and capabilities to be successful in negotiating budget needs for nursing with the chief financial officer and other executives.

At other times Ashlee's head is filled with visions of what she could accomplish as a CNO. Although she had considered returning to school for her PhD in nursing, she delayed those plans for personal reasons. Now she really regrets that decision. Although the position description for the CNO indicated that a PhD was preferred, Ashlee wondered if the applicants with a PhD would have preferential consideration. On the other hand she realizes that she has an excellent reputation in the organization as a visionary leader, and her department is nearly always in compliance with the organization's performance goals and other important metrics such as HCAPS scores and nursing-sensitive indicators. Ashlee knows that although she has experienced many past successes, she would need to stretch her own capabilities to be successful in the CNO role. Being a positive person, she tries to envision herself in the role and rehearses in her mind the steps that she would need to take to lead the nursing division successfully. It is a huge risk and opportunity, and she is feeling the weight of her own advice to others in coaching them to stretch and expand themselves in assuming new roles. She has often told others to allow themselves to become vulnerable to grow personally and professionally. Now she remembers her own advice to others, and her advice is cogent to her as well.

Ashlee's colleague applies for the CNO role, and she learns that there are at least two other outside applicants who have previous experience as CNOs at other organizations. One of these outside applicants also has a PhD in Nursing Administration. Now Ashlee is all the more conflicted as she considers her own decision and evaluates her own capabilities for the role. She decides to talk over this important decision with trusted friends and colleagues inside and outside of the organization. Many encourage her to step forward and apply for the position even though she is comfortable in her current role. Realizing that she doesn't have much time to ponder this decision, Ashlee finally decides that she should throw her "hat into the ring," and she applies for the position.

After talking with the Human Resources representative, Ashlee is slated to interview with members of the executive team, physicians, nursing director representatives, and other divisional leaders. She also meets individually with the CEO and the COO, and then in a group interview with the entire executive team. Ashlee tries to prepare herself for the individual and group interviews by reviewing the vision and strategy of the hospital and updating her knowledge of some of the current financial challenges faced by the hospital in the new healthcare economic environment. Ashlee has a strong vision of nursing and its role in maximizing the patient-centered experience of patients and families who are served by the hospital. She discusses her goals of improving nurse–physician relationships in an effort to ensure positive patient outcomes and opportunities for change that would not only improve the nursing work environment, but would also enhance the organization's success in meeting the hospital's goals.

In the interviews, Ashlee discloses a lot about herself, her personal goals, and her goals for nursing. She indicates that she has a very positive relationship with many of the leaders in the organization. One of the more difficult questions that she has to address is to describe an innovation she has done to achieve a desired program or goal for her department. Ashlee carefully considers before she speaks, but then describes an example of planning and implementing a program where nurses and physicians round together and include the patient in the discussion of the plan of care. She indicates that at first physicians were very reluctant to participate in the collaborative rounds, and she describes the strategy that she used to first listen to their concerns and those of the nurses. She discusses how she identified champions of the change process and used the nurse and physician champions to facilitate the acceptance of the process by those who were more reticent. She also describes how she measured the change using a collaborative behavior scale and nurse and physician satisfaction scale before and after the implementation of the collaborative rounding approach. Ashlee suggests to the interviewers that she believes strongly that measuring the results of change is critical to demonstrate the effectiveness of the change to others, building trust for future changes. The implementation of the collaborative rounding process resulted in an improvement in patient satisfaction scores and in collaborative behavior, nurse satisfaction, and physician satisfaction scores.

In one of the interviews, Ashlee is asked whether she truthfully feels that she has the capabilities to fulfill the role of the CNO because she doesn't have experience as a CNO. At first Ashlee is a bit intimidated by the question, but she thinks carefully before she answers. She explains she is highly successful in her current role and is viewed as a visionary leader in the overall hospital organization. She also indicates that she would have some learning and developmental needs, but she feels confident that she could work with her executive colleagues, the nursing leaders in the organization, and her peers to enhance her skills and competencies in the role. She thinks that it is best to be honest about her development needs in the new role but indicates that she is willing and able to advance herself and to provide value to the organization as a new CNO. After the interviews are completed, Ashlee wonders whether she should have expanded on her past successes rather than being so open and honest about her development needs for the new role. She silently hopes that she has not lost the position because of her honesty, but she feels that it is important that the selection team sees her as an individual who could carefully assess her own strengths and weaknesses for such an important position.

Questions

1. What do you think about Ashlee's decision to apply for the CNO role?
2. How would you have answered the question if you were Ashlee and were asked about your capabilities to fill the CNO role?
3. How did Ashlee show her vulnerability as a leader in considering the CNO role and in her answers to the interview groups?
4. What are the areas of vulnerability that Ashlee will face as a new CNO?
5. What do you perceive to be Ashlee's areas of strength and areas that need development?
6. What challenges and obstacles do you think that Ashlee might encounter if she were selected for the role of CNO?
7. If you were on the interview team, how would you vote when Ashlee is considered against her competitors for the role?
8. Would you have preference for an applicant who had past experience as a CNO, an applicant who had a PhD in nursing, or an inside applicant who had experience with the hospital and the current nursing division's vision for the future?

References

Abrahamson, E. (2000, July–August). Change without pain. *Harvard Business Review*, 75–79.

Capra, F. (1982). *The turning point: Science, society and the rising culture*. New York, NY: Simon and Schuster.

Chamorro-Premuzic, T. (2012). The dark side of charisma. HBR Blog network. Retrieved from http://blogs .hbr.org/2012/11/the-dark-side-of-charisma/

Cleveland, H. (1972). *The future executive: A guide for tomorrow's managers*. New York, NY: Harper & Row

George, B. (2004). The journey to authenticity. *Leader to Leader, 31*, 29–35.

Gill, R. (2011). *Theory and practice of leadership* (2nd ed.). Los Angeles, CA: Sage.

Graham, P. (Ed.). (1995). *Mary Parker Follett—Prophet of management: A celebration of writings from the 1920s*. Boston, MA: Harvard Business School Press.

Hock, D. (1999). *Birth of the chaordic age*. San Francisco, CA: Berrett-Kohler.

Kellner-Rogers, M. (1999). Changing the way we change: Lessons from complexity. *Inner Edge, 1*(6), 18–22.

Kouzes, J. M. (2000, October). Link me to your leader. *Business2.com, 10*, 292–295.

Kurtsman, J. (2010). *Common purpose: How great leaders get organizations to achieve the extraordinary*. San Francisco, CA: Jossey-Bass.

Lencioni, P. (1998). *The five temptations of a CEO*. San Francisco, CA: Jossey-Bass.

Porter-O'Grady, T., & Malloch, K. (2011). Quantum leadership: Advancing innovation, transforming healthcare. Sudbury, MA: Jones & Bartlett Learning.

Torbert, W. R. (2000). Exercising vulnerable power. *Inner Edge, 3*(4), 19–22.

Uhl-Bein, M., & Marion, R. (2008). *Complexity leadership: Part 1: Conceptual foundations*. Charlotte, NC: Information Age.

Weber, D. (2000, September). The lack of diversity at the top. *Health Forum Journal*.

Weick, K., & Sutcliffe, K. (2001). *Managing the unexpected: Assuring high performance in an age of complexity*. San Francisco, CA: Jossey-Bass.

Suggested Readings

Axelrod, D. (2000). *Elizabeth I CEO: Strategic lessons from the leader who built an empire*. Paramus, NJ: Prentice Hall.

Bell, C. R. (2005). The vulnerable leader. *Leader to Leader, 35*, 19–23.

Bly, R. (Ed. and Trans.). (1981). *Selected poems of Rainer Maria Rilke*. New York, NY.

Cranley, L. A., Doran, D. M., Tourangeau, A. E., Kushniruk, A., & Nagle, L. (2012). Recognizing and responding to uncertainty: A grounded theory of nurses' uncertainty. *Worldviews of Evidence-Based Nursing, 9*(3), 149–158.

Crenshaw, J. T., & Yoder-Wise, P. S. (2013, February 24–27). Creating an environment for innovation: The risk-taking leadership competency. *Nurse Leader*.

Cukan, A. (n.d.). Caregiving: Fighting a culture of fear. Retrieved from http://www.upi.com/ Health_News/2006/02/14/Caregiving-Fighting-a-culture-of-fear/UPI-38431139947951/

Krass, P. (Ed.). (1998). *The book of leadership wisdom: Classic writings by legendary business leaders*. New York, NY: Wiley.

Malloch, K. (1999). The performance measurement matrix: A framework to optimize decision making. *Journal of Nursing Quality, 13*(3), 1–12.

Margolis, J. D., & Stoltz, P. G. (2010, January–February). How to bounce back from adversity. *Harvard Business Review*, 87–92.

Murphy, L. G. (2012). Authentic leadership: Becoming and remaining an authentic nurse leader. *Journal of Nursing Administration, 42*(11), 507–512.

Porter-O'Grady, T., & Malloch, K. (2012). *Leadership in nursing practice: Changing the landscape of health care.* Burlington, MA: Jones & Bartlett Learning.

Quinn, R. E. (1996). *Deep change: Discovering the leader within.* San Francisco: Jossey-Bass.

Rooke, D., & Torbert, W. R. (2005, April). Transformation of leadership. *Harvard Business Review*, 67–76.

Rosen, R. H. (2008, Fall). Embracing uncertainty and anxiety. *Leader to Leader*, 34–38.

Shirey, M. R. (2012). How resilient are your team members? *Journal of Nursing Administration, 42*(12), 551–553.

Werbach, K. (2000, May–June). Syndication: The emerging model for business in the Internet era. *Harvard Business Review*, 85–93.

Youngblood, M. D. (1997). *Life at the edge of chaos: Creating the quantum organization.* Dallas, TX: Perceval.

Quiz Questions

Select the best answer for each of the following questions.

1. Vulnerability is an essential leadership trait for the quantum leader. Which of the following is its major effect?
    a. To expose the leader's weaknesses to others in the organization
    b. To improve the leader's ability to manage information
    c. To reduce the leader's authority and control
    d. To improve the leader's ability to uncover multiple perspectives on an issue

2. Uncertainty in organizations results in a wide range of reactions from leaders. What do most leaders in quantum organizations believe about uncertainty?
    a. Uncertainty is normal.
    b. Uncertainty is the cause of errors.
    c. Uncertainty is a deterrent to creativity.
    d. Uncertainty is surmountable.

3. Nonlinear evaluation of work is the norm for quantum healthcare organizations. What does the nonlinear evaluation of a work process look at?
    a. The cause-and-effect relationships of the process
    b. Outcomes that occur repeatedly
    c. Multiple outcomes
    d. Multiple process participants and multiple outcomes

4. The recognition that uncertainty and chaos are present in all organizations is changing the nature of strategic planning. Which one of the following tactics can be used to increase the utility of the planning process?
    a. Decreasing the time frame under consideration
    b. Tinkering
    c. Adding team members with different perspectives
    d. Increasing the attention given to specific measurable goals and objectives

5. Complexity communication leads to several important results. Which one of the following is a result?

a. An increased focus on the sending of information
b. Collective mindfulness
c. Greater participation of team members
d. More risk taking

6. New strategies are needed for leaders to provide health care in an environment that is unpredictable and changing rapidly. What is the strategy of open communication designed to do?

a. Prevent hasty decisions
b. Increase team member participation in meetings
c. Increase trust in the decision-making process
d. Eliminate confidential information

7. A leader's understanding of his or her personal boundaries, privacy needs, and self-disclosure limits is an important new tool in the leader's toolbox. What does this tool allow the leader to do?

a. Set limits with employees
b. Share feelings and expectations in a meaningful way
c. Develop a clear sense of his or her identity as a precursor to relationship building
d. Avoid conflict and support team processes

8. A leader's relationships or social connections have increased in importance as a means to which end?

a. Facilitate the work of the organization
b. Increase the leader's visibility
c. Interpret information
d. Manage conflict

9. Privacy is a continuing concern for healthcare leaders. How is it best controlled?

a. By government agencies
b. By each individual
c. By eliminating communication on the Internet
d. By developing coded communication

10. Syndication is a new way of using healthcare resources creatively and cost-effectively. What is one of its main disadvantages?

a. Syndication is expensive.
b. Syndication requires an increased number of employees.
c. Syndication has not been used extensively in the healthcare field.
d. Syndication results in the sharing of information.

CHAPTER NINE

Healing Brokenness:
Error as Opportunity

It is often the best people that make the worst mistakes—error is not the
monopoly of an unfortunate few. We cannot change the human condition,
but we can change the conditions under which humans work.

—*James T. Reason*

Reproduced from Reason, J. (2000 March 18) Human error: models and
management. British Medical Journal, 320: 768, 2000 with permission from
BMJ Publishing Group Ltd.

Chapter Objectives

At the completion of this chapter, the reader will be able to

- Describe the concept of error as an opportunity to improve healthcare outcomes.
- Describe the advantages and disadvantages of mandatory reporting and disclosure of errors.
- Compare the advantages and disadvantages of managing error solely from a systems perspective
  with managing error from an individual perspective.
- Describe the advantages and disadvantages of remediation and discipline as interventions for
  minimizing error.
- Show how healthcare leadership errors can be transformed into practices supportive of the
  quantum organization.

Given the complexity of the healthcare system and the chaos emerging from the challenges of healthcare reform, workforce shortages, and reimbursement limitations, it is not
surprising that health professionals continue to commit significant medical errors and
that healthcare leaders frequently feel challenged beyond their ability to cope. As a result,
healthcare leaders and professionals are generally fearful of making the wrong decision or
doing the wrong thing. Yet the potential for errors or breakdowns in the care of patients
is always present. Breakdowns can be caused by poor healthcare provider performance,
the unavailability of essential resources, and systemic problems. In the best case scenario,
good systems design and proper staffing serve to minimize errors and crises. Healthcare
leaders have the ultimate responsibility for making decisions that create safe clinical

practice conditions and for responding to public pressure to improve medical care and reduce errors. This chapter presents new perspectives on both clinical and leadership error and describes opportunities for reducing the incidence of error in current systems.

Error in General

The reality is that if human beings are involved, mistakes occur sooner or later. Big mistakes, little mistakes, mistakes of consequence with adverse outcomes, and mistakes of little consequence occur every day. To be sure, not every error results in harm. Further, errors have many sources, from human incompetence to systemic problems. Near-misses are also of concern. Although a near-miss, by its nature, does not result in full-scale harm, the surrounding events offer a rich source of data to be studied as a means of avoiding similar situations in the future. Discussing near-misses allows an organization to assess specific products or procedures and develop recommendations for improvement.

Given the inevitability of error, reacting to mistakes punitively is unlikely to minimize their occurrence, even though our culture leads us to expect the assignment of blame, correction of the situation, and, in most cases, punishment of those who made the mistakes. Punishment and blame are also meted out to those who come in second. For example, when there is a loser in a competition, even the competition between healthcare organizations for market share, people tend to seek a scapegoat, someone to blame for the lack of success. Winning is everything in our society, and coming in second place or losing a competition is not viewed as acceptable.

> ### Point to Ponder
>
> Consider what would have happened if you had allowed shame and embarrassment to overwhelm you when you fell as a baby while trying to learn how to walk. You would still be crawling!

Our drive to be the best, to have the most, and to be in control has led to substantial achievements, but it does not always bring about the best outcome for an organization and in some cases results in failure. When the outcome is less than optimal, the leaders and employees are held accountable, despite the fact that few leaders and employees, if any, ever achieve perfect success.

The constant attaching of blame to individuals creates a climate of shame and guilt and decreases the candid reporting and discussion of mistakes. Unfortunately, the main approach to error, not only in health care but in society at large, is to punish supposed offenders. Given that punishment usually has the effect of quashing the human spirit, it is curious that leaders, or anyone else, continue to view mistakes as failures rather than as opportunities for improvement. In some cases, leaders use punishment for the purpose of retaining and reinforcing their power within the organization. In other cases, they simply believe that it is the right thing to do and to do anything less would tarnish their reputation for effectiveness. Whatever the rationale, punishment of error makers not only fails to produce the desired result (the elimination of error), but the negative impact of the punishment dissuades the employees from doing more than the minimum because they fear making more mistakes and suffering additional punishment. In short, the mistakes themselves become less of a problem than the societal response to the mistakes.

> **Point to Ponder**
>
> Being foolish does not mean that one is inherently good or evil—just foolish!

Error as Foolishness

In attempting to gain an understanding of behaviors related to error, it is helpful to reflect on our cultural roots and values. According to the view of many cultures, humanity begins in a state of perfection, but the journey of life is filled with temptation and distractions. Understandably, humans eventually partake of the tree of knowledge of good and evil (Kaye, 2000).

Consider the two spiritual traditions of Judeo-Christianity and Buddhism. Both espouse the view that human nature is fundamentally perfect but that people soon stray from their natural state of perfection and make mistakes. They become distracted and tempted by many things, especially worldly goods. Not surprisingly, people follow their desires, lose their awareness of perfection, ignore their inner voice of wisdom, and give in to temptation. Sometimes a person risks everything for one more possession—another automobile, boat, computer, or vacation—and thereby negates his or her sense of personal wholeness.

Although not everyone is an adherent of a particular spiritual tradition, looking at errors from the perspective of such traditions can help people understand the phenomenon of error in a more positive way, a way that humanizes the error factor. By recognizing that mistakes are expressions of inescapable foolishness rather than malice, people can let them go, avoid taking them personally, and prevent them from casting a shadow over a lifetime career. Further, when people accept their fallibility and view their own mistakes in this way, they are more likely to respond to the mistakes of others with understanding rather than anger or resentment.

Leaders, like other people, find it a challenge to overcome the human tendency to hold a grudge when someone makes an error. Yet leaders must learn to forgive others when mistakes are made and begin to coach others to learn from the mistakes. When leaders move beyond resentment, they encourage employees to expect to be treated with

Group Discussion

Reflect on a recent error that resulted in serious harm to your organization. How was the situation managed? Did the questions asked focus on identifying someone to blame, such as these: What is wrong here? Who was responsible for this? Or did the questions enable the organization and the provider to learn more about the situation and be better positioned to avoid recurrences of the error? Better questions for investigating an error include these: Why is this error occurring again and again? Am I missing a lesson here? How can I turn this situation into an opportunity for growth and learning for myself and the team?

Exhibit 9-1   Asking Better Questions

Do Ask
- Why do you think this error occurred?
- Is there a way to avoid this occurring again in the future?
- What can the team learn from this situation?

Do Not Ask
- Why did this happen?
- What did you do wrong?
- Who is responsible for this error?

---

understanding and kindness. It is unhealthy when employees are in constant fear of mistreatment as the result of errors.

By perceiving errors as foolishness rather than as failures, leaders open the door to a new approach to managing errors. Rather than punishing those who commit errors, they treat errors as opportunities for improvement. **Exhibit 9-1** lists appropriate questions to ask when an error has occurred. One good example of the way errors can lead to positive outcomes is the story of the invention of Post-it notes: The disaster of a newly created glue that did not work as planned was turned into a great success—the creation of easily removable stick-on notes. As this example shows, mistakes may bring good fortune, and learning to trust the potential of mistakes to create new opportunities is the only way to move from the toxicity of a blameful culture to the productivity of an accountability culture.

Recognizing and Recovering from Error

Nearly every spiritual tradition includes avenues to recognize and recover from error. The intent of each tradition is to learn from mistakes, to identify actions that decrease the chance of repeating the same mistakes, and to improve performance as a result. For organizations to survive and thrive, they must develop traditions that support employees in recognizing errors and rectifying their effects. This includes allowing employees to take responsibility for the impact of their actions and maintaining openness in the workplace, which is critical for reporting and discussing errors and using them as opportunities for improvement (**Exhibit 9-2**).

Exhibit 9-2   Recovering from Error

- Recognize the lack of provider or leader preparation to manage errors as opportunities.
- Develop strategies to cope with the sense of failure, disappointment, and remorse that often follows errors.
- Create a coaching script for leaders to address serious errors. The process of dealing with a serious error includes
  - Identifying critical events
  - Identifying opportunities for individual improvement
  - Identifying opportunities for system improvement
  - Following up on these steps by implementing changes
- Following an error, ask the individual how he or she thinks it will affect future practice.

Coaching employees through the error recovery process ranges from simple one-time dialogue sessions to long-term counseling and frequent reassurance. A mistake that results in significant harm or in the filing of a lawsuit has the potential to destroy the career of an otherwise exceptionally competent healthcare provider. If the person has a hard time coping with the sense of failure, disappointment, and remorse, he or she also will have a hard time learning how to prevent a recurrence of the mistake. Getting stuck in personal grief or remorse or assigning blame to others does not prevent a repeat performance. In fact, by focusing on the negative emotions felt, the person is distracted from taking measures to solve the problem that led to the mistake. On the other hand, by focusing on what others could or should have done, the person may allay his or her feelings of remorse but may begin to feel powerless or even victimized. The ideal strategy is to accept as much responsibility for the mistake as is warranted and then go on to explore measures for changing the system in a way that reduces the chance of repeating the mistake.

Given the need for openness, effective coping strategies, and support for moving on, the work of the leader is clear. If mistakes are to be treated as opportunities for improvement, healthcare leaders must meet the challenge and create new structures and processes that support dialogue about errors and ongoing follow-up. The overall strategy includes

- Acknowledging the sense of remorse or failure a person who committed an error might feel
- Seeking clarification from that person and providing social support
- Attempting to discover the sources of the problem
- Taking concrete actions to prevent future repetitions

In addition, healthcare leaders must create or strengthen support structures for those in litigation because all too often these individuals are subtly ostracized by the healthcare team.

Errors in Healthcare Service

Healthcare Providers and Error

No provider ever intends to make an error or harm a patient. Health care is about helping others to manage their health, relieving pain and distress, restoring functionality, or assisting in a peaceful death. Healthcare providers feel a sense of satisfaction and accomplishment when a patient experiences relief, a patient's functionality is improved, or a terminally ill patient dies tranquilly. They feel the opposite—discontent and guilt—when their care results in unanticipated bad outcomes. In such a situation, the essence of their healing work has not been realized. Learning to understand the role of the human error factor is one of the greatest challenges for providers.

Expecting Perfection

Health care, by its very nature, is uncertain and imperfect. The variability in perceptions and in the interpretations of clinical data by both patients and providers means that many decisions are partially accidental. Further, medicine is inherently experimental

---

Exhibit 9-3   Two Strategies for Handling Errors

Expecting Perfection
- Is unrealistic but is considered the proper attitude
- Creates unrealistic expectations
- Fails to consider the wide variability in patient situations
- Positions providers as scapegoats for lack of success

Honoring Excellence
- Takes into account the trial-and-error nature of health care
- Supports the evolution to best practices
- Supports continual improvement processes
- Respects the nature of human interactions
- Reinforces a positive culture of excellence

---

in that each patient has a unique set of characteristics (e.g., age, weight, metabolism, existing conditions, and behavior patterns). Regardless of the number of participants in a clinical trial, when a drug is given to a particular patient, it may or may not act according to the established standards. There is never total assurance in health care, and when the uncertainty of care is denied, when perfection is expected, care providers become the scapegoats (**Exhibit 9-3**). Although the mind may understand and tolerate error, the human heart is most unforgiving when things do not go well.

Additional complexity has been introduced with healthcare reform, an effort to improve quality and reduce costs. The anticipated significant overhaul of the current system to achieve the desired patient-driven, continuum-based care system is evolving and outcomes are unknown. It is important to note that when decision makers do not have day-to-day contact with patients, they can confuse what produces dissatisfaction with what is truly erroneous. The health professionals providing the care—those closest to the patients—were expected to practice within the established norms, regardless of their goodness of fit with the specific patient clinical situations. This approach, unconditional adherence to standards, simply does not lead to good care overall.

Honoring Excellence

In many cases, leaders work diligently to preserve the status quo and avoid tinkering with current processes for fear of making mistakes. When mistakes do occur, leaders usually act to rectify the situation immediately and return to the status quo ante. Unfortunately, their fear of disrupting existing routines discourages creativity and motivates employees to refrain from rocking the boat as well. In other words, their drive to sustain the perceived perfect present quashes their own spirit and the spirit of the employees, obstructing the investigation of potential improvements. Indeed, the fear of failure or retribution that employees feel causes them to essentially "retire on the job" and reduces their productivity. The reality is that trial and error are necessary for improvements to be discovered and implemented.

When things do not go as planned, the best response is to look for the message in the error and use the information received to chart a change in course (see Exhibit 9-3). Overcoming the common obstacles to an open culture, fear of punishment for self-reporting, and fear of retaliation for reporting others' errors, must be part of the strategy to honor excellence (HealthLeaders Media, 2013). It is through the continual remodeling of care that best practices or templates for excellence are uncovered. When leaders believe that perfection has already been achieved, they view modifications as inappropriate and a waste of time, thereby hindering the emergence of true excellence.

Learning to appreciate errors as a catalyst for change and improvement opens the door to unexpected opportunities. Errors allow leaders to look at things differently and even revise their plans in light of their new perspective. Quantum leaders examine mistakes or misfires carefully and work to minimize or eliminate feelings of shame and embarrassment—the traditional response to mistakes. Growing from our experiences requires a mindset that recognizes human fallibility and uncertainty. Our expectations should not be based on perfectionism.

Further, an important organizational dynamic emerges when leaders acknowledge that being right all the time is not even a possibility. If leaders are not highly invested in always being right, they find their employees appreciate their attitude and are more likely to approach them with new ideas.

Public Reaction to Error

Significant attention has been given to medical errors. The Institute of Medicine (IOM) report on errors, titled *To Err Is Human* (Kohn, Corrigan, & Donaldson, 2000), elevated not only the healthcare community's awareness of this issue but also the public's awareness because the reported statistics have implications for every single American. The report raised new issues, proposed solutions, and challenged health professionals and the public at large to work to reduce medical errors by at least 50% in the next 5 years. More recently, Finkelman and Kenner (2009) have reinforced the five core competencies of IOM. **Exhibit 9-4** lists the broad goals identified by a coalition of organizations as essential to reform the healthcare system.

Exhibit 9-4   National Quality Strategy's Six Priorities

1. Making care safer by reducing harm caused in the delivery of care.
2. Ensuring that each person and family are engaged as partners in their care.
3. Promoting effective communication and coordination of care.
4. Promoting the most effective prevention and treatment practices for the leading causes of mortality, starting with cardiovascular disease.
5. Working with communities to promote wide use of best practices to enable healthy living.
6. Making quality care more affordable for individuals, families, employers, and governments by developing and spreading new healthcare delivery models.

The National Priorities Partnership is a partnership of 52 major national organizations with a shared vision to achieve better health and a safe, equitable, and value-driven healthcare system.

Source: U.S. Department of Health and Human Services. (2012). *National strategy for quality improvement in health care.* Retrieved from http://www.ahrq.gov/workingforquality/nqs/nqs2012annlrpt.pdf

These competencies support quantum leadership notions that mandatory reporting is consistent with the idea that errors are opportunities for improvement, as is the recommendation to establish a national resource for error research, including research into standards and best practices. Putting these recommendations into effect requires the commitment of leaders and their trust that the open approach will work in the long term.

The IOM competencies and multiple reports unfortunately do not clarify the locus of accountability for error. Recommendations for using a multifocal, evidence-driven approach are strongly encouraged. Both internal and external oversight mechanisms are recommended. Management of errors internally—in fact, nearest the point of service (or the point of error)—offers the best opportunity for continuing improvement, especially if there is a national repository of data on safety and supporting practices. External control reinforces the blame approach to error management.

Finally, mandatory reporting may be a blessing for the public but could be seen as a curse by care providers. Although the consumers must be given information to assist them in choosing providers and services, not all errors provide pertinent information or help in making such decisions. More specific approaches that support error as opportunity are needed, although negligence must of course be reported.

Mandatory Error Reporting

The reporting of every minor incident to a state or national board does not necessarily enhance the protection of the public. Mandatory reporting serves to inform the public of errors but can obstruct the use of errors as opportunities for improvement. Because of the threat represented by reporting to a public body, care providers may be unwilling to declare their errors, particularly minor ones. Further, minor incidents in which patients are not placed at risk of harm and care providers' competence is not put into question usually can be handled inside the organization. Most healthcare leaders believe that if mechanisms are in place to take corrective action, remediate deficits, and detect patterns of behavior, no additional benefit is gained from the mandatory reporting of minor incidents. In fact, punishing a provider for a minor error adds to the bureaucratic burden and results in costs to the organization. The approach favored here, of using errors as opportunities for improvement, can best be supported by informing the public of significant

Group Discussion

A colleague in nursing reports the following incident to you: "I recently gave a patient the wrong medication. The patient was not affected, and I did not write an incident report because I did not want it noted in my personnel file or reported to the state board of nursing. This type of mistake happens often because most facilities are understaffed." How would you handle this situation? Do you agree with the nurse? What changes could be made to the system to support the reporting of this type of error and create opportunities to learn from the commission of errors? When should a medication error be reported to the board of nursing?

errors and care provider negligence but withholding information about minor errors so that these can be brought out into the open within the organization and be used as vehicles for improvement.

Disclosure

Not only is mandatory reporting a complicating factor in error management, so too is the expectation of disclosure. Morally, disclosure is the right thing to do. The ethics manual of the American College of Physicians states that physicians should disclose to patients information about procedural or judgment errors made during care if such information is material to patients' well-being. The ethics manual notes that errors do not necessarily constitute improper, negligent, or unethical behavior, but failure to disclose them may.

The disclosure of errors provides the chance to recognize brokenness. In addition, depending on the circumstances, the person who commits an error may have an obligation to apologize for it or offer reparation. Although professional codes do not clearly state when an apology or reparation is expected, care providers in every discipline, not just physicians, may find themselves in a situation where some sort of acknowledgment of error is morally required. Other ethical issues arise with respect to disclosure. For example, care providers have argued that nondisclosure may be appropriate if the harm from disclosure exceeds the harm from nondisclosure or if the error is inconsequential and disclosure does not empower the patient.

The disclosure of an error raises certain practical issues, especially the timing of the disclosure, where and how to make it, to whom to make it, and what to expect as a consequence. However noble and right it is to disclose errors, the current litigious culture makes it nearly impossible for care providers to willingly divulge their mistakes, a problem not addressed in the IOM report. Their fear of malpractice suits and their resulting tendency to remain silent about errors could easily keep care providers from moving beyond the status quo of error management. In addition, the malpractice system is unlikely to change in the near future, and alternative methods of dispute resolution are unlikely to be instituted. On the other hand, changes in how errors are dealt with should not wait until the legal system is corrected.

For one thing, care providers should be educated in how to disclose errors and how to maintain a relationship with a patient after an injury caused by a medical error. Not only are leaders challenged to create a culture that supports disclosure, but in many cases they need to provide educational processes for developing postdisclosure management skills. The acquiring of the skills necessary to handle disclosure appropriately requires incredible effort from every member of the healthcare team and patience for the expertise to emerge. The following is a set of guidelines for discussing errors (Wu, Cavanaugh, McPhee, Lo, & Micco, 1997):

- Treat the situation as bad news.
- Begin by saying that you regret that you have made a mistake.
- Describe what happened and the decisions made.
- Describe the course of events using nontechnical language.
- State the nature of the mistake.
- Describe the corrective action and any consequences.
- Express personal regret and apology.
- Listen to them—accept, empathize, and answer questions.

Care Provider Disenfranchisement

In addition to the fear of litigation, barriers to the disclosure of medical errors include shame, emotional upset, early denial, grief, and dread of the patient's reaction. It is painfully obvious that medical errors harm not only the patient but also the care provider. Feelings of guilt and worry about potential job loss and professional isolation are all too common. When a serious error occurs, the fear of repercussion demoralizes even the most competent care provider. The frustration and demoralization that follow the making of an error negatively affect productivity and future practice not only for the person who committed the error but for other providers in the practice environment. These providers may feel relief that they did not commit the error but realize that it is all too probable that they will commit errors in the future and be faced with similar emotional upset.

Transforming a Punitive Culture

Efforts to decrease negative reactions to errors have been undertaken both within and outside healthcare organizations, including the Institute for Healthcare Improvement and The Joint Commission. Regardless of the source of the initiative to transform a punitive safety culture, leaders must embark on the purposeful and deliberate work of changing expectations and behaviors to support patient safety, the reporting of errors, and the management of the employee in a way that reflects the realities of healthcare errors rather than condemnation of an individual. The work of culture transformation does not occur quickly; time is required to establish new behaviors and build the necessary trust among individuals. Progress is directly related to the collective ability of the team to learn from mistakes.

Once errors are perceived as opportunities, they can be managed using several new approaches. These new approaches, including modified interventions for addressing errors, are consistent with a new mental model of error that is more positive and reinforces the quest for excellence rather than perfection.

System Versus Individual Errors

Identifying and understanding the source of an error or set of errors are essential first steps in identifying breakdowns and opportunities for improvement (**Exhibit 9-5**). Unfortunately, the information needed to achieve this step is commonly lacking, partially because those responsible for the errors are reluctant to volunteer what they know. An incomplete analysis of the situation stalls the process and can lead to inappropriate recommendations. The quality of the information surrounding an error affects the quality and sustainability of the follow-up interventions. Once all the information is collected, the source of error can be localized, and the interactions between the individual and the system and their role in causing the less-than-desirable outcome can be examined.

> **Key Point**
>
> When an error occurs, do not react immediately. Take a deep breath and share your feelings. Learn to ask questions to gain as much information as possible about the error. Avoid the tendency to criticize.

Exhibit 9-5   Key Concepts

- *Adverse event:* An injury caused by medical management rather than by the underlying disease or condition of the patient
- *Accident:* An event that involves damage to a defined system that disrupts the ongoing or future output of that system (Kohn et al., 2000)
- *Breakdown:* Situations that unfold in undesirable ways as the result of team members' performance, the unavailability of essential resources, and system problems (Benner, Malloch, & Sheets, 2010)
- *Error:* The failure of a planned action to be completed as intended (error of execution) or the use of a wrong plan to achieve an aim (error of planning) (Kohn et al., 2000)
- *Mistake:* An error in action, opinion, or judgment caused by poor reasoning, carelessness, or insufficient knowledge
- *Safety:* Freedom from accidental injury

Much rhetoric has been devoted to system-related causes of medical errors, partly as a result of the significant publicity generated by the 2001 IOM report on patient safety and medical errors. The media, policymakers, healthcare providers, and the public have all expressed concern and urged that something be done, and consequently healthcare leaders are expected to pay special attention to the system-related problems. Although the IOM report emphasized the importance of system-related factors for reducing the incidence of errors, such as safety systems, job design, and medication administration, the solution does not lie in an either/or approach (**Exhibit 9-6**).

Although the problem is not one of bad people working in health care but of good people working in bad systems, those bad systems are created by people—people who have the capacity to fix them. Further, the systems approach has the disadvantage that it

- Decreases attention to particular aspects of care, especially in the area of relationships
- Flattens out beneficial variations in practice
- Promotes a false and distorting vision of medicine as solely technical
- Weakens the moral commitment of professionals (Benner et al., 2010)

Exhibit 9-6   Comparison of Individual and System Accountability

Individual	System
• Professional/legal mandates	• Human factors research
• Emphasizes individual factors	• Emphasizes structure and organizational factors
• Emphasizes individual expertise, thoroughness, and accountability	• Emphasizes standards, automation, and redundancy
• Views individual as locus of responsibility for errors	• Views the system as locus of responsibility for errors
• Aims to assign blame and/or extract compensation	• Aims to decrease guilt and increase honesty in reporting

361

In other words, including both system-related factors and individual behavior in error analysis is important if leaders are to develop new approaches to error management that are effective and sustainable.

Further, neither assigning blame by itself nor locating the source of error by itself is likely to minimize the incidence of mistakes. Although each approach may have advantages in the short term, neither leads to positive outcomes for the system or the individuals in the long term. First, neither the organization nor the individual has total control over the events surrounding an error. Second, using a systems approach by itself is liable to create new patient care risks by minimizing the significance of the individual customization of care and of professionalism, stifling innovation, discounting the relational aspects of practice, mitigating the power of personal responsibility, and spreading responsibility too thinly. Conversely, the individual responsibility model separates care providers from the community.

Remediation Versus Discipline

The way in which the accountability of health professionals is defined by state licensing boards tends to push leaders toward instituting disciplinary action against individuals who make errors. However, the overall effectiveness of disciplining for improving practice or minimizing errors has not been substantiated. Further, state licensing boards have different reporting requirements. Some states, for instance, require only the reporting of significant errors that resulted in harm, whereas others require the reporting of all errors, including minor ones. The value of reporting minor errors with low risk for harm does not appear to be worth the trauma caused to the care providers.

Drawing the disciplinary line, according to Marx (2001), is the real challenge in determining when to remediate and learn from mistakes and when to discipline. He describes four behavioral categories helpful in making this decision: human error, negligence, intentional rule violations, and reckless conduct. Human error needs to be separated out from the categories for remediation because it is about individual behavior that inadvertently caused or could cause an undesirable outcome.

The strategy of using remediation first and discipline when more than human error is involved deserves consideration (**Exhibit 9-7**). Remediation (counseling and guidance provided in a timely manner) serves to protect the care provider's dignity and minimizes shame. In addition, remediation is consistent with the treatment of errors as opportunities for learning new, more effective behaviors.

Exhibit 9-7   Remediation Guidelines

Consider remediation when
- The potential risk of physical, emotional, or financial harm to the client resulting from the incident is very low.
- The incident is a singular event with no pattern of poor practice.
- The employee exhibits a conscientious approach to and accountability for his or her practice.
- The employee appears to have the knowledge and skill to practice safely.

This strategy also makes both the system and the individual accountable for addressing errors. The person who committed the error is expected to participate in the analysis of the error and identify alternative approaches that will reduce the chance of a recurrence. The other

> ### Point to Ponder
>
> Learn from the mistakes of others; you can't live long enough to make them all yourself.
> —Anonymous

members of the team or work group also review the error and contribute to the list of recommendations. These individuals thereby gain insights that will help them avoid similar errors. In other words, all the members learn not only from their mistakes but from the mistakes of others, which is invaluable for the individual members, the team, and the organization as a whole.

Finally, the strategy puts the leader of the organization in the position to manage errors without additional reporting to an outside agency. This is an advantage because the leader is best suited to manage minor errors and work with the providers to ensure that these errors are not repeated. Although not traditionally labeled remediators, most leaders are skilled in remediation techniques, especially the giving of feedback. By discussing the situation in private first, by being specific and focusing on the facts, and by following up to increase the chances of success, the leader can reduce minor errors without causing the providers to feel unnecessary shame and guilt.

Errors that carry a significant risk of physical, emotional, or financial harm or errors that show a pattern of recurrence require greater scrutiny and management. The leader should still refrain from using discipline until the system-related and individual issues are evaluated and a pattern of incompetence and/or negligence has been identified. The goal, in the "error as opportunity" approach, is always to learn from errors by focusing on the relationship between the individual and the system and by implementing appropriate revisions in the work processes. Discipline should be the intervention of last resort.

Healthcare Leadership: Errors and Opportunities

Everyone acknowledges that learning comes not only from the successful performance of an activity or practice, but also from mistakes—from breakdowns or situations that did not go well. But most people are reluctant to reveal their failures, especially at work in front of others. And this in itself is an error. The reluctance to talk about mistakes means the whole team risks losing vital pieces of information that can be derived from looking at the mistakes carefully. Even worse, the likelihood that others will repeat the same mistakes increases dramatically.

Clinical errors do not occur in isolation. As noted in the IOM reports, an organization's system—its structures and processes—has a large impact on the incidence of errors. Indeed, the system not only is the most important influence on the type and number of errors that are committed but also provides the greatest opportunity for improvement. It is through understanding the errors of the past that leaders can redesign the future to support the practices that minimize system breakdowns and individual mistakes.

Unfortunately, the recognition of errors is not a simple or obvious process. Habitual routines often obviate the need to recognize errors, and it is true that changing what has become established involves some short-term costs. Habitual routines are familiar, comfortable, and usually temporarily successful. However, long-term survival must be the focus. The desire of most leaders to experience stability in their work life makes it difficult for them to admit that the system is not working as well as it could be and that it needs to be revised. Quantum leaders realize that routine practices, standard operating procedures, and traditional protocols seldom meet organizational needs for any extended length of time. Constant tinkering with processes is always necessary to ensure continuous goodness of fit with the environment.

Traditional leaders tend to put a premium on "being right." They want to be seen as a competent, comprehensive resource and thereby win the respect of the employees. In contrast, quantum leaders and their teams must learn to become comfortable with quickly acknowledging the existence of outdated processes, suboptimal choices, and leadership mistakes and to move on regardless of the investment. They must identify current practices that are not working or have become obstacles to providing healthcare services and then tinker with them so they function better. In most cases, these practices should not be looked on as errors but rather as outdated. They simply no longer fit the organization's needs and currently fail to result in the desired outcomes, no matter how effective they were in the past (Ricks, 2012).

The remainder of the chapter consists of a discussion of five leadership errors, associated opportunities for change, and specific strategies for supporting the desired improvements. The purpose here is not to criticize or negate the work of leaders but rather to focus on common problems and stretch creative thinking to support our journey into the Information Age, where error is opportunity. The five errors are as follows:

1. Failure to shift to value-based healthcare services
2. Failure to own healthcare products
3. Fragmented leadership
4. Dehumanization of healthcare providers
5. Demanding the impossible

Error 1: Failure to Shift to Value-Based Healthcare Services

Dramatic changes in health care have occurred over the last 30 years, most notably in the area of reimbursement. Unfortunately, few if any healthcare structures have changed to the extent needed to ensure the delivery of high-quality healthcare services.

Financial resources have become the focus of clinical decision making. Financial officers work diligently to maximize reimbursement and reduce expenses, whereas care providers do their best to deliver the comprehensive care expected by consumers. Many healthcare leaders continue to believe that good financial performance supports clinical quality in the same way as in the past. The role of finance has become so important, in fact, that in many organizations the chief financial officer has a line position and controls processes and operations, whereas the medical director holds a staff position and offers input and suggestions but is impotent to control patient care services. Such changes in authority and decision making, although perhaps not reflected in the organizational chart, are otherwise explicitly recognized.

For many healthcare providers, these role changes interfere with the real work of the organization, and they view healthcare leadership these days as more like dealership. Health plan contract negotiations are based almost solely on actuarial data and the expectation that patients will use the least amount of services available. Further, although recognizing that both productivity and a healthy financial base are essential for survival, care providers find it disconcerting that these are to be achieved at the expense of patient care quality. In short, healthcare organizations have failed to adapt the healthcare system to the changing supply-and-demand factors and marketplace values, and this failure is the source of the incredible chaos being experienced by leaders, care providers, payers, and the public.

Before the advent of prospective payment systems, the issue of value was only a minor one. Expenses were covered by payers interested in increasing the access to healthcare services. Leaders worked to expand the types and numbers of services they offered to keep their organizations competitive. With this model, there is no accountability and no control. Not surprisingly, resources ran out, and the public rebelled against escalating healthcare expenditures. The imperative for leaders continues to be to reconnect the system with the marketplace and reestablish a balance between service (the providing of assistance), quality, and cost.

The separation of marketplace value and clinical outcomes was tolerable when no connection was expected in the marketplace. Consumers received the services provided, and the payers reimbursed providers as billed. Healthcare value in the retrospective payment system was determined by the provider, not by the patient. It is important to note that provider behavior was not intended to diminish the importance of fiscal issues. There was simply no demand for real fiscal accountability. Providers were expected to provide the best of everything. They delivered as many healthcare services as possible. Functional, role, and clinical issues were of central concern, not financial issues. In fact, discussion of financial issues by care providers was considered inappropriate and was discouraged.

Opportunity 1: Practice Within the Marketplace

As they begin the journey of shifting organizational work to support marketplace values, leaders need to keep in mind how health care got to its current state of chaos. The main causal factor is the current imbalance between the types and amount of services being provided and the dollars available for their purchase. In fact, the lack of dollars has created serious instability in the marketplace. In many organizations, changes are being implemented to shift the focus back to the provision of healthcare services within the marketplace parameters. Unfortunately, not all organizations have begun the work of transformation, and some have yet to identify the needed revisions.

Every healthcare leader must critically assess the services his or her organization provides to ensure that they are consistent with the organization's mission. Fixing marketplace errors requires a shift from managing for profit to managing for the organizational mission of delivering value-based health care. The process of fitting care to the available dollars cannot begin without an understanding of the value that is being bartered. Reducing or controlling services without a clear notion of the value each discipline contributes to clinical outcomes is like taking a shot in the dark. At best, it is an example of irresponsible leadership.

What Is Value?

It is not uncommon for leaders to be unsure of the real value of the services provided by healthcare providers in their organizations. Some providers are not sure of this themselves. Evidence must show that resources are being used efficiently to bring about clear improvements in patient conditions, increase the ability of the patients to manage their own health, and add to the patients' knowledge of their conditions and/or healthy behaviors. This is quite different from providing services as defined in a standards manual.

Determining the value of healthcare services is an integral part of quantum leadership. This value, which is defined by means of an equation containing the three elements of cost, quality, and service, is never simply a matter of dollars (Malloch & Porter-O'Grady, 1999). Instead, its calculation takes into account what is actually gained and what are the real costs. The exact equation is expressed thus: healthcare value = resources (funds and labor and supplies) + quality (appropriateness of interventions) + service (satisfaction and effective relationships).

Finding the value of a healthcare service requires healthcare leaders and care providers to ask the following questions:

- What is the actual service provided?
- How do organizational processes support this service?
- What are the interactions between these processes?
- What impact does the service have on the patients and the community?

The answers to these questions guide leaders and healthcare providers toward wise choices—toward clinical decisions that are the most cost-effective and result in the highest quality care being provided at the lowest cost (Pappas, 2013). The challenge for leaders is to reframe the healthcare quality issue as a value question. Again, value is defined as the result of an interactive process involving cost, quality, and service. The cost of health care in the marketplace is determined by both the available resources and reimbursement; the quality of the service is determined by the outcome of the service (i.e., how delivery of the service changes the patient's state of health); and service, which is the rendering of assistance, is partly a function of the time and manner of provision.

Within this framework, the marketplace phenomenon becomes apparent. The value equation is out of balance in that too much care is being provided given the level of available dollars—or too few resources are being applied to health care. The greatest opportunity or leverage point for changing the value equation begins with the element of service, not the cost or quality. If there are limited resources, questions such as this arise: Should the response to every sign or symptom be some type of intervention, particularly if it results in minimal or no improvement in the patient's clinical condition? What an incredibly difficult challenge it is for providers and leaders to deal with the issue of rationing, especially those schooled in the philosophy that increased access to health care is always in the public's interest. Indeed, rationing of healthcare services has traditionally been seen as incongruent with the American spirit. Of course, the reality is that it has occurred throughout history; it is just more obvious when the issue moves beyond the closed ranks of health professionals to the community at large.

The Metrics of Value-Based Health Care

To determine the value of health care, leaders and providers are faced with deciding what should be measured. What are the metrics of success? What constitutes value for the consumer? How are all the metrics interrelated? Current financial management is concerned with statistics such as net income margin, net present value, return on equity, return on investment, and return on assets. These metrics are unfamiliar to clinicians and are very different from the metrics they see as vital, such as responsiveness to treatment, level of pain management, and wound healing.

Traditionally, the financial mind-set has focused on return on investment for dollars spent. This measure has limited applicability in health care. In a return-on-investment analysis, the cost-to-benefit ratio shows the worth of spending dollars to make dollars. If the benefits of a healthcare program or service can be priced in dollars, then a cost-to-benefit analysis is appropriate, and the alternative that leads to the greatest dollar benefits for the cost has a good claim to be chosen. However, many healthcare decisions and services involve far more than simply generating income. In fact, healthcare dollars are often spent on a clinical problem to improve the outcomes of patient care, and ascribing a monetary value to a health outcome is a complex, if not impossible, task. Another issue is that cost-to-benefit analysis is not sensitive to healthcare objectives, including the psychological benefits of improved health, the psychological and physiological benefits of clean air and water, and so on.

Increasingly, healthcare leaders are switching to cost-effectiveness analysis (Buerhaus, 1998). Instead of measuring benefits and costs in dollars, a cost-effectiveness analysis uses units such as years of life saved to measure health outcomes and dollars to measure the cost of the treatment. Although a cost-effectiveness analysis cannot determine whether a single program's benefits outweigh its costs, it can be used to compare alternative programs.

It is nearly impossible to draw conclusions about services on the basis of a single metric. Multiple influencing factors must be considered in reaching decisions on allocating resources. Healthcare leaders are best advised to develop a matrix of metrics in which multiple essential indicators are considered in the evaluation of resource use. Cost-effectiveness should be measured in the aggregate from the multiple perspectives of quality, productivity, and cost and from the patient, care provider, and organization levels. Blending the cultures of finance and health care is challenging at best, but it can be made somewhat more manageable if everyone understands the common ground shared by finance and health professionals—they are all dependent on their checkbooks and their health, neither of which is able to exist effectively without the other.

Eliminating Non-Valued-Added Services

Most healthcare providers assume that every service provided is an essential service and that there are no opportunities for changing service patterns. They believe that if a service did not make a difference to the health of patients—did not add value in terms of increased well-being—they would not be providing it. Yet most providers have not examined each service to determine whether it really does affect the clinical conditions of patients, enhance patients' understanding of their conditions, or increase their ability to manage their own health. In many cases, services are provided to conform to standards but without improving patient outcomes.

Consider a patient who suffers from chronic uncontrolled diabetes. The patient is regularly hospitalized for stabilization and treatment. During each hospitalization, the patient receives diabetic education and attends two information sessions, in accordance with the established standard of care. Despite the instruction, the patient and family have never been able to commit to the required dietary changes, and they do not plan to make any changes. In this case, the diabetic education has failed to make a difference in terms of clinical stability, knowledge of the disease, or ability to manage the patient's health; consequently, it is a non-value-added service. Given the overwhelming workload of the providers, the service should be provided to this patient in an abbreviated form or possibly not at all. The patient medical record should reflect the reality of the situation, namely, that continuing education was considered but not implemented because of the lack of expected clinical effect.

When services that fail to add value are discovered, the leader must support the team in eliminating them, a daunting task at best. Fear of the unknown often overrides the need to change, feeding organizational inertia and reinforcing assumptions that the current way is the right and only way to do the work. Limited resources and concern about short-term costs can further impede progress. The leader's challenge is to create a culture in which all members are expected to continually seek better and more efficient ways of providing services and to eliminate practices that are no longer effective.

Once the leader identifies what actual services are delivered, what outcomes they produce, and what their costs are, the dialogue with managed care organizations changes dramatically. If the managed care organization negotiators want to decrease premiums, the leader can now translate the reduction into a decrease in services. Conversely, the leader can request premium increases to match improvements in patient outcomes. No longer is it expected that services remain the same despite a reduction in available dollars. Further, the amount of negotiating power is determined by the value produced rather than the number of individuals around the table or their negotiating tenacity. Decisions should be made from a consumer value perspective.

Group Discussion

Consider the impact of an organization-wide directive focused on increasing personal and professional accountability. Each clinician is asked to recommend the elimination of two current policies that he or she believes are within the scope of their licensure and professional accountability. Would the value of health care increase or decrease as a result of this approach and expectation? Who might oppose the approach and who might favor it?

Team-Based Health Care

For healthcare services and leadership practices to receive the kind of critical examination that is needed, the leader and the other team members must undergo a renewal of team spirit and show a willingness to challenge the status quo and expose the sacred cows of health care. No provider should decide alone what to do for patients. Engaging in dialogue with each other is the only way providers can ensure their value-based goals are achieved. In addition, dialogue between providers minimizes the potential for system breakdown and error. As collaboration increases, the team becomes more competent in frontline quality management and system repair. It is then able to monitor service value and to act as the agent in monitoring and managing system breakdowns. The quantum leader must create the context in which the necessary communication skills are both valued and expected.

Regardless of past practices, every decision made by a provider should take into account the choices and decisions of others. In practice, providers seldom act as a team in implementing interventions and evaluating care, and each provider delivers the kind of care that those within the provider's discipline believe is best (as indicated by the discipline's established practice standards). To combat unilateral decision making and ensure a good fit between decisions made along the continuum of care, providers and patients must exhibit a strong pattern of communication and interaction.

Error 2: Failure to Own Healthcare Products

The increasing involvement of external agencies in determining appropriate healthcare services sounds an alarm for even the most inexperienced healthcare leader. Regardless of perceived past failures of healthcare organizations to manage internal processes, the return of healthcare oversight and management to the point of service is needed to minimize bureaucracy and support the shift toward using errors as opportunities for improvement rather than punishment.

Perhaps the chaos of the transition from a retrospective payment system to a fixed payment system has blurred the expectations of all stakeholders. The expectation for healthcare systems is that processes are in place to ensure that services are both effective and provided within the marketplace parameters. The oversight of staffing, scheduling, pain management, advance directives, and so on by external agencies interferes with the performance and accountability of the internal leadership, yet the public call for organizations to meet the core responsibilities of error management, safe staffing, and pain management reinforces the notion that healthcare leaders have not previously been held sufficiently accountable.

Besides dealing with unclear expectations and uncertainty, healthcare leaders face intense financial pressures that distort the order of their stewardship obligations, which should be service first, survival second, and profit third. They also often are placed in ethical dilemmas in which the right decision is hard to determine, let alone carry out. As evidence of this, fraud and abuse stories have become all too common in the press. It seems that the prevalence of such stories is partly explained by the fact that leaders are in the position of desperately searching for financial revenues and sometimes choose questionable methods. Of course, not only is fraud, when uncovered, detrimental to the reputation of the organization, but the intense scrutiny that follows its discovery creates an atmosphere of mistrust between care providers, payers, and the government. Yet, although fraud is a criminal matter that must be addressed in the court system, many issues are better managed internally. The challenge for leaders is to determine which issues are best managed internally and which issues must be managed externally.

Opportunity 2: Moving from External Oversight to Internal Accountability

There is a pronounced need for less external regulation and more professional accountability within organizations. The locus of accountability for clinical quality lies within each profession, and the content is defined by its standards. The accountability for an organization's systems, structures, and processes rests with the leaders, and the content is defined by the organization's mission, vision, and values. The control or oversight of the organization's services and leadership rests with the governing board because its members understand the needs and expectations of the community being served much better than any external accrediting agency could. It should not be necessary for business and government agencies to force or direct care providers and organizations to address issues such as the high incidence of medical errors or perform their essential duties as providers of health care.

Living Accountability

Accountability-based health care is an essential foundation for the "error as opportunity" approach recommended in this chapter. To ensure accountability for system processes, expectations for performance must be clearly defined for and shared by all members of the organization, and performance that meets the stated expectations must be recognized and rewarded routinely. In addition, incompetence or failure to live the expected behaviors must be dealt with in a timely manner. All too often leaders ignore incompetence because they want to avoid confrontation. Hoping that the problem simply disappears is unrealistic and damaging to the morale of the organization, for it has the effect of lowering the performance standards. Quantum leaders are competent not only at managing incompetence but also at coaching other team members in managing incompetence. They know that managing incompetence is strongly associated with improved organizational performance and increased employee morale as well as decreased errors.

Political Competence

Developing political skills is essential for all members of the quantum organization. In the past, healthcare leaders have played a role in devising and implementing health-related policies at the local, state, and national levels, but as organizations increase the extent of their team-based activities, political competence is a requirement for all employees involved in providing services.

Political competence is defined by Longest (1998) as the dual capacity to accurately assess the impact of public policies on one's area of responsibility and to influence public policy making at both the state and local levels. For each healthcare service offered by an organization, the organization's leaders must understand the service and try to determine the expected impact of public policies and the policies of accrediting organizations and health plans on the service. Further, each member of the organization must understand

Group Discussion

Healthcare providers are under pressure to discharge patients according to protocols and guidelines. When patients fall outside the guidelines, the providers must advocate for lengthier stays with insurance companies and, when their requests are denied, are put in the untenable position of discharging patients under unsafe conditions. As leader of the surgical unit, you believe patients are often being discharged prematurely, especially patients who are unsteady and not voiding well. In this situation what is your obligation as leader? What information should you be communicating, and when and to whom should you be communicating it? What changes in practice are recommended? What rationale for these changes is likely to garner the most support?

the internal policies that apply to the provision of services and know when to communicate concerns to the organization's leaders, when to use positional power to exert influence on policymakers, and when to remove or mitigate barriers to care to ensure that the services are provided.

Politically competent healthcare providers are also able to assist regulators and legislators in creating solutions and to describe the clinical and economic value of healthcare services to patients, purchasers, and policy analysts. Organizational policies and procedures are designed to incorporate professional standards, define expectations, and enhance service quality. When policies exist that are inconsistent with standards, contradict expectations, or impede service quality, politically competent providers can communicate the issues of concern and facilitate the revision of the policies.

Error 3: Fragmented Leadership

Traditional healthcare organizations rely on clinical professionals to deliver the services defined by the mission, and they rely on management professionals to make the service processes more efficient and effective. Given that the clinical and management professions have different knowledge bases and values, clinicians and managers are sometimes at odds with each other. However, their differences have become increasingly problematic for the delivery of healthcare services as the environment has been affected by burdensome new payer constraints, increasing competition for a larger share of diminishing resources, and a lack of qualified healthcare workers. Indeed, the internal competition between clinicians and managers has negatively affected productivity and, more important, discouraged innovation.

Because of the ongoing financial pressure and competition experienced by healthcare organizations, patient care often loses out to financial priorities. In fact, left with few opportunities for reducing expenses, healthcare leaders often end up searching for ways of managing the demand for healthcare services rather than managing expenses.

Most healthcare leaders are experts on healthcare infrastructure and marketplace principles. Very few are experts on clinical care and marketplace principles. As a result, many organizations are struggling because their leaders do not have clinical competence and are making decisions solely from a financial perspective. No longer can healthcare organizations afford leaders incapable of integrating patient care needs and financial survival.

Opportunity 3: Holographic Leadership

The strategy of minimizing competition between financial and clinical priorities and increasing collaboration demands a new model of healthcare leadership. Leaders in quantum healthcare organizations need to be competent and knowledgeable in both health care and marketplace management. The position of chief executive or patient care administrator should be occupied by someone who has advanced clinical training (e.g., a physician, nurse, social worker, or physical therapist) and has expertise in the management of these clinical services. The chief executive's knowledge base should include an understanding of how services are provided, what their outcomes are, how to estimate costs, and how to determine the availability of reimbursement. A background in the business end of health care is not by itself sufficient for leading a twenty-first-century healthcare organization, and neither is experience as a clinical provider.

As the healthcare environment changes, so too does the set of critical leadership competencies. The new competencies reflect an integrated or holographic perspective on the healthcare experience that encompasses the technical, relational, and intentional aspects of patient care. The quantum healthcare leader must have a clear understanding of the procedural work of providers and must possess the skills to connect providers to the service and system infrastructure in such a way as to ensure value-based care is delivered within the limits of the available resources. Health care provided without a specific intention or without effective relationships between providers is fragmented care, and fragmented care is no longer acceptable or affordable.

Necessarily, all operational or line positions in health care require knowledge, skills, and abilities that jointly reflect a holographic healthcare perspective. Operational positions are held by healthcare employees accountable for ensuring that the value equation is balanced. Staff positions are those positions that support the work of the organization but do not require clinical competence. In many ways, this model should suit those who were in traditional staff positions but were pushed into operational roles without being

Group Discussion

Imagine a healthcare organization in which the leaders were competent in both clinical and management disciplines. Speculate on how the organization would be structured. What roles would be added or eliminated? Would the patient care outcomes likely be different? In what way? Would job satisfaction be affected? Summarize the advantages and disadvantages of this model.

given adequate training. Such professionals (e.g., finance officers) are now expected to do what they do best without the additional burden of making decisions in areas in which they lack expertise. Experts in planning, human resources, and finance are ideally suited for staff or consultant positions, and together they can participate as team members in a shared leadership team model.

Leaders at the beginning of the new millennium must determine the most effective and efficient processes to achieve the three goals of high-quality patient care, organizational viability, and respectable profits. Given that healthcare economists focus on the supply and demand for services, reimbursement mechanisms, productivity, the impact of technology, workforce issues, market dynamics, and health-related public policy, it is incumbent upon care providers to provide a clear description of the healthcare services and their outcomes, the time and skill level requirements for each service, and the cost of providing each service so that the economists can analyze the aforementioned factors and their relationships accurately.

Error 4: Dehumanization of Healthcare Providers

The financial pressure experienced by healthcare organizations not only has affected the type and number of services afforded patients but also has altered the way organizational leaders are managing healthcare providers. In some cases the providers perceive their treatment as uncaring and ruthless and see themselves as pawns. As evidence, providers can point to regular rounds of staff reductions, staffing by ratios, elimination of continuing education programs, and the use of hiring bonuses.

Workforce Reductions

The elimination of leadership and care provider positions with little or no warning has seriously marred the morale of the healthcare workforce. Competent leaders and care providers are finding it increasingly difficult to rebound and find new employment. Regardless of how the termination is handled, they find it nearly impossible to live with the notion that "it's not personal, it's business" when their livelihood has been dramatically altered.

The hidden costs that result from the disruption of relationships in the workplace have yet to be measured. One hidden cost is the loss of departing employees' knowledge of the job and the other workers and the organization. Another is the reduction in needed

Group Discussion

Some leaders focus on processes alone, others on outcomes alone, still others on both processes and outcomes. What are the consequences for the organization when the leader is process oriented? When the leader is outcome oriented? When the leader is both process and outcome oriented? Compare the differing effects of the three approaches. What are the advantages and disadvantages of each? Which approach fits best with holographic leadership?

competence and experience, which, if severe enough, can lead to a phenomenon known as failure to rescue (described later). Further, because length of employment usually determines who gets let go, newly hired employees with up-to-date skills and knowledge are eliminated in favor of employees who have minimal or outdated competencies.

To understand the harm that can occur from workforce reductions, consider the critical surveillance role played by nurses. Indeed, their vigilance is essential to rescuing many patients who have experienced a complication. In such a situation nurses must first recognize that a complication has occurred or is impending, and then they must intervene rapidly to ensure the patient's survival. When nurse staffing levels are reduced, the ability of the nurses on the floor to recognize a potential or an actual problem is compromised, sometimes to the extent that they fail to save a patient who might otherwise have survived.

Another common effect of decreasing the number of competent registered nurses is the implementation of mandatory overtime. In fact, more than 70% of hospitals in the United States have formal mandatory overtime requirements. Making healthcare providers put in extra hours can push them beyond their physical limits and reduce their ability to perform competently. Tired and overworked care providers are poorly suited for the level of clinical surveillance required for quality patient care.

Finally, in addition to reductions in the absolute number of nurses employed, licensed personnel are being replaced with unlicensed care providers, thereby diluting the skill mix. As a cost-saving measure, the shift to employing fewer licensed care providers has not been particularly successful. Not only do the overall number of hours of care increase when the licensed hours are decreased, but the level of surveillance also declines dramatically. There is no substitute for having a reasonable number of highly trained nurses provide care to the patients.

Staffing by Ratios

Staffing levels are closely tied to the incidence of medical errors. The potential of inappropriate staffing to cause an increase in the number of medical errors is generally recognized but not always taken into account in an organization's decision making. There is little evidence to use in determining the necessary level of staffing to ensure that the quality of patient care is maintained, organizational goals are met, and the providers' working conditions are acceptable. Studies intended to assess the effects of different ratios of patients to registered nurses are numerous and conflicting. Thus, historical averages of hours of care provided for each patient are typically used as the basis of daily staffing.

The problem is that this technique wrongly assumes that the needs of all patients are essentially the same and, more important, that the skills of nurses are comparable. Instead, patient needs vary widely, as do levels of nursing competence. Indeed, if a historically based ratio is used, such as four patients to one nurse, the chance of a match between patient care needs and on-the-job personnel is low. For example, on some days the correct ratio for meeting patient needs adequately might be three to one, whereas on other days it might be five to one. Frustration increases for both patients and providers when there is no adjustment in staffing, up or down, to meet the identified needs.

Evidence-based staffing confronts leaders with two challenges. First, although providers often dislike ratio staffing, they have difficulty when assignment ratios vary among colleagues. For example, nurses expect to be given reasonable workloads, but even when patient acuity is lower than average, they still resist accepting an assignment with a higher than average patient-to-nurse ratio. Getting nurses to understand and accept assignments based on workload instead of numbers is a challenge for leaders—and an opportunity.

The second challenge is to determine which healthcare interventions contribute to meeting patient care needs and how effective they are. The main problem is that the nature and types of interventions vary widely from organization to organization and from provider to provider. Valid and reliable information that demonstrates the value of each provider's contribution is sorely needed because it improves the dialogue between care providers and leaders and helps them find meaningful solutions to managing the workload.

Developmental Freeze

Equally demoralizing for providers is the inconsistency of leadership support for continuing education aimed at giving them skills they need to function effectively in the changing marketplace. Elimination of funding for continuing education programs, both internal and external, commonly occurs when resources become strained. The strategy of requiring employees to attend seminars on vacation time at personal expense and limiting out-of-state travel reimbursement sends a strong negative message as to the value of continuous learning to the organization.

In addition, these restrictions increase the probability of failure-to-rescue incidents and other crises. The unavoidable breakdowns that occur in providing patient care and in the organization's systems require quick responses to prevent the breakdowns from developing into full-blown catastrophes. Most educational programs focus on giving providers the knowledge and skills they require to meet current standards of practice, but few offer learning opportunities that would allow providers to develop the proper skills for responding to imminent breakdowns. As the environment changes, so do the skills and interventions needed to manage developing crises, and continuous learning is a requisite for gaining the competence to address the kind of breakdowns that are likely to occur in the present.

Hiring Bonuses

In desperation, leaders sometimes use economic enticements to recruit needed healthcare providers. The practice of offering sign-on bonuses is based on two assumptions—that individuals usually act in ways they believe will make them better off and that individuals generally believe better off means more money. The reality is that each person has his or her own preference map and that dangling cash before healthcare providers does not always induce the desired behaviors. Besides money, providers want respect, involvement in decision making, and good relationships with colleagues, among other things. The bonus model, by treating providers as shallow and materialistic, has the effect of disparaging them. Some providers, of course, respond to the enticement of a financial bonus in given situations, but most are motivated by a combination of social, emotional, and material needs, not just led by the dollar.

Sign-on bonuses also send the wrong message to existing staff, especially long-time employees, who likely feel resentment because they have not gotten bonuses for their loyalty. Sign-on bonuses therefore tend to reduce employee morale and create a revolving door, which can seriously affect patient care. Further, there is no way the sign-on bonuses can neutralize the cost of turnover, which is between $5,000 and $50,000 per nurse. The assumption of sign-on bonuses is that healthcare providers are for sale to the highest bidder and are willing to go across the street for dollars. They thus cause competition among healthcare organizations as well.

Opportunity 4: Revaluing Healthcare Providers as Vital Capital

The healthcare marketplace can hardly support guarantees of lifetime employment for anyone. Yet there are other options besides discarding employees whenever the marketplace demands change. In fact, some of these options, by respecting the dignity of the individual and encouraging creativity and innovation, are more likely to improve an organization's long-term performance than are cyclical episodes of mass layoffs. The challenge for leaders is to make hiring and firing decisions from a broad perspective that takes into account multiple performance indicators, not merely the monthly cash flow or short-term costs. In particular, these decisions should be based on a full consideration of the effects of staff reductions and restructuring on patient care outcomes and on the ability of care providers to provide healthcare services efficiently and effectively.

Given the increasing documentation that experienced and credentialed employees have a positive impact on patient outcomes, other approaches to managing the workforce are indicated. The first step is to shift to a type of evidence-based decision making that considers not only financial indicators but also the intellectual capital profile of the employees. The second step is to look at both short- and long-term effects of resource decisions. **Exhibit 9-8** contains a list of studies that show the impact of staffing on patient outcomes and healthcare provider satisfaction.

Evidence-Based Staffing

Effective staffing is a matter not just of numbers but of mix. It requires developing new and creative strategies to manage the combination of predictable and unpredictable workloads and the availability and supply of experienced and competent healthcare providers. Given that at least 80% of the healthcare workload is predictable and repeatable, one challenge is to develop a workforce suitable for this portion of the workload. Core staffing must meet the identified range of care needs on a shift-by-shift and day-to-day basis. The second challenge is to handle the remaining 20% of the workload—the unpredictable portion. Because the services needed are unpredictable, it is futile to attempt to plan for and manage this portion. People generally do not call ahead and schedule trauma, deliveries, and medical emergencies with any sensitivity to the time of day or the availability of care providers. The goal therefore is to build enough flexibility into the staffing to ensure appropriate care providers are on hand to respond quickly to an unscheduled event. Meeting these two challenges requires two very different philosophies regarding staff availability and compensation.

Exhibit 9-8   Nurse Staffing and Patient Outcomes: Selected References

Aiken, L., Clarke, S. P., Cheuny, R. B., Sloane, D. M., & Silber, J. H. (2003). Education levels of hospital nurses and patient mortality. *Journal of the American Medical Association, 290,* 12.

Aiken, L., Clarke, S. P., Sloane, D. M., Sochalsi, J., & Silber, J. H. (2002). Hospital nurse staffing and patient mortality, nurse burnout, and job dissatisfaction. *Journal of the American Medical Association, 288,* 1987–1993.

Allen, S., Fiorini, P., & Dickey, M. (2010). A streamlined clinical advancement program improves RN participation and retention. *Journal of Nursing Administration, 40*(7/8), 316–322.

American Nurses Association. (2012). *Principles for nurse staffing.* Silver Spring, MD: Author.

Bae, S. (2012). Nursing overtime: Why, how much, and under what working conditions. *Nursing Economic$, 30*(2), 60–71.

Behner, K. G., Fogg, L. F., Fournier, L. C., Frankenbach, J. T., & Robertson, S. B. (1990). Nursing resource management: Analyzing the relationship between costs and quality in staffing decisions. *Health Care Management Review, 15*(4), 63–71.

Blegen, M., Goode, C., & Reed, L. (1998). Nurse staffing and patient outcomes. *Nursing Research, 47*(1), 43–50.

Blegen, M., Goode, C., Spetz, J., Vaughn, T., & Park, S. (2011). Nurse staffing effects on patient outcomes: Safety-net and non-safety-net hospital. *Medical Care, 49*(4), 406–414.

Boev, C. (2012). The relationship between nurses' perception of work environment and patient satisfaction in adult critical care. *Journal of Nursing Scholarship, 44*(4), 368–375.

Bolton, L. B., Jones, D., Aydin, C., Donaldson, N., Brown, D. S., Lowe, M., . . . Harms, D. (2001). A response to California's mandated nursing ratios. *Journal of Nursing Scholarship, 33,* 179–184.

Buerhaus, P. (2010). What is the harm in imposing mandatory hospital nurse staffing regulations? *and* It's time to stop the regulation of hospital nurse staffing dead in its tracks. *Nursing Economic$, 28*(2), 87–93, 110–113.

Buerhaus, P. I., Staiger, D. O., & Auerbach, D. I. (2009). *The future of the nursing workforce in the United States.* Sudbury, MA: Jones and Bartlett.

Buffington, A., Zwink, J., & Fink, R. (2012). Factors affecting nurse retention at an academic Magnet hospital. *Journal of Nursing Administration, 42*(5), 273–281.

Cairns, L., Hoffmann, R., Dudjak, L., & Lorenz, H. (2013). Utilizing bedside shift report to improve the effectiveness of shift handoff. *Journal of Nursing Administration, 43*(4), 160–165.

Carlson, S. (2013). Make it a habit: 2 weeks to bedside report. *Nursing Management, 44*(3), 554.

Cathro, H. (2013). A practical guide to making patient assignments in acute care. *Journal of Nursing Administration, 43*(1), 6–9.

Cho, S. K., Ketefian, S., Barkauskas, V. H., & Smith, D. G. (2003). The effects of nurse staffing on adverse events, morbidity, mortality and medical costs. *Nursing Research, 52*(2), 71–79.

Cimiotti, J., Haas, J., Saiman, L., & Larson, E. (2006). Impact of staffing on bloodstream infections in the neonatal intensive care unit. *Archives of Pediatric & Adolescent Medicine, 160*(8), 832–836.

Clancy, T., in Fitzpatrick, T., & Brooks, B. (2010). The nurse leader as logistician: Optimizing human capital. *Journal of Nursing Administration, 40*(2), 69–74.

(Continued)

Exhibit 9-8   Continued

Clarke, S., & Donaldson, N. (2007). Nurse staffing and patient care quality and safety. In R. G. Hughes (Ed.), *Patient safety and quality: An evidence-based handbook for nurses* (AHRQ Publication No. 07-0015). Rockville, MD: Agency for Healthcare Research and Quality.

Coffman, J. M., Seago, J. A., & Spetz, J. (2002). Minimum nurse-to-patient ratios in acute care hospitals in California. *Health Affairs, 21*(5), 53–63.

Cornell, P., & Riordan, M. (2011). Barriers to critical thinking: Workflow interruptions and task switching among nurses. *Journal of Nursing Administration, 41*(10), 407–414.

Demir, D., & Rodwell, J. (2012). Psychosocial antecedents and consequences of workplace aggression for hospital nurses. *Journal of Nursing Scholarship, 44*(4), 376–384.

DesRoches, C., Miralles, P., Buerhaus, P., Hess, R., & Donelan, K. (2011). Health information technology in the workplace: Findings from a 2010 national survey of registered nurses. *The Journal of Nursing Administration, 41*(9), 357–364.

Eastabrooks, C. A., Midodzi, W. K., Cummings, G. G., Ricker, K. L., & Giovannetti, P. (2005). The impact of hospital nursing characteristics on 30-day mortality. *Nursing Research, 54*(2), 74–84.

Eggenberger, T. (2012). Exploring the charge nurse role: Holding the frontline. *Journal of Nursing Administration, 42*(11), 502–506.

Friese, C., & Himes-Ferris, L. (2013). Nursing practice environments and job outcomes in ambulatory oncology settings. *Journal of Nursing Administration, 43*(3), 149–154.

Frith, K., Anderson, E., Tseng, F., & Fong, E. (2012). Nurse staffing is an important strategy to prevent medication errors in community hospitals. *Nursing Economic$, 30*(5), 288–294.

Good, E., & Bishop, P. (2011). Willing to walk: A creative strategy to minimize stress related to floating. *Journal of Nursing Administration, 41*(5), 231–234.

Gran-Moravec, M. B., & Hughes, C. M. (2005). Nursing time allocation and other considerations for staffing. *Nursing and Health Sciences, 7,* 126–133.

Hall, L., Peterson, J., Lalonde, M., Cripps, L., & Dales, L. (2011). Strategies for retaining midcareer nurses. *Journal of Nursing Administration, 41*(12), 531–537.

Hamilton, K. E., Redshaw, M. N. E., & Tarnow-Mordi, W. (2007). Nurse staffing in relation to risk-adjusted mortality in neonatal care. *Archives of Disease in Childhood. Fetal and Neonatal Edition, 92*(2), F99–F103.

Hardin, D. (2012). Strategies for nurse leaders to address aggressive and violent events. *Journal of Nursing Administration, 42*(1), 5–8.

Harper, E. (2012). Staffing based on evidence: Can health information technology make it possible? *Nursing Economic$, 30*(5), 262–267.

Hickey, P., Gauvreau, K., & Connor, J. (2010). The relationship of nurse staffing, skill mix, and Magnet recognition to institutional volume and mortality for congenital heart surgery. *Journal of Nursing Administration, 40*(5), 226–232.

Institute of Medicine. (2010). *The future of nursing: Leading change, advancing health.* Washington, DC: National Academies Press.

Exhibit 9-8   Continued

Kalisch, B., & Lee, K. (2012). Congruence of perceptions among nursing leaders and staff regarding missed nursing care and teamwork. *Journal of Nursing Administration, 42*(10), 473–477.

Needleman, J., Buerhaus, P., Mattke, S., Stewart, M., & Zelevinky, K. (2002). Nurse staffing in hospitals: Is there a business case for quality? *Health Affairs, 25*(1), 204–211.

Pappas, S. H. (2013). Value, a nursing outcome. *Nursing Administration Quarterly, 37*(2), 122–128.

Patrician, P., Loan, L., McCarthy, M., Fridman, M., Donaldson, N., Bingham, M., & Brosch, L. (2011). The association of shift-level nurse staffing with adverse patient events. *Journal of Nursing Administration, 41*(2), 64–70.

Prestia, A., & Dyess, S. (2012). Maximizing caring relationships between nursing assistants and patients: Care partners. *Journal of Nursing Administration, 42*(30), 144–147.

Salin, S., Kaunonen, M., & Aalto, P. (2012). Explaining patient satisfaction with outpatient care using data based nurse staffing indicators. *Journal of Nursing Administration, 42*(12), 592–597.

Trepanier, S., Early, S., Ulrich, B., & Cherry, B. (2012). New graduate nurse residency program: A cost-benefit analysis based on turnover the contract labor usage. *Nursing Economic$, 30*(4), 207–214.

Unruh, L. (2003). Licensed nurse staffing and adverse events in hospitals. *Medical Care, 1*(1), 142–152.

Unruh, L., & Fottler, M. (2006). Patient turnover and nursing staff adequacy. *Health Services Research, 41,* 599–612.

U.S. Department of Health and Human Services. Nurse staffing and patient outcomes in hospitals. Retrieved from http://www.ahrq.gov/research/findings/factsheets/services/nursestaffing/index.html

To regain the respect and support of employees, leaders must learn to manage employees continuously and in real time rather than implement regular rounds of layoffs. On the other hand, employees have a corresponding obligation to ensure that their skills and abilities are appropriate to the needs of the organization. When there is a gap between the organization's needs and what the employees are able to offer, change is indicated. How this change is managed is crucial for the organization. Leaders and employees must enter into a dialogue to reach a clear understanding of the organization's responsibility to support employee skill enhancement and the employees' responsibility to obtain the desired skills. Regardless, group layoffs that come as a "surprise" serve no useful purpose in the long term. Early collaborative dialogue between employees and leaders on how to respond to changing needs leads to a more stable workforce and greater employee satisfaction.

Staffing for Patient Needs

Attempts to devise accepted national standards for nurse-to-patient ratios have yet to produce meaningful recommendations, and with good reason: Facility case mix indices, reimbursement plans, and available support services vary widely. Further, the standards would set average numbers for meeting patient care needs, and these needs, by virtue of

Group Discussion

In many organizations, when staff reductions are needed, those with least seniority are eliminated rather than those with greater seniority. Seldom is consideration given to the specific skills and credentials of those who are let go. Review the following research data and create a plan to manage the next round of staff reductions in your organization.

- Compared with other healthcare providers, certified nurses report fewer adverse events, have higher patient satisfaction ratings, and are more effective communicators and collaborators with other providers.
- An extra hour of nursing care is related to fewer urinary tract infections, a decrease in pneumonia, and a decrease in the probability of postoperative blood clots.
- As the number of medical residents, registered nurses, registered pharmacists, medical technologists, and total hospital personnel per occupied bed increases, mortality rates decrease.

Should the plan take into account employee longevity? If so, how? What effects on patient outcomes should the new model be expected to have? Who will support the new model and who will oppose it?

their unpredictability, cannot be met by using average numbers for daily staffing. In most organizations, daily patient needs vary at least 20% above and below the average, and it is possible that at no time do the actual needs exactly equal the average. In fact, using average numbers in planning the daily staffing discounts the range of nursing activities that are needed to respond to different case mixes.

Revising the nurse-to-patient ratio daily is essential for minimizing discrepancies between patient needs and provider capacities. In some organizations, valid and reliable patient classification systems have been used to determine patient care needs on a shift-by-shift basis. The information gathered becomes the basis for daily staffing and long-term scheduling. Once a representative sample of patient care needs that reflect the full range of needs is determined, the average nurse-to-patient ratios can be calculated. These ratios serve as standards, although they can become problematic when used for shift-to-shift staffing because they are not sensitive to fluctuations in patient needs, technology, and procedures required.

In determining daily patient care needs and the proper number and mix of providers, leaders need to consider the dynamic interaction of the economic factors, technology, and labor availability. The greatest hope for developing valid standards lies in understanding the interrelationships of nurse-to-patient ratios and patient needs (acuity).

Shared Accountability for Learning

Healthcare providers have an interest in continuing to acquire more knowledge and develop new skills throughout their career life, and the organizations that employ them share this interest. In fact, investing in their employees is a way for organizations to invest in the future, and therefore it makes sense for any organization to create programs that recognize the continuing education efforts of its providers. The providers, on the other hand, should be willing to make a commitment to continue working for the organization as a quid pro quo. It is not unreasonable for an organization to expect a promise of 5 years of employment in return for tuition support for a higher education degree. Similarly, if an organization compensates an employee for attending a conference or pays the registration fees, the employee should be expected to share new information with the healthcare team. The terms of any agreement must be determined before the investment.

In cases where employees pay for their own continuing education and show improvement in their performance because of their educational efforts, they can rightly expect the organization to recognize their increased ability through some form of compensation, such as an increase in salary. Employees should not suppose the organization will reward educational efforts that fail to affect their performance.

Error 5: Demanding the Impossible

Healthcare provider assignments are increasingly complex and sometimes overwhelming. Indeed, feasible assignments are the exception rather than the norm. Providers, nurses in particular, frequently are demoralized by being asked to do more than they are capable of, and for many the gap between what is being requested and what is possible has grown wider.

The limitations and inflexibility of current staffing and scheduling systems, coupled with the pressure to minimize costs, have prevented leaders from adequately supporting providers who have been given arduous assignments. At best, these providers receive encouragement and sympathy; at worst, they are berated for their inability to manage the workload. Although not the intent of leaders, the result is that employees feel abandoned and mistreated, they seek assistance outside of the organization, and the relationship between the employees and leaders becomes increasingly adversarial.

It is disconcerting for the profession and the community at large to observe providers who believe themselves abandoned by the leaders of the organizations for which they work. Exhortations to do one's best are no longer able to counter the professional discouragement felt by providers. As a result some providers have become openly critical of the health professions, discouraging others from joining or even leaving themselves for another.

Opportunity 5: Managing the Needs–Resources Gap as a Team

Even using the most reliable and valid patient classification systems, leaders rarely match actual patient care needs and staff resources, including hours of staff time. Because some gap between needs and resources is almost inevitable, the challenge for leaders is to create effective systems for managing the gap.

Providers and consumers must engage in a dialogue to identify more precisely clinical care needs, desired outcomes of services, and available resources. In addition, if they discover a gap between needs and resources, they must reevaluate these. Attempting to provide all services regardless of the available resources, as has been the practice in the past, is irresponsible.

Much of the difficulty in identifying and managing the needs–resources gap stems from the failure of society to decide whether health care is a right or a privilege. Until society reaches a verdict on this issue, confusion will reign. As clearly as can be determined, health care is a cross between a right and a privilege—a right when you fit the parameters of the government and a privilege when there is limited access and nonemergency services are involved.

Several strategies offer help in minimizing the gap between healthcare needs and staff resources:

- Ensure that the system used to estimate patient care needs is valid and reliable.
- Eliminate non-valued-added services. After carefully examining all services to determine how they affect outcomes, eliminate those that generally fail to have a positive effect.
- Delay noncritical functions until staff resources are available. Some interventions, to be effective, depend on the delivery of services at precise times. Other interventions are not time sensitive and can be delayed without compromising the overall treatment. Most medications cannot be delayed, but daily treatments can be moved to the next shift.
- Reexamine previous efforts to call in additional care providers, and move staff from unit to unit to uncover opportunities for putting personnel to better use.

Currently, the responsibility of managing the needs–resources gap is placed on individual providers, increasing their feelings of abandonment. Further, providers are often expected to administer decisions made elsewhere and on the basis of economic factors—decisions that frequently put patients and families at risk. The preceding strategies can be used by individual providers to the best of their ability. The most common strategy is to eliminate or delay services, and each provider uses his or her personal criteria in deciding whether to use them because open discussion of the associated issues has been discouraged. Failure of providers to manage their assignments is generally viewed as a sign of incompetence rather than as a sign of system overload. The challenge faced by healthcare leaders is to shift management of the needs–resources gap from the individual to the healthcare team—and ultimately to the community, if need be. Accountability for managing the gap must be elevated to the collective level so that healthcare providers, healthcare leaders, and the community can work together to find solutions.

Group Discussion

Consider a situation in which a unit is short two nurses. Using the principles of variance management, develop a plan to address the gap. Answer the following questions: When should the discussion about the gap occur? Who should be present? Identify the strategies that will be used (e.g., eliminate non-emergency-related work, request nurses to work overtime, stop admissions). How will the actions taken be documented? What future discussion will occur to avoid the same situation or to prepare for managing a similar situation?

Conclusion

It is not errors that are the problem but how we respond to errors when we forget that errors are natural—natural as long as there is any shred of humanness present. By keeping in mind that errors are natural, we are more likely to recognize that errors, besides causing inconvenience or hardship, offer opportunities for improvement. Unfortunately, most leaders view errors as solely harmful and believe it is their responsibility to discipline those who commit them. They therefore look for someone to blame and possibly punish, and this is the problem. The punitive approach to error management encourages secrecy and discourages analysis of the situation and development of strategies to avoid repeat errors.

Any changes to the current system have the potential to threaten the established power base of leaders. The structure of power and the organizational culture often bias the perspectives of those who benefit from the existing system. Alterations in the organization's structure and the roles of its members may increase the power of some members and reduce the power of others. Some resist reward systems or metrics that diminish their status and authority within the organization. Nevertheless, shifting from a culture of blame to an open culture in which error is perceived as an opportunity for improvement requires leaders to reconsider how power is perceived and used in the organization. Punitive power becomes passé and intolerable, whereas the power of dialogue emerges as the propulsive force driving the organization toward success.

Managing errors as opportunities and improving our services without debasing our values and subverting our commitment to public safety remain important challenges. The presentation of the five leadership errors discussed in this chapter is intended to heighten readers' awareness that many long-held practices may no longer be effective. The opportunities discussed are just a few of the many available to creative healthcare leaders—opportunities waiting only for discovery and testing. One of the opportunities that is currently prevalent, the opportunity to reframe the work of health care using a value-based model, can only serve to enhance a system in which partnerships among patients, families, and providers work to empower the patients to manage their own health.

Finally, even when things are going wrong and mistakes abound, trust in your journey and look for the lesson to be learned. Find the gift in the goof!

Case Study 9-1

So, What Is Really Broken Here?

Central Valley Hospital is a well-respected community hospital that provides a comprehensive array of medical and surgical services and maternal newborn services. The hospital has been recognized with Planetree and Magnet designations and is viewed in the community as one of the top hospitals for excellent services. Employees generally view the culture of the hospital as very positive, and management has prescribed to a multifocal strategy to enhance employee, physician, and patient satisfaction. The mission statement, values, and behavioral standards are posted openly where they can be seen by all, and every employee's performance expectations and performance appraisal include an evaluation of how that person lives the expected values and behavioral standards. The values include integrity, trust, honesty, professionalism, patient centeredness, and excellence.

Central Valley has an active Quality department that reviews all patient and organizational outcomes and meets with department leaders to discuss ways of continually improving outcomes. There is significant emphasis on "excellence," and managers at all levels of the organization are evaluated on their ability not only to meet financial budget targets, but also to meet various quality indicators and national benchmarks.

Reyna is a manager in a 32-bed general medical unit, and she has approximately 150 part-time and full-time employees who report to her. Reyna reports to the vice president of medical surgical services, who in turn reports to the chief nursing officer (CNO). Reyna has a bachelor of science degree in nursing and is currently in her second year of the graduate program in nursing with an emphasis on nursing administration. She has enjoyed her classes on leadership theories and their application in the healthcare setting, financial management, quality and program evaluation, and a practicum that focused on just culture, patient safety, and quality improvement using tools such as Lean and Six Sigma. Reyna tries to apply much of what she learns in the school setting to her daily work.

Every year Central Valley disseminates the results of the employee opinion, physician satisfaction, and patient satisfaction surveys to the management team. Feedback regarding the national benchmarking quality indicators such as NDNQI and CalNOC data is shared with the nursing management team. Reyna and her nurse manager colleagues appreciate the openness of the organization in sharing the results with them, but talking among themselves they realize how much stress is created when they receive results that do not meet expected standards. Reyna is faced with a decline in scores on the patient satisfaction, employee satisfaction, and culture of safety surveys. She attributes the decline of patient satisfaction to recent changes in the dietary department that have resulted in delays in tray delivery and a remodeling project on the unit that has created unexpected noise during the day.

She has also evaluated potential causes of the decline in employee satisfaction and identified a trend that has occurred annually with lower employee satisfaction scores during the months of July through October. During these months, the patient census and average patient acuity are higher than all other months in the year. Reyna does all possible to ensure adequate staffing and ensures that she is visible and available to the staff more than usual during these times. She is surprised to see the decline in the culture of safety scores, and she begins to investigate potential reasons for the decline by talking with the staff to get their perspective on why they scored specific items so low. Reyna feels that she is held accountable for scores without being in control of all of the factors that cause staff and patients to score the surveys so low.

At a recent nursing leadership meeting, the directors announced that all managers who did not meet the targeted levels on the patient satisfaction, physician satisfaction, employee opinion survey, and the culture of safety survey must prepare a report outlining their strategy to correct the problems and ensure that the next survey demonstrates an improvement.

In her meeting with the director, the director is even more critical about Reyna's performance as a nurse manager in allowing these declines to occur. She tells Reyna that her performance is under scrutiny and that there needs to be corrective action taken immediately to improve the scores; Reyna must demonstrate changes immediately on the unit to improve the situation. Needless to say, Reyna feels completely deflated at the end of the meeting and feels unfairly blamed and unsupported by her director. When she reflects back on her classes on just culture and leadership, she questions her director's approach with her. She feels that her director should do more to support her and give her encouragement and direction in improving the survey scores and in changing the potential causes of the problems that contribute to the dissatisfaction of staff and patients. When she discusses the situation with her colleagues, those that report to her same director experience the same concerns. Other managers with different directors indicate that their directors partner with them in identifying methods to continually improve scores on all quality indicators.

When Reyna reviews the items on the various surveys with her staff, she discovers that the staff do not have a clear understanding of the meaning of some of the questions. After discussing some of the items on both the employee opinion survey and the culture of safety survey, the staff inform her that they would have scored the items differently if they understood the meaning of the items. She begins to wonder whether patients felt the same way about their patient satisfaction survey or their overall satisfaction rate was unfairly weighted with their discontent with the noise factor and the late meal trays as contrasted to their overall level of satisfaction with their nursing care.

Reyna feels more frustrated than ever being held accountable for survey scores that contained items that are not in her control to change and improve. She also is frustrated with the attitude of her director, who seems to blame her for the scores and offers no insight or assistance in resolving the underlying problems that are reflected in the survey scores. Reyna feels powerless and victimized in the situation. As she prepares her report to submit strategies for improving the scores, she includes the discussions with her staff about their interpretation of the wording on some of the items and outlines how she and her staff would partner in improving the workplace environment to ultimately improve the survey scores. Reyna also includes the plans that she and her staff had developed together to enhance patient satisfaction. Reyna had met with the manager of the Dietary department to negotiate a solution to prevent late tray delivery, which she believes is a major contributor to patient dissatisfaction. Despite her report and strategies to improve survey scores, Reyna dreads meeting with her director and feels that she could not trust her to evaluate her fairly or to manage her up to the CNO or other executives in the hospital. Reyna believes that her director is neither living the values of the hospital nor demonstrating the principles of just culture in blaming the managers rather than partnering with them to correct situations that contribute to lower survey scores.

Questions

1. How do you feel that the director's actions influenced the culture of her department and her nurse managers' work performance?
2. If blame should be placed for the low survey scores on the patient satisfaction survey, the employee opinion survey, and the culture of safety survey, who should be blamed for the decline in scores?
3. If you were Reyna, what actions would you take to improve the scores on these three surveys?

4. If you were the director of the department, what might you do differently to facilitate improvement in the survey scores?
5. Managers are frequently held accountable for outcomes over which they do not have direct control. How can leaders influence managers in these situations to remain motivated and to continually improve the outcomes?

Case Study 9-2

It Could Have Happened to Anyone?

The phone rings at 2 a.m., and Judy is immediately awakened from her sleep. As she listens to the voice on the other end, she suddenly feels sickened with the news. The assistant manager of the unit informs her that a patient has been given a large dose of insulin that was intended for a different patient. The nurse failed to check the receiving patient's armband or call the patient by name prior to administering the insulin. Because it was in the middle of the night, the patient was groggy and did not question why he was receiving medication. Now the patient was in severe hypoglycemia, hypotensive, and exhibiting cardiac arrhythmias. The patient was transferred to the intensive care unit, and the family was called and informed of the error. The assistant manager reported that the nurse was one of the more senior and experienced nurses who had an impeccable work ethic and a reputation for being one of the best nurses on the unit. She shared that the nurse was absolutely devastated about the error and nearly hysterical. The patient's physician was very angry on the phone when the error was reported to him, and he was on his way to the hospital. Judy told the assistant manager that she would come to the hospital right away to meet with the patient's family, physician, and the nurse. Before she left home, Judy phoned the department director, who also indicated that he would come in to the hospital to assist in any way possible.

When Judy arrived at the hospital, she was informed that the patient had just expired and that his family was on their way to the hospital. The patient's physician was in the ICU talking with the other physicians and nurses who tried to resuscitate the patient. The ICU physician indicated that although the overdose of insulin contributed to the death, the patient's underlying condition made it impossible to correct the hypoglycemia and to save the patient.

After speaking to the physicians, Judy went to her own unit to speak with the nurse who made the medication error. She could only imagine how devastated the nurse was feeling, so she approached her gently and with compassion in her voice and mannerisms. Judy listened to the nurse as she tearfully recounted the story of going into the patient's room and administering the medication. She acknowledged that she had not checked the patient's armband because she didn't want to disturb the patient, who was sleeping. This was her first night to care for the patient who received the insulin and the patient next door who was supposed to receive the insulin. Both of the patients were men in their 70s who had the same diagnosis and who actually had similar physical characteristics and facial features. Both men had been admitted during the day and were assigned to adjacent rooms. To make matters worse their last names were similar. The nurse could hardly speak for the tears, and she was shaking uncontrollably. The assistant manager completed the forms necessary to report the incident to the hospital's quality and risk management departments. After the nurse signed documentation, Judy suggested that she ask a family member to come and drive her home. Judy was concerned for the nurse's safety because she was completely distraught. She told her that it would be necessary for her to take several administrative days off, but she should be available to speak with the hospital attorneys and risk management.

After leaving the nurse, Judy went back to the ICU to meet with the patient's family. When she arrived there, the department director was already engaged with the family, who were both angry and devastated with the news of how the patient had been given the wrong medication inadvertently and had expired. Since the department director and social services were working with the family, Judy returned to her unit to meet with her staff and the assistant manager.

Everybody on the unit was affected by the event, and many of the nurses were in tears. The assistant manager was also feeling the pressure of the situation and was trying to coordinate the care of the remaining patients on the unit. After working to stabilize the emotions on the unit, Judy met with the department director, the CNO, the physicians, and the attorney for risk management. The required phone calls and paperwork were completed notifying the Health Department of the medication error and the patient's death. Everyone realized that the Health Department would conduct a thorough investigation of the situation, review the hospital's policies and procedures related to medication administration, and inquire as to how nurse competencies were assessed and reviewed. The hospital attorney indicated that he and the risk management team would continue to meet with the family and suggested that social work or a clinical psychologist be involved in the meetings. The CEO met with the public relations department to prepare an official hospital statement about the situation because reporters from the community television stations were already calling and requesting information about the patient's death.

Questions

1. If you are Judy, what steps would you take with your nursing staff to stabilize their emotions about the situation?
2. What should Judy do to heal the brokenness on the unit and to prevent the potential reoccurrence?
3. What steps should Judy or the hospital's leaders take with the nurse who administered the wrong medication to the patient? Should this employee be terminated as a result of the error?
4. Identify both the individual errors and the system errors that contributed to the medication error.
5. What work needs to be done by the hospital's leadership to manage the internal and external (public) reaction to the error and the patient's death?
6. What should leadership do to help the hospital recover from this error?

References

Benner, P., Malloch, K., & Sheets, V. (Eds.). (2010). Overview: NCSBN practice breakdown initiative. In *Nursing pathways for patient safety: Expert panel on practice breakdown*. Philadelphia, PA: Elsevier.

Buerhaus, P. (1998). Milton Weinstein's insights on the development, use, and methodologic problems in cost-effectiveness analysis. *Image: Journal of Nursing Scholarship, 30*, 223–227.

Finkelman, A., & Kenner, C. (2009). *Teaching IOM: Implications of the Institute of Medicine reports for nursing education* (2nd ed.). Silver Spring, MD: ANA.

HealthLeaders Media. (2013, July). Safety stumbling blocks. Advancing clinical quality from data to decisions. Retrieved from http://content.hcpro.com/pdf/content/293611.pdf

Institute of Medicine. (2001). *Informing the future: Critical issues in health*. Washington, DC: National Academies Press.

Kaye, L. (2000). The spiritual roots of mistakes. *Inner Edge, 3*(2), 5–7.

Kohn, L. T., Corrigan, J. M., & Donaldson, M. S. (Eds.). (2000). *To err is human: Building a safer health system*. Washington, DC: National Academies Press.

Longest, B. (1998). Managerial competence at senior levels of integrated delivery systems. *Journal of Healthcare Management, 43*, 115–135.

Malloch, K., & Porter-O'Grady, T. (1999). Partnership economics: Nursing's challenge in a quantum age. *Nursing Economics, 17*, 299–307.

Marx, D. (2001). Patient safety and the "just culture": A primer for healthcare executives. Retrieved from http://www.psnet.ahrq.gov/resource.aspx?resourceID=1582

Pappas, S. H. (2013). Value, a nursing outcome. *Nursing Administration Quaterly, 37*(2), 122–128.

Ricks, T. E. (2012). What ever happened to accountability? *Harvard Business Review, 90*(10), 93–98.

Wu, A. W., Cavanaugh, T. A., McPhee, S. J., Lo, B., & Micco, G. P. (1997). To tell the truth: Ethical and practical issues in disclosing medical mistakes to patients. *Journal of General Internal Medicine, 12*, 770–775.

Suggested Readings

Ariely, D. (2010). Good decisions, Bad outcomes. *Harvard Business Review, 88*(11), 40.

Benner, P. (2000). *Error in medicine: A complex sorrow*. Paper presented at conference, University of California–Berkeley, March 11–12.

Benner, P., Kyriakidis, P. H., & Stannard, R. D. (2001). *Clinical wisdom and interventions in critical care: A thinking-in-action approach*. Philadelphia, PA: Saunders.

Berkow, S., Jaggi, T., & Fogelson, R. (2007). Fourteen unit attributes to guide staffing. *Journal of Nursing Administration, 37*(3), 150–155.

Buerhaus, P. I. (2009). Avoiding mandatory hospital nurse staffing ratios: An economic commentary. *Nursing Outlook, 57*(2), 107–112.

Chang, Y., & Mark, B. A. (2009). Antecedents of severe and nonsevere medication errors. *Journal of Nursing Scholarship, 41*(1), 70–78.

Chuang, Y., Ginsburg, L., & Berta, W. B. (2007). Learning from preventable adverse events in healthcare organizations: Development of a multilevel model of learning and propositions. *Health Care Management Review, 32*(4), 330–340.

Clancy, C. (2009, September–October). Patient safety: One decade after *To Err Is Human*. *Patient Safety and Quality Healthcare*, 8–10.

Committee on Quality Health Care in America, Institute of Medicine. (2001). *Crossing the quality chasm: A new health system for the 21st century*. Washington, DC: National Academy Press.

Ebright, P. R., Urden, L., Patterson, E., & Chalko, B. (2004). Themes surrounding novice nurse near-miss and adverse-event situations. *Journal of Nursing Administration, 34*(11), 531–538.

Fagin, C. M. (2001). *When care becomes a burden: Diminishing access to adequate nursing*. New York, NY: Milbank Memorial Fund.

Hofmann, P. B. (2005, January/February). Responsibility for unsuccessful promotions. *Healthcare Executive*, 32–36.

Hyun, S., Bakken, S., Douglas, K., & Stone, P. W. (2008). Evidence-based staffing: Potential roles for informatics. *Nursing Economic$, 26*(3), 151–158, 173.

Institute of Medicine. (2004). *Keeping patients safe: Transforming the work environment of nurses.* Washington, DC: National Academies Press.

Kalish, B. J., Landstrom, G., & Williams, R. A. (2009). Missed nursing care: Errors of omission. *Nursing Outlook, 57,* 3–9.

Lachman, V. D. (Ed.). (2006). *Applied ethics in nursing.* New York, NY: Springer.

Reason, J. (2000). Human error: Models and management. *British Medical Journal, 320,* 768–770.

Rosner, F., Berger, J. T., Kark, P., Potash, J., & Bennett, A. J. (2000). Disclosure and prevention of medical errors. *Archives in Internal Medicine, 160,* 2089–2092.

Silber, J. H., Williams, S. V., Krakauer, H., & Schwartz, J. S. (1992). Hospital and patient characteristics associated with death after surgery: A study of adverse occurrence and failure to rescue. *Medical Care, 30,* 615–629.

Watson, J. (2006, January–March). Caring theory as an ethical guide to administrative and clinical practices. *Nursing Administration Quarterly, 30*(1), 48–55.

Williams, L. L. (2006, January–March). The fair factor in matters of trust. *Nursing Administration Quarterly, 30*(1), 30–37.

Quiz Questions

Select the best answer for each of the following questions.

1. Marketplace value incorporates the essential factors affecting health care. Which of these factors is not included in the marketplace value equation?
   a. Available reimbursement
   b. Time and type of provider
   c. Return on investment
   d. Appropriateness of clinical service

2. Errors in health care are inevitable. Given the nature of the interactions between providers, patients, technology, and the environment, errors should be _____.
   a. Expected and tolerated
   b. Managed by the team
   c. Viewed as opportunities for learning and improvement
   d. Eliminated at all costs

3. Disclosure and mandatory reporting of errors are both recommended as strategies for managing errors in health care. Why are these two behaviors incompatible?
   a. Mandatory reporting removes the safety from disclosure and makes providers unwilling to admit to their errors.
   b. Disclosure of errors implies failure.
   c. Malpractice cases do not allow disclosure of errors.
   d. The goal of mandatory reporting of errors is to establish blame, whereas the goal of disclosing errors is to generate an open dialogue.

389

4. To shift from external regulation to internal accountability, which of the following does an organization require?

   a. An increase in the number of committees

   b. Elimination of licensing requirements

   c. The commitment of the leadership to monitor and manage the meeting of healthcare standards

   d. Support from The Joint Commission

5. Cost-effectiveness analysis has been proposed as more appropriate than cost-to-benefit analysis for evaluating healthcare services. Which of the following demonstrate its advantages?

   a. It takes into account health outcomes and the cost of treatment.

   b. It takes into account the cost of treatment and the cost of health outcomes.

   c. It takes into account the cost of the service and the savings achieved.

   d. It uses units such as years of life saved instead of dollars to measure health outcomes.

6. Why have providers not been able to manage the gap (variance) between patient needs and healthcare resources effectively?

   a. It is difficult to determine the actual variance.

   b. The interventions selected by an individual provider to manage the variance are not known to the others on the healthcare team.

   c. The individual provider feels abandoned by the system.

   d. Ownership of the problem and the solution rests with the healthcare team.

7. What does staffing by ratio (the ratio of patients to providers) require?

   a. Sufficient funding

   b. A valid and reliable baseline of patient care needs

   c. Historical trend data to support the ratio

   d. Approval of the legislature

8. How do holographic leadership and fragmented leadership differ?

   a. Philosophically

   b. In the skills required of leaders

   c. In the leaders' scope of responsibilities

   d. In the degree of financial expertise required of leaders

9. The process of recovering from the negative consequences of committing a medical error has not been discussed openly in the past, most likely for which of the following reasons?

   a. The emphasis of healthcare education and practice is on doing things right.

   b. The threat of lawsuits forces providers to keep silent about the errors they commit.

   c. Most providers do not need guidance in learning to live with errors.

   d. Most providers receive help confidentially.

10. Managed care is believed to increase the incidence of error. If this is true, the reason probably is that managed care _____.

   a. Removes clinical decision making from the point of service

   b. Leads to a lack of funding to support quality care

   c. Encourages the use of noncredentialed providers

   d. Is more productive and leads to more patients being treated

CHAPTER TEN

The Fully Engaged Leader: Integrated Capacity for Success

The illiterate of the 21st century will not be those who cannot read and write, but those who cannot learn, unlearn, and relearn.
—*Alvin Toffler*

Chapter Objectives

www

At the completion of this chapter, the reader will be able to

· Understand the attributes of the fully engaged leader and the relationship of engagement to organizational outcomes.
· Review the theoretical underpinnings of the emotional aspects of leadership and the challenges of integrating these concepts into leadership development.
· Explain the role of self-awareness, compassion, passionate optimism, and impulse control in the development of emotional competence.
· Describe the stages of acquiring emotional competence for the individual and for the team.
· Discuss the challenges of measuring and documenting the organizational impact of emotional competence.

Fully engaged leaders perhaps best portray the notion of complexity in the relationships they form as they transform work and the workplace, help others own their change, undertake the right change processes, and integrate the rules of engagement for the postindustrial age. Engaged leaders act and reflect on the events and processes of leading that emphasize the short term and integrate the long-term needs of the community.

Leader success depends on a wide range of variables that relate to the work to be done, the skills and abilities of the leader and the team, the needs of the team members, the resources available, and the motivation of all those involved. This list is not all-inclusive, and it continually evolves. The right stuff of leadership may indeed have common characteristics and behaviors, but the reality is that each leader has a unique combination of characteristics, values, behaviors, and ability to get the work done. Most leaders develop their personal essence on the basis of education, experience, mental intelligence, emotional intelligence, and the ability to form meaningful relationships. This chapter presents the emerging profile of the fully engaged leader to demonstrate a greater appreciation of the complexity of leadership and the significance of engagement as a leader characteristic and to stimulate discussion of the potential impact of engaged behaviors on organizational performance. A brief review of the emotional intelligence literature and processes to develop engagement and a discussion of team emotional competence are also presented.

To support the work of the organization, leaders must have not only technical management skills but also skills in managing emotions—theirs as well as those of other individuals in the organization. Emotionally competent leaders exhibit a high regard for colleagues and subordinates, an understanding of basic motivations, as well as basic justice, a willingness to take responsibility, a willingness to correct faulty situations, and a willingness to take positive, quick, and aggressive action when indicated.

Quantum leaders recognize that they have no more control over organizational outcomes than do police officers over the movement of a large crowd. The officers may be able to herd the crowd in a certain direction for a period of time, but their control over the crowd is only temporary and cursory. As noted in previous chapters, leaders can no longer rely on command-and-control leadership methods. They are being challenged to shift to behaviors that support team building and shared decision making and allow all team members to gain an understanding of the work.

Leaders must replace traditional leadership methods with coaching, mentoring, and facilitating. To do this, they must gain an understanding of the emotions and attitudes of all members of the organization and communicate this understanding to everyone else. Only when all members have an appreciation for each other's emotions and share an understanding of the goals of the organization can the real work be accomplished. In short, integrating emotional competence into the leadership model has a substantial impact on the quality of the work processes and their outcomes.

Managing the feeling side of the organization requires emotional competence. For leaders, emotional competence encompasses the abilities to identify, understand, use, and regulate the emotions that arise during the course of their work. Emotions in organizations are similar to emotions experienced in all walks of life and are seldom unique to the workplace or to an individual. Although it is difficult to separate emotions by setting, this chapter attempts to focus on the typical emotional experience in the workplace and the behaviors that organizational leaders tend to use.

Underpinnings of Emotional Competence

The worldview of the quantum leader differs significantly from the traditional Newtonian worldview. Leadership theory in quantum organizations takes into account the realities of dissipative (transforming or chaotic) systems. In these systems, structures that exchange energy and matter with their environment, form spontaneously. Given that healthcare organizations experience continuous and complex interactions during the formation of the new structures, competence in managing the feeling side of work becomes essential. Following is a description of five quantum organization characteristics that reflect the emotional realities of human systems.

Holism

Quantum organizations are holistic rather than fragmented, which means they recognize the connectedness between work processes and individuals. Holism, as an organizational value, supports the organization's integration with the world and is inconsistent with organizational structures made up of distinct departments and processes.

Intrinsic Motivation

A quantum organization operates on the principle that human beings, by their very nature, are internally motivated. In other words, the leaders of a quantum organization use a theory Y style of management, or a style that assumes that employees are ambitious and self-motivated, and fully recognize the creativity, capability, and motivation of all members of the organization. Further, the leaders do not structure the organization hierarchically, with chains of command encompassing many levels of superiors and subordinates, and they do not believe that the members are inherently lazy and uncreative and always in need of specific directions to be productive. They believe, instead, that for members to show initiative, ownership, and high productivity, the only requisites are positive support and a context for performance. Quantum leaders also believe that collective wisdom is most likely to emerge when all members are treated as if they are internally motivated to act in the organization's best interests. The belief is that individuals who are valued and encouraged to thrive create a synergistic cooperative that itself thrives.

Emergent Leadership

According to quantum leadership theory, organizational leadership emerges from the combined active engagement of all members of the organization. Thus as the engagement of individuals in the work of the organization increases, the leadership also increases. In this view, leadership is not attached to individuals but rather occurs in the space between individuals. It is not something done by one person (the leader) to many others (the followers), and it is not a role reserved for the people at the top of the organization.

The model of leadership as emergent differs importantly from the dyadic model of leadership, which is based on hierarchical (superior–subordinate) relationships (Allen, 2000). In this latter model, leadership is treated as a solution to particular organizational problems, specifically problems of performance. An organization that uses the dyadic model tends to be equilibrium seeking and structure preserving; certainty and stability are important goals, but leadership does not expect control to be complete because they know that some degree of change is unpredictable or uncontrollable and that change in structure results in energy loss. High levels of performance occur only when a leader of superior capability defines and directs the work to be done.

> ### Key Point
>
> Leadership occurs in the space between individuals working together. It is an emergent property of their relationships, and not the management or direction of work by individuals placed in superior positions.

Treating leadership as emergent fits well with the belief that individuals are intrinsically motivated, creative, and capable. It also fits well with dissipative models of leadership, which are discussed next.

Dissipative Leadership

Whereas the traditional dyadic model of leadership considers disruption as an anomaly that should be eliminated as soon as possible, the dissipative model views change and the disruption it brings as necessary for survival and growth (Barker, 1998). Because of the complex nature of today's society, simplistic problem-solving models based on linear command and control are no longer adequate tools for managing change. Administrative or leadership theory must be revised, therefore, to reflect the current nature of organizations as complex, dynamic, dissipative systems. Change is not merely a problem to be solved; change is.

The dissipative model of leadership rightly treats change as normal. It also favors transferring leadership responsibilities to a group process in which no specific person is in charge but every person is assumed to occupy a leadership role to some degree. It views leadership as a dynamic community-building process rather than a means for achieving organizational goals—as a process of change where the ethics (rules of conduct) of individuals are integrated into the mores (customs accepted without question) of a community. Further, in this model leadership becomes a form of participative democracy in which the actions of individuals are motivated by their own wants and needs and directed toward a perceived collective good. The focus is on the intrinsic and foundational values of individuals and the group rather than on causes and effects; leadership, in this view, is the emergent property of relationships, not the management of work by individuals placed in superior positions.

Integrated Leadership

The quantum leadership model recognizes emotional competence as an important skill, especially for leaders of healthcare organizations. Quantum leaders must possess not only intellect, analytical ability, technical skills, and appropriate experience, they must also possess the ability to understand and manage relationships, including their emotional dimension. To be fully effective, they must first master the required technical work skills, second, understand and intentionally choose those work processes most likely to achieve the desired outcomes, and third, be able to form and sustain relationships—and they must do all this in an organization in which the interdependence of individuals and work processes is recognized (**Figure 10-1**).

Traditional leadership job descriptions generally do well defining the necessary product- or service-specific knowledge, skills, and abilities. As for the second requirement, choosing the appropriate work processes, leaders often find it difficult to determine which interventions or processes achieve the organization's goals efficiently. The object is to define and commit to value-based interventions. Too often organizations use long-established processes that are outdated and do not contribute to reaching the desired outcomes in any way.

Consider the myriad times healthcare providers monitor and record vital signs and no intervention follows. Why perform these activities with such frequency? Perhaps it

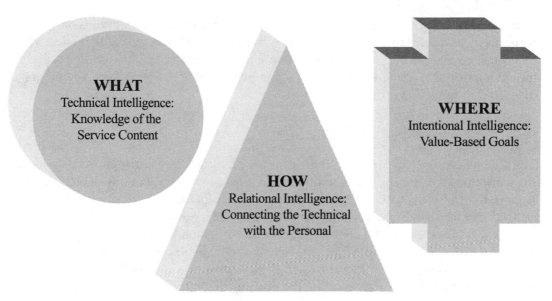

Figure 10-1 The Components of Leadership Effectiveness.

is just because "we've always done it this way." The reality is that taking vital signs, although it requires skilled providers, seldom contributes to the outcome. Indeed, the need to show that taking vital signs frequently has real benefits for patients deserves consideration. Providers are reluctant to give up long-held practices for fear of losing critical data and the legal ramifications, but given the serious shortage of healthcare workers, any and all practices that do not obviously contribute to better patient outcomes should be evaluated for elimination. Leaders, especially in this new age, must ensure that resources are appropriately allocated and that the work of each individual is aligned with the goals of the customers and the organization. In fact, all members of the organization must become skilled in selecting interventions that further the organization's mission.

Purposeful (intentional) use of time, labor, and equipment is closely related to the third requisite, developing and sustaining relationships to support work processes. Proficiency at building rapport among members of the organization

Key Point

Principles of emotional competence:
- The individual members of an organization are interconnected and interrelated.
- The individual members perceive their work as natural and a source of fulfillment and growth.
- Creativity is inherent in the individual and in the collective wisdom of each team.
- The individual members are motivated to contribute to meaningful goals and focus on self-esteem and self-actualization.
- Leadership emerges from the combined active engagement of all members of the organization, not from the activities of a single individual.

is increasingly seen as an essential leadership skill; effective relationships, it is now recognized, can substantially improve performance. It is also recognized that effective relationships require the participants to have some understanding of naturally occurring human emotions. The nature of emotional competence required by leaders (and others) is discussed in the following section.

Nature of Emotional Competence

Traditional leaders tend to look on the meaning or feeling side of leadership as its soft side, the work that is often subjective and difficult to teach or measure. Emotional competence is more than a list of attributes. It is a collection of perceptions, behaviors, knowledge, and values that, for instance, enable a leader to manage meaning between individuals and groups within an organization. For healthcare leaders, emotional competence involves the interpretation and translation of personal feelings into the processes of the workplace. The key concepts of cognition, competence, emotion, intelligence, and volition are defined in **Exhibit 10-1** to assist in understanding the essence of emotional competence. The characteristics and behaviors that make up emotional competence include the following:

- Self-awareness
- Mindfulness
- Openness
- Impulse control
- Personal humility
- Appreciation of ambiguity and paradox
- Appreciation of knowledge
- Willpower
- Compassion
- Passionate optimism
- Resilience

At times leaders become overfocused on the style and behaviors of leadership to the extent where members' style (Myers-Briggs type or DiSC) is identified on the employee

---

Exhibit 10-1   Key Concepts

- *Cognition:*   Pertains to mental processes of perception, memory, judgment, and reasoning.
- *Competence:* The state of having suitable or sufficient skill, knowledge, and experience for some purpose.
- *Emotion:*   The affective side of consciousness in which joy, sorrow, fear, and so on are experienced. Emotions are distinguished from cognitive and volitional states of consciousness.
- *Intelligence:* The capacity for learning, reasoning, and understanding; aptitude in grasping truths, relationships, facts, or meanings; mental alertness and quickness of understanding.
- *Volition:*   The act of willing, choosing, or resolving; the exercise of the will.

---

badge. Both leaders and employees become focused on the style of decision making at the expense of the desired outcomes. Although it is certainly relevant to know, for example, that some individuals are ENTJs (extraversion, intuition, thinking, judging types) and make decisions more quickly than others, this information is one piece of data and does not take into consideration the current context of events and interactions. When there is a need to respond quickly to ensure patient safety, the end goal of patient safety must be primary, while individual styles are secondary or in some situations irrelevant. The fact that one's primary behavior or decision-making style reflects the need for time to process is secondary to the contextual realities of the situation. The fully engaged leader ensures focus is on the desired, value-based outcomes that support quality patient care service and that information specific to style is supportive but not the driver of processes.

Many scholars continue to offer guidelines for leadership, but there is no widely accepted, standard template of behaviors for effective leadership. Outcomes of good leadership, such as the achievement of clinical outcomes, employee satisfaction, and fiscal stability, which integrate and reflect the unique values, beliefs, and skills of the organization, have been identified more consistently than behaviors have. Regardless of the approach or theoretical underpinning selected by the leader to guide the development of interpersonal or soft skills, the process of development must always be directed to the outcomes; processes must never overtake the significance of the desired outcomes. As previously noted, working to identify one's decision-making style and focusing on the need for expression of that style in deference to achieving organizational goals are inappropriate. The goal is to understand one's style, integrate it into the group decision-making process, and achieve the desired goal (Gill, 2011).

Although it is difficult to describe or measure the soft stuff in the business world, its absence is usually very obvious. When negative outcomes result from the lack of the soft side of leadership, for instance, these can be described very clearly by nearly every leader. They include the negative consequences of disregarding others as unique individuals, discounting the feelings of others, and being abrasive to or ignoring others, all of which tend to cause alienation and loss of support. A leader may accomplish the technical side of a task quickly and in an exemplary manner, but a failure to consider the feelings of those involved usually prevents the outcome from being sustainable and diminishes the commitment and motivation of the team in the future.

Self-Knowledge

When leaders know what works for themselves it enhances their ability to understand what works for others in similar situations. In fact, self-knowledge is an important pillar of emotional competence. To achieve self-knowledge, leaders need to understand the quality of consciousness they bring to the workplace and recognize that, although they cannot always control events, they can control their thoughts.

They also need to realize that individuals each have unique patterns and perceptual filters that affect their interactions with others. This is not to suggest that every individual requires a psychoanalytical evaluation. The point is that leaders need to appreciate that they each have a preferred style of interacting, have their own sources of motivation and energy, and have unique ways of perceiving information and determining which types of

TABLE 10-1   Behavioral Assessment Categories

Emotional Competence				
Source	*Categories*			
Astrology	Water	Fire	Air	Earth
Hippocrates	Melancholy	Sanguine	Phlegmatic	Choleric
Jung	Feeler	Intuitor	Thinker	Sensor
Merrill, Wilson, and Allessandra	Amiable	Expressive	Analytical	Driver
Performax	Steadiness	Influence	Compliance	Dominance
Cathcart and Allessandra	Relater	Socializer	Thinker	Director

information to consider. Leaders (and others) also have different communication styles (e.g., open, confrontational, assertive, and withholding) and different decision-making styles (e.g., autocratic, collaborative, participative, and consensus building). Numerous assessment tools are available to help leaders determine their degree of assertiveness, their type of creativity, and their styles of collaborating and communicating. (**Table 10-1** presents examples of behavioral assessment categories.)

Self-knowledge is also about developing an understanding of and appreciation for ambiguity and paradox. Although uncertainty or ambiguity can have a positive value, not everyone is comfortable with the lack of clear and certain pathways. Learning to live with paradox or seemingly contradictory ideas becomes a significant challenge for the leader trained and experienced in the command-and-control leadership model. Yet leaders today must recognize that paradoxical situations are a normal part of the organizational landscape and do not necessarily have to be resolved through compromise. For example, contradictions and uncertainty create opportunities for leaders to explore perspectives that differ from theirs and to be confronted with new ideas and feelings. In short, far from being calamitous, paradox, much like conflict, offers formerly hidden benefits to the organization that is open to profit from it.

The leadership role as it relates to relationships has a paradoxical aspect. Although people generally have a need to belong to a group for support and for reference, research indicates that effective leaders, despite spending most of the work time in contact with others, tend to have minimal need to belong to a specific group. Leaders instead tend to be self-reliant and are comfortable acting as a dissenting voice or challenging the status quo. This is not to say that leaders do not create and sustain meaningful relationships. Rather, recognizing that integrating subjective meanings into the leadership data set is essential for achieving optimal outcomes, emotionally competent leaders use both personal relationship data and organizational data to inform their decisions. Note, however, that this is very different from aligning with specific partisan perspectives or choosing sides in decision making.

Collins (2001) found that powerful leaders often possess a paradoxical mixture of personal humility and professional will. The combination of humble unpretentiousness and fierce, even stoic, resolve is at odds with the traditional image of leaders as larger than life. Yet this union of modesty and willfulness has some obvious merits as a leadership style, especially for leaders in the coming age. Among other things, leaders who are both modest and willful tend to act with a clearly expressed openness to others, place people and their feelings first, recognize the positive and negative aspects of the current reality, sustain their faith in the organization's potential for success, channel their energy into the organization, and are disposed to develop successors rather than leave the issue of succession unresolved. They appreciate the traps inherent in short-term success and false optimism, and they are inclined to foster organizational learning because of their healthy skepticism of their own accomplishments. Besides documenting this unusual combination of leadership values and priorities, recent research has shown that overwhelming improvements in organizational performance can result.

Openness to New Ideas

Leaders who understand their own decision-making and communication styles find it easier to appreciate other perspectives. They thus can take better advantage of the fact that every healthcare organization, because of its range of individuals, teams, and disciplines, is a repository of multiple viewpoints on everything needed to create cost-effective services, from the content of the services to the processes for designing and delivering them.

In addition, such leaders, by considering other viewpoints, can achieve a high level of emotional competence, which includes the ability to listen to what others have to say and integrate what is important into the organization's collective wisdom. Sometimes, because of the fast-paced, results-oriented environment in which they function, leaders are forced to learn how to maintain suffering silence, which is a form of listening in which the emotions that obstruct listening and the objective evaluation of ideas are suppressed.

Valuing Knowledge

For leaders of quantum organizations, self-knowledge and openness to the opinions of others are closely related to the perception that new information is essential for growth. Necessarily, besides developing a thirst for new knowledge, leaders also must acquire the ability to filter out insignificant information. In the current data-rich age, far too much information is available on the Internet, and more passes through every leader's hands. Filtering and managing new information nonetheless reinforce the undeniable passion of leaders to make a difference.

The greater a leader's self-knowledge and openness to new ideas, the greater the leader's confidence in making decisions. Emotionally competent leaders make decisions readily and enthusiastically, not because they believe they are always correct but because they understand that there is always a risk of error and that progress cannot be made without taking action. In fact, they strongly believe that unsuccessful outcomes or errors are opportunities for improvement and not something to be avoided or eliminated.

Compassion

Compassion is another main pillar of emotional competence. In health care the emotional intensity surrounding trauma, birth, suffering, and dying makes compassionate service the intended norm. Providers and patients have indeed come to recognize the importance of understanding and sharing one another's feelings, including joy, sorrow,

> ### Point to Ponder
>
> Without feelings of deep sympathy and sorrow for others struck by misfortune and a genuine desire to alleviate suffering, patient care service would be no more than a robotic endeavor for caregivers.

and all the emotions in between. Further, compassion fosters the kind of personal involvement that is necessary for providers and patients to develop strong and effective relationships and for providers to apply their objective (technical) knowledge and skills.

Interestingly, the powerful urge of providers to alleviate patient distress cannot prevent them from objectifying patients when they discuss patient issues. The patient becomes "the gallbladder on Hall 1"—a medical condition instead of a person. In contrast, providers who are emotionally competent learn to integrate the objectivity of the gallbladder disease with the subjectivity of the patient and to perceive the patient's unique needs and feelings about the disease and its impact on the patient's functionality. The patient remains a person and is not referred to as a room number or a diagnosis.

In many ways, compassionate patient care is similar to compassionate leadership. For instance, the leader attempts to integrate the subjective, which here encompasses the relationships between the members of the organization, and the objective, which encompasses the work to be accomplished. In addition, although the leader should sympathize with an employee who has suffered a misfortune, he or she should refrain from attempting to resolve the employee's issues. Offering guidance and reassurance is appropriate and consistent with the principle of personal accountability, but attempting to manage another's situation is paternalistic and disempowering. The emotionally competent leader develops the ability to express sincere sympathy when an employee experiences adversity but does not cross the line into paternalism. The challenge is to integrate the subjective and the objective—to remain personal in the relationship with the employee while also considering the organization's needs and the employee's accountability for doing his or her job. In meeting this challenge, the leader avoids objectifying the employee (e.g., treating the employee as an attendance problem).

Consider this common situation. An employee with repeated absences is disciplined by a leader on the basis of an established attendance policy. The leader's goal may be compassionate leadership, yet the objective policy is allowed to get in the way. To act with compassion, the leader needs to inject subjectivity into the equation, which can be done by exploring the surrounding events (the context of the absences) and the employee's feelings. Compassionate leadership emerges when the leader looks at both the personal information and the objective needs of the organization to find an equitable solution. This is not to say that it is okay not to hold the employee accountable for meeting the expectations of the organization. In fact, compassionate leadership is a broad enough concept to include dismissing the employee if the employee fails to make a sincere effort to do his or her job.

As shown by this example, compassionate leadership is sometimes hard to achieve. It is especially hard to achieve in a traditional organization, where workforce numbers and productivity targets are determined by the chief executive officer (CEO) and handed down to managers for implementation. In difficult times the CEO usually mandates a reduction in the workforce using one of two approaches. In the first approach, the CEO keeps distant from the process, causing the employees to view him or her as callous. In reality the CEO may be very compassionate, but by not becoming directly involved in the process he or she inadvertently appears indifferent. In the second approach, the CEO, having identified the workforce reductions to be implemented, remains involved and available during the communication and early implementation stages. As a result, the employees perceive the CEO as compassionate and caring.

Presence

For any leader, being present—especially being available following any decision that has positive or negative implications for others—shows that the leader is connected with the employees and is willing to participate with them in a common journey. Leaders with a low degree of emotional competence tend to be visible in the workplace after announcements of pay raises or new benefits packages and noticeably out of town when decisions that negatively affect members of the organization are first publicized. Involvement in managing the impact of all decisions shows that the leader is committed to the employees, is willing to claim ownership of the decisions, and is sensitive to the varied meanings of the decisions for the employees. Absence, by contrast, conveys that the leader is uninterested in the impact of difficult decisions on others and is afraid of claiming the decisions. Leaders must realize that it is not only their technical skills or verbal communication that makes a difference; it is also their ability to show that there is someone at the top who cares about what is happening.

Group Discussion

Imagine that in the midst of a recent blizzard, a healthcare organization experiences a serious staffing shortage. Because the storm is forecast to continue, the employees who are at work wonder whether they should inform the leadership team of the shortage. At what point, if at all, should they contact the senior leaders? When should the senior leaders be required to be present at the organization? How would the leaders' actions likely affect the willingness of others to attempt to come to work? What impact would the leaders' presence have on the employees' morale? How long will the employees remember the presence or absence of the leaders?

Employees who are facing layoffs will search for the linkage between the (objective) financial goals of the organization and the (subjective) impact of the workforce reduction on their lives. In such a situation, the employees interpret the leader's physical presence and availability for dialogue as compassionate leadership. Note that this does not negate the importance of the role of middle managers; yet employees facing adversity seek to connect their subjective reality (e.g., the reality of being out of work) with the personal (subjective) responses of the chief decision maker.

Mindfulness

The emotionally competent leader is mindful of recurring situations, the past reactions of members of the organization, and the implications of these reactions. As a result, the leader is able to identify certain patterns of behavior and develop skill in understanding and interpreting these situations as guidelines for future behavior. In essence, the leader interprets the emotional reactions of individuals in recurring situations and ensures that he or she is present when another such situation arises. For example, a disaster of any kind requires the physical presence of the leader to support the employees emotionally. Seldom is the presence of the leader needed—or even desired—for the technical work of a disaster. Yet the leader should have no question as to the significance of his or her presence when employees are emotionally affected.

Nonverbal Emotional Competence

A leader's physical stance and actions transmit nonverbal messages and can arouse positive or negative emotions. Imagine a group of people standing together in such a way as to invite new participants. Now imagine a group standing close to each other in a closed circle and speaking in hushed tones. The message sent by this arrangement is that newcomers are not welcome. Again, an extended arm, a handshake, and the offering of physical space are friendly behaviors, whereas turning one's back to an approaching person, folding one's arms, and speaking in hushed tones are inhospitable behaviors. The former convey feelings of acceptance, whereas the latter are rejecting and exclusionary. Or consider the unexpected entry of a competitor into a group of highly antagonistic opponents. The conversation may stop altogether or verbal confrontation may ensue, depending on the emotional state of all the parties. Emotional reactions are pervasive in any situation in which people are present, and dealing with these reactions requires great compassion and self-awareness.

Passionate Optimism

In this time of chaos and unending challenges, healthcare leaders often find it difficult to remain enthusiastic about the work to be done, and they may find it easier to see the cup as half empty rather than as half full. They may therefore need the refreshment afforded by reminiscing about the beginning of their careers, when their deep concern for patient care was the driving force of all their actions. During this earlier period, besides acting out of altruism, they undoubtedly believed they could truly make a difference. In fact, as new professionals, they were focused on understanding the seriousness of each patient's condition and identifying the treatment most likely to result in a favorable outcome. In spite of the challenges, hopefulness was their modus operandi. Emotionally competent leaders retain the passion of their early healthcare experiences and work diligently to guide others in developing and cherishing the same spirit of passionate optimism. This is not to say that they are immune to discouragement or unrealistic about the future. All leaders experience disappointment and disillusionment, but emotionally competent leaders recognize that successes and failures are both normal and that times of disappointment eventually give way to times of breakthrough and achievement.

Maintaining a positive mind-set means holding positive images rather than negative images and viewing all situations as blessings and/or opportunities. When the results are not desired or anticipated, leaders should look for lessons to be learned and value the information gained. A positive mind-set stands in sharp contrast to a pessimistic worldview, which fosters passivity and a general unwillingness to take appropriate action in the face of adversity. Pessimism depletes the life force of all involved. Even in the worst of circumstances, leaders are challenged to find positive meaning for themselves and the members of the organization. And when positive meaning cannot be found, the most logical source of encouragement becomes each individual's support system, including family and friends.

Resilience

Few leaders have acquired the skill set needed to manage personal disappointments and to coach others in the management of their disappointments. Traditionally, individuals who receive bad news are expected to deal with it outside of the workplace. Yet when a team jointly addresses the disappointments of individual team members, productivity is likely to be enhanced and work disruption minimized. Further, allowing time for the team to process disappointments and create effective coping strategies strengthens the emotional competence of the team.

Passion Through Balance

Creating or restoring passion for work typically has a subtle impact at the outset, but eventually the results become very obvious. Passion often emerges from situations that seem overwhelming. Given the current rate of change and innovation, few can keep pace to their satisfaction. There is far too much knowledge available and not enough time or skill to winnow out the unneeded information. Reestablishing a proper balance requires a new filter for consciousness, a filter that allows leaders to sift through information and select only what is pertinent to the issue at hand. Also, leaders can find new comfort in accepting their limitations and the impossibility of reviewing all there is to know. They can also find comfort in realizing that if out-of-the-ordinary information is needed, it probably is available through the Internet. Establishing a balance between information input and available time is one component of the total equation, and it helps in creating the space needed for passionate optimism. Establishing a balance between work and personal life is another prerequisite for passionate optimism.

> **Point to Ponder**
>
> Thoughts on resilience:
> - Resilience is the capacity to cope with unanticipated dangers after they have become manifest and to learn to bounce back.
> - To be resilient means being able to come away from the event with an even greater capacity to prevent and contain future errors.
> - Resilience is the capacity for improvisation, which allows the organization to expand exponentially not only with the range of actions in its repertoire but also the range of potential threats it can foresee.
>
> —Karl Weick and Kathleen Sutcliffe
>
> *Source*: Weick, K., & Sutcliffe, K. (2000, Summer) High reliability: The power of mindfulness. *Leader to Leader, 21*, 33–38. Copyright (c) 2000 by John Wiley & Sons. Reproduced with permission of Wiley Inc.

Passion is more easily sustained when the conflict between personal life and work life is minimal. Emotionally competent leaders act to ensure that employees do not feel they have to hang their personal values at the door when they come to work. Although the purpose of their activities is to assist the organization in meeting its goals, only when these goals are congruent with the employees' personal values will their enthusiasm survive. If there is a conflict between goals and values, the best strategy is to bring the conflict and the employees' feelings into view and work to minimize the conflict. Failure to address such conflicts quickly depletes the energy of the organization.

Noted leadership expert and philosopher Peter Russell postulated that in the past it was difficult for people to develop passion and happiness because they had scant material possessions and few career options (Russell, 1993). For example, in preindustrial times 97% of Americans worked on the land. Life was hard and food was scarce. There was no central heating, and the water was not always healthy to drink.

Today, in contrast, grocery stores offer a bounty of food, department stores are filled with clothing and other goods, and hot or cool air is available with the push of a button. If we are unhappy or lack passion, therefore, the probable reason, rather than the absence of something external, is that we are experiencing an inner lack of meaning or sense of personal purpose. Society tells us that to overcome our unhappiness we must do something to meet an external need—buy new clothes or a new car or eat a well-prepared meal—but the void remains. As a consequence, people increasingly recognize that what they are missing is meaning in their life. Meanwhile, the drive for more technology and more material goods continues to accelerate. The challenge is not to negate the value of material well-being, but to make a place for passion—to use emotional competence to create a balance between the material and the emotional sides of life.

Impulse Control

Full emotional competence includes impulse control, or self-regulation—the ability to temper negative emotions. Emotionally competent leaders know how to share feelings appropriately and maintain dignity. Managing emotions is not the same as lacking emotions. Even the most emotionally competent leader experiences feelings of anger and frustration, but he or she is able to mediate and reframe them to minimize the misuse of energy. The common expectation is that the fundamentals of impulse control were developed in childhood and that anger and frustration are thus managed in a healthy way. Unfortunately, not every individual grew up in a family in which healthy impulse control strategies were handed down. Many instead learned patterns of behavior that were obstacles to personal growth and accountability, such as conflict avoidance and assumption of a victim attitude. These individuals need new skills and behaviors to function in high-stress environments.

As the need for emotional competence becomes more apparent, organizations are developing personal growth and development programs not only for leaders but for all employees and even members of the community. Not surprisingly, attendees of such programs identify nonworkplace roles, such as that of parent, spouse, friend, and community member, to which the skills they learn can be profitably applied.

Leaders are expected to achieve personal impulse control and also to acquire the skills to coach others to develop and maintain impulse control. By generally remaining composed and positive in attitude, leaders are better able to support group processes and contribute to the accomplishment of the organizational work. They can still express strong and passionate feelings, but they keep themselves from losing control. Maintaining their cool also allows them to better manage other individuals who become emotionally upset or agitated. If someone does begin to get overly excited, an emotionally competent leader can respond in such a way as to deescalate the loss of control and minimize the chance of emotional fireworks.

Interestingly, self-control manifests largely in the absence of obvious outbursts. Being unfazed under stress and handling a hostile person without lashing out in return are indications of self-regulation and the ability to manage negative emotions. Controlled emotional behavior avoids misinterpretation of events through the lens of anger and minimizes the chance that a benign comment will lead to skewed perceptions through hostility.

Related Concepts

Several concepts related to emotional competence—emotional intelligence, character, and integrity—are helpful in understanding its underpinnings and significance. Although none is equivalent to or subsumed under the concept of emotional intelligence, each applies to the same set of phenomena. For example, although the concept of character is much broader than the concept of emotional competence, a person's character—the traits that form that person's nature—directly affects the person's ability to become emotionally competent. In general, an emotionally competent leader possesses a high level of emotional intelligence, a strong character, uncompromising integrity, a strong moral conscience, and an optimistic outlook on life.

Emotional Intelligence

Goleman (1998) has done groundbreaking research on the nature of emotional intelligence and its importance as a factor in achieving personal excellence. Emotional intelligence, according to Goleman, determines our potential for learning the practical skills of emotional competence. The five elements that make up emotional intelligence are as follows:

1. Self-awareness is the ability to recognize and understand one's moods, emotions, and drives, as well as their effect on others.
2. Self-regulation is the ability to handle emotions so they facilitate rather than interfere with the work to be done. People with this ability are conscientious, able to delay gratification to pursue goals, able to control or redirect disruptive impulses and moods, and prone to suspend judgment and to think before acting.
3. Motivation is a passion to engage in work for reasons that go beyond money or status. It leads to a propensity to pursue goals with energy and to persevere in the face of setbacks and frustrations.
4. Empathy is the ability to understand the emotional makeup of other people. It allows a person to develop rapport with a broad diversity of people and to treat them according to their own emotional reactions.
5. Social skill is a proficiency in managing relationships and building networks. People with this skill can read social situations accurately and find common ground and build rapport.

Recent variations in the descriptions of emotional intelligence (EI) have raised concerns for some scholars. Some believe that the significance of EI has been overstated because of the lack of evidence supporting the relationship between emotional intelligence and workplace success (Vitello-Cicciu, 2002). Despite the criticisms of the lack of conceptual clarity and overriding behaviors, the basic notion of EI continues to enlighten many leaders about the complexities of emotions and their impact on the workplace. By its nature, emotional intelligence is a complex phenomenon subsuming theories of emotion, motivation, behavior, intelligence, organizational behavior, and neuroscience. The intersections and overlapping of one's feelings, sense of purpose, knowledge, and attitude vary widely and often unpredictably. New perspectives and new approaches to further engagement and expertise in relationship building can still be learned from the study of the emotional intelligence literature.

Emotional competence, like other kinds of competence, is the possession of certain skills, learned or unlearned. As indicated previously, emotional intelligence, like other kinds of intelligence, is the potential to learn new skills. Thus, a person who has emotional intelligence has the potential to learn how to be emotionally competent, whereas a person who has emotional competence already possesses a fair number of the appropriate skills.

Character

The term *character* is ambiguous. First, it can refer to the aggregate of features and traits that form the individual nature of a given person. The term has that meaning in such sentences as "What is her character?" and "He has a bad character." The term can also be used as a synonym for moral fortitude, as when we tell someone, "Show some character." To say that a person has character in this latter sense is to say that the person has the moral fortitude and discipline to exemplify the highest virtues of his or her time.

Integrity

Integrity is the quality of being morally upright and always acting openly and honestly. Individuals who have integrity consistently act on their own values in all situations and do not hide critical information, break promises, or fail to fulfill commitments. Commitment to the journey that requires leaders to be emotionally competent and fully engaged is not always valued. Significant pressures emphasize the technical work of strategic planning, budgeting, and controlling. Time and energy to develop relationships or the soft side of leadership are viewed as luxuries, given that they are not believed to be necessarily related to the net income margin. Developing the people skills of leadership—regardless of which label or attribute is attached to them—provides the most effective vehicle for sustained learning to occur through the recognized power of the collective emotions of the team. It is through people's full engagement with their work that the measurable, sustainable results of satisfaction, quality outcomes, and strong net income margins are achieved. Organizations continue to struggle not only to recognize the quantifiable value of emotional competence but also to inexorably link these attributes to technical leadership processes. Continual reinforcement and demonstration of these relationships is a never-ending process for engaged and enlightened leaders.

Emotional Risks of Leadership

All leadership decisions are inherently uncertain and have the potential for error. But even if a leader fully understands that mistakes are unavoidable and accepts that he or she will make some wrong decisions, the emotional impact of making an error can be devastating. Historically, leadership education programs have offered participants little preparation for managing miscalculations and missteps. The emphasis has been on success, not failure.

The emotional effects of failure that leaders face on a daily basis cannot be eliminated. They can only be managed. In essence, the reputation of the leader is continually at stake. To manage emotional risk, leaders need a high level of emotional competence, including self-awareness, compassion, passionate optimism, and resilience. They typically must use their emotional competence to deal with issues such as lack of feedback, inconsistency in the reactions of stakeholders, and employment insecurity, all of which have the power to cause confusion and emotional turmoil.

Lack of Feedback

Honest feedback given to a leader and recognition for work accomplished fuel the leader's passion for doing his or her job. Both are highly valued and sought after by most leaders (and also by most employees). On the reverse side, a lack of performance feedback causes stress and undermines the leader's confidence. So does a lack of acknowledgment from a supervisor, whether positive or negative. Not knowing where he or she stands with the supervisor is emotionally draining.

In addition, the more uncertain the leader becomes about his or her performance (because of the lack of feedback), the more likely the leader is to lose confidence in his or her decision-making ability and the more likely the supervisor is to continue to withhold feedback, leading to a cycle of uncertainty and negative emotions. Failure to create the ideal team, to achieve clinical goals, or to meet financial targets results in damage to a leader's ego. In such cases, timely feedback is critical to reversing negative outcomes, learning from the undesired outcomes, and relieving the leader's emotional stress.

Inconsistent Feedback

Imagine that the patient care standards committee develops a plan for patient restraint management with the intent of ensuring patient safety and meeting regulatory requirements. When the plan is presented to the medical staff committees, the medical committee quickly reviews and approves the plan, but the surgical committee recommends numerous revisions and withholds its endorsement. The leader of the patient care standards committee, faced with such different stakeholder responses, is likely to feel confused as well as less confident in his or her abilities. Yet the leader should keep in mind that, all too often, actions that are successful in one situation are disastrous in others, with no apparent explanation. In other words, the wide-ranging responses that different individuals or groups can have to the same action might appear as an impenetrable mystery that challenges a leader's ability to lead, but in such situations it is healthy to avoid being overly self-critical and to minimize the emotional insult. The best strategy is to focus on the context of the actions and reactions and to recognize that the values and goals of the stakeholders can vary widely, resulting in widely differing responses. In the case at hand, the leader's task includes not just creating an appropriate plan but understanding and managing the context in which the plan is proposed.

Employment Insecurity

In the typical organization, leaders serve at the will of the organization and can be removed without much notice or explanation. An employment contract helps in managing the processes of separation, but it cannot prevent the emotional damage that results from the removal. Regardless of the health of the individual's ego, the experience is devastating. Expecting a leader to view the discharge as a business decision and not as a personal judgment is insulting and dishonest. Whenever someone's professional relationships are severed, membership in an organizational team is canceled, or income is eliminated, it is, in fact, very personal.

Being discharged from a job or position often results in serious emotional trauma. In fact, heightened sensitivity to the experience can be seen as the downside of emotional competence. If the leader avoided all feelings and emotions, he or she actually could view the discharge simply as a business issue. The reality is that situations that negatively affect any part of an individual's life are personal and often painful. Compounding the problem for healthcare leaders is that people in health care are expected to provide care rather than receive care. Thus, it is very difficult for them to handle being in need of support, sympathy, and compassion.

Although the emotional effects of uncertainty and employment insecurity are not unique to health care, the values of providers, especially the importance they place on caregiving, cause them to have heightened emotional sensitivity and often heightened vulnerability to emotional upset. Among the consequences are that providers, especially those who are emotionally incompetent, are predisposed to experience great stress, suffer a loss of confidence and passion, and feel incredible turmoil and disappointment. The solution to being exposed to emotional risk is to develop significant emotional competence. In addition, a leader undergoing an employment crisis can mitigate the resulting depression and sense of devastation by keeping in mind his or her skills and abilities and past performance and achievements.

Benefits of Emotional Competence in Health Care

The soft stuff—meaning and emotions—does make a difference in health care. That is not a controversial claim. But leaders are often unsure how the value of the soft stuff can be substantiated and translated into organizational effectiveness and a better bottom line. Traditionally, leaders have examined care delivery from a purely technical perspective. However, the processes involved in providing care encompass both technical (quantitative) and human-related (qualitative) attributes. Thus, a holistic perspective, one that includes quantitative and qualitative measures, is needed for evaluating care delivery.

Leaders know that technical skills are necessary for producing products and services and are essential for success. Leaders also know that defined goal-directed (intentional) behaviors are essential. More recently, they have begun to realize that the relationships among members of the organization have an impact on effectiveness. Yet all too often they fail to see the interconnections between the technical aspect of work, the intentional aspect of work, and the relationships among the workers. Only when leaders integrate the workers' essential technical skills, their goal-directed activities, and their ability to form meaningful relationships does optimal organizational effectiveness result (see Figure 10-1). In addition, treating the work to be accomplished as a nonreducible unit of service shifts the evaluation focus from the parts to the whole, where it properly belongs.

Group Discussion

The three components of integrated leadership—the technical, relational, and intentional—offer a framework for optimizing the use of resources. In a recent committee meeting, a new benefit for child care was introduced and added to the benefits package at the request of an influential board member. The benefit offers a fixed per diem reimbursement amount to pay for child care provided to the children of employees. It is uncertain whether employees are interested in or will use this benefit. It is also uncertain how the value of this benefit will be assessed. Analyze the addition of this benefit from the perspective of the three components of integrated leadership. That is, identify the technical, relational, and intentional considerations that pertain to it. Based on the discussion of these considerations, recommend whether to add the benefit or reject its inclusion into the benefits package.

The value of emotional competence is evident in nearly every interaction in an organization. For instance, effective leaders possess a high degree of self-awareness, compassion for others, self-control, resilience, and passionate optimism, and this powerful combination enables them to achieve the most challenging goals and enlist others in completing the organization's work. Yet it is difficult not only for the leaders themselves to measure the value of passion and emotional competence but also for board members, who tend to neglect these in the selection of CEOs, especially where the financial stakes are substantial.

Focused Hiring

Increasing evidence exists that choosing a leader should involve more than finding the candidate with the best history of financial performance, stock pricing, expense management, merger experience, and workforce reductions. Many boards, however, still believe that if a candidate's achievements are notable, especially in the financial area, they cannot go wrong in hiring that candidate. The problem with this strategy is that many hard-nosed number crunchers are emotionally inept, and because they are—because they fail to listen to others, develop meaningful relationships, share honest feelings, and empathize with others—their leadership can harm organizational performance rather than improve it. In particular, their way of handling subordinates might easily cause an increase in turnover and a decrease in market share and net income. Cases in which this has occurred confirm a relationship between the emotional competence of an organization's leader (soft stuff) and the organization's financial measures (hard stuff).

The cost of turnover continues to be a challenge. In many job categories the cost of turnover and replacement for one position exceeds $50,000. With healthcare annual turnover rates averaging 15% to 20%, the annualized costs are significant. In addition, although many organizations assume the greatest turnover is at the staff level, in fact the greatest turnover is at the middle management level.

Researchers found that the staged encounters of the formal interview process seldom reveal the real nature of any job applicant. Finding an applicant with the right fit requires spending extensive time evaluating the most promising candidates before hiring. Then, once the candidate with the greatest potential for success is selected, extensive time is required to integrate him or her into the organization. Recent evidence indicates that the more time spent with the candidates before hiring, the more likely the candidate with the best fit is hired, the less likely that person is to leave the organization, and, as the new hire becomes more acculturated over the first year, the greater the job satisfaction he or she experiences. New interviewing processes and different types of questions are needed to identify the chemistry between an applicant and the members of the organization (**Exhibit 10-2**).

Exhibit 10-2   Interviewing for Emotional Competence

These questions are asked of both the candidate and the representatives in the current work environment. Interviewing team members compare responses for consistency and fit with the organization.

Directions: Select the most appropriate response.

	Strongly Disagree	Disagree	Agree	Strongly Agree
1. Does the candidate have the ability to manage disappointment?	❑	❑	❑	❑
2. Does the candidate listen to others' ideas?	❑	❑	❑	❑
3. Does the candidate value the contributions of team members?	❑	❑	❑	❑
4. Does the candidate hold others accountable for their performance and promises?	❑	❑	❑	❑
5. Is the candidate comfortable delegating important tasks to others?	❑	❑	❑	❑
6. Does the candidate energize others?	❑	❑	❑	❑
7. Does the candidate spend time communicating the organization's vision and purpose?	❑	❑	❑	❑
8. Do members of the organization trust the promises of the candidate?	❑	❑	❑	❑
9. Is the candidate interested in the concerns of employees?	❑	❑	❑	❑
10. Does the candidate share information willingly and in a timely manner?	❑	❑	❑	❑

Improved Succession Planning

Another opportunity for leaders to use emotional competence is in succession planning. Currently, there seems to be a lack of qualified or committed candidates for healthcare leadership positions, and consequently organizations are wise to increase their efforts to ensure that the integrated skill sets of all management hires, not just the top leaders, are consistent with their needs. Because lower-level managers become candidates for leadership positions in the future, the skill sets and characteristics desired for these positions should be clearly defined and shared within the organization.

Successful leaders have a tendency to encourage their heirs apparent to model their behaviors, failing to recognize these behaviors will become outdated by the time current leaders resign. The challenges of each upcoming generation are different, and so the best strategy is to create new pathways bridging the generations rather than to expect later generations to conform to the values of earlier ones. Attempts to clone current leaders can only hold back organizations from moving into the future. As an example, retirement-age leaders who are currently instilling the principles of the command-and-control model into their likely successors may prevent the new leaders from traveling the same pathway as their peers (i.e., keep them from using more participative models, focusing on short-term goals, and eliminating middle-management positions through technological innovations).

The incongruence of traditional healthcare leadership values with the values of the emerging generation of leaders may explain the common concern that talented leaders are being attracted to industries other than health care. Generational management is about understanding the meaning of the work for individuals of different generations. It is a form of diversity management—integrating the different beliefs and values of different age groups and not negating the beliefs and values of the emerging generation or attempting to make them conform to those of past generations. Emotionally competent succession planning allows current and aspiring leaders to make the skill sets of emotional competence, specifically self-awareness and passionate optimism, a permanent part of the organization. It ensures that the feelings of individuals in the organization and the community are not suppressed out of concern for marketplace values.

Higher Productivity

Significant opportunities for increased productivity exist when emotional competence becomes an attribute not just of individual members but of the entire team. Given that the real work of an organization occurs within a team framework, the greater the ability of team members to truly work together, the greater the positive impact on organizational performance. Note that working together involves more than cooperation, participation, and commitment to goals. The team members must exhibit self-awareness, compassion, passionate optimism, and impulse regulation if they are to achieve their desired outcomes. According to Druskat and Wolff (2001), team success lies in the fundamental conditions that allow effective task processes to emerge and cause members to engage in these processes wholeheartedly. Three conditions—trust among members, a sense of group identity, and a sense of group efficacy—are essential to effectiveness. Without these, teams simply go through the motions of cooperating and participating, and members hold back rather than fully engage, reducing the level of effectiveness.

Healthcare teams that recognize the interconnectedness of members and acknowledge the unique contributions of each to the delivery of services make substantial contributions to the achievement of organizational goals. Specifically, they help improve patient care outcomes, implement strategies in a shorter time, apply new knowledge as it becomes available, use organizational resources more productively, problem solve more creatively, and manage work processes more effectively. According to Orsburn, Moran, Musselwhite, and Zenter (1990), most organizations experience a 20% to 40% increase in productivity when employees are deeply involved in their work.

Selecting and mentoring individuals for team membership using the principles of emotional competence reinforce the benefits of effective teams. The goal is to select members who are not just team players but who also bring to the team varied interests and skills. To do this, it is helpful to look at the results of self-assessment exercises used to assist members in learning about themselves and other team members. These exercises can provide information about behavior patterns and the filters people use in their interactions with others. Understanding the unique characteristics of different team members facilitates the team's work and makes it timelier. Information on the following usually can be easily obtained:

- *Decision-making style:* Some individuals consider information and ideas objectively and logically, whereas others tend to be more subjective and value oriented.
- *Motivation:* Some individuals are energized by dealing with the outside world and thrive on personal interactions, whereas others are more comfortable thinking and reflecting and are disinclined to share an idea until comfortable with it.
- *Values:* Some individuals require facts and step-by-step processes and focus on the present, whereas others are more comfortable with insights and intuitions and focus on the future.
- *Orientation to outside information:* Many individuals strive for control and want as much information as they can get, whereas others tend to be comfortable with little information and letting things happen.

If all the team members are aware of each other's behavior patterns, interests, and background, the team will work together more effectively and plan for future membership. For instance, if a behavior pattern is missing from the team (e.g., the reflective pattern mentioned under "motivation" in the previous list), the team can try to identify candidates who possess it. The team can also target candidates likely to offer a range of ideas or have the skills to facilitate the team's work.

In addition to providing guidance in the selection of members, emotional competence increases the probability that team members will hear each other's concerns and understand each other's feelings. By taking time to consider matters from each member's perspective before making a decision, the team, besides being able to incorporate the different perspectives into the final decision, recognizes each member's importance, thereby improving the members' morale and willingness to cooperate. This process is very different from calling for a majority vote in the interest of expedience. Teams with high levels of emotional competence understand that consideration of the views of each member is a requisite of sustainable decisions. They try to obtain a consensus rather than majority agreement to ensure that all team members are behind the decision. The intent is never to remove the emotion from the process, but rather to give every member a hearing to create trust and ultimately foster greater participation among members.

Group Discussion

Giving feedback upward is the same as giving feedback downward or sideways (to peers), provided you establish an explicit contract with your boss to do so. The CEO of your organization has scheduled a leadership retreat at a time when the staffing is seriously low. The topic of staffing does not appear to be of interest to the senior leaders or at least is of less concern to them than other topics. Together with your team, create a plan to discuss this situation with the CEO. The goal is to give feedback to the CEO, a person with more power, authority, and/or experience than you. In the best case scenario, the feedback will enhance the effectiveness of the retreat and ultimately improve the organization's performance. The risk is that the feedback may be rejected by the CEO and may negatively affect your relationship with the CEO. You can use the following list of steps to guide your preparation for the "coaching upward" meeting:

1. Describe the situation (topic).
2. Agree on the specific objective of the session.
3. Share your assessment of the situation. Why is a change needed? How will the CEO benefit from the change? How will the organization benefit from the change?
4. Validate your assumptions with the CEO. Ask for comments.
5. Invite suggestions from the CEO.
6. Suggest possible solutions. Cover the full range of options.
7. Select a course of action.
8. Agree on the course of action. Identify the time frame for the expected change.
9. Identify specific steps to achieve the change.
10. Commit to action. Thank the CEO for his or her willingness to examine the issues and work to make the organization more effective.

Coaching Upward

Coaching is a valued method of developing skills, but it traditionally has been used almost exclusively by superiors to assist those below them. The most challenging type of coaching—and the one ordinarily overlooked—involves providing feedback to those individuals with greater authority. As the members of an organization become more emotionally competent, coaching upward becomes less challenging and is embraced more readily. Once the halo of infallibility is removed from the most powerful positions in the organization, those in other positions can use the skills of coaching upward to give appropriate feedback, often averting serious negative outcomes as a result.

People generally appreciate constructive, timely, and sensitively delivered feedback that can be put to practical use. Despite this, people who give feedback frequently are tentative and unsure that what they are doing is appropriate. Giving feedback completes the circle of communication and further advances the work of the organization in a positive manner.

Developing Emotional Competence

Effective and accomplished leaders are often referred to as "born leaders" based on the belief that leadership skills are inherent or learned at an early age. Although some leaders may indeed have natural leadership ability, those who are not born leaders can acquire the necessary skills, including those that make up emotional competence. These latter skills, however, cannot be obtained by attending a one-day workshop. Rather, their development requires focused coaching, time, and experience.

Exhibit 10-3 presents a five-stage model of development based on the Dreyfus and Dreyfus (1996) skill acquisition model as a framework for understanding how leaders obtain emotional competence incrementally. Each of the five skill levels is described to assist readers in assessing their own level of emotional competence and in continuing to mature toward the highest skill level. The following subsections describe the levels of emotional competence in more detail, and behaviors that demonstrate emotional incompetence that individuals sometimes exhibit and should seek to eliminate are discussed in an upcoming section.

Novice Stage

In the first stage, the individual, despite having formal education in leadership, has no experience in the application of leadership knowledge and skills. The novice is a detached observer of the processes of leadership and, in regard to emotional competence, has at most a personal awareness of interaction styles and behavior patterns.

Advanced Beginner Stage

The advanced beginner is finally engaged in a leadership role, testing the knowledge and skills gained during formal education. The focus is on developing competence in coaching and mentoring and in relationship building. Although the advanced beginner's level of self-awareness is increasing, his or her main goal is to demonstrate personal competence and ensure satisfactory work. The advanced beginner is starting to think about group processes and how to integrate the emotions of others but is not always certain of the connections between an event and another's emotional reaction.

The advanced beginner spends little time or attention on understanding the reactions of others in the setting. Also, he or she is not always open to the ideas of others and tends to be judgmental. The advanced beginner is starting to become more confident as a decision maker but is discouraged easily and is not always optimistic about the future.

Competent Stage

In the third stage, the individual is more experienced as a leader and is beginning to develop compassion for others. The individual can think about issues and simultaneously have feelings and acknowledge the feelings of others. He or she also now develops the ability to be present physically and mentally, attend to conversations with authenticity, and listen to and ask questions of team members with sensitivity to their emotions.

The individual is increasingly compassionate and open to the ideas of others and is less judgmental than previously. He or she also exhibits a greater ability to control impulses and begins to feel comfortable challenging the status quo.

Exhibit 10-3   Individual Emotional Competence Skill Levels and Behaviors

- Novice (detached observer)
  - Formally educated in the principles of emotional competence
  - Aware of personal interaction styles and behavior patterns
  - Has not held a formal leadership position
- Advanced beginner (active participant)
  - Has increasing self-awareness but limited openness to the ideas of others
  - Tends to be judgmental
  - Has increasing confidence in ability to participate and make decisions
  - Begins to think and feel simultaneously; not always certain of the meaning of events or if there is a connection between an event and another's emotional reaction
  - Is easily discouraged and not always optimistic about the future
- Competent (integrated with the process)
  - Has emerging compassion for others
  - Exhibits authentic presence in teamwork; listens actively and critically to others
  - Is able to think and feel simultaneously and acknowledge the feelings of others
  - Gives both positive and negative feedback (a requirement of effective communication)
  - Is increasingly open to others' ideas
  - Gains comfort in challenging the status quo
  - Begins to develop the ability to control impulses
- Proficient (therapeutic engagement)
  - Has emerging sense of optimism and ability to manage negative emotions
  - Is able to read or experience chemistry between people (e.g., recognizes allies, identifies who to trust, and recognizes nonsupport or hostility)
  - Understands the meaning of relationships
  - Has a positive but realistic attitude; believes in the team's ability to accomplish the work to be done
  - Believes integrity is an essential characteristic
  - Has emerging passion for the process and the relationships among team members
  - Inspires others with passionate spirit and commitment
  - Begins to develop resilience to negative events
  - Exhibits increasing impulse control
- Expert (dialogic engagement)
  - Demonstrates self-awareness and utilizes self-assessment information to improve personal performance and to support and understand team members
  - Possesses strong resilience to the negative realities of the workplace and coaches others in developing similar skills; able to manage difficult information
  - Is able to think and feel simultaneously
  - Is open to others' ideas and viewpoints
  - Actively seeks opinions from team members on their task processes, progress, and performance
  - Actively coaches and mentors new members as well as current members
  - Exhibits well-developed impulse control

Proficient Stage

Team leaders often hit an invisible wall at the competent stage and do not make it to the proficient stage. If this happens, the teamwork becomes rote and frequently is ineffective. Long-standing teams that meet without adding value to healthcare outcomes fit this category.

A team leader who reaches the proficient stage is noticeably more comfortable in the role and has a better grasp of the influence of relationships on team activities. The proficient leader can think and feel simultaneously and read the chemistry among people, recognize allies, identify who to trust, and sense where nonsupport or hostility is present. This leader is beginning to develop the ability to manage negative feelings and is generally optimistic, including about the team's ability to accomplish its work. Only rarely is the individual discouraged or negative about the future. Passionate optimism—the integration of a positive outlook and wholehearted commitment—becomes the norm. Finally, the proficient leader has increasing control over impulses and is developing resilience in the face of difficulties or crises.

Expert Stage

The leader at the expert stage uses self-assessment information to improve personal performance and to support the other members of the team. Thinking and feeling simultaneously is the only way the expert leader knows how to act. As an accomplished team member, the expert leader not only is open to new ideas but also seeks input from others. The expert leader actively coaches and mentors new members as well as current members in developing expert emotional competence skills. As a passionate optimist, the expert leader is highly resilient and at the same time possesses sophisticated impulse control.

Emotionally Incompetent Behaviors

In journeying toward full emotional competence, people exhibit behaviors indicative of emotional incompetence. Given that incompetence is often easier to describe than competence, the following examples of emotional incompetence are presented as a means of indicating what emotional competence is.

Acting as Devil's Advocate

All too often, people consider an issue or situation from the self-appointed position of devil's advocate. In most such cases, people assume this perspective for lack of self-awareness and understanding of their own point of view. They hide behind the role for any number of reasons—usually known only to them. Common reasons include lack of information, inability to support an idea while unsure how to express nonsupport, and desire to block the decision-making process.

Displaying a Bad Attitude

People who have a difficult time participating in work processes often display negative behaviors ranging from grumbling to shirking. They usually do not understand that such behaviors impede progress and decrease the overall morale of the group, or, if they do, they might refuse to acknowledge the effects of their actions on others or dismiss their behavior by claiming, "That's just the way I am."

Displaying a Superior Attitude

An individual with a superior attitude responds to comments with indignation and criticism. The individual also usually does not recognize the adversarial nature of his or her responses and their impact on others but views them as a necessary means for getting the entire group to understand its inadequacies.

Tolerating Errors

Tolerating errors or undesirable behaviors implies these are accepted. In many cases, the tolerance results from the inability of those in charge to react and correct the errors or behaviors and/or the organizational culture's lack of support for managing problematic behaviors. When an individual fails to meet the relevant behavioral standards, managers and others in the organization must use the situation as an opportunity to reinforce the organizational culture and build better relationships.

Failing to Balance Work and Relaxation

Often leaders find themselves spending more time at work and less time at home, believing that the operation of the organization is more important than other priorities. Further, they commonly believe their presence is required for productivity to occur. They thus wind up spending excessive hours at work and neglect the other parts of their lives, including recreating with family and friends. The focus on work tasks is characteristic of the advanced beginner level of emotional competence, whereas achieving a balance between work and family and community is characteristic of the expert level.

Team Emotional Competence

In creating team-level emotional competence, a team builds on the skills of the individual members and extends the focus to itself as a collective. The assumption is that the members have at least a basic understanding of team processes such as goal setting, agenda management, and communication. It is through these processes that the team members begin to feel confidence in each other and in the team as a whole, reinforcing successful team behaviors. Team emotional competence, like the individual variety, usually is developed incrementally in a five-stage process (**Exhibit 10-4**).

Novice Stage

A novice team consists of individuals coming together for the first time for a newly defined purpose. The members know very little, if anything, about each other and typically do not share common feelings or values—or if they do, they are not aware of their commonalities at this point. A novice team's focus is on understanding the purpose of the team and setting the ground rules.

Exhibit 10-4   Team Emotional Competence Skill Levels and Behaviors

- Novice (detached observer)
  - Team is newly formed and consists of independent participants.
  - Members have no prior relationships with or knowledge of behavior patterns and emotions of other members.
- Advanced beginner (active participant)
  - Group guidelines are developed and understood by members (this transition stage reflects the shift from the use of individual power to integrated goals and unified or shared support for goals).
  - Group cohesion is beginning to develop.
  - Team is mainly focused on meeting processes.
  - Team behavior patterns are beginning to emerge.
  - At times, the team is overwhelmed and easily discouraged.
- Competent (integrated with the process)
  - Members are increasingly self-aware and sensitive to communication dynamics between members.
  - Team establishes realistic ground rules.
  - Members understand each other's skills and emotions.
  - Team routinely requests feedback from every member at the beginning and the end of the meetings.
  - Outcomes of the team's work are evident.
- Proficient (therapeutic engagement)
  - Team members understand the goals of the team and the relationship of their work to that of other teams in the organization.
  - Team members seek feedback from others in the organization following team meetings and bring feedback to the next meeting.
  - Team is passionate about its work and optimistic that it can make a difference.
  - Team shows tolerance for character failings.
- Expert (dialogic engagement)
  - Team members understand the team's goals and how they relate to the organization and community at large.
  - Team consists of experienced and mature members.
  - Team is able to integrate local and national regulations into its work.
  - Team often makes recommendations and moves beyond its specific assigned tasks to create better options for the organization.
  - Team terminates itself when it is unable to add further value to the organization.

Advanced Beginner Stage

In this stage, the team becomes more cohesive through establishing how to carry out meeting tasks such as setting agendas, recording the minutes, and ensuring that the ground rules are defined and followed. Jockeying for power often occurs at this level, but it tends to end once the team develops feedback skills and gets into the habit of recognizing the contributions of each member. The team makes a conscious and deliberate effort to (1) shift from valuing power as traditionally used to foster empowerment and (2) develop an awareness of the behavior patterns of each member. However, the members evidence little openness toward substantive ideas and dialogue. Their focus is on task completion and agenda management. They also are discouraged easily and are uncertain as to their ability to create meaningful change.

Competent Stage

A competent team is a compassionate team, and its compassion is reflected in its willingness to discuss every member's issues of concern. The team members have moved from trying to acquire individual power to acting as an authentic collective. They not only show themselves capable of thinking and feeling simultaneously, but also acknowledge each other's feelings and integrate them into the team's overall work. In addition, they set and follow ground rules that are realistic and support the team's work. The coaching and mentoring they do with each other are intended to foster behaviors that aid the team, rather than to develop skills that are useful only outside of the team. Finally, the team's level of trust in itself grows, and the members begin to challenge the status quo and consider alternatives to the way things are currently done.

As with individual emotional competence, there is often an invisible wall between the competent and proficient stages. Teams at the competent stage can meet the requirements for standard success but find it impossible to become passionately optimistic while re-creating the future or to maintain resilience in the face of negative events. They accomplish the assigned work but seldom move beyond the assigned boundaries.

Proficient Stage

As the emotional skills of the team mature, the team develops a sense of passionate optimism about the future. A proficient team differs from a competent team in considering the needs and priorities of the whole organization as integral to its work. All the members are aware of and understand each other's behavior patterns and use these patterns in developing a consensus on issues, encouraging each other to discuss difficult issues, and addressing the emotions that these issues tend raise. At this stage, the team members recognize each other's character failings as inevitable and work to restore the integrity of relationships.

Expert Stage

For a team to arrive at the expert level of emotional competence is a highly desirable but rare event. An expert team is purposefully coached and mentored and requires ongoing support and validation if it is to be sustained. At this level of performance, the team not only embodies all the characteristics of the proficient team but also considers the needs and priorities of the organization and the healthcare community and ensures that proposed team actions are congruent with the organization's culture and politics.

The members are aware of individual, team, and organizational emotions as an interactive whole. As a team, they have established norms that strengthen their ability to respond effectively to the kind of emotional challenges a group confronts on a regular basis. These norms are directed toward three goals: creating resources for working with emotions, fostering an affirmative environment, and encouraging proactive problem solving. In addition, the expert team embodies resilience to the realities of the environment. Finally, the team members, besides being individually aware of their inward- and outward-directed emotions and able to regulate them, jointly develop a level of group mindfulness.

Causes of Team Dysfunction

Teams that have existed for a long time commonly acquire behavior patterns that can render them inefficient or nonproductive. For instance, they often leave assignments incomplete, allow malcontents to continue griping, pay scant notice to habitual tardiness and absenteeism, and go off on tangents that have little to do with their intended work. Each team has a natural life span, and when its work is completed it should be disbanded or assigned another project.

It is also important to realize that a team may move along the developmental trajectory at an irregular rate and may even regress, such as when its membership and goals change. Further, it is common for a team's development to inexplicably halt before the proficiency stage, in which case the team never gets to the point of integrating its work with that of the organization, much less with the environment or the community at large.

To see how team development can be arrested, consider the breach between senior healthcare leaders and point-of-service providers that occurred after the implementation of managed care. As the reimbursement systems changed and the actual dollars paid to organizations decreased dramatically, significant expense reductions were needed. Nonetheless, in many cases the actual work increased. The point-of-service workers ranted and raved about the impact on quality and staff morale, yet the leaders demanded more and more expense reductions as external reimbursement continued to decline. The rift between staff and management widened, with little hope of relief.

Before the reimbursement levels were reduced, healthcare teams, although not yet at the proficiency level, were aware of the needs and feelings of all individuals, and their emotional performance could be rated as competent. Their work had two focuses: providing high-quality patient care and maximizing reimbursement. When reimbursement decreased, the teams fell even further short of taking into account the goals of all members (or the goals of the organization as a whole) and thus never reached the proficiency level.

In many ways the course of events described resembles Levy's (2001) Nut Island effect. The Nut Island story is about a team of competent, highly committed employees who performed a vital behind-the-scenes task. The team was adept at organizing and managing itself. Its self-sufficiency was taken for granted by senior management, and when it asked for help or tried to warn of impending trouble, it was ignored or put off because senior management, looking at its history of success, would assume it could handle the current situation. Consequently, an adversarial relationship began to develop between senior management and the team. Unfortunately, the team reacted in a way that worsened the problem. The team made it a priority to stay out of management's line of sight, which led it to deny or minimize problems and avoid asking for help. Eventually, the team began to make up its own rules to enable it to fulfill its own mission—apart from the mission of the organization as a whole.

At this point, both senior management and the team had distorted views that were very difficult to correct. The team members believed they were the only ones who really understood their work and were unwilling to listen to outsiders attempting to help solve their problems. Management remained disconnected, believing that no news was good news. Only a significant external event could change the course of events. Neither the senior managers nor the team members considered the meaning of their work within the context of the entire organization or the marketplace. As a result, the team's level of emotional competence decreased dramatically.

Connecting with Generations of Workers

Workforce composition has always included different generations of workers and varying beliefs, values, and expectations. The emotionally competent leader recognizes the impact of each generation and works to understand the defining characteristics of each and ensure that all are respected. Too often, the generation of the leader is proffered as the only acceptable behavior for all generations. Each generation is characterized by historical, political, and social events that share core values, work ethics, and economic movements of its members. The collective personality of each generation serves as a reference point from which to comprehend how life experiences affect core values and influence one's work. Generalizations of worker profiles should be avoided, given that the traits are often overlapping between generations and anecdotal. Current workforces include four generations: matures or traditionalists born between 1922 and 1945; baby boomers born between 1946 and 1964; generation Xers born between 1965 and 1978; and generation Yers born between 1979 and the present (Hart, 2006).

Group Discussion

The Nut Island story (described in the text) encompasses a number of issues, including lack of teamwork, insensitivity to a team's context, and disharmony between the feelings of individuals in the local setting (the team members) and individuals at the system level (the senior managers). Can you use this story to elucidate adversarial relationships that exist between leaders and departments in your organization? If so, identify at least three strategies to mitigate the friction or hostility between the parties using emotional competence as the framework. What outcomes would you select as measures of the effectiveness of these strategies?

Measuring Emotional Competence

Most healthcare organizations know how to measure and document clinical outcomes, financial results, and market share. Most, however, are very uncomfortable assessing factors such as behavior patterns, compassion, passionate optimism, and impulse control. The reality is that individuals tend to measure what they are comfortable with and ignore those areas they are not comfortable measuring. Given that at least four characteristics have been identified that reflect emotional competence, individuals and groups have the opportunity to measure their level of competence in handling their own and others' feelings.

Exhibit 10-5   Reputation Assessment and Management Survey

1. Am I trustworthy?
2. To what extent do I trust others?
3. Do I practice what I preach?
4. Do I tell people who need to know what I am thinking and why I am acting in a particular way?
5. Am I dependable?
6. Do I listen nondefensively?
7. Am I able to find the grain of truth embedded in a criticism?
8. Am I visible and available when things are not going well?
9. Am I perceived as a hard worker?
10. Do I value the contributions of team members?

> **Point to Ponder**
>
> The way to gain a good reputation is to endeavor to be what you desire to appear.
>
> —Socrates

First, individual leaders should consider developing a reputation assessment and management survey (**Exhibit 10-5**) to help them formally manage their reputations. Many forward-thinking leaders have done reputation management informally on the assumption that how others perceive them influences their ability to affect organizational operations. By creating a personal sensitivity process for gathering accurate feedback, a leader can learn about his or her effect on others and gain useful information for developing a reputation management plan. Both self-perceptions and the perceptions of others provide a helpful perspective on one's effectiveness.

Self-knowledge allows leaders to begin the journey toward the highest level of emotional competence. In many organizations, leaders use a 360-degree evaluation to gain additional information about their leadership abilities. Although feedback from superiors, peers, and subordinates is important, the source of the feedback must be identified to reinforce the importance of trust and honest communication. Further, such assessments need to contain items for measuring behaviors and characteristics that reflect emotional competence, including self-awareness, compassion, passionate optimism, self-regulation, and resilience.

To help measure the emotional competence of teams, specific items related to self-awareness, compassion, passionate optimism, self-regulation, and resilience should be included in employee satisfaction and patient satisfaction surveys. The integration of individual and team information provides an overview of the emotional competence of the organization.

Conclusion

We live in complex times. To be successful, we need to think and feel simultaneously and to acknowledge our feelings and those of others. The goal of the quantum leader is to learn as much as possible from the past and gracefully and soundly move to more appropriate methods of managing the work of organizations. These methods include acting in ways that are sensitive to people's emotions to increase their active engagement with their work.

The ability to manage feelings is a skill no leader can be without. The first step toward gaining this skill is to understand what is important not only to oneself but also to others in the organization. Ignoring the feelings and behaviors of others is a sure way to impede progress. Although progress is usually incremental at best, quantum leaders always have an eye on the future while holding onto their passionate optimism as a sacred gift.

Case Study 10-1

www

Managing a Team When the Stakes Are High

Mary is the director of case management and has six managers who report to her. In Mary's hospital and healthcare system, case management has a direct interface with the financial department, and Mary reports directly to the chief financial officer (CFO). She also interfaces with the payer side of the business, which includes contract negotiations with various state and federal payers, HMOs, insurers, self-insured employer groups, and the hospital's own self-insured/managed care group. In interfacing with these various groups over the years, Mary has improved her competencies in interprofessional collaboration and negotiation. It hasn't always been easy balancing the needs of the patients with the financial demands of the payer groups, but Mary has astute business skills that position her well in hard-nosed discussions related to cost, profits, quality, and more demand than the system can supply.

The skills of the managers who report to Mary are quite varied. Two of the six have earned their master's degree in nursing and are relatively new to their roles and case management. One of the other direct reports has an MBA and came from the payer side of the business. The other three have been in their roles for a number of years, and although they perform well, they rarely show the initiative to "think outside the box" or advocate for patients when the patient need is not strictly within the prescribed guidelines. These three individuals work well together, but they do not seem to interface well with the other members of their team. When Mary meets with them individually, she hears stories of how they do not trust the other three, who have more education than they do but less experience in case management. In the meetings Mary observes these three and notices that they rarely speak up or contribute unless they are directly asked a question. Their body language and eye contact clearly indicate that they are disengaged from the rest of the group.

On the other hand, the three members of the team with more advanced education and less experience have many questions and need reassurance about their decisions with patients who need special considerations. Although they are eager to make patient-centered decisions, they are uncertain how far they can push the limits in negotiating with payers for additional coverage or equipment for patients. The manager with the MBA is very confident in his skills and is highly regarded by Mary's boss, the CFO. The manager speaks the "financial language" with ease, which impresses the CFO. The two of them often joke and laugh with one another, and clearly a strong relationship has formed. Mary not only observes her manager's very confident demeanor, she also recognizes that he demonstrates a very superior attitude when working with the others on her team. Because of his financial background, he often acts as the devil's advocate when innovative ideas are brought forward for discussion within the group. He has absolutely no tolerance for the three more senior individuals, whom he regards as being unprepared for their roles because of their lack of a master's degree and specifically their lack of financial knowledge. For the most part it seems as if he disregards much of what they say when they occasionally speak up in the team meetings. He often laughs when others are speaking or becomes engaged in other activities such as reading his emails or texts on his mobile phone.

One of the less experienced managers is very sensitive emotionally, and when pushed, it almost seems as if she is ready to cry in the team meetings. Of course, it doesn't take long for the MBA manager to take advantage of her vulnerability and relate to her in ways that increase her level of discomfort. He nitpicks every presentation she makes to the point that it drives her to tears, which appears to be very entertaining to him. Mary has assessed that the sensitive manager has the competencies and knowledge necessary to be successful in the role, but her inability to keep her emotions in control seems to detract from how others perceive her competencies. The CFO has frequently made comments to Mary about how this sensitive manager is the weakest member of the team, which requires Mary to advocate for her on several occasions. The CFO has put subtle pressure on Mary to terminate this individual because he perceives her to be very weak and incompetent. Mary has coached the manager frequently in their individual meetings about her need to develop a stronger "business face" and has tried to determine the underlying cause of the manager's lack of self-confidence because she has significant knowledge and understanding of case management. She has asked the manager to engage in some self-assessment and self-reflection related to her emotional intelligence and to work with the hospital's Employee Resource Center to develop ways to improve her self-confidence and to adapt her behavior in ways that would make her less vulnerable in group situations.

With new requirements and stricter guidelines in place with the hospital's designation as an accountable care organization, Mary's department is pressured to achieve better financial outcomes while also improving patient satisfaction levels. Her department is also held responsible for preventing 30-day readmissions that will penalize the hospital's reimbursement from Medicare. Mary realizes that her only hope for success is to improve the individual functioning of each of her direct reports and to improve the team's ability to work as a high-performing team. It is clear that every member of the team is at a different level of knowledge and experience in case management and at very different levels of emotional intelligence. When Mary assesses her team, she recognizes that she has one bully in the group who is overconfident about his own skills, completely unaware of how he comes across to others, but highly skilled in his financial understanding and case management. At the other end of the continuum, she has an individual who has the knowledge and skills of case management but who lacks self-confidence and is highly sensitive to any criticism or questioning of her knowledge base. The three less educated case managers have formed a subgroup that refuses to engage with the other members of the team because they do not trust the others. It appears that Mary only has one strong manager, who is less experienced in case management, but who demonstrates a high level of emotional intelligence, desire to learn the role, and willingness to engage with all members of the team including the bully. It's clear to Mary that the team is completely dysfunctional and that she needs to develop a strategy to help this group either develop as a highly functioning team or replace some of its members with new individuals who are more willing to work as a team to meet the organization's goals.

Questions

1. How do you feel about Mary's assessment of her direct reports' job competencies and emotional competencies and their ability to work together as a team?
2. If you were Mary, what steps would you take to improve the team's level of functioning?
3. How should Mary manage the bully on her team given that he has the most expert knowledge of the financial side of case management and is highly regarded by Mary's boss, the chief financial officer?
4. What should Mary do to help the manager who is emotionally sensitive and easily brought to tears in the team meetings?
5. If you were Mary, how would you manage the three more experienced individuals who have opted out of the team's membership and who are boycotting any participation in the team meetings?
6. Mary highly values the one manager, who has job knowledge but less experience and who displays the highest level of emotional intelligence. How could Mary ensure her continuing success in her individual role and use her to facilitate growth for the team?
7. Using Goldman's conceptual model of the four elements of emotional intelligence, describe Mary's level of emotional intelligence.

Case Study 10-2

I See You and You See Me, But Do I See Me?

It is absolutely clear to Bob that his colleague Karen has no clue as to how she comes across to others. The two of them are directors in a large metropolitan hospital, and competition among all the directors for resources, recognition from the chief nursing officer (CNO), and the potential for promotion is fierce. Bob really likes Karen and would love to help her gain more insight into her interactions with others and how she perceives herself in these interactions. He has watched her time and again in the Directors Council interrupting others, using sarcastic language, and demonstrating counterproductive body language and facial expressions when others present their perspectives on controversial issues. In Bob's opinion, Karen is a very effective leader for her managers, but he wonders whether she exhibits some of the same behaviors in her meetings with her managers. It seems like Karen's managers are satisfied in their roles and have a good relationship with Karen, but Bob can't be sure. He really is uncertain whether he should speak to Karen about how she is being perceived in the Directors Council, or whether he should just let it go because it isn't really his issue. On the other hand, because of their friendship, Bob feels compelled to try to help Karen gain more self-awareness and read the faces of other individuals around the table for feedback on how they are reacting to her comments and how they perceive her.

The entire director team recently participated in a 360-degree analysis of their individual skills, competencies, and behaviors in their respective roles. Input from their peers, subordinates, and supervisors was received, analyzed, and developed into an overall analysis of their strengths and areas that need to be developed for them to be successful in their roles. Bob is not certain how Karen fared with the 360-degree analysis, but he suspects that some of their peers may have been critical of her behaviors. He wonders whether he should ask Karen to join him for coffee to discuss their respective assessments, but he is not sure if she would value his openness about the situation. Bob is clear that he is not willing to discuss the matter with their boss, the CNO, because he does not perceive her to be a good leader. Although it would be her role to coach Karen and encourage her to use the hospital's resources to improve her self-awareness, Bob fears that the CNO would use the information against Karen.

Bob has spent considerable time reviewing his own results from the 360-degree assessment and has reflected on the positive and negative feedback regarding his own skills competencies. He was pleased that his subordinates perceived him as being a very authentic leader who is committed to the employees, engages them in decisions, and is physically present in both crisis and positive situations. His subordinates perceive him to be very open and easy to engage in conversation and indicated that he values them in their roles as nurses. Although he could not determine where the input came from among the executive team, he was highly rated for his resilience and nimbleness in managing crises and other difficult situations. He seemed to be highly regarded for his character and integrity among his colleagues as well as his subordinates and supervisors. An area that was noted for further development included the need to improve his ability to find a balance between his work and personal life because he was perceived to be a "workaholic," which had affected his personal life adversely. Those who knew Bob well realized that he had recently gone through a separation with his significant other. Other areas that Bob needed to improve were his ability to listen nondefensively when others were critical of his proposals and his ability to identify and develop some of his subordinates for a viable succession plan. Bob recognizes that he has a tendency to do everything himself instead of encouraging others to participate in activities to gain knowledge and experience to prepare them for future leadership roles. Although Bob was busy taking notes about how he could improve his own performance, he was constantly reminded of his dear friend Karen and his uncertainty about how he could most effectively help her to gain more self-awareness and improved emotional intelligence.

Questions

1. How do you think Bob can most effectively help Karen, or do you think that it is none of his business?
2. What level of emotional intelligence do you think that Bob demonstrates in his work with his subordinates, supervisors, and colleagues?
3. What level of emotional intelligence do you think that Karen demonstrates with her colleagues on the Directors Council and with her direct reports?
4. Based on the information provided in this case, how would you assess the CNO's level of emotional intelligence? Based on your assessment, should Bob realistically use her as a resource to coach Karen?
5. Develop a script that Bob might use to talk with Karen and give her feedback about her interactions with her colleagues on the Directors Council.

References

Allen, K. E. (2000). Leadership as an emergent property of individual and group interaction. *Inner Edge*, 3(6), 20–21.

Barker, R. A. (1998). The future of leadership research. *Futures Research Quarterly*, 14(1), 5–16.

Collins, J. (2001). Level 5 leadership: The triumph of humility and fierce resolve. *Harvard Business Review*, 79(1), 67–76.

Dreyfus, H. L., & Dreyfus, S. E. (1996). The relationship of theory and practice in the acquisition of skill. In P. Benner, C. Tanner, & C. A. Chesla (Eds.), *Expertise in nursing practice: Caring, clinical judgment, and ethics* (pp. 29–47). New York, NY: Springer.

Druskat, V. U., & Wolff, S. B. (2001). Building the emotional intelligence of groups. *Harvard Business Review*, 79(3), 81–90.

Gill, R. (2011). *Theory and practice of leadership* (2nd ed.). Thousand Oaks, CA: Sage.

Goleman, D. (1998). *Working with emotional intelligence*. New York, NY: Bantam.

Hart, S. M. (2006). Generational diversity: Impact on recruitment and retention of registered nurses. *Journal of Nursing Administration*, 36(1), 10–12.

Levy, P. F. (2001). The Nut Island effect: When good teams go wrong. *Harvard Business Review*, 79(3), 51–59.

Orsburn, J. D., Moran, J., Musselwhite, E., & Zenter, J. H. (1990). *Self-directed work teams*. Homewood, IL: Business One Irwin.

Russel, P. (1993). *The white hole in time: Our future evolution and the meaning of now*. New York, NY: Harper Collins.

Vitello-Cicciu, J. M. (2002). Exploring emotional intelligence: Implications for nursing leaders. *Journal of Nursing Administration*, 32(4), 203–210.

Suggested Readings

Barsh, J., Cranston, S., & Craske, R. A. (2008). Centered leadership: How talented women thrive. *McKinsey Quarterly*. Retrieved from http://www.mckinsey.com/insights/leading_in_the_21st_century/centered_leadership_how_talented_women_thrive

Bennis, W., & O'Toole, J. (2000). Don't hire the wrong CEO. *Harvard Business Review*, 78(5), 171–176.

Brousseau, K. R., Driver, M. J., Hourihan, G., & Larsson, R. (2006). The seasoned executive's decision-making style. *Harvard Business Review*, 84(2), 111–121.

Buchanan, L. (2004). The young and the restful. *Harvard Business Review, 82*(4), 25.

Contu, D. (2009). Why teams don't work. *Harvard Business Review, 87*(5), 99–105.

Davis, P. D., Hensley, S. L., Muzik, L., Comeau, O., Bell, L., Carroll, A. R., . . . Douglas, M. K. (2012). Enhancing RN professional engagement and contribution: An innovative competency and clinical advancement program. *Nurse Leader, 10*(3), 34–39.

Duchscher, J. E. B. (2004). Multigenerational nurses in the workplace. *Journal of Nursing Administration, 34*(11), 493–501.

Dyer, W. (1976). *Your erroneous zones.* New York, NY: HarperCollins.

Forsyth, S., & Parish, M. (1999). The practical side of emotional intelligence. *Inner Edge, 1*(5) 9–11.

Grayson, M. A. (2005). Generation X, Y, Zzzz. *Journal of Nursing Administration, 35*(7/8), 326–327.

Hansen, M. T. (2009). When internal collaboration is bad for your company. *Harvard Business Review, 87*(4), 83–88.

Hansen, M. T., & von Oetinger, B. (2001). Introducing T-shaped managers: Knowledge management's next generation. *Harvard Business Review, 79*(3), 107–116.

Jones, C., & Gates, M. (2007). The costs and benefits of nurse turnover: A business case for nurse retention. *Online Journal of Issues in Nursing, 12*(3), 2.

Lancaster, L. C., & Stilman, D. (2002). *When generations collide: Who they are, why they clash, how to solve the generational puzzle at work.* New York, NY: HarperCollins.

Mecklenburg, G. A. (2001). Career performance: How are we doing? *Journal of Healthcare Management, 46*(1), 8–13.

Menkes, J. (2005). Hiring for smarts. *Harvard Business Review, 83*(11), 100–108.

Porter-O'Grady, T., & Wilson, C. K. (1998). *The health care team book.* St. Louis, MO: Mosby.

Safian, R. (2012, November). Secrets of the flux leader. *Fast Company,* 96–107.

Sandberg, J. (2001). Understanding competence at work. *Harvard Business Review, 79*(3), 24–28.

Smola, K. W., & Sutton, C. D. (2002). Generational differences: Revisiting generational work values for the new millennium. *Journal of Organizational Behavior, 23*, 363–382.

Vestal, K. (2005). The ugly truth: Some managers are just inept. *Nurse Leader, 3*(4), 11, 16.

Vestal, K. (2012). Which matters: Employee satisfaction or employee engagement? *Nurse Leader, 10*(4), 10–11.

Weick, K., & Sutcliffe, K. (2000, Summer). High reliability: The power of mindfulness. *Leader to Leader, 21*, 33–38.

Wheeler, P. A. (2005, January/February). The importance of interpersonal skills. *Healthcare Executive,* 44–45.

Quiz Questions

Select the best answer for each of the following questions.

1. Emotional competence is based on specific principles. Which one of the following is not consistent with these principles?

   a. Holism

   b. Newtonian principles

   c. Theory Y behaviors

   d. Emergent leadership

2. Leaders have resisted the notion that emotional competence is an essential leadership characteristic. What is the most likely reason for this resistance?

   a. The difficulty of measuring and evaluating the impact of emotional competence
   b. The lack of theoretical support for the concept of emotional competence
   c. The cost of integrating emotionally competent behaviors into an organization
   d. The lack of employee support for the idea that emotional competence is important

3. Which are the four attributes specific to emotional competence?

   a. Self-awareness, integrity, passionate optimism, and compassion
   b. Self-awareness, passionate optimism, character, and impulse control
   c. Self-awareness, compassion, passionate optimism, and emotional intelligence
   d. Self-awareness, compassion, passionate optimism, and character

4. Integrated leadership is a synergistic combination of technical, relational, and intentional skills. What does this combination lead to?

   a. Emotionally competent individuals and leaders
   b. Optimal resource use and positive patient outcomes
   c. Additional costs to the organization
   d. Improved employee satisfaction

5. Self-awareness—the understanding of one's behavior patterns and preferences—is a fundamental characteristic of emotional competence. Among other benefits, which of the following does it lead to?

   a. Passionate optimism and compassion
   b. Impulse control
   c. Openness to others and an appreciation of paradox
   d. Character and integrity

6. The emotional risks of leadership are ever present and cannot be ignored. Which of the following is a source of emotional risk faced by leaders?

   a. The lack of timely feedback
   b. The lack of an employment contract
   c. Unacceptable levels of employee dissatisfaction
   d. Sharing decision making with team members

7. Emergent leadership is one of the underpinnings of emotional competence. How does emergent leadership differ from the dyadic model of leadership?

   a. The organizational chart for emergent leadership is a matrix.
   b. Emergent leadership eliminates the need for a CEO.
   c. Emergent leadership is based on the principle that high levels of organizational performance depend on the presence of a strong leader who defines the work of the organization.
   d. Emergent leadership is based on the principle that high levels of organizational performance depend on the engagement of the members in the work of the organization.

8. Impulse control is one of the hallmarks of the emotionally competent individual. How does an individual develop this skill?

   a. The person reframes negative feelings when necessary to maximize the use of his or her energy.
   b. The person learns how to apologize sincerely.
   c. The person recognizes conflict as normative.
   d. The person works to eliminate emotions in the workplace.

9. Focused hiring is a way of selecting new employees that _____.

   a. Eliminates the need for external search firms
   b. Decreases leadership turnover
   c. Focuses on the fit between the candidates and the organization
   d. Identifies the candidate with the greatest potential for integrating into the organization successfully

10. Individual emotional competence develops gradually through the novice, advanced beginner, competence, and proficiency stages to finally arrive at the level of expertise. What can individuals who have reached the competence stage do?

    a. Think and feel simultaneously while considering the opinions of others
    b. Project passionate optimism for the work of their profession
    c. Control their impulses effectively
    d. Coach others in the development of emotional competence

11. Team emotional competence develops through the same five stages as individual emotional competence. What can a team that has reached emotional proficiency do?

    a. Understand the skills and emotions of all team members
    b. Orient its work toward meeting the needs of the community
    c. Orient its work toward meeting the goals and needs of the organization
    d. Integrate local and national regulations into its work

CHAPTER ELEVEN

Toxic Organizations and People: The Leader as Transformer

The workplace can be a positive crucible, not a mind-bending and spirit-shattering one.

—William Lundin and Kathleen Lundin,
Reprinted with permission of the publisher. From The healing manager: How to build quality relationships and productive cultures at work, copyright (c) 1993 by Lundin, W., & Lundin, K., Berrett-Koehler Publishers, Inc., San Francisco, CA. All rights reserved. www.bkconnection.com

Chapter Objectives

At the completion of this chapter, the reader will be able to

· Identify the common sources of toxicity and dysfunction in healthcare organizations.
· Analyze long-standing leadership behaviors that negatively affect organizations.
· Describe the negative impact of system toxic practice on employee performance.
· Describe the negative impact of career entrenchment and career entrapment on organizational effectiveness.
· Critique the 10 principles for minimizing organizational toxicity.

Continually changing, complex organizations are often engaged in restructuring, downsizing, and merging. Organizational leaders find themselves increasingly challenged by dysfunctional and toxic situations. Healthcare organizations, as any other, are microcosms of society. The potential for the expression of positive and helpful behaviors or negative and interfering ones always exists. There is no screen for dysfunctional behaviors when hiring, except for the most obvious. Dysfunctional behaviors come in various degrees and affect organizational effectiveness in a range of ways.

This chapter discusses dysfunctional behaviors that typically impair healthcare organizations, including antisocial behaviors, toxic mentoring, and neurotic and self-defeating behaviors. It also discusses organizational practices that are prone to dysfunction and organizational characteristics that reinforce dysfunction. To mitigate the negative impact of dysfunctional behaviors, the chapter presents 10 principles designed to minimize organizational toxicity. These principles focus on reversing the dysfunctional behaviors of leaders and guiding them toward more appropriate practices that can transform dysfunction into health. Specifically, leaders need to become more self-aware, become more consistent in word and behavior, listen better, empower employees, and create new models for reward and recognition.

Increasingly, health professionals ask themselves the following questions: If healing is my profession and contribution to society, why do I feel so bad? Why are so many of my colleagues more discouraged with their work than ever before? Shortages of available workers, declining enrollments in colleges and universities, and the unstable financing system all continue to fuel the disfranchisement of health professionals. Employees are reluctant to trust one another and must be coaxed to interact. More often, they engage in labor union activity as a means of mediating their pain. Care providers frequently are conflicted over whether to give care or withhold it. Many believe the care that is given is substandard, incomplete, and sometimes even harmful. The environment these problems create tends to kill cooperation and creativity.

The complaints of colleagues, along with the newspaper headlines, might suggest that healthcare organizations are more toxic and in greater distress than are many of the patients receiving healthcare services. Far too many health professionals, particularly leaders and point-of-service workers, are missing the energy and collaborative spirit that mirror health. Their psyches have been assaulted too severely and for too long by neurotic leadership styles, dysfunctional group processes, inappropriate superior–subordinate bonding, and abandonment. These unfortunate toxicogenic practices need to be swiftly reversed because they are destroying the vitality of healthcare organizations.

Some may be tempted to attribute the distress of healthcare workers solely to changes in reimbursement policy and to look for the solution in a more palatable financing structure. The reality, however, is that the toxicity of healthcare organizations is not just a matter of reimbursement. Indeed, the silver lining of the prospective payment and managed care models may be that they can help expose the subtle yet pervasive toxins currently harming the healthcare system.

Healthcare organizations, for example, have been plagued by a delivery model in which (mostly male) physicians have almost total control, not to mention disempowering practices, a mentality of personal entitlement, and resistance to change. These factors, along with the increasing challenge of financing care and a philosophy of things first and people second, cause organizational toxicity and nullify the essential values of healing and restoration of health. The job of organizational leaders is to identify the toxic behaviors and develop strategies to minimize their effects. Rather than attempting to determine who the guilty parties are—individuals or organizations (or both)—the challenge is to move forward and create the kind of culture that will lead to organizational health.

Some of the main differences between toxic and healthy organizations concern the issues of control, conflict, and adaptability. For example, an organization in which the level of toxicity is high can be characterized in this way:

- The employees are widely subject to forces outside their control.
- Because of their lack of control, the employees are more susceptible to illness.

Group Discussion

At the next team meeting, ask employees to identify at least two toxic behaviors in the organization they believe should be changed. Consider the following questions: Can you clearly and objectively define the problem? If you were in charge, how would you change behaviors to make them less toxic? What indicators would you use to measure the change in behaviors?

- The leaders and employees try to decrease conflict rather than accept it as normal and useful.
- The employees tend to become stuck and lose their ability to change.

The following is true of a healthy organization:

- The organization depends on group process and shared decision making to accomplish its work.
- The employees are basically relaxed rather than stressed.
- The leaders and employees recognize conflict as normal and treat instances of conflict as opportunities for gaining information and planning and implementing improvements.
- Individuals and groups become facile at adapting to changing circumstances.

Healing Is Our Business?

Paradoxically, the working conditions in healthcare organizations are generally not healthy. Many leaders are aware that changes need to be made, but not all leaders understand that the cures for the toxicity in the healthcare system should come from within the system, in particular, from the health professionals who create and manage the system. If a better system is to be built, it must rest on the fundamental values of healers—restoring wholeness and a state of harmonious energy.

The principles that apply to the health of individuals also apply to the health of organizations. In the case of individuals, health is "harmony between the most basic cell and its environment in which there is abundant energy and the basic unit is effectively performing the function appropriate to its location in time and space" (King, 1989, p. 30). To function properly, each individual cell requires a sufficient supply of nutrients and an efficient system of cleansing or waste removal (**Figure 11-1**).

An organization likewise requires nutrients (inputs) to provide health care: dollars, medical supplies, and human resources, for example. A healthy organization, like a healthy individual, can be described as an entity harmoniously connected with its environment and thus able to take advantage of the environment's available energy. All life requires a continual replenishment of inputs. A shortage or oversupply of inputs can result in negative outcomes. Too much food results in obesity (**Figure 11-2**), and too little results in the loss of mass and energy; the result in both cases is an impairment of the

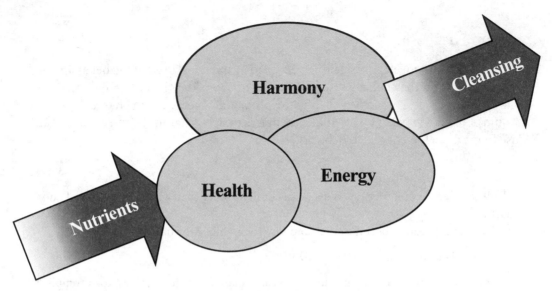

Figure 11-1 Adequate Nutrients and Adequate Cleansing Result in a Balance of Health, Harmony, and Energy.

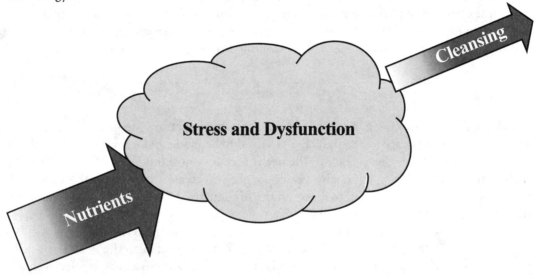

Figure 11-2 Excess Nutrients Lead to Obesity and to Stress and Dysfunction.

entity's ability to function (**Figure 11-3**). Similarly, a surfeit of employees or unrestrained financial resources lead to a lack of accountability and cause dysfunction. When there are no parameters on resource availability or use, there is no accountability—until the resources run out!

All organizations also require the removal of waste products in an effective and timely manner. When an organization is unable to remove waste, the buildup of toxins begins to impede functioning. At some point, enough "cells" are affected to cause a symptom and bring the problem to conscious attention. For instance, the organization, by retaining

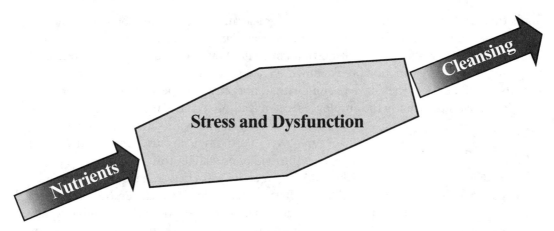

Figure 11-3 Inadequate Nutrients Lead to Loss of Mass and Energy and to Stress and Dysfunction.

policies and practices that no longer serve a purpose or add value, becomes toxic from the buildup of these. The goal may be to preserve tradition, but the result is inappropriate resource use leading to dysfunction.

Whether the problem is under- or oversupply of nutrients or disturbance of the cleansing processes, an entity (an organism or organization) experiences decreased effectiveness and possibly distress. When an organization is unable to remove waste, the toxins begin to build up and impede functioning. Indeed, if an organization retains less-than-adequate employees or ineffective equipment, the processes needed for transformation are ineffective and non-value-added work continues to drain resources and act as a serious obstacle to doing the work that needs to be done. If the flow of nutrients to an organism is constrained or the organism's cleansing processes are inhibited, the organism experiences tension. In an organization, constriction in the flow of inputs (money, materials, or health professionals) impedes the work processes and causes dysfunction and damage.

The stress that results from balancing nutrients and cleansing occurs as a natural effect of resistance to change. Resistance, like stress, is not bad in and of itself. It enables us to sense our environment and to grow by working through challenges and accomplishing

Group Discussion

In both organisms and organizations, there is a healthy middle ground between an overabundance and a deficiency of inputs. From this perspective, consider whether there is a shortage of healthcare workers in your organization. Ask team members the following questions: Is there an excess of employees who are less-than-average performers? Is there a shortage of employees with appropriate skills to meet the contemporary needs of the organization? What are the missing skill sets? Develop a plan that focuses on improving the skills and increasing the number of employees. What indicators of organizational performance will be used to measure progress?

goals that stretch our talents and capacities for learning. But for these benefits to accrue, a dynamic balance between resistance and nonresistance must be maintained. Distress comes from rigid resistance, the kind that continues beyond the point of effectiveness and into the range where function breaks down. When practices that produce no obvious value are sustained because they have become ritual, not only does performance suffer, but toxicity accelerates among the employees, often leading to the demise of the organization.

> ### Key Point
>
> If you are not the master of your spirit and permit yourself to be demeaned, you are going to get sick unless something changes.
> —William Lundin and Kathleen Lundin, *The Healing Manager: How to Build Quality Relationships and Productive Cultures at Work*

Toxicity in an organization can affect employees both physically and emotionally. Indeed, the field of psychoneuroimmunology has documented links between feeling states and physiological responses. The emotions associated with caring—namely, hope, love, and joy—have been identified as ingredients in the remission of disease, whereas loss of hope or love and the failure to adequately cope with stress have been identified as factors in both the onset and exacerbation of the symptoms of major illness. In other words, the lack of caring or nurturing may be a primary causative factor in disease. Surely, there is a relationship between the lack of organizational caring and nurturing and the level of organizational toxicity.

Organizational toxicity is often unnoticed at the onset but slowly emerges as cynicism, declining morale, loss of creativity, and lower productivity. If its emotional component is not addressed, it can leave a toxic residue, preventing a complete return of function. The broken spirit never heals. That is, the unresolved or buried anger and resentment remain and thwart organizational efforts.

Often, the organizational response to toxicity mirrors the primitive response of granuloma formation. In a case of granuloma formation, the body does not deal with the underlying injury but instead walls it off with a fibrous deposit of cells. The injury merely appears to be mended, and no additional healing occurs. So too can an organization seal off a dysfunctional component while believing that it is taking proper corrective action. Unfortunately, this response prevents the organization from developing strategies for avoiding similar types of dysfunction in the future and also impedes work processes that should involve the dysfunctional component. The unresolved organizational conflict, like a granuloma, persists and affects every related decision in the future.

Toxic Behaviors

When an organization provides services in ways that subtly work against its stated goals, it violates its fundamental covenant with its employees and the community. At the same time, the organization's leaders and other members reinforce negative beliefs about the organization and further entrench the dysfunctional behaviors. The resulting toxic interactions become destructive to effective relationships.

Toxic or hostile work environments are recognizable not just by the presence of screaming, flaring tempers, and abusive language, but also by the less noticeable but often more damaging quiet demoralization that occurs. Unilateral decision making, the ignoring of requests, and the avoidance of unpleasant issues cause substantial toxicity, specifically, employee discontent. Furthermore, although chronically angry individuals and controlling supervisors regularly reinforce the toxicity, careless insensitivity to the impact of one's actions on others is one of the main causes. Leaders do not always stop and think!

The organizational culture, which of course has an enormous impact on decision making, leadership style, strategy formation, and organizational change, can be influenced in subtle and complex ways by invisible long-standing psychological forces hidden from the individuals who experience them. These covert forces all too often produce organizational outcomes that appear to be extremely irrational and dysfunctional.

Healthcare leaders are seldom satisfied with the structures, processes, and outcomes of their organization. It is the complex, long-standing interdependencies between stakeholders that create both healthy behaviors and toxic behaviors difficult to untangle and remedy. Toxic behaviors within an organization seldom are the result of one individual process gone awry but rather are the culmination of many dysfunctions that form a syndrome of organizational pathology. Similar patterns of strategic and structural defects can be as dramatic and bold as they are toxic. If one top executive uses a neurotic leadership style, others adopt similar behaviors. The result is a poorly functioning self-defeating organization.

This is not to deny that some mildly dysfunctional traits and behaviors can occur in moderation without causing significant difficulties. Most individuals exhibit low levels of shyness and depression and have a few irrational fears and suspicions. Major problems occur when these dysfunctional traits and behaviors dominate relationships between individuals.

Following, 10 sources of organizational toxicity are presented to help the readers gain an understanding of its dynamics and formulate strategies to decrease it (**Exhibit 11-1**). Note that the distinction between the toxic behaviors of individuals and organizational toxicity is artificial because the work of individuals acting as a team is in fact the work of the organization.

Exhibit 11-1   Ten Sources of Organizational Toxicity

1. Vertical authority structure
2. Inequitable reward and recognition practices
3. Abuse of power
4. Lack of respect for the workforce
5. Failure to manage unmotivated employees
6. Tolerance of antisocial behavior
7. Toxic mentoring
8. Inconsistency and dishonesty
9. Imbalance between work and personal life
10. Advocacy gone awry

Vertical Authority Structure

The structure of an organization, including its authority and decision-making parameters, can be a source of organizational toxicity. A vertical organizational structure, for example, frequently reinforces negative behaviors and serves as a defense against personal involvement. Leaders of vertically structured organizations tend to believe there is "an enemy out there" that must be managed, and they become driven by anger, fear, and suspicion. A vertical structure, besides encompassing a rigid hierarchy of authority, restricts communication because directives must be handed down from the chief executive level to the staff through multiple layers of middle managers. Employees are discouraged from engaging in accountable behaviors, healthy dialogue, and creative thinking.

> ## Group Discussion: Complexity Leadership
>
> The authority and decision-making structures in an organization can be paralyzing to progress and timely integration of evidence into practice. Describe the approval processes and number of individuals involved and the timeline for approval for the last four policies that affected your work. Once this information is identified, develop a strategy to eliminate non-value-added steps and propose a new process for the organization. What are the obstacles to eliminating all clinical policies and holding each licensed clinician accountable for state-of-the-art practice within the organization?

In addition, traditional vertical organizations require clear localization of decision making at the higher levels. Leaders often become obsessively vigilant because of their belief that subordinates and competitors cannot be trusted. Their paranoia also leads to the centralization of power and to excessive control over individuals and decision making. These organizations suffer from too much leadership, too many rigid procedures, too much documentation, and too much attention paid to keeping on schedule. Leaders in a vertical organization typically fear change and steadfastly defend ritualistic behaviors out of a desire for security.

The corporate culture in a traditional vertical organization typically suppresses individual creativity. Managed like a monarchy, this type of organization infantilizes its employees by expecting near-blind obedience. The rare exceptions tend to be organizations that have adopted a shared leadership model as a needed replacement for the traditional command-and-control model.

Vertical organizations recognize that creative people are expressive people but do not allow employees to be expressive at work. They believe that emotional outbursts should be saved for the home. Later, when their emotions recede, the employees are supposed to produce new ideas. This expectation leads to a waste of talent—talent for the original thinking that organizations so desperately need for survival and success. Furthermore, as a result of the suppression of emotions at work, employees develop a desire to be managed, nourished, and protected by a leader, and their misplaced awe for the leader can lead to depression and guilt.

In a vertical organization, the different types of vice president—senior vice president, executive vice president, assistant vice president—connote varying degrees of authority and reflect an imbalance of power within the executive team. The practice of having several levels of vice presidencies may be intended to allow for progression through the executive ranks, but in reality it minimizes the opportunity to create a mutually valuing and cooperative setting.

The separation of individuals into departments and divisions rather than functional units further reinforces power differentials. In this model, the core processes are specific to each department and are focused more on meeting departmental needs than on creating and delivering products and services to meet customer needs.

Reorganization within a vertical organization often results in mazelike reporting networks in which managers manage other managers and set precise communication expectations. If reorganization is a recurring phenomenon, the frequent changes in team size and membership hinder the development of expert team behaviors. Also, the threat of losing organizational positions because of anticipated mergers and acquisitions has in some cases caused senior leaders to move in opposite directions, harbor personal agendas, and be minimally compatible with each other. As for the employees of a vertical organization, when greater productivity is expected at the same time that resources are decreased, they unsurprisingly become angry and disillusioned. The survivors of layoffs are frequently less productive, develop poor job attitudes, and often voluntarily follow their discharged coworkers into unemployment or to other organizations. Yet the essential vertical structure is retained regardless of the frequency of the shuffling or the complexity of the rearrangements. Power is retained at the top and distributed through departmental leaders.

Inequitable Reward and Recognition Practices

Another toxin found in most organizations is inequitable pay. It is important to note that few people are ever satisfied with their level of compensation. Nonetheless, although always desirous of more money, most individuals recognize that resources are limited and are only seeking equitable compensation. Compensation practices become toxic when rewards and recognition are inequitable or inconsistent.

Severely compressed pay ranges, particularly in nursing, limit financial growth while making other disciplines, such as law, engineering, and technological fields, more attractive. Also, limitations on annual compensation packages result in equal but minimal increases for all employees. Employees who do the requisite work without extending themselves, attend only mandatory continuing education programs, and miss work occasionally (although staying within the normal range) are awarded the same 3% increase as are employees who receive numerous thank-you letters from patients, attend external continuing education programs, have perfect attendance, and participate on committees.

The challenge of using limited available dollars to pay employees appropriately for their different levels of effort is rarely taken up by leaders. Rather than awarding 0% to mediocre employees and 10% to exemplary employees, leaders use the across-the-board approach so that everyone gets something. Seldom are other rewards, such as preferred scheduling, used as alternatives for rewarding excellent performers.

Group Discussion

Compressed pay ranges and limited dollars for reward and recognition continue to challenge leaders in their efforts to recognize staff. In collaboration with members of your team, revise the current reward and recognition system or create an entirely new one. Make sure the system you design

- Separates the compensation process from the performance evaluation process
- Awards nothing to employees who have a mediocre performance rating
- Includes nonmonetary rewards, such as preferred scheduling, weekend or holiday preferences, and inclusion in decision making
- Uses objective measures of performance to determine the effect of nonmonetary programs on employee satisfaction and turnover and on patient outcomes

Compensation continues to be highly subjective, particularly at the senior level. Compensation for leaders is often based more on market standards than on their performance as team members. Consequently, compensation practices can cause severe division, infighting, jealousy, and mistrust, particularly when the senior executive's compensation is 20 times greater than that of the entry-level employee.

Abuse of Power

The third toxin is abuse of power. Because the highest turnover occurs at the middle management level, leaders scramble to fill positions at this level, often selecting expert nurses with little or no management experience. In such cases, reports of the new "manager from hell" may soon begin to circulate. In short, the wrong person has been promoted to a leadership position and then, with title and power in hand, runs into trouble. Nearly every organization faces the problem of quickly finding candidates with adequate experience to fill leadership positions and guiding them to become effective managers. Indeed, the toxicity mainly results not from the appointment of inexperienced managers, but from the failure to intervene early in the process of assisting appointees to develop the skills needed for their positions.

When a new manager belittles staff members in front of patients or other staff members, communicates by memo rather than face to face, changes policies without input from others, and is rude and thoughtless, the staff soon runs out of patience. Some staff members may attempt to communicate the issues to the manager and the manager's supervisor, but any dialogue among the staff, the new manager, and the supervisor typically results in assigning blame—of the new manager by the staff and of the staff by the new manager. Eventually, the staff members resign or transfer to other areas without making clear that their reason for changing employment was the lack of collegiality and of a respectful and caring work environment. The senior managers generally assume the staff members were seeking better salaries, better schedules, or shorter commutes to work—easily recognizable concrete reasons—and fail to recognize the true reason, allowing the toxicity to continue and intensify.

Mandatory Overtime

Another example of abuse of power is mandatory overtime. Although health care by its very nature involves the delivery of vital services that cannot be turned off and on in line with the availability of staff, mandatory overtime in a predominantly female profession raises significant issues, such as the difficulty of meeting both professional and family responsibilities. Nurses often feel exhausted and discouraged when they leave work, powerless to effect changes to ensure safe patient care and overburdened by the overtime they are expected to put in. Like the shoemaker's children who had no shoes, healthcare workers have no health—or are being slowly stripped of the healthy balance between work and personal life they once had.

Intolerance Toward Diversity

Because communication technology and supersonic travel have made the world smaller, the diverse peoples of the world are able to share ideas and learn new approaches to a multiplicity of tasks. Yet healthcare organizations have commonly failed to integrate the multiple cultures of their staff members and patients (e.g., by not giving due consideration to their dietary habits and religious beliefs). Many have also been reluctant to actively seek diverse perspectives by including representatives from all gender and age groups in essential work teams. Instead, stereotypical executives—male and middle aged—continue to develop strategic, human resource, and budgetary plans. Thus, despite educational programs designed to minimize discriminatory practices, more proactive efforts to increase the diversity of the workforce are needed. This is especially important given that the communities served by the predominantly white healthcare workforce are on average more than 30% nonwhite.

Lack of Respect for the Workforce

Leaders of healthcare organizations have been known to view staff members as expendable nuisances—as the cost of doing business. They have been known to objectify their employees and give them little or no consideration. Leaders may fall into such attitudes out of fear of dependency and an associated sense of vulnerability. For instance, when they see dependency in their subordinates they may experience anxiety, causing them to reject their subordinates.

Employees often feel like foster children, powerless and completely dependent. They never know what they are going to get until they are hired. If an employee does not like the organization, he or she, like an unhappy child, can daydream and pretend not even to be there. Or the employee can run away and live on the street (resign and remain unemployed). Or the employee can hope that a nice gentleman with a big heart will appear with the offer of a better job!

Lack of respect takes many forms, from obvious rudeness to subtle discourtesy. It can include not responding to employee requests, dismissing new ideas with a smile, refusing to discuss issues that are important to employees, and exhibiting a general lack of manners, such as failing to say "thank you."

To be sure, the price of incivility is high. According to Porath and Pearson (2013), incivility hurts both morale and the bottom line. Data specific to decreased work effort, decreased time spent at work, decreased quality of work, lost time avoiding the offender, and taking their frustration out on others have been quantified and examined from numerous perspectives.

Failure to Manage Unmotivated Employees

The fifth toxin is one that haunts even the best leaders. Finding the time and energy to work with unmotivated career employees can be overwhelming. The difficulty is not in recognizing less-than-optimal performance but in continuing to work with these employees despite minimal success at guiding them to do better. The lifetime career syndrome—lackluster performance by career employees unexcited or burnt out by their jobs—is one of the impediments to efficiency that leaders are required to deal with regularly.

New expectations regarding employment have emerged during the last 20 years. Organizations are not prepared to enter into lifelong partnerships with individuals. No longer can an individual expect a durable commitment as a condition of employment. The trend is for the terms of employment to be congruent with the needs and financial resources of the hiring organization. When these needs or resources change, the employee's services are likely to be terminated.

Of course, terminating the services of long-term employees has never been an easy task. Many employees stay with an organization out of desperation, but do not remain committed to it in the way management would like. Rather than firing these employees, managers often continue to invest in them in the hope that the support given to them will reverse their attitudes.

Many organizations are in fact burdened with workers who want to leave but, for a variety of reasons, stay nonetheless. Department managers and directors often whisper among themselves, cursing the organization's flaws, but stay on because they are afraid to leave or because the pay, if little else, is excellent. Furthermore, if they left, they would have to sacrifice imminent salary increases, paid holidays and vacations, and retirement benefits. Yet they do not identify with or feel emotionally attached to their current position and do nothing about changing the situation.

Research by Carson and Carson (1997) confirmed that career entrenchment and career entrapment are actual phenomena of organizational life. Career entrenchment is the tendency to stay in a vocation because of the investment already made, psychological preservation, and a perception of few career opportunities. Entrenched or entrapped employees have an established way of life, usually have good salaries, and know the challenges of the workplace. Leaving their jobs would create uncertainty as well as loss of identity and loss of income. Career entrenchment perpetuates itself because when an employee becomes reconciled to staying in a career despite unhappiness with it, the employee is likely to invest further in the career, becoming more entrenched.

Individuals who are dissatisfied with their career usually engage in one of four coping strategies to manage the associated stress: leave the career, openly discuss entrenchment with their employer, remain loyal to the organization while hoping for improvement in the future, or retire on the job (**Exhibit 11-2**).

Exhibit 11-2   Career Entrapment Strategies

Exit: An active strategy in which an individual leaves a career to change fields, retire, or withdraw from the labor force.

Voice: An active strategy in which an individual constructively tries to improve conditions through verbalization of concerns.

Loyalty: A passive strategy in which an individual passively but optimistically waits for conditions to improve.

Neglect: A passive strategy in which an individual allows conditions to deteriorate through reduced interest and effort, tardiness or absenteeism, increased errors, and ineffective use of working time.

Source: Carson, K.D., and P. Carson. 1997. The Academy of Management Executives 11, no. 2: 62–76. Copyright 1997 by the Academy of Management.

People choose to enter a career based on their interests, preferences, and evaluation of opportunities. Once a person has selected a career, he or she then invests money and effort to achieve success. Typically, the person will periodically look at whether the career chosen truly offers adequate opportunities for meeting the person's needs and achieving his or her goals. If it appears to do that, the person will continue to invest in the career. On the other hand, if it does not, the person may change careers, especially if the level of investment to date has been low (a high level of investment might incline the person to remain in the career to justify the investment).

A career change also can be involuntary, as when an employee's job becomes obsolete or the employee is underutilized. Career changes sometimes cause only minimal disruption in lifestyle and sometimes major upheavals. For a person to see a potential new career as viable, he or she must perceive the career as desirable, be willing to invest in the career, and have a reasonable opportunity to enter it.

Group Discussion

Which came first, the lack of interest in nursing or the toxic conditions in the workplace? Together, the serious nursing shortage, the reluctance of nurses to recruit others into nursing, unmanageable workloads, the lack of valid and reliable workload systems to measure patient care needs, compressed pay scales, and the increased attractiveness of other professions have broadened the challenge of maintaining a viable healthcare workforce. Create a flow chart of the nursing supply that reflects these conditions and any others that you believe affect the shortage. Where are the leverage points for increasing the supply? Where would you begin? What resources are needed? What outcomes are to be expected from the interventions you recommend?

Most individuals attempt to select careers that match their personal interests. When a good match does not occur, the individual, besides having little passion for the work and being unsatisfied, is likely to be ineffective on the job. Unfortunately, whether a career is really congruent with an individual's personal interests is not always immediately evident, and thus mismatches and their negative consequences cannot always be avoided.

In the steady-state career prototype, an individual selects a career in late adolescence or early adulthood using a minimal amount of information, is trained in the career, and maintains the necessary performance skills for remaining in the career. Interestingly, some careers in which a high proportion of the professionals fit the steady-state model, including nursing, teaching, social work, and law enforcement, often result in burnout. Daily confrontation with human suffering and death in conjunction with lack of autonomy, heavy caseloads, court-ordered mandates, inadequate salaries, and frequent interpersonal conflicts understandably cause many individuals in these careers to want to escape.

Career entrapment occurs when a person is deeply entrenched in a career because of prior investment in career development, psychological attachments, and a sense of obligation. Among other things, the emotional bonds forged in coworker relationships and the intimacy of a mentor–protégé relationship may be difficult to give up. As the career tenure lengthens, the person spends greater energy rationalizing the decision to stay and convincing himself or herself that success is within reach. The person also may experience social pressure to continue in the current field or have a low propensity for risk taking (a career change obviously carries risks, including the risk that the new career may be no more fulfilling than the last).

Paradoxically, whereas dismal labor and market conditions and high unemployment negatively affect turnover, they can positively affect the process of changing careers. The pressures of depressed economic conditions often provide the impetus for entrapped or entrenched employees to seek other employment opportunities. Further, an economic crisis can cause an organization to retrain employees, thus providing them a chance to escape unfulfilling positions.

Individuals who experience career dissatisfaction and distress are susceptible to anxiety, anger, and depression. The anguish of boredom and tedium associated with work tasks often lead to rumination, resentment, melancholy, and an accompanying sense of hopelessness, with negative consequences for the organization.

Leaders often have to manage individuals they don't particularly like. Not every member of the team is friendly, thoughtful, and courteous. In fact, according to Gallo (2013) in a *Harvard Business Review* blog, many team members are irritating; they perform their work adequately, but are not easy to work with. Such interpersonal issues should not always be looked at as negative but rather as an opportunity to seek out the positive in the individual(s), reflect on the annoying behavior (it can be something that reminds you of another negative situation), or be sure your evaluation standards of performance are not biased against the unlikable individuals.

Tolerance of Antisocial Behavior

Much has been written about deviant or antisocial behaviors in the workplace. Bullying, sexual harassment, dishonesty, rumor mongering, withholding effort, and stealing are of obvious concern because they reduce group effectiveness, among other consequences. Of these, bulllying has been the most identified and studied across the globe (Branch, Ramsay, & Barker, 2013). In addition, the failure of leaders to recognize antisocial behaviors as inappropriate and try to minimize these behaviors has a negative impact on the social climate and the general moral conduct of employees.

According to Robinson and O'Leary-Kelly (1998), the social context largely determines how employees think and feel about aspects of their work environment and how they behave. In particular, a positive relationship exists between a given individual's level of antisocial behavior and the level of antisocial behavior of his or her coworkers. This should come as no surprise because individual group members working in a shared social environment receive similar social cues (cues perhaps indicating that certain types and levels of antisocial behavior are acceptable). In addition, when a new employee enters an established group, the extent of the group's antisocial behavior affects how likely the newcomer is to develop similar behaviors. Typically, the newcomer adjusts his or her personal behavior to fit the work environment or eventually leaves the organization. Indeed, the longer an employee remains in a group, the greater the chance he or she will behave in accordance with the group's standards of behavior.

Another factor that affects the level of a group's antisocial behavior is the degree of task interdependence (i.e., the extent to which the group members must coordinate their individual efforts). Enhanced interaction allows the members to more easily acquire the social information that determines their subsequent behavior. In other words, the higher the level of interaction, the greater the likelihood that group members will take each other as role models.

Of course, in any workgroup it is always possible that some members perceive themselves to be significantly different in some important way from the majority, feel dissatisfied with their poor fit, and want to withdraw from the group. In the case of antisocial behaviors, because these, by definition, violate social mores, it is even likely that some group members feel alienated by antisocial behaviors prevalent in the workgroup as a whole. To be sure, nothing is more destructive than leadership failure to manage the obvious negative and destructive behaviors in an organization. Employees hear value-based proclamations for performance and integrity; what is observed is contradictory to those values and beliefs.

Research efforts to increase understanding of these antisocial behaviors, including cyberbullying, and identify reliable formal and informal approaches to prevention and interventions are continuing at both local and national levels (Branch et al., 2013).

Toxic Mentoring

Mentoring has long been extolled as a means of guiding the development of inexperienced employees, but not all mentoring results in the growth of the mentee. Some leaders in fact believe that mentoring is an ill-conceived method of continuing past practices—ill-conceived because it obstructs necessary adaptations to changes in the work environment, the marketplace, and society at large. In their view, rather than seeking out a wise elder as a guide to corporate life, an aspiring leader should read a lot, listen a lot, work a lot, and observe a lot. That way, according to Geneen (1997), the young leader learns a lot on his or her own and is not spoon-fed antiquated wisdom gained from someone else's past. It is worth noting here that the workplaces of America are filled with industrious and upright citizens on a treadmill to nowhere because they are so intent on playing it safe.

Toxic mentoring can also result when an aspiring leader seeks to please an experienced leader that he or she has idealized. If the mentor (the experienced leader) does not assist the mentee in developing his or her own identity and leadership style, the mentee could be misled into following the established path of the mentor. The main danger here is that once the mentor is no longer on hand as a guide, the mentee might become empty and powerless and unable to progress.

Another hazard of mentoring occurs when an experienced leader idealizes an aspiring leader and places unrealistic hopes on him or her. The mentor then gives the mentee overly ambitious assignments that frequently remain uncompleted. Finally, some mentors attempt to transfer their defense mechanisms to their mentees or at least convince them of the need to approach situations from a defensive and hostile posture rather than a posture of openness and inquiry. In such cases, the mentoring process is more a cloning process than a means of growth and development.

Often, leaders espousing transformational or servant leadership can be quite harmful. When leaders use strategies to create purpose, community building, and empowerment and the processes include abuse of power, a sense of self-importance, use of fear tactics, and being somewhat isolated, the leadership becomes harmful to not only mentees, but also everyone in the organization (Mohr, 2013).

The point that aspiring leaders must keep in mind is the need to take the initiative rather than travel the same old route, to be decisive rather than defer to a higher authority, to expose themselves to failure rather than make peace with mediocrity, and to seize opportunities rather than retreat from them.

From a somewhat different perspective, toxic mentoring exemplifies the negative side of transferring one's experiences. It is impossible to approach new people or situations with a blank sheet, so we use our past experiences, positive or negative, and the stereotypes we have inherited to fill the pages (**Exhibit 11-3**). A good mentor tries to keep the

---

Exhibit 11-3   Toxic Stereotypes

1. Female leaders cannot understand financial situations and cannot sustain company solvency.
2. Older leaders cannot be effective because they do not have technical competence.
3. Younger leaders cannot hold senior leadership positions because they do not have enough experience.
4. Members of our church will make better leaders because we know we can count on them.
5. Avoid members of certain ethnic groups when selecting new leaders because some are too expressive.
6. Overweight leaders will never concentrate on the business of the day.
7. Avoid selecting leaders for your committee who require too much time to make decisions because they think too slowly.

---

slate as clean as possible. The mentee needs to make personal assessments and form personal opinions using his or her own emerging leadership lens.

Toxic mentors typically base perceptions not only on current practices but also on early childhood experiences. They make judgments about individuals and situations before examining the circumstances and the available data. They often put forth negative profiles of individuals that include derogatory references to the individuals' gender, age, culture, mental capacity, physical stature, or religion.

Effective mentoring is truly circular in nature. Sharing experiences from the past with aspiring leaders is as important as sharing experiences with colleagues and superiors. Mentoring upward, sideways, and downward reinforces the importance of lifelong learning and makes the point that wisdom and insight are not limited to those with tenure. The healthy mentor encourages self-assessment, open and nonjudgmental examination of issues, and reevaluation of decisions as new information becomes available.

Rather than selecting and promoting others of their own image, experienced leaders need to ensure that aspiring leaders gain an appreciation of the substantial personality differences that leaders can exhibit and the importance of diversity in personality and methodology for creating optimal solutions.

Inconsistency and Dishonesty

Leaders frequently add to the toxicity in an organization by being inconsistent in word and action and by telling white lies. In general, employees respect and are willing to follow leaders who act in accordance with their values, principles, and beliefs. When a company identifies balancing work and leisure as a goal, it usually focuses on the employees' time at work and develops initiatives giving employees work-hour flexibility. But if the company at the same time is not filling vacancies and is asking employees to do more with less, the added flexibility is counteracted by the extra 5 or 10 hours of work that each employee must put in weekly. The company's message becomes ambiguous, and, worse, when the employees complain, management sees them as ungrateful, making the employees feel that the executives just don't get it.

Ambiguous or contradictory messages are quite common and usually sow confusion. The recipients of these messages begin to feel angry, insecure, and entrapped. For instance, if one employee has a clearly superior performance review but is given the same compensation as mediocre performers, the contradictory message—performance both counts (because it is measured) and does not count (because superior performance is not compensated)—likely demoralizes the employee with the outstanding record.

Although people are ordinarily uncomfortable with conflict, their discomfort reduces their opportunities to learn more about the differing positions and viewpoints of colleagues. This in and of itself is enough to support the notion that conflict should be considered normal, but there is another very important reason. People's lack of comfort with conflict and confronting the truth has resulted in the "white lies of leadership" syndrome. White lies, in fact, have become all too common in performance reviews, the selection of candidates for positions, and explanations for downsizing given to employees (Malloch, 2001).

The performance review process continues to be a struggle for most leaders, especially identifying strengths and areas for improvement in an honest and meaningful way.

Reviewers find it difficult to discuss inadequate performance openly and kindly, particularly if the deficiencies have been persistent and have never been addressed. Leaders generally wish for performance problems to disappear from lack of attention so that they do not have to deal with the issue or engage in uncomfortable dialogue. To avoid confrontation, leaders sometimes rate mediocre behavior as above standard—or to equalize the distribution of a limited compensation package, they routinely rate the performance of all employees as above standard. Regardless of their intent, these types of misevaluations are forms of dishonesty.

Truth telling is also difficult when a job candidate is not picked for the position. Unselected candidates are often told the chosen candidate had better credentials, more experience, or more education. Although this may be true, there is usually more to the decision. Factors such as personal appearance, aggressiveness in the interview, or nonsupport from a colleague often play a role in the selection process, but information about such issues is rarely shared, preventing the candidate from learning how to better prepare for the next interview. Holding back critical comments, even if done out of kindness, takes control away from employees and can be seen as a form of autocratic leadership behavior.

Finally, leaders often tell white lies when explaining decisions to downsize or eliminate positions. Most often they claim the decisions are not personal or about the employees' competence but rather based on financial considerations. The truth is that downsizing is often used to weed out mediocre or dissident employees. It is also used as a way to cover the effects of poor management, such as when leaders fail to adapt to incremental changes in the marketplace or neglect to retrain employees to meet emerging needs. Nothing is more destructive to the morale of an organization than the chronic recycling of human beings, especially in an industry that espouses health as its service.

Imbalance Between Work and Personal Life

For many people, the boundary between work life and personal life has all but collapsed with the advent of the Internet. Technology has opened new doors to new experiences, and the condition of being without something to do is almost inconceivable. Individuals today spend much of their time learning new ideas or deciding what to do next. Being in demand is a sign of importance and value, and new communication technologies allow people to seek out and contact each other in new ways. iPads, pagers, and home shopping networks increase the role of scheduling in our lives and divide our days into ever smaller segments. Yet there is evidence that technological advances are not really increasing efficiency. It is important to realize that technology is not always adept at solving nontechnical problems—a better timepiece does not eliminate chronic lateness.

Perhaps high-speed living is toxic to human beings. So much time can be put into arrivals and departures that not enough is left over for the experiences themselves. Raising children, developing relationships, and creating art are not tasks that lend themselves to being done speedily and efficiently. The high-speed world of technology has separated individuals from contemplation and slow-knowing—the process of reflecting creatively rather than relying on the mere analytical horsepower of technology. The amazing data-analyzing capabilities of computers have turned contemplation into a seemingly old-fashioned pastime. The focus is on problem solving. Dwelling on issues to see whether they might lead to deeper issues is seen as inefficient and self-indulgent.

What we know is that neither technology nor efficiency can acquire more time for anyone. Time is not something one had or lost; it is what one lives in. For most of us, there is never enough time. The real challenge is to develop a balance between work and personal life and to work to maintain the desired balance.

The challenge of finding enough time to function effectively in work and at home is even greater for female leaders. Because organizations desire the senior management profile to reflect the composition of the marketplace, they are on the lookout for competent women to hire. The problem experienced by female leaders is that women remain the primary family man-

> ### Point to Ponder
>
> Extremes of up and down are interrelated. Excessiveness ushers in disorder and disaster, which lead to burnout and fatigue as we walk the way of personal destruction. In leading others there is nothing better than moderation. Leisure is good, yet too much can lead to restlessness and boredom. Work is important and beneficial, yet in abundance it can cause havoc in other aspects of life. Avoid the temptations of overdoing and overextending, no matter how enticing and attractive the pulls and lures might be.
>
> Brief quote from p. 155 from MENTORING: THE ART OF GIVING AND RECEIVING WISDOM by CHUNGLIANG AL HUANG and JERRY LYNCH. Copyright (c) 1995 by Chungliang Al Huang and Jerry Lynch. Reprinted by permission of HarperCollins Publishers

agers and spend nearly twice as many hours on household and childcare responsibilities as men do. The conflicts of interest created by playing a leadership role and acting as a mother make it nearly impossible for women to remain as executives without failing to meet their full responsibilities in one or both areas and suffering a noticeable lack of balance between work and personal life. More flexibility in the workplace and an increase in the participation of males in child rearing are needed to end the male orientation of the workplace and bring about a true partnership.

Interestingly, some people believe the main challenge is not too much work but overstimulation. According to this view, there are too many demands and not enough sensible priority setting. If people had a healthy selfishness, they could step back from the minutiae of their work lives and find a good balance between responsibilities—one that allows them to be true to their personal values.

Some individuals have proposed the practice of "unplugging" for various lengths of time to restore balance and create time for thinking and reflection. Taking a digital vacation, according to Baradunde Thurston in a *Fast Company* article, was well worth the effort. Thurston faced his FOMO (fear of missing out) and prepared for a lengthy digital vacation. He informed key colleagues of his plan, identified the special things he wanted to do while away, and then deactivated his iPhone and social media services. Although this may seem quite severe, organizations are adopting other practices to begin to mediate the overconnected syndrome. These include limiting connections with the workplace in the evenings and on weekends and not bringing smartphones into meetings.

Reactive Advocacy Gone Awry

Health professionals find solace in serving patients and acting as advocates for them, but advocacy, when it is reactive, can sometimes be a source of toxicity. Consider the following scenario. The family of a patient in a critical care unit recognized that all interventions were futile and informed the nurses and attending physician they wished to cease treatment. Keeping the patient comfortable was their only goal at this time. On the next shift, the consulting physician examined the patient and determined that he needed respiratory support. The physician then proceeded to intubate the patient. Given the power and reputation of the physician, no staff member challenged his actions, even though they were contrary to the family's wishes.

On the next shift, the returning nurse realized that the wishes of the family had been violated and called the attending physician, who in turn removed the respiratory support. The nurse expressed a feeling of accomplishment, although she was concerned about receiving a tongue-lashing from the consulting physician because she had gone over his head.

Advocacy leadership in health care is a proactive process. Its purpose is to create the conditions for patients to receive the care they desire. It involves much more than removing the barriers as they are identified; in fact, the goal of advocacy leadership is to avoid having barriers in the first place. Unfortunately, reactive advocacy is the kind of advocacy that has become commonplace in our world of ambiguous values. When traditional leaders take action to alleviate unhealthy situations, they feel accomplished and complete, despite often failing to identify or address the basic problems.

Consider the following. To thrive in the global economy, the United States requires a democratized workforce. Despite coming far in a journey that began with slavery and the cruel exploitation of child and immigrant labor, the country still has numerous organizations in which most workers are alienated and apathetic. Further, our social institutions, including our schools and churches, have notably failed to fill the values void that pervades all sectors of society. The workplace, according to Lundin and Lundin (1993), may be the logical place to fill this void. It may be, but healthcare organizations often operate on the assumption that health care is a commodity rather than a service, presenting their leaders with the challenge of designing and implementing strategies to cure them of their toxicity.

Widely touted theories of transformational leadership are based on the belief that leaders have the power needed to transform a low-performing organization into a high-performing organization. This belief is itself based on the classical model of system control, which is inconsistent with the concept of organizational transformation. If one knocks down an anthill and rebuilds it, that is restructuring, not transformation. If the ants sprout wings and move to the trees, that is transformation. Thus, a quantum leader who is truly a transformer needs to approach the organization from a very different perspective—in other words, to avoid change strategies that amount to merely rearranging current structures, policies, procedures, and reward systems. Rather, a transforming leader creates a new and improved system that allows individuals to contribute to their fullest potential to deliver the most effective health care possible. And there can be no idea of asserting control in the traditional sense.

Some individuals are closer to being naturally gifted healing leaders than others, but almost everyone can be helped to reach their full potential for care and compassion. People can and do change. They find capacities they did not know they had. The fact is that healing traits are dormant within everyone. These traits are expressed in times of great joy, happiness, love, or compassion, when the spirit of caring and optimism overpowers any negative feelings.

The final challenge for quantum leaders is to avoid the obvious trap of believing that organizations are inherently toxic and that their job is to eradicate toxic behaviors wherever they are found. Their main focus should instead be on recognizing new beliefs and behaviors, understanding their implications, and integrating those that appear to be beneficial into current practice.

The solution to the problems that plague health care today lies in building bridges between the disciplines and recognizing the imperative to practice in such a way that environment–health connections receive primary consideration. Physical healing takes place through a multifaceted process in which the fabric of the body repairs and regenerates itself. So too can organizations heal.

Ten Principles for Minimizing Toxic Behavior in Organizations

The first step in minimizing the negative effects of dysfunctional behaviors is to recognize that these behaviors exist and that their elimination requires a commitment to discarding the toxic past and redefining what should be. One of the reasons that effective organizational change is often so difficult is that it involves taking authority, status, prestige, and security away from those in power, threatening their self-image and provoking resistance. But there is no other choice because many of the toxins originate in misplaced authority and power.

For the work of transformation to begin, the organizational culture must support, as its main value, the common good rather than self-interest. Organizations steeped in bureaucracy and paternalism experience a difficult transformation requiring persistent effort. For others the journey may be somewhat less complex and traumatic. The model of seven evolving levels of organizational culture described by Barrett (1995) can serve as a guideline for organizations in monitoring their progress on the journey toward supporting the common good (**Exhibit 11-4**). Although these levels are progressive, an organization might regress at different times in the journey.

> ### Key Point
>
> Healing manager: A person who helps others grow emotionally and intellectually—the emotional pathway from chaotic relationships to total quality relationships.
>

Exhibit 11-5 contains a list of 10 principles useful for combating toxicity in an organization. By following these rules, discussed subsequently, leaders can reduce the potency of the sources of toxicity described earlier or eliminate them entirely.

Principle 1: Know Thyself

For the leader of an organization, the most important rule for minimizing dysfunction is to know what he or she stands for and what behaviors he or she finds unacceptable. Barrett (1995) makes the point that whatever a person identifies with, that person cares for.

Exhibit 11-4   Seven Levels of Corporate Culture

1. *Survival consciousness:* The organization is focused on profits and typically uses an autocratic, uncaring, and fear-driven culture.
2. *Relationship consciousness:* This is a benevolent, paternalistic culture with a focus on internal communications. Fears at this level can lead to internal competition, blame, and manipulative culture.
3. *Self-esteem consciousness:* The focus is on a desire to be the biggest or the best. Hierarchical power structure with goals of order, efficiency, productivity, and quality. Strong results orientation.
4. *Transformation:* The focus is on self-discovery, vision, mission, and awareness of values. Beginning of focus on equality and diversity.
5. *Organization consciousness:* The focus is on integrity, trust, creativity, intuition, innovation, freedom, and generosity. Efforts abound to create conditions for cohesion, community spirit, and mutual accountability.
6. *Community consciousness:* Voluntary environmental and social audits and support for local community and businesses. The search is for long-term sustainability.
7. *Global/unity consciousness:* The organization contributes to resolving social, human rights, and environmental issues beyond the local community. The focus is on ethics and a search for truth and wisdom.

Source: Barrett, Richard. *Liberating the Corporate Soul*, pp. 61–67. Copyright (c) 2011. Reprinted by permission of Routledge/Taylor & Francis Books (UK).

Exhibit 11-5   Ten Principles for Minimizing Dysfunctional Behaviors

1. Know thyself.
2. Walk the talk.
3. Be willing to listen.
4. Value the truth of the whole.
5. Empower employees.
6. Build relationships on respect.
7. Act as an agent of transformation.
8. Screen job candidates for dysfunction.
9. Expect accountability.
10. Reward value-adding behaviors.

When people identify with family members, they give them support. When they identify with their environment, they protect and nurture it. When they identify with their organization, they give it their very best. Further, when they enlarge their sense of self by identifying with their organization, they develop a greater sense of responsibility toward it and link its welfare with theirs.

Knowing yourself is more than identifying your patterns of decision making. It includes identifying your values, your outlook on life, and the importance you place on integrity and the work ethic. The leader who believes that employees are basically honest, hard working, and optimistic about the future is quite different from the leader who believes that employees do only what they absolutely must, tend to be less than truthful, and are typically negative about the future.

Leaders need to listen to what others have to say about them and to look carefully at their style of communication and the way they treat point-of-service workers. The words others say about them are not always easy to swallow but cannot be ignored. As leaders, they are honor-bound to respond and make the changes necessary to improve their reputation. Interestingly, most leaders listen to negative feedback up to a point and permit some change. The goal, however, is to pass through a make-or-break threshold of anxiety about having to change, trust others, and renounce autocratic behavior. Getting through this threshold helps everyone in the organization, whereas backing away from making the necessary changes allows the damage to continue.

Leaders should look at themselves, confront their emotions, and acknowledge the pain and resentment of employees. For how much of the pain are they accountable? When an intimidating senior manager says to an employee, "I want to know how you see me," the employee might be reluctant to answer honestly out of fear of retaliation. If a leader discovers that others are afraid of being open, he or she must make the effort to eliminate the toxic behaviors that cause their fear, such as yelling, criticism, and negative feedback.

> ### Point to Ponder
>
> Passion is manifested in a commitment of energy and a personal investment in an effort so strongly felt that adversity cannot diminish the effort. Passion sees the leader through those inevitable times of toughness, darkness, and slow change.
>
> —Tim Porter-O'Grady, "A Call for Leaders"

Personal assessment often allows leaders to gain an appreciation of unexplained discrepancies between how they are viewed by colleagues and by family and friends. At work even though people look the same, what they become in the eyes of others is seldom the same as how they are perceived in their personal life. It is possible, for example, for an individual to be considered competent outside of the workplace but incompetent at work—or vice versa. Although self-assessment and dialogue with others can clarify paradoxical perceptions, they cannot eliminate the disparities.

As leaders journey through the self-assessment process, they may find that meditation is useful for relaxing and regaining a healthy balance. Relaxation is not just the relief of tension but the foundation of self-healing abilities. By learning to relax, people build confidence in their ability to control their body, feelings, and thoughts. They become aware of having more choices in how to react and how to feel. They also become more aware of what kinds of things, people, and thoughts tend to produce tension—an important first step in learning to deal with these sources of tension constructively. In addition, relaxation interrupts habitual negative thought patterns and clears the mind.

Principle 2: Walk the Talk

The second rule for reducing toxicity is to walk the talk—to act in accordance with expressed values. If leaders did in fact walk their talk and consequently did listen to employees, would it be necessary to have suggestion boxes? If they really had an open-door policy, would they have to sell it so emphatically? Building trust between two individuals requires the words and actions of each to be congruent. The trust that leaders acquire by walking their talk encourages innovative behaviors by employees, minimizes the potential for discrepancies between expectations and reality, reinforces their perceived integrity, strengthens the confidence that employees have in the appropriateness of future interactions, and reinforces the bond between the leaders and employees.

In times of chaos, the importance of constancy of values increases. Although the healthcare environment and marketplace present regular challenges for health professionals, the mission and values of health care remain unchanged. The values of respect, compassion, confidentiality, patient advocacy, accountability, competence, continuing knowledge development, supportive work environments, and collaboration remain constant beacons of light for those who work in the field.

Creating a team (or committee) to act as the conscience of the organization could assist all employees in evaluating their success at walking the talk. The committee, an extension of the traditional ethics committee, would provide an ongoing critique of leadership decision making to ensure that the decisions chosen are consistent with the values and norms of the organization. In addition, it could give careful consideration to potential conflicts between formally stated organizational values and unavoidable financial or business pressures, as well as issues related to all types of harassment, coercion, and discrimination.

As an example, recent downsizing efforts, despite organizations' professed respect for the dignity of all individuals, resulted in a significant loss of dignity by the employees who were laid off. If instead these organizations had used their power appropriately, acted to protect human rights and dignity, and taken organizational and societal issues into consideration at the outset of their decision making, they could have responded to the financial pressures in a way that minimized the negative impact on employees and thus minimized the resulting organizational toxicity.

Given that the traditional contract between employers and employees—in which long-term job security is traded for loyalty—is becoming extinct, a new contract needs to be fashioned to ensure that employees are not victimized or wind up working in a trustless environment. In other words, the employer–employee relationship needs to be reconceived. Although it is true that promises of long-term employment and associated benefits are inappropriate in the current marketplace, employers and employees should openly and honestly discuss the nature of the work, expected changes that affect the work, and ways in which employees can remain useful to the organization. If an employee leaves the organization, the termination of employment should be the result of a mutual decision rather than a unilateral act by either the employer or the employee.

Principle 3: Be Willing to Listen

Active listening is not just a matter of hearing, for instance, employees' feelings of loss, anger, or survivor guilt; it also encompasses taking these feelings to heart and not dismissing them as merely trivial. The leader who is an expert at listening believes that every employee is a source of unique information critical to the organization's success.

Shared leadership is one leadership model that is especially conducive to active listening—and to healthy dialogue. Also conducive to active listening is the horizontal organizational model, in which teams of individuals are involved in organization-wide, cross-functional core processes.

Group Discussion

If you could whisper one thing in the ear of your organization's leader, what would it be? Would it concern specific toxic behaviors? Look at what other people in your group would want to whisper. Would their questions and comments be like these?

- Why don't you react to that behavior?
- Give us a sign that you understand and truly care about employees in our organization.
- Why don't you fire that person?
- How do I know whether you are satisfied with my performance?

Consider the differences and similarities in the questions and comments and identify at least two strategies to correct the problems you have identified.

Listening is an essential part of effective problem solving and decision making. Leaders in quantum organizations use active and critical listening skills to gain a full understanding of problem situations. To acquire the depth of understanding they need, they must explore multiple issues and gather myriad data, both of which begin with critical listening.

Principle 4: Value the Truth of the Whole

The power to be gained from understanding both sides of an issue often goes unappreciated. Instead, an individual will strive to have others believe and support a particular point of view—his or her own. In the quantum organization, understanding multiple perspectives and balancing differing opinions are particularly helpful for arriving at optimal decisions. The challenge for the quantum leader is to cherish the fruitful opposition between order and creativity and to escape the grip of either/or thinking. Multiple perspectives are essential for understanding the whole. Often, the whole truth is a paradoxical joining of apparent opposites, and if the whole truth is desired, the opposites need to be embraced as a unit.

Perhaps one of the most challenging tasks involved in arriving at the truth is error management. Errors, although always part of the whole reality of a situation, have been historically cast aside, leaving only the successes to be remembered. Learning to integrate errors and absorb their lessons promises to be a long and arduous journey.

The emotional pain that is caused when an error is committed is often contagious and leads to self-defeating behaviors. Employees begin to have doubts about their own competence, and new mistakes appear to come out of nowhere. All too often these mistakes result from insidious lapses in judgment that occur when knowledge is steeped in the apathy and immobilization of emotional pain. Open and honest management of the whole of the situation—successes and errors—serves to reinforce positive practices and minimizes the potential for continuing errors and patient injury.

Finally, the leadership team should have room for a whole constellation of personality styles to ensure the effectiveness of its decision-making practices. Healthy organizations typically seek to include a broad variety of leadership personality styles so that multiple perspectives can be considered and no single one can dominate in the creation of strategies and structures, thereby minimizing the potential for groupthink.

Principle 5: Empower Employees

Leaders of quantum organizations work to empower employees and ensure they have the freedom to make suggestions, grow and mature, and become sensitized to themselves and others. The corporate social democracy they practice is much different from the corporate elitism associated with centralized power. Instead of the chief executive and managers thinking for everyone, all individuals in the organization think. Instead of a mission statement being handed down, all employees should participate in the creation of the organization's vision, mission, and values because they do the work and deserve the right to define these critical elements.

Leadership expertise is easily identified in action but difficult to describe in its richness. The wisdom of leaders is similar to the clinical wisdom of clinicians described by Benner, Hooper-Kyriakidis, and Stannard (1999). It includes the essential skills of grasp (comprehension), inquiry, and forethought. Leaders who want to serve as transformers need to acquire this wisdom.

Obtaining these skills requires significant leadership experience. Leaders who have this level of experience become expert at problem identification and solving and can act in situations that are ambiguous, underdetermined, unexpected, and/or markedly different from their preconceptions. Grasping involves making qualitative distinctions, doing detective work, recognizing changes, and developing relevant knowledge bases. Inquiry involves knowing what questions to ask. Expert leaders learn to use their knowledge, experience, and intuition to anticipate crises, risks, and vulnerabilities that may affect the organization or its employees.

For example, in implementing a program, the timing of events is often crucial to success. During a period when employees are demoralized from downsizing in other local organizations, a wise leader would not choose to reduce benefits and cause additional stress. Although it is possible to view this decision as motivated by expedience, political cowardice, or unrealistic optimism, it is more likely to be based on a grasp of the organization's entire context and a realization that traumatizing employees further is counterproductive in the long run.

Forethought is another component of leadership wisdom that emerges after significant experience dealing with common situations and unanticipated events. It is basically the ability to anticipate likely eventualities and to take the appropriate actions—an ability seldom articulated despite the fact that it is pervasive in the everyday actions of expert leaders. These leaders subconsciously project possible situations that may result from particular conditions. Then, by being extra attentive and by using their ability to recognize patterns and sense the relevance of events, they are able to prepare the organization for the most probable of these situations.

Empowering employees is a career-long journey of mentoring. The goal is to transfer leadership wisdom not only to aspiring leaders but to all employees. Along this journey, expert leaders provide tools for employees to do their jobs well and to help them feel successful. They try to create a culture of respect based on the belief that employees who feel successful and appreciated in the workplace truly leave their work, both physically and mentally, at the end of the day and are thus better able to manage their time and achieve and maintain a healthy balance between work and personal life.

Principle 6: Build Relationships on Respect

Each and every interaction among employees and between employees and patients should be directed toward achieving therapeutic outcomes. No relationships characterized by disrespectful behavior, insulting language, or emotional harm can be tolerated. Respect for employees is an expectation that is never open to discussion. No individual ever has the permission to be rude or abusive to any other individual. The fundamental right of every person to be treated in a manner that reflects the inherent value of human beings is the guiding principle of all human relationships.

Following are rules that leaders should keep in mind to help ensure that their relationships with employees and the relationships among employees are essentially therapeutic:

- Behave so as to preserve every person's dignity.
- Encourage employees to talk with each other to learn more about each other's opinions before reaching a conclusion.
- Encourage self-improvement.
- Give employees feedback on their performance.
- Be open to new ideas.
- Encourage employees to do their best.
- Compensate employees fairly for the work they do.

These next rules apply to the relationships between care providers and patients. Because their purpose is likewise to help ensure that these relationships are fundamentally therapeutic, they need to be followed by the care providers:

- Probe to uncover the rationale for any decision that a patient makes.
- Recognize that family members and friends can have a significant impact on a patient's ability to manage his or her own health.
- Consider a patient's cultural beliefs before providing care.
- Consider a patient's spiritual beliefs before providing care.
- Empower patients to avoid unnecessary dependency or overtreatment.
- Recognize that clinical and behavioral outcomes affect each other.
- Support a patient's choice to use culturally based healing practices.
- Be fully present and listen to each patient.
- Assist each patient to develop or sustain his or her ability to cope with life situations.
- Identify each patient's feelings about his or her illness and expectations for recovery.
- Encourage patients to participate in self-care programs.
- Recognize that a patient's choices should guide the plan of care.

Principle 7: Act as an Agent of Transformation

Quantum leaders encourage employees to be self-reliant and to take charge of their careers, not only their current jobs. They assist employees in overcoming the negative effects of career entrenchment or entrapment, such as dissatisfaction and ineffectiveness. Quantum leaders also

- Encourage employees to voice concerns and work collaboratively to identify and address dissatisfaction.
- Do not threaten retaliation when employees express negative emotions or opinions.
- Recognize discrepancy between ideal career progression and reality.
- Seek to transform career pathways into a progressive career management program.
- Recognize that employee loyalty has advantages and disadvantages (e.g., loyalty can be merely passive and result in skill atrophy, boredom, and depression).

In addition, quantum leaders encourage employees to engage in extra-role activities that are not directly compensated but that can decrease employee stress while simultaneously benefiting the organization. Acting as a mentor outside the organization is an example of extra-role citizenship work that can decrease the frustration of entrenched employees while reducing stress and meeting affiliation needs.

Quantum leaders understand that entrenched employees who attempt to cope with their career issues through loyalty or by acting as a constructive voice do contribute to workforce stability and reduce turnover costs. These employees often can be jarred from their entrenchment by giving them the opportunity to be involved in special projects, by permitting job rotation, by facilitating downward or lateral moves, by training them in cross-functional roles, and by allowing temporary reassignments (**Exhibit 11-6**).

Career development programs can assist employees in using the "constructive voice" approach to dealing with career entrenchment. Retraining and redeployment programs further assist employees in managing their careers and thereby help the organization sustain its viability. Employees in organizations that avoid career management are less likely to discuss career issues affecting their performance.

Finally, when all else fails, it may be necessary to remove an employee who has retired on the job. Employees who have lost the motivation to develop and grow become increasingly less productive and focus on noncareer activities at the expense of the organization. They therefore need to be counseled to seek employment opportunities outside of the organization.

Exhibit 11-6   Organizational Strategies to Minimize Career Entrenchment

- Offer generous severance pay packages to fund employees' explorations into new careers.
- Offer tuition reimbursements and time off for employees to attend classes while still employed.
- Give employees time to rotate to other positions in the organization so that they might explore another career option within the relatively safe confines of the organization.
- Discourage linear career paths and emphasize psychological success.
- Ensure that employees do not feel as though they are violating the organization's trust as they investigate new career options.
- Allow employees who leave in good standing to return if their new career plans fail.

Exhibit 11-7   Interviewing to Minimize Toxicity

1. Tell me about your preferences for assignments, delegating, and managing authority.
2. How frequently do you believe feedback and updating of work are needed?
3. What is your major frustration in your current job? What are the major frustrations in the jobs performed by those you have supervised?
4. What would make you comfortable in overriding my authority and decisions?
5. What type of people and financial support do you require to ensure that your job is done well?
6. What are the perceived strengths and weaknesses of this organization?

Principle 8: Screen Job Candidates for Dysfunction

New employees represent a significant investment for the organization, and job candidates require more scrutiny than they currently receive. To help in screening job candidates, leaders should identify specific dysfunctional behaviors that have a negative impact on organizational performance and, with the assistance of human resource experts, should develop new approaches to interviewing and selecting employees. The 10 principles for minimizing toxic behaviors under discussion in this section are likely to be useful in these endeavors, as are the 6 questions presented in **Exhibit 11-7**. In addition, these questions are appropriate for ongoing use to prevent or decrease dysfunction among current employees. Getting regular feedback from employees about their assignment preferences and current frustrations assists leaders in developing a good working relationship with them.

Principle 9: Expect Accountability

Accountability is more than the background against which everyday decisions are made. In fact, the way in which accountability is created, negotiated, communicated, and evaluated lies at the heart of an organization's operations. Unfortunately, years of entitlement philosophies have created workers who park their brains at the door and are comfortable with being rewarded for simply showing up. According to Connors, Smith, and Hickman (1994), the concept of accountability has been poorly defined in the popular press and in the literature on business. Consequently, most people believe accountability is something that happens to them or is inflicted upon them. They perceive it as a heavy burden, although they also view it as something that is applied only when something goes wrong or when someone else is trying to pinpoint the blame for a problem. Instead, Connors and colleagues suggest the following definition of accountability:

> An attitude of continually asking "what else can I do to rise above my circumstances and achieve the results I desire?" It is the process of seeing it, owning it, solving it, and doing it. It requires a level of ownership that includes making, keeping, and proactively answering for personal commitments. It is a perspective that embraces both current and future efforts, rather than reactive and historical explanations.

Accountability systems, to function properly, require the clear delineation of individual behaviors and supporting management practices. Both individual accountability and system accountability are necessary to support the values of integrity and transformation and to foster therapeutic relationships. Individuals in a quantum organization are not threatened by the expectation for accountability but rather need accountability to perform at a high level.

Principle 10: Reward Value-Adding Behaviors

The opportunity now exists for leaders to shift the focus from return on investment to cost-effectiveness and to create new rules that lay the groundwork for value-based reward and recognition programs. First and foremost, healthcare leaders are called on by the economic community to use resources in a way that ensures healthcare value. Care providers can no longer give the best of everything without any financial accounting.

Healthcare leaders and providers are now required to examine services within the value equation. If resources are limited, does every patient symptom require intervention, particularly if little or no improvement in the patient's clinical condition is likely to result? Just to ask this question is a challenge for providers and leaders schooled in an environment characterized by increasing growth of and access to the healthcare system. Provision of as many services as possible was the sign of the successful leader. Unfortunately, there was no accountability and no control in the fee-for-service payment system. The result is well known: the exhaustion of resources.

Healthcare services need to be appropriate to the conditions being treated, focused on outcomes, and consistent with the wishes of the patients and families being served. The buyers and users of health care want to know they are getting value for the resources expended. They want to know that something good or better will happen because of the purchase of healthcare services—that the users' health will be improved. They also are demanding that the choices made by care providers are rational and based on evidence.

Given the expectations of buyers and users, healthcare leaders need to create an organizational context that supports the desired services and directs the rewards and recognition of the organization toward efforts that can meet these expectations. In addition, the success of care providers in improving the health of patients or community members and in managing their own health needs to be recognized and rewarded.

In a quantum healthcare organization, the care providers work to ensure that the patients

- Experience an improvement in their clinical condition, possibly including increased physical functioning, greater tolerance of activity, improved ambulation, and/or reduced pain
- Improve their ability to care for themselves, including performing wound care, taking medications on schedule, maintaining a nutritious diet, and eliminating properly
- Learn more about their condition and its treatment, including their own treatment regime, appropriate procedures, potential complications, and emergency interventions
- Are aware of the elements of a healthy lifestyle, including proper nutrition, weight management, activity, stress management, sleep, safety, infection control, and disease screening

The main tasks of the leaders of a quantum healthcare organization include

- Hiring and developing a workforce capable of achieving the patient outcomes listed previously
- Retaining and continuing to develop the care providers needed to meet the organization's future needs
- Creating a system in which providers and leaders can influence the context of care provision based on their understanding of what is needed and what they are capable of doing (e.g., providers and leaders both need to actively intervene to improve communication, understand potential situations likely to unfold, and alter the context as necessary)
- Fostering therapeutic relationships among leaders, providers, and patients that focus on the values and beliefs of the patients, develop the inner capacities of the patients and providers, involve patients in decision making, and make room for self-responsibility

Organizations might find it helpful to use the topic of organizational toxins and ways of minimizing behavioral dysfunction as the theme of a leadership retreat. In such a retreat, the participants could be challenged to identify toxins in their department or the organization as a whole and then consider strategies to reduce the toxicity using the preceding principles.

Conclusion

To counteract the toxicity that currently exists in healthcare organizations, leaders need to return humanity to the workplace. There is nothing easy, however, about creating the proper context for providing healthcare services. An organization is an open system consisting of inputs, throughputs, and outputs, all of which can be healthy or toxic. The work of delivering care is complex and emotional. Care providers deal with human beings at their most vulnerable, which requires of the providers a high level of personal involvement and commitment.

What is terrifying about dysfunctional organizations is that employee emotional pain is accepted as a natural phenomenon. Employees are expected to live with discomfort as a condition of employment. The real mystery is the continual denial by leaders of a connection between employee pain and service quality. It seems to escape many leaders that employee dissatisfaction leads inevitably to patient dissatisfaction and that, conversely, there is a correlation between contented employees and gratified patients. Even when they accept this correlation, leaders find it difficult to create the conditions and practices that increase both employee and patient satisfaction.

The aim of leadership is not to create a workers' paradise but rather to engender an organizational culture that allows for organizational transformation and for the employees' performance to live and grow. It is the obligation of the leader of a healthcare organization to push toward organizational health so that the will of the patient is respected. To do this, the leader needs to demonstrate a willingness and ability to cultivate self-transformations, as well as transformations in others, on a continuing basis.

The obligations of leaders and employees are interconnected. Neither group can be successful without both of them meeting their responsibilities. Leadership is never an either/or situation. Further, leadership is a rational service performed by rational people directed toward achieving sensible organizational objectives. However, these rational people carry with them past experiences laden with neurotic styles, negative transference, superior–subordinate entanglements, and untenable strategies. Not surprisingly, unless the leaders recognize this and foster appropriate behaviors, the result is persistent dysfunction.

Finally, leaders need to forget about ever finding enough time. There is never enough time for all the things individuals want to do. Rather, the challenge is to find a healthy balance between the things of importance: work, family, and hobbies.

Case Study 11-1

Toxic Incivility at the Unit Level

Jeannie Walker just accepted a job as nurse manager for the ortho-neuro unit of a large community hospital. She just graduated with her master's degree in nursing with an emphasis on nursing leadership in healthcare settings. Excited about the new role and opportunities to influence positive changes on a nursing unit, Jeannie wasn't at all concerned when the human resources officer mentioned that the last three managers on the ortho-neuro unit left the position after 12 to 18 months. Jeannie had lots of clinical experience, and now armed with all that she had learned in graduate school, she was confident that she would be able to handle the management of the 32-bed unit with a staff consisting of 120 full- and part-time employees. The human resources officer had told her that half of the staff were long-term employees, but the other half were fairly new to the unit. There seemed to be a lot of turnover among newer employees, but the long-term employees had worked on the unit an average of 20 years. Jeannie had aspirations of leading her unit in collaborative governance and hopefully influencing other directors and managers to begin the Magnet journey.

During her first few weeks in the role, Jeannie discovered a lot of facts about the staff and the care delivery model. With a nurse-to-patient ratio of one nurse to four patients and one nursing assistant for every eight patients, the unit seemed to be reasonably staffed for the expected workload required for patient care. She also discovered that only 35% of the nurses were prepared at the baccalaureate level, 55% had attained an associate's degree, and 10% had a diploma in nursing. There was a strong ethnic mix as well, with nearly 30% of the nurses educated in foreign countries such as the Philippines (20%) and India (10%) and others who were second-generation immigrants from the Philippines (30%), Middle East (10%), Canada (7%), and Germany (3%) educated in the United States. The remaining 20% were American born and educated. Jeannie also discovered that the unit was experiencing a higher than hospital and national average rate for hospital-acquired infections (HAIs), patient falls, and medication errors. Nurse satisfaction levels were the lowest of all of the nursing units at the hospital, and if this wasn't enough, the patient and physician satisfaction levels were also lower than the hospital average. Jeannie was surprised with such quality indicators, but she attributed such poor performance to the need for a consistent, strong, and visionary leader who would inspire the staff to work together and improve these quality indicators. She felt up to the challenge to transform this staff and voiced this commitment to excellence to nurses at her first staff meeting. After an energetic and inspiring "state of the union" address accompanied by her vision for the future, Jeannie was a bit surprised that the staff remained absolutely stoic and had no response to her plans to create a collaborative governance structure with unit councils providing staff input into decisions affecting nursing and patient care. Perhaps it was because she was new?

Over the course of a few months, Jeannie tried to establish a Unit Practice Council (UPC) and a Research and Evidence-Based Practice (REBP) Council, but few of the staff volunteered to participate on either of the councils. Jeannie sought a handful of nurses who she believed would be strong leaders and talked with them about her vision for empowering the nurses through council involvement. She was shocked to hear a resounding "no" from the nurses, who shared that they were afraid to participate. The repetitive answer from many of the nurses was "I only want to do my job and go home." As Jeannie inquired more and more, she discovered that the staff were extremely fractionated into cultural groups who did not like to integrate or communicate any more than absolutely necessary with other cultural groups. Not only were the nurses in firm social cliques, but the more senior nurses on both shifts had first preference for scheduling, patient assignments, and lunch breaks. They refused to take assignments to orient new personnel or to be preceptors for nursing students. Because they were such a powerful group, they seemed to make the decisions for all of the staff. If any of the nurses from other cultural groups voiced a complaint, they were the ones who were canceled first for scheduled or overtime shifts or received the most difficult patients for an assignment.

Jeannie learned that there was often open conflict among the nurses with name calling, accusations, threats, and retaliations. Evening shift nurses accused day shift nurses of being "lazy," not completing patient care assignments, or leaving the bulk of work to the evening/night shift nurses. Day shift nurses complained that night nurses were "sleeping on the job" and not properly assessing patients or documenting appropriately. To make matters worse, several of the physicians joined in with their own complaints and accusations that "these nurses are the worst of any unit in the entire hospital," "they don't know anything about ortho-neuro patients," and "they call all hours of the night for trivial things." After a few weeks of hearing all the complaints from multiple sources, seeing the negative unit quality indicators, and refereeing a number of conflicts among nurses and physicians, Jeannie felt completely overwhelmed. She mentioned to a comanager, "I feel like the man in the circus who spins plates on a bunch of poles all at once. He has to keep dancing around just to keep a plate from following down and breaking."

Jeannie tried many of the ideas she had learned in class about managing interpersonal conflict, using change theories as a framework for change, and leading intergenerational and intercultural work groups. She met with nurses individually and in groups. She tried to create a shared vision of what the future could be. She reread Chapter 11 in *Quantum Leadership* and tried to remember class discussions of others who had witnessed similar situations in their clinical experiences. She remained confident that collaborative governance would be the best option for correcting many of the problems on the unit.

The entire unit of nurses seemed reluctant to change and seemed to have absolutely no interest in a collaborative governance structure. Because the hospital was under a union collective bargaining contract for nursing, the union shop steward, Angelina, asked for a meeting with Jeannie.

Angelina explained that the nurses as a collective whole didn't support moving to a collaborative governance structure, nor did they want input into unit decisions. "This is the job of management and not of staff nurses," Angelina explained, and she advised Jeannie to cease from trying to change the unit.

Jeannie faces huge and complex challenges with her new role as nurse manager. It is clear to her that change is critically needed to ensure optimal patient outcomes and to create a work environment that is safe and healthy for the nursing staff.

Questions

1. Using the principles discussed in this chapter, describe the stakeholders in this case; then, take on the perspective of each stakeholder group and analyze the case from that perspective. How would you transform this unit from a toxic work environment to a healthy, supportive work environment?
2. Identify the players who are the power holders and how they use that power to influence the whole unit.
3. Describe the various issues that complicate the case. How are these issues interrelated?
4. Take on the role of Jeannie, and describe how you might manage this situation and transform the unit.

References

Barrett, R. (1995). *A guide to liberating your soul.* Alexandria, VA: Unfoldment.

Benner, P., Hooper-Kyriakidis, P., & Stannard, D. (1999). *Clinical wisdom and interventions in critical care: A thinking-in-action approach.* Philadelphia, PA: Saunders.

Branch, S., Ramsay, S., & Barker, M. (2013). Workplace bullying, mobbing and general harassment: A review. *International Journal of Management Reviews, 15*(3), 280–299.

Carson, K. D., & Carson, P. P. (1997). Career entrenchment: A quiet march toward occupational death. *Academy of Management Executives, 11*(2), 62–76.

Connors, R., Smith, T., & Hickman, E. (1994). *The Oz principle: Getting results through individual and organizational accountability.* Englewood Cliffs, NJ: Prentice Hall.

Gallo, A. (2013). How to manage someone you don't like. HBR Blog Network. Retrieved from http://blogs .hbr.org/2013/08/how-to-manage-someone-you-dont/

Geneen, H. (1997). *The synergy myth.* New York, NY: St. Martin's.

Huang, C. A., & Lynch, J. (1995). *Mentoring: The Tao of giving and receiving wisdom.* San Francisco, CA: Harper Collins.

King, S. K. (1989). Removing distress to reveal health. In R. Carlson & B. Shield (Eds.), *Healers on healing.* Los Angeles, CA: Jeremy P. Tarcher.

Lundin, W., & Lundin, K. (1993). *The healing manager: How to build quality relationships and productive cultures at work.* San Francisco, CA: Berrett-Koehler.

Malloch, K. (2001). The white lies of leadership. *Nursing Administration Quarterly, 25*(3), 61–68.

Mohr, J. M. (2013). Wolf in sheep's clothing: Harmful leadership with a moral façade. *Journal of Leadership Studies, 7*(1), 18–32.

Porath, C., & Pearson, C. (2013). The price of incivility: Lack of respect hurts morale—and the bottom line. *Harvard Business Review, 91*(1), 115–121.

Porter-O'Grady, T. (2000). A call for leaders. *SSM, 6*(10), 10–12.

Robinson, S. L., & O'Leary-Kelly, A. M. (1998). Monkey see, monkey do: The influence of work groups on the antisocial behavior of employees. *Academy of Management Journal, 41,* 658–672.

Suggested Readings

Carlson, R., & Shield, B. (Eds.). (1989). *Healers on healing.* Los Angeles, CA: Jeremy P. Tarcher.

Hardy, R. E., & Schwartz, R. (1996). *The self-defeating organization: How smart companies can stop out-smarting themselves.* Reading, MA: Addison-Wesley.

Kets de Vries, M. F. R., & Miller, D. (1984). *The neurotic organization.* San Francisco, CA: Jossey-Bass.

Palmer, P. J. (1998). *The courage to teach: Exploring the inner landscape of a teacher's life.* San Francisco, CA: Jossey-Bass.

Rosenstein, A. H., & O'Daniel, M. (2005). Disruptive behavior and clinical outcomes: Perceptions of nurses and physicians. *Nursing Management, 36*(1), 18–28.

Thurston, B. (2013, July/August). #Unplug. *Fast Company,* 73–75.

Quiz Questions

Select the best answer for each of the following questions.

1. How can toxic behaviors in healthcare organizations be described?
   a. They are behaviors and practices that work against the delivery of healthcare services.
   b. They are engaged in specifically by individuals fearful of accountability.
   c. They can be remedied easily once the toxins are identified.
   d. They result from established rituals rather than faulty communication.

2. Much like physical toxins that cause illness in individuals, toxic behaviors cause illness in organizations. Which of the following is true of both human illness and organizational illness?
   a. Illness results from an imbalance in the amount and type of nutrients and cleansing activities.
   b. Additional nutrients lead to the restoration of health.
   c. Routine cleansing of waste is an effective means of restoring health.
   d. Health is the absence of dysfunction.

3. What are toxic behaviors in healthcare organizations caused by?
   a. Decreased financial support resulting from the advent of managed care
   b. The personal characteristics of the leaders and employees coupled with the realities of the marketplace
   c. A lack of leadership development
   d. Poor parenting during the leaders' developmental years

4. Why are vertical organizations often considered toxic?

   a. The departments do not communicate with each other.
   b. The customer (or patient) is not the first concern.
   c. The vigilance of the senior leaders is not appreciated by the employees and other leaders.
   d. Authority and decision making are localized at the top.

5. How can mandatory overtime as a management practice used in healthcare organizations be characterized?

   a. It is an appropriate means of responding to staffing needs where life and death situations frequently occur.
   b. It shows an unjustifiable lack of consideration for the need of employees to balance work and personal life.
   c. It is a matter best handled through legislation at the state level.
   d. It should be up to each organization to use as it sees fit.

6. An employee who feels entrenched or entrapped may well experience hope when?

   a. When the organization brings in a new leadership team
   b. When the employee is released from the expectation that he or she will perform community service
   c. When the employee is rotated to a different position to explore another career option within the confines of the organization
   d. When a new employee benefits package is implemented

7. Tolerance of antisocial behaviors has a negative impact on the social climate and general moral conduct of employees. When can antisocial behaviors be minimized?

   a. When group interaction is encouraged and work tasks are shared
   b. When individual members of the group confront the offending employees
   c. When these behaviors are discouraged by the organization's leader
   d. When employees with a history of antisocial behavior are not allowed to join groups in which antisocial behavior is absent

8. How can individual accountability best be described?

   a. It is the ability to give the reasons for one's actions upon request.
   b. It is something that happens to or is inflicted upon an individual.
   c. It is ownership of one's behaviors.
   d. It is the process of seeing it, owning it, solving it, and doing it.

9. If leaders are inconsistent in word and action, employees _____.

   a. Wonder whether their decisions will be respected
   b. View regular communication as unimportant
   c. Feel a lack of support from the leaders
   d. Feel entrapped, angry, and insecure

10. The importance of therapeutic relationships between employees and leaders is not always recognized. What is the expected outcome of such relationships?

a. Improved communication and more productive interaction

b. More accurate medical documentation

c. Preservation of confidentiality

d. Improved job satisfaction

11. Advocacy is often misunderstood by leaders, especially when efforts are expended to repair a broken system. Which of the following is the best way to view patient advocacy?

a. As the process of creating the necessary conditions for patients to receive the care they desire

b. As the proper responsibility of an ombudsman within the healthcare facility

c. As a means of quickly addressing the situations in which patient requests were not honored

d. As a desirable but often unattained phenomenon

12. Self-assessment is an essential task for a leader who wants to transform his or her organization. For this type of leader, what is the goal of self-assessment?

a. To create a sense of identity with the organization and motivate the leader to do his or her very best

b. To discover both positive and negative behaviors that affect performance

c. To share personal flaws with other employees

d. To identify continuing education needs

CHAPTER TWELVE

Coaching for Unending Change: Transforming the Membership Community

We can succeed only by concert. It is not "can any of us imagine better?" but, "can we all do better?" The dogmas of the quiet past are inadequate to the stormy present. The occasion is piled high with difficulty, and we must rise with the occasion. As our case is new, so we must think anew, and act anew.

—*Abraham Lincoln, 1862*

Chapter Objectives

At the completion of this chapter, the reader will be able to

- Recognize the key elements of coaching within a fast-paced organization in highly charged and changing times.
- Translate the characteristics of transformational coaching into the planning and implementation of new skill formation.
- Describe the needs of teams in a system and explain the importance of team leadership.
- Identify the fundamentals of the learning organization and the dynamics of learning leadership.
- Name the steps of revolutionary and innovation coaching and how it applies to the role of the leader.

In the highly complex contemporary environment of most healthcare organizations, understanding how the role of leadership is both challenged and transformed by the emerging principles of complexity leadership is critical to thriving and succeeding. In this accelerating age of complexity, no role has been more greatly challenged. The role of leader requires a whole new frame for expression. Much of the work of leaders now is directed toward helping others confront the vagaries of major changes occurring in the work and structure of the workplace. Leaders must exhibit a new set of skills to create the conditions for a new accountable care environment that ties effective service quality directly to

> **Key Point**
>
> Leadership requires a level of self-knowledge and vulnerability that makes the growth experience visible to others.

positive health outcomes. The mental models and performance expectations of staff require heavy retooling to ensure they can thrive in the new work environment. Leaders will learn some of the elements of leading in this new environment and the steps necessary to get staff engaged and motivated to change and grow in a context demanding a different way of delivering health care.

Leadership is not so much who you are as what you do with who you are. Leadership is not a state of being. It is instead a set of internal tools possessed by a person with the energy and skill to use them well. Much of the work of leadership in this new century consists of transferring new skills to the people who live and work in organizations.

Because this is a time of great change, increasing complexity, and fast-moving advances in technology, with higher expectations for health in an accountable care environment, people find it increasingly difficult to meet the growing number of new demands. Social and technological forces conspire to create the conditions that affect how people work, relate, and plan for their own future. In this process the role of leaders is to live the positive experience of change and master the ability to engage the questions and challenges that accompany change. Staff members are watching closely to see how leaders embrace and engage the challenges of change. By observing how leaders do this, staff members create a vision for their own adjustment to change. The leaders' role modeling of adjustment to change encourages staff to adapt to change and demonstrates the necessary techniques.

From Responsibility to Accountability

In the coming age of accountable care, responsibility is no longer the key element of work performance. Historically, a worker's performance was judged to be acceptable if the worker simply did well what he or she was supposed to do. For the performance to be evaluated as excellent, the worker had to do this work and do it exceptionally well. In the twentieth-century workplace, the focus on responsibility was prevalent in every aspect of the definition of work and the measurement of performance.

This focus was structured in the workplace in several ways. First, job descriptions were often laundry lists of functions and activities. In other words, they zeroed in on the activities of work rather than their product. Second, performance evaluations reviewed the work someone did—the functions of work and the ability of the person to do the work. The person's behavior and ability to get along with others were included in the list of "competencies." How well the person did the work, not whether the work was worthwhile, determined whether the person was to be specially rewarded. Third, the evaluation of work tended to concentrate on the quality of the work processes—how the work was done and how many errors were committed. It also looked at efficiency, or the amount of time the worker spent in delivering a service or product as compared with the average.

Slavish attachment to process has been an earmark of the twentieth-century workplace. Process improvement, process evaluation, process measurement, process effectiveness—these all concern what workers do rather than what they achieve. One reason for this may be that, in health care, the relationship between outcome and process has never been well understood.

In this twenty-first-century accountable care environment, work is now viewed from the perspective of its outcomes.

> ### Point to Ponder
>
> Accountability requires that people have ownership over their work. Consequently, the organization must recognize that it does not control the work that people do but simply provides the context within which they do it.

Research has shown that focusing on outcomes alters work processes and the elements of the work. Indeed, it is now clear that all processes gain their meaning from their results or products. In other words, a process is considered valuable to the extent it relates "tightly" to the desired outcome. Much effort is now being expended on investigating the goodness of fit between work processes and their intended outcomes and improving the fit where possible.

In short, it is the Age of Accountability. The major role of leaders is to move people and organizations from responsibility to accountability—from a narrow focus on processes to a perspective that encompasses processes and results (**Exhibit 12-1**). In the Age of Accountability, leaders are expected to ensure that all components of the fit between processes and results come together into a complete vision of the work and its products. Among other tasks, they need to define expected outcomes for all actions and activities and to establish aggregate performance measures for evaluating the work performed by teams.

This movement toward the appreciation of outcomes requires a tremendous reorientation of the work and the workers. For the whole of the twentieth century, the emphasis was on functions and work processes, whereas now it is on creating sustainability in a time of rapid technological change. Focusing on work processes is no longer a viable strategy because they have such short life spans. The appropriate goal is to define the critical integration between means and ends, products and processes. This must be done with an understanding that sustainability is not resident in the work or even the incremental product of a given process or time. Sustainability instead results from a continuum of

---

Exhibit 12-1   Responsibility Versus Accountability

Responsibility (Twentieth Century)	Accountability (Twenty-First Century)
• Process	• Product
• Action	• Result
• Work	• Outcome
• Do	• Accomplish
• Task	• Difference
• Function	• Fit
• Job	• Role
• Incremental	• Sustainable
• Externally generated	• Internally generated

efforts that, when connected together, indicate the journey to be taken to improve the conditions or quality of life. In fact, this is the definitive foundation of the movement from volume-based health services to value-driven health outcomes.

Accountability is internally generated. It arises first and foremost within. Specifically, accountability is the result of a person's commitment to advancing, improving, growing, adapting, and enhancing his or her life experience. Accountability is generated out of the energy that a person brings to the exercise of living, whether at work or in other realms of life. In addition, accountability depends on individuals' having complete ownership of what they are and what they do and their commitment to apply their talents, energies, and skills in ways that make the circumstances of life better for themselves and others.

> **Key Point**
>
> In an organization, the leader is responsible for creating a sustainable structure for work and ensuring a good fit between the organization's goals and processes. Congruence here guarantees that the system functions as it should.

In an organization, in particular, accountability depends on members joining in a concerted, collective effort to achieve the organization's ends. If each person brings his or her energy, gifts, skills, and knowledge to bear fully on the work to be done, the outcomes of that work are ensured. Everyone in the workplace has a right to expect a commitment from all to apply themselves and use their skills and talents to the fullest. Furthermore, everyone has a right to expect that each team member (or employee in a group work context) will have a positive relationship with the other members and exhibit energy and commitment to the work and its products.

Leaders are obligated to make certain that the processes and structures needed to support ownership of the work are fully present. Each of the three main components—structure, relationship, and process—should be directed toward facilitating ownership so that the organization's work can be sustained and advanced. If the energy and desire of the worker cannot be maintained, it is impossible to sustain and advance the work of the organization.

Leaders must understand and apply the principles of human action and interaction. Human beings are dynamic and complex beings. When colleagues' commitment and motivation are at high levels, conflicts and other challenges arise. The work processes in place must be designed with the understanding that such challenges are normal and to be expected. They should also be designed to anticipate these challenges and address them in a way that increases the probability of good outcomes and sustains the work and the relationships among the employees.

In accountability-based organizations, leaders must recognize that the vagaries of human behavior and relationship are normal. Leaders must be aware of the whole spectrum of human dynamics and be capable of managing these dynamics. They must have tools and techniques to maintain the energy and focus of the workplace and its members in a way that advances the work and the achievement of desirable outcomes.

One of these techniques is to establish the expectation that principles are consistently applied and that accountability is maintained. If this is made clear to all members of the organization, along with a commitment not to permit behavior inconsistent with this expectation, the members will try to live up to the expectation and act appropriately. In accountability-based work processes, members articulate and enumerate the range of acceptable practices and behaviors, and processes for creating consistency are available to help members address those issues outside the agreed framework. Membership in a work group, like membership in any other collaborative enterprise, requires that the expressed expectations for the members are fulfilled; otherwise, the goals of the group are threatened or only partially achieved.

In regard to accountability, certain patterns of behavior reflect negative characteristics that ultimately impede personal expression and team interaction in the workplace (Brewer & Sanford, 2011; Hickey & Kritek, 2012; Lencioni, 2008). Which ones fall below the line and which above depend on the particular culture and context of the workplace. Members must clearly outline the two sets of behaviors to form a framework

> ### Point to Ponder
>
> Typically, approximately 90% of the leadership role is devoted to managing relationships. If a leader determines that managing relationships takes up a much smaller percentage of work time than that, the leader may need to reassess her or his priorities.

for the principles that determine the rules of engagement in the work relationship. The structure and process of leading and managing must be designed to ensure that the above-the-line behaviors are sustained. When the below-the-line behaviors emerge, the processes and methodologies in place must "click in" so that these behaviors can be addressed quickly and effectively. Quick response to behavioral variances is essential to prevent subsequent and sometimes irresolvable problems.

It must be remembered that accountability really means something. So often in the past decade accountability lost its central meaning and its impact on organizations and people. The financial scandals of the 1990s and the 2000s highlighted just how little understanding of accountability really exists. Accountability assumes that the leader accepts the full responsibility of that which occurs under the auspices of his or her leadership. It doesn't matter whether someone else "did the deed"; it only matters that the leader claims accountability for the actions of those for whom he or she holds leadership responsibility.

Accountability has three major elements: the right to decide and act, the power to decide and act, and the competence to decide and act. Productive accountability requires all three to be present in the role of the leader. Failure to exercise any of the three elements always results in a failure of accountability. Personal and organizational conflict result when any one of these elements is missing from the expression of accountability. Persons and organizations suffer when there is a failure to integrate or appropriately express these components of accountability in the best interest of persons and organizations.

The dynamics of relationship and work are highly complex and variable. Although it might seem beneficial for the framework for human behavior in the workplace to be permanent and unchanging, a permanent framework, besides being impractical, is inappropriate. It is within the course of relationships and interpersonal demands that the vagaries of life always have an impact. Personal patterns of behavior and changing patterns of interaction challenge the best work environment.

> ## Group Discussion
>
> Often, *responsibility* and *accountability* are used interchangeably, but they have different meanings. Based on the analysis of accountability in this chapter, compare how to change behavior in an accountability-based organization and how to change it in a responsibility-based organization.

Good leaders "read" work situations. They assess the demands and the dynamics of intersecting and interacting variables and judge how they affect the work being done and the relationships among the workers. They know that these variables create challenges for work relationships and functions—challenges that they are required to address. Research in the area of accountable behavior and organizational considerations is ongoing. Thus, leaders need to review this research periodically to gain up-to-date information on how to ensure that work processes result in desired outcomes.

Transforming Work and the Transforming Worker

During the current era, the major leadership task is to change the mental model of and framework for work. In all segments of society, work and the workplace are changing too fast for most people to keep up. Leaders, therefore, must guide the transformation of work and help people adjust as required.

For transformation to occur, a fundamental change in thinking must take place. Workers, for example, must completely reconceptualize their roles. Most people are satisfied with establishing a pattern of work and a set of rituals. Eventually, they become so accustomed to the pattern and rituals they see them as essential to the work. Indeed, they begin to see the work from within these patterns and rituals and ultimately become suspicious of anything that threatens what has become normal for them. Despite the fact that their adherence to patterns and rituals may impede necessary changes, leaders, who are agents of change, should not criticize them.

Leaders who try to bring about certain changes often become so unhappy with people's attachment to rituals that the rituals become the visible representation of people's unwillingness to change. After all, people's attachment to the routines of work ensures that the work gets done and meets certain standards of performance. Their attachment may obstruct improvements in quality, but it does virtually guarantee performance of the work activities.

> ### Key Point
>
> A whole body of research demonstrates that an open, inclusive, and accountable structure for work creates extra opportunities for creativity and innovation.

In times of transformation, leaders look to establish new patterns of work, even if the patterns soon need to be revised because of further rapidly changing circumstances. In addition, leaders often want workers to establish the same kind of attachment to a new pattern even though they complained when the workers were attached to the old patterns.

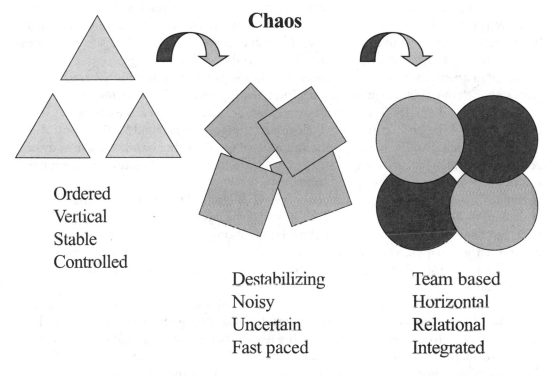

20th-Century Work　　　　　**21st-Century Work**

Chaos

Ordered
Vertical
Stable
Controlled

Destabilizing　　　　Team based
Noisy　　　　　　　Horizontal
Uncertain　　　　　Relational
Fast paced　　　　　Integrated

Figure 12-1　Transition from Twentieth-Century Work. The transition involves moving through the stages of change from predominantly vertical organizations to more horizontal systems.

There are also organizational dangers to transformative thinking. This type of thinking is characterized by a willingness to seriously question all current processes and can threaten organizational stability. During transformation, leaders engage the staff and other stakeholders in a dialogue and hear what would normally not be expressed. In fact, to make the transformation succeed, the leaders must be open to new ideas and be willing to listen to all kinds of responses from all stakeholders. Even the thinking that underpins the changes must be subject to questioning and exploration if the implementation of new ideas is to be appropriately rigorous and thorough. The environment necessary to support transformative thinking creates a level of challenge and instability that even leaders may not be comfortable with (**Figure 12-1** and **Exhibit 12-2**).

Exhibit 12-2　　Causes of Transformation

- Destabilized environment
- Noise
- Culture of change
- Loss
- Emerging reality

- New financial realities
- Demand for new behaviors
- Work process changes
- Shifting technology

The process of transformation requires an environment in which creativity and change are embraced. In other words, discourse, deliberation, dialogue, consensus building, and experimentation must be viewed as safe and appropriate strategies. Leaders must create this environment before they can expect to see innovation and engagement with change become routine in their units or services. If the staff members do not feel safe in the presence of change, they certainly will not feel comfortable making change.

Living in an environment of horizontal relationships and accountability-based controls rather than management-driven decision making and vertical controls is a different experience for all parties. The former type of environment, however, is essential for transformative thinking and acting. Very little research suggests that rigid vertical control structures lead naturally to change and innovation. On the other hand, a whole body of research indicates that an open, inclusive, and accountable work structure creates numerous opportunities for creativity and innovation.

Biology has lessons for organizational survival. Biological research shows that growth and adaptation are required for life to continue. If the environment changes noticeably because of some cataclysmic event or the accumulation of small alterations, plants and animals either adapt or cease to exist. Indeed, past changes form the foundation for future changes, and adaptation to earlier changes determines the level of adjustment to future changes.

The same is true of organizations and other forms of social life. Even minor changes can upset the delicate balance that allows certain kinds of organizations to thrive and can turn the environment instead into a threatening place. For organizations to survive in this world, many of the processes and behaviors, rituals and routines that have their foundation in Industrial Age models of leadership thinking must be replaced by new processes and behaviors grounded in understanding of complex organizational dynamics. The transition requires true leadership and a transformational format for radically altering everything that workers know and do.

Group Discussion

In the emerging world of health care, the major leadership task is to transform people's attitudes and insights regarding the changes that are required of them. On a flip chart, list changes that affect what healthcare providers must now do in a reformed system and list attitudes toward the demand for change. Order the attitudes based on their potential influence, and discuss how a healthcare leader could alter the two most important to smooth the transition to new ways of working.

Evolution and Revolution

The only difference between evolution and revolution is the rate of change—the amount of time it takes for changes to occur. Certainly, the social digital transformation, because of its high rate of innovation, is undergoing a revolution, but the resulting changes in society are occurring at more of an evolutionary pace. It takes much longer to incorporate social and behavioral changes than to implement technological advances. Yet both types of change must be accommodated, and people need to adjust at a fast rate and a more studied rate. The challenge is to know which is occurring and to attach the right rate of accommodation to the process.

Leaders in an organization need to recognize the demand for change in enough time to respond correctly—at the right time and in the right format. Of course, leaders cannot know all changes far enough in advance to allow appropriate and timely responses. Nonetheless, the chance of responding correctly is increased if leaders assess the probability of reasonably likely changes and consider the expected effects. By anticipating the kind of changes that will occur, developing an understanding of their conditions and circumstances, and passing this understanding on to the staff, leaders ensure that the staff can react appropriately. In short, leaders must be signpost readers and articulate trends clearly enough to create a picture of their impact. Contemporary trends in accountable care require significant and specific changes in the context and content of clinical practice, representing the shifting requisites of a growing accountable care environment (Naylor & Kurtzman, 2010; Porter-O'Grady, 2013; Shomaker, 2011).

Leaders must also be transformational agents. In coaching staff members to embrace necessary changes, leaders must show the same tone, enthusiasm, and skill in adaptation they expect from others. Seeing the signposts is simply the first step in transferring the information to the staff in a way that puts accountability for response into their hands. Leaders must be able to see systemness and complexity as normal conditions of change and adaptation. Through expressing their accountability for witnessing and previewing the potential for change, leaders prepare the staff to deal with the right change at the right time and in the right circumstances.

Transformational coaching requires leaders to engage in an array of activities that move employees through the process of responding to essential changes in a way that embraces the changes and achieves desired outcomes. In fact, leaders are responsible for creating a system of response to essential changes and then creating a structure and process for these changes to occur as lived or operational experience. Transformational coaching is more of a system than a process, and in applying the components of this system leaders can ensure a dynamic, ongoing framework for adaptation and engagement.

The Learning Organization

An organization's ability to adapt to change depends on how open and responsive the social and organizational context is to change and to the dynamic processes of learning. If the organization values change and learning, the vagaries of change will be less traumatic and incidentally dynamic. Research has uncovered the rules of engagement for creating a true learning context.

Chris Argyris (2006), in a review of the research, indicated some basic criteria for success at any level of organizational learning and change. The focus must first be on behaviors and attitudes. Identifying the fundamentals of behavior and the factors that influence specific behaviors is critical for creating a context and process for change. Once these behaviors and attitudes are identified, the focus switches to the vagaries that affect particular behaviors or recurrent patterns of behavior and through them affect the way work is done or the way it is adapted to new realities (Argote, 2013).

The system developed for addressing behaviors must include a mechanism for reducing the number of continuing counterproductive activities and self-fulfilling patterns of behavior that keep participants from fully engaging with the changes they must make. Behaviors that are inconsistent with both norms and expectations find room to exist if not addressed quickly and efficiently. They even stand a chance of becoming the norm and in any case can compromise the environment and participants in a way that obstructs adaptation to the necessary changes. The noise that results creates a further impediment to the participants' ability to engage with the changes and thrive.

Focusing on the behavior of participants gives leaders an image of the mental and emotional "maps" in operation. Leaders can then use these maps as a beginning point for the process of making meaningful and sustainable change. They need to look critically at the participants' mental maps to determine the pattern of response they have helped to create. In fact, this pattern of response—the participants' theory-in-use—has a more dramatic impact on the participants' engagement with essential change than do the behaviors themselves.

When leaders approach participants to discuss their mental maps, they do need to be cautious. These maps form the contextual framework out of which behavior flows. The theory-in-use is simply the conceptual constant that the person draws on to explain, justify, and retain sufficient commitment or energy to a particular course of action. In this highly individual context, the person seeks to provide a solid values or belief foundation that can give meaning to a position or a specific action. Often, the theory-in-use is identified as the rationale or justification the person uses for his or her actions. This theory-in-use has only an inferential relationship to the truth. It relates more to the individual's sense of truth or interpretation or application of truth than to anything that may actually be true. Regardless, it is vitally important to the person. It is the theory-in-use out of which that person acts, and it gives a reason for the action. In this issue, leaders find that much of a theory-in-use cannot be discussed, for it concerns who the participants perceive themselves to be, even to the point of being perceived as a part of their identity. A person's role and sense of self in the role and the person's relationships with others and the organization create a foundation for the person's pattern of behaviors. However, because every person's theory-in-use is expressed in his or her pattern of behaviors, the patterns of all participants must be directly addressed if the behaviors necessary to learning, adaptation, and meaningful change are ever to be evidenced in the organization. This awareness of a person's theory-in-use helps the leader understand and address particular behaviors and gives a clearer context to an individual's personal struggle with change.

Almost every organization fails to maintain adaptability over time. The main reason is that organizations, although they might change what people do, usually fall short of changing how they think. Because the conditions of change are now so prevalent, not to change the thinking of people has ceased to be an option. Nurses, for example, must learn to practice in a world where institutional models of practice, hospital stays, and long-term patient relationships no longer define nursing practice. Nurses who complain of a lack of time for patient care have failed to realize that their grievances reflect an outmoded mental model of nursing. Hospital-based stays will continue to shorten, the aged

> ## Point to Ponder
>
> Failure to thrive is not uncommon in times of great change. The main reason is that organizations, although they might change what people do, usually fall short of changing how they think.

will be cared for in ways that do not require their institutionalization, new pharmaceuticals and gene-based treatments will radically alter how patients are treated, and so on. In this instance, the role of leaders is to assail the old mental model and create a fluid enough foundation for nurses' expectations that they give up their old expectations and acquire new ones.

Physicians also need to be aware that the circumstances that brought them into medicine no longer exist. The unilateral, responsible, but nonaccountable practice modalities that once defined medicine are disappearing, to be replaced by accountability-based, outcome-oriented, health-focused, rational, complex, and multifocal modalities. Discussions of the healthcare system are rife with the dissatisfaction expressed by physicians who say they can no longer practice the medicine they know. What they have failed to recognize is that the twentieth-century manual and mechanical model of medicine has died. The one that is emerging, driven by all the improvements and enhancements in therapy and treatment, and growing emphasis on ensuring healthy populations, has altered forever what medicine is and how it will be practiced. For physicians and others to enthusiastically and energetically engage with the changes affecting medical practices, leaders must confront their mental models directly and in a manner that allows the stakeholders to identify the discrepancies between what they believe and the current reality.

Effective adaptability also includes leaders developing the ability to predict changes before they actually occur. This predictive skill is now as much a part of the skill set of the leader as any other recognized leadership skill. Predictive capacity calls the leader to synthesize data and information about the convergence of forces and to define the resulting conditions or circumstances. Such skill becomes less optional for leaders as the pace of change quickens and the significance of each change increases the impact on people and groups. The scope of global changes and the broad landscape of change events now call leaders to visualize the groundswell of particular events and to link it to other elements to help prepare organization members for the onset and impact of changes far in advance of experiencing them.

Over the past 35 years, shared governance has enumerated the structural components and context necessary to create the scaffolding for sustainable change and full participation (Porter-O'Grady, 2007, 2009). Now we are joining a host of contemporary leaders in declaring the importance of empowerment, shared decision making, self-direction, and shared governance and urge the replacement of traditional organizational and management constructs with currently relevant models of workplace organization.

To gain a fuller understanding of how to adapt to the changes that are occurring, leaders must create an environment that fosters learning. In doing this, they should keep the following in mind:

- Learning must be oriented to the actual experience of the learners in their own environment.
- The purpose of learning is to ensure growth, improvement, and adaptability.
- People need to be empowered to take charge of the design of their own learning and to alter their roles and behaviors in response to what they discover.
- The organization must be willing to allow experimentation and risk taking so that innovation becomes a constant.
- Learning requires time, and the organization must therefore allow staff the time it needs to pursue new knowledge.
- Learning should not be accidental or incremental; an infrastructure for learning should be developed to ensure that innovation and new learning are considered an ongoing part of the way of doing business in any environment.
- People need to feel they are growing and improving. Therefore, learning should always be directed toward giving people new skills that are relevant to their job activities.

Learning can be single loop or double loop. In single-loop learning, the learning process is implemented as designed, and the outcome is achieved as anticipated. Single-loop learning deals with the apparent, the visible, and the symptomatic. In double-loop learning, the governing variables, the driving forces, the root causes, or the foundations for action are understood and applied to the process. In addition, the participants are familiar with the process of learning and incorporate it into their own learning activities as an ongoing part of delivering health services. Double-loop learning is essential to sustainable solutions and enduring results.

For learning to occur, especially double-loop learning, participants must understand their own theory-in-use (or automatic reasoning processes). Most people bring their own reasoning processes and preexisting notions to any learning situation and even look for information that validates their preexisting notions. The mother of one of the authors is a smoker of many years. When confronted with the fact that long-term smoking leads inevitably to illness and death, she invariably identifies those rare creatures who are long-lived, lifelong smokers. When reminded that she can name these people because so few are still alive, the logic escapes her. Her theory-in-use forces her to identify the circumstances in which her premises and beliefs can be confirmed and reinforced, giving her, in her own mind, no reason to change her pattern of behavior.

Everyone has preexisting notions and a propensity to try to validate them. Leaders (or anyone else acting as a coach) must recognize

> **Key Point**
>
> Being open to the dynamic processes of learning and change is a requisite of adaptability. The leader is always testing the system to see how much the staff engage with the demands of change and how quickly their roles adjust to new performance expectations and the chaos and vagaries of changing the way work is done.

Group Discussion

How many of us really know why we believe what we do or act as we do? The members of the group should each identify a statement about their professional work that they believe and two reasons for believing it. What is the theory-in-use in the application of this belief? Do others understand the statement in the same way? Is it really rational to believe the statement? Helping others change means knowing your own rituals and routines and the rational basis for acting on them.

the importance of identifying and describing these notions clearly enough to address them and use them as vehicles for personal learning and change. The goal of coaching is to help people acquire new ideas that validate the experience of change and more accurately reflect the prevailing reality, ensuring they have a place in it.

Newer concepts of triple-loop learning encourage a system that supports the questioning of premises, the clarification of beliefs, and the foundation of new learning. The infrastructure of the organization and the configuration of leadership expectations must now be aligned to ensure that past or current notions or concepts of the work do not become impediments to questioning the prevailing beliefs, practices, rituals, and routines. This becomes necessary to ensure that the organization does not become irrelevant or so inculcated in its own story and practices that it fails to see a different world and role ahead.

The final step in the learning process is to generalize what has been learned and reinforce it through applied action. Using new knowledge is the best way to incorporate it into the foundation on which the processes of work are built. Furthermore, integrating new knowledge into the foundation leads to additional new learning and to additional revision of the foundation, allowing workers to achieve higher levels of performance and personal satisfaction.

Point to Ponder

Adults learn most easily when they can apply what they have learned. The best approach is to teach them on the job so that they can apply their new knowledge then and there. Likewise, they accept changes most easily when they can act on the changes immediately.

Leaders need to understand that for double- and triple-loop learning to occur, they must create a culture that promotes the necessary processes and risk taking. This means that every role at every level of the organization—from the very highest levels of authority to the point of service—must be involved to some degree in the learning process and make use of available learning tools (**Exhibit 12-3**). In other words, the organization must live the learning process in everything it does. When an organization fails to embrace learning, often the reason is that a genuine culture of learning and adaptation was not designed and structured into the life of the organization. Dynamic adaptation and learning are simply unsustainable in any organization that does not have a vibrant learning culture.

Exhibit 12-3   Action Learning Tools

- Case studies
- Clinical exemplars
- Comparative modeling
- Computerized scenarios
- Group practice sessions
- PowerPoint presentations

- Satellite interactive sessions
- Simulation practice models
- Storyboards
- Video presentations
- Virtual classrooms

All learning is essentially individual. It begins at the personal level before it can become organization-wide. Therefore, each member of an organization must be expected to engage in learning activities, and the structure of the organization should even make it impossible for members to survive without pursuing new knowledge. The need for all members to become more knowledgeable is especially great now because of the reconfiguration of systems and enterprises that is occurring. Leaders, through coaching, can help staff change the language in use and find the right questions to ask—those that reflect the current reality; it is in this reality that the answers lie.

People are so strongly socialized by their past relationships and experiences that it is difficult to alter behaviors resulting from their socialization. When people come to work, their socialized behaviors come with them and are acted out. Leaders must recognize that socialization is a critical factor with regard to change and make sure it is incorporated into the structure and dynamic of learning. By engaging employees in a discussion of the effects of socialization on their behaviors and incorporating that discussion into the learning equation, leaders are more likely to foster the personal changes necessary to generate the shifts in work processes and outcomes.

Organizing for Transformation

Leaders know that behaviors do not change accidentally or on request. The context or culture of the organization or unit plays a major role in determining what behaviors occur and how they become modified. The leader of a unit, for instance, must have in place a uniformly applied set of expectations to ensure that the patterns of behavior are consistent. Further, the expectations and associated patterns of behavior must be congruent with the environmental demands that drive the work of the unit to ensure that responses to the demands are quick and appropriate. Finally, the interplay between behavior and structure must be such that the prevailing operational processes reflect it and can use this intersection as a way of advancing organizational effectiveness.

Another essential leadership task is to establish, together with the unit's members, some basic foundations for the unit's functions. To do this, the leader must continuously assess the patterns of relationship, interaction, and personal and professional behavior within the context of the expectations defined for them. In the culture of adaptation, clearly understood and consistently applied processes assure each participant that the agreed parameters are up front and continuously applied.

The leader should be aware that the purpose of these processes and structures is not to keep people happy. In many organizations, the goal of keeping people happy actually has become an impediment to making them happy. In fact, the knowledge that the leader expects employees to be happy can create conditions that ensure they are not.

Happiness is not something that can be achieved through organizational means; it is instead a personal matter. What is within the leader's purview is keeping employees motivated, invested, involved, and satisfied with what they are doing. The leader's best chance of creating an environment in which employees are all of these things is to set expectations that are high but not so high as to prevent the employees from consistently meeting and even surpassing them. These expectations and the structures and processes developed to ensure they can be met form the framework for advancing the organization's goals and those of the people who make it up.

The leader is also responsible for ensuring that certain basic requirements for learning and adaptation are in place:

- The members of the unit must be informed of the prevailing rules for personal behavior, personal interaction, and problem identification.
- Innovation must be an expectation of the workplace and of organizational learning to ensure that workers understand that contributing to their own change and that of the system is an expectation of work.
- There must be a mechanism for calling the parties to the table when a problem occurs or an issue arises. This mechanism must become the unit's normal means for first responding to problems and issues.
- There must be a routine mechanism for discussing and critically reviewing each issue that affects the staff. The purpose of this mechanism is to give the relevant parties an opportunity to play an active part in the deliberations and decision making intended to resolve the issue.
- Shared decision-making models should be used for empowering staff members and giving them a role in dealing with issues for which they are accountable.
- There must be a forum and a method of resolution for conflicts between members, concepts, plans, or processes. These conflicts should be addressed as quickly as possible. In the case of conflicts between individuals, the goal is to return the parties to a productive and active relationship with each other. If a good working relationship cannot be established, there must be a mechanism for separating the parties.
- Staff should be involved in the strategic and tactical activities of leadership. In particular, they should participate in decisions that define their future, thereby gaining ownership of their work.

Besides building appropriate processes and structures, the leader is responsible for

> **Key Point**
>
> When gathering people together, the first step is to clarify the rules of engagement. Although this can be tiresome, people must be reminded of the expectations regarding interaction and communication. Deliberations break down most often because the parameters for dialogue were not determined, reinforced, and followed.

stimulating the members of the unit to achieve high levels of performance. This can be done through building a shared vision and helping the members see that their work is a significant part of a great enterprise. The leader must realize that everyone wants to be a part of something important and make a meaningful and sustainable difference. The leader keeps the members as focused on the purpose of their work as on its processes. The members should not become so fixed on the work itself that they lose sight of why they are doing it.

Structure is a critical element in the creation of a meaningful and motivating work environment because it provides the context for behavior and sets the parameters for how the processes of work unfold. A good structure enhances personal interaction, problem solving, learning, and adaptation and keeps alive the human dynamics that energize and give meaning to the work. In the absence of such a structure, none of this can be ensured (**Figure 12-2**).

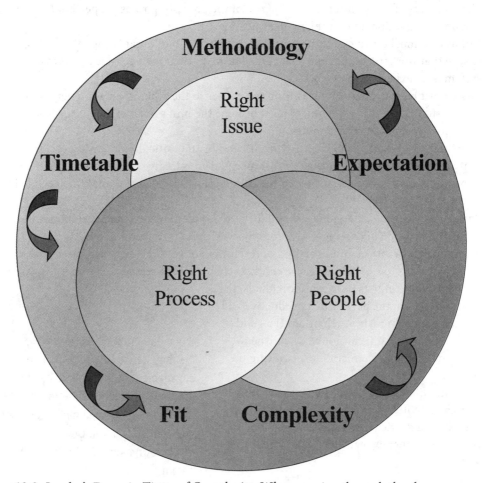

Figure 12-2 Leader's Focus in Times of Complexity. When moving through the change process, leaders must focus on core elements.

Dealing with the Lack of Time

"Not enough time" is perhaps the most widely heard mantra in the workplace today. In the past few years, it seems as if work has expanded and time has been compressed. Although time has not literally shrunk, dramatic changes during this period have affected people's perception of both time and work.

First, in general, work has become more complex. Although the purpose of a job may remain the same, what it takes to do it has changed radically. There is simply more to the job than there used to be. In health care, for example, managing the continuum of care so that the proper services are provided in a timely fashion requires communication and interaction with a whole host of professionals and use of numerous resources that are new on the scene. The need to do work speedily and effectively has also increased the intensity of the work and made time even more of a concern.

Leaders and staff need to look at the issue of time differently. For many years, work was viewed as a process that had no beginning or end. As a result, it became an end in itself, and the usual goal was simply to be efficient and do what had to be done on time. The issues are now more profound and require a different mental model for their resolution. Rather than looking for more resources or time, leaders are confronted with the questions about who should be used and how they should be used—questions about being different in a world that is changing before our very eyes. The fact is that resources, human and other, are not available in the same numbers and format they once were. The questions are no longer about more of anything. Looking for more resources, people, or time is not likely to help get more of any. The issue is no longer about doing more with less; instead, questions are about doing and being different in a changing world.

> **Point to Ponder**
>
> Leaders can have a big impact on problem solving merely by eliminating the word *more* from the dialogue. As long as people believe that more resources—more money, time, people, capital, equipment, and so on—will solve their problems, they will not put enough imagination and creativity into the mix to discover sustainable solutions. An abundance of resources can often be the enemy of imagination and creativity.

In other words, leaders need to challenge the prevailing framework. For instance, in addition to realizing that resources are finite and not as readily available as before, leaders must repeatedly point out to the staff that the value of work is embedded in outcomes, not processes. They must also recognize that nurses and physicians are challenged with having to validate their treatment decisions by providing evidence that their choices were less costly or less resource intensive than comparably effective treatments or had better results than other possible treatments could have had. For most of their years in practice, health professionals never had to prove a functional relationship between what they did and what resulted. Today, there is no future for healthcare decisions and actions for which such a relationship cannot be demonstrated.

Work in this new era requires more flexibility and fluidity than previously. The old notion that work should have fixed time and function parameters is no longer realistic.

With wireless technology, a healthcare provider can be anywhere and still be reached for advice or follow-up. When does a provider's job really begin, and when does it really end? It is now the responsibility of the individual to determine his or her workload and availability and the extent of the work period. In the past people went to a workplace, did their jobs, and went home. Today, jobs go with the jobholders wherever they go, and no parameters define the jobs more narrowly.

Leaders must now begin to apply tools to staffing that allow the planning and utilization of staff to be more flexible. They must also consider job candidates with an eye to their skill sets and personality characteristics to ensure they increase the organization's adaptability. The notion of goodness of fit applies to people just as it does to roles. Scheduling around workload is now a critical method of staffing. So is contracting for workload—bringing staff members on board based on an agreed workload and paying them for the workload rather than for time and function. These methods give staff members more control over their work life and over their life outside work.

The revolution in communications gives staff members more documentation and information-gathering options, not to mention unprecedented access to each other. The hands-free earpiece or headset allows providers to connect with others at a wide variety of times rather than just during a few set periods (e.g., rounds). Finding someone, reading the chart, and documenting information have become easier with the new telephone and personal digital assistant devices now common in the workplace.

Because of the increase in specialization, health professionals have become more interdependent. No one can be an expert in everything, and the members of a healthcare team must identify and make use of each other's expertise, fashioning a strong clinical network in the process. The leader of the team helps the other members become more self-reliant, where appropriate, and more interdependent. Rather than being a manager in the traditional sense, the leader is instead a colleague who creates the possibilities and conditions for real advancement and learning.

Time and resource problems do not always have easy solutions, and what might work in one part of an organization might fail outright in another. The organization's leader should realize that all problem solving is ultimately local and that those individuals who own a problem must be the ones to discover and implement its solution. Therefore, the leader needs to push staff members to find their own solutions and to identify processes that work for them and can be sustained in their environment. The key here is ownership. Those in administrative areas of the organization do not know how to resolve all the difficulties that arise at the point of work. Rather, the staff members know how to handle problems there, and the leader's job is to make them understand that they are expected to own the problems that arise, apply the appropriate methods and tools to solve them, and then use the necessary means to evaluate the outcomes and sustain whatever benefits they have achieved. The leader, of course, keeps his or her eye on the results, knowing that outcomes drive all processes and that all processes are disciplined by sustainable outcomes.

Leaders are often required to play the role of coach, and they bring to this role not only insight and skill but passion as well. In fact, by exhibiting energy and drive, they encourage others to stay invested in their own activities and commitments. They act as living examples of the excitement that results from engagement with the challenges of the times.

486

Coaches, including leaders acting as guides or counselors to staff members, find their greatest reward in helping others develop and move in the direction they need to go. They become invested in the achievements of those they are helping to learn and experience the learners' gains as gains of their own. Issues that arise in coaching and that leaders acting as coaches in a team situation need to keep in mind are as follows:

> **Key Point**
>
> Staff members must be allowed to find solutions to their own problems. The role of the leader is not to solve problems for others, but to make certain that staff members have the insights and skills necessary to problem solve. A leader's one absolute unforgivable act is to take ownership for other people's problems.

- *Having a genuine interest in people means supporting their growth.* Every team leader therefore needs to make sure other members know and feel the obligation to advance themselves and become full participants in the process of learning and adapting. The individual team members are accountable for thriving, and the leader must always keep this truth in front of the team members' eyes.

- *Coaching team members is not the same as raising children.* The team members are always fully accountable for their own development. The leader provides assistance in the form of tools and support but does not take on the burden of accountability for the other members' growth and advancement. The leader's role is to remind the team members of relevant expectations and parameters for action and to support them in meeting those expectations.

- *When coaching other members of a team, the leader does not take possession of their work.* Also, the leader does not own the staff's relationships and interactions or the outcomes of their efforts. The leader is alert to staff attempts to transfer ownership and must ensure that ownership remains where it belongs. The leader is like a circuit rider, moving continuously around the periphery of the team, observing, interacting, assessing, and identifying. When issues, deficits, or concerns arise, the leader is ready to transfer skills, insights, and tools to the team members in a clear way to ensure they have what they need to deal with their problems and advance their own work.

- *The team leader is not in control of the lives of the other team members or the circumstances in which they do their work.* The leader is their colleague rather than their manager, and the coaching role is one of partnership. The team leader's job is to keep the other members connected, invested, and aware and to help them develop to the point where they can operate with little outside intervention. In a transformational time, the leader is always pushing at the edges, helping the other members recognize the changes that are occurring, the issues that are arising, and the best methods for resolving them. The leader is in back, pushing the team into its reality, not in front, pulling it into his or her reality.

- *The leader is the chief learner on the team.* By modeling her or his commitment to the "way of learning" as a way of living, the leader helps create a learning culture and shows others how to embark on their own journey. The leader is always curious, searching, reading signposts, transferring information, raising issues, and pushing the parameters. The leader sees learning as a dynamic, as an essential constituent of living and relating, and becomes for the team a visual representation of learning in action.

In these times, because the work of transforming organizations is so critical, leaders in their role as coaches must exhibit the attitudes and behaviors of change and adaptation. In living the process of change, they perhaps do more to further the ability of others to handle change than they do through explicit instruction. People need to see leaders dealing with change so that they have someone rather than something to identify with. They look to leaders to humanize the experience of change by growing and adapting themselves. By seeing others who are successfully adjusting to change, they become more comfortable carrying out their own personal journey of transformation.

The Leader as Revolutionary

As mentioned repeatedly, the healthcare system is at a critical juncture. New thinking, different models and processes of accountable care and service, and whole new technologies are pushing the system toward a huge transformation. Yet there is so much in the way—a long history of now outmoded patterns, rituals, routines, and infrastructure. To help carry out the transformation, each leader must become a revolutionary in residence.

> **Point to Ponder**
>
> The only real difference between evolution and revolution is the pace of change.

The skills of revolution are different from those of evolution, because, in a revolutionary context, time is compressed, it is already too late, the options to thrive are significantly threatened, and leaders and personnel are almost paralyzed by their circumstances. In this case the leader of an organization has the job of initiating a number of processes so that the organization as a whole can engage with the radical changes occurring and implement adaptations in a timely fashion. Of course, the leader cannot do it alone. A coalition of like-minded revolutionaries is necessary for substantive change to occur. Indeed, the leader, acting as a transformational revolutionary, seeks to widen the circle of "conspirators" until the whole organization is conspiring to transform itself and its processes to meet current demands. This section describes several steps a revolutionary leader goes through to ensure that adaptation becomes the modus operandi of the system.

Create an Argument for Revolution

The organizational leader must create a vision of the transformation because what the transformation is and does are critical to mobilizing people. The leader thus gathers like-minded leaders within the organization to make a statement about the efforts required by the transformation—essentially a vision statement. This translational skill set is now essential for leaders to be able to refine changes in the social, political, and economic environments in a language and manner that can be understood at the point of service. The forces at play, the impact of events, the changing circumstances, the altered financial configurations—all these jointly determine how the current mental model should be revised and what needs to be done. The organizational leader then collects data to validate and refine the vision statement. The statement must show a clear connection

Group Discussion

As a group, identify one major change currently under way in health transformation that directly affects the delivery of patient care. Make sure that the change is significant and radical. Using a flip chart, create a plan for revolution around the identified change. Identify the various constituencies and conspiracies that are necessary for building momentum. Evaluate whether the plan is revolutionary and how and where to implement it.

between the conditions and the response and indicate why the conditions are so compelling as to make nonresponding a nonchoice. The vision statement must not only describe the conditions but also explain the response, citing the critical factors that influence the organization's position in the future.

Develop a Charter for the Future

After clarifying the conditions demanding transformation, the leader and his or her coconspirators must develop an agenda for the future. This can be likened to a map of the territory through which the system must now travel (the trajectory of change). The goal at this stage is not to devise a detailed program for change but to articulate the themes and signposts indicating the organization's proper direction. The charter should consist of a simple and clear point-by-point enumeration of the factors and themes of "becoming." It should contain engaging terminology so that key words and phrases such as "creating a sustainable partnership" or "building the health journey" can be pulled out and used to generate energy and enterprise throughout the organization. It should also indicate obstacles in the way of achieving the goals for which the conspirators need all of their commitment to overcome.

Build the Conspiracy

The transformation process has no meaning and will die an ignoble death if the conspiracy does not continuously expand. The charter starts to gain life when the organization embraces it as its work. The role of the leader is to make sure that commitment to the transformation moves outward into the far reaches of the organization. All the key players, informal and formal, at all places in the organization must embrace the charter, take ownership of it, and move it to the next levels of application. No formal mechanism of generation is required. Those who "get it" are brought on board when they are ready, and then they do their part to find and lead others who can get it as well. As might be guessed, the various organizational committees, from medical staff committees to management councils, are great vehicles for publicizing the vision and expanding the conspiracy.

This kind of revolution must be fully transparent. Everyone eventually must be on board to help in the creation of a preferred future. The work of the conspiracy is merely to stimulate this journey for all members of the organization, from those at the point of service to those in the boardroom. Joining the conspiracy to operational processes already under way is a good mechanism for getting the charter on the table of those who most need to engage with it.

Be Strategic and Patient

There are no enemies in this revolution—only those not yet part of it. The conspirators must understand which stakeholders they need to bring on board to give the charter both life and legs. They must also understand when to approach these individuals and groups or include the charter in their work.

Further, they should know the local politics of communication and action and identify which strategies are best for addressing specific challenges and circumstances. Getting specific individuals to perform certain required actions (because of their relationships, positions, or skills) is a part of the strategic process of managing the charter and guiding it through the political landscape. Indeed, one-on-one interactions with key players are as important as group meetings. In approaching key players, the conspirators need to translate the charter into their language to obtain their acceptance and advocacy. Key players have to be able to see how the process benefits them and advances their own opportunities and circumstances—that is part of the political process.

Seek Out Significant Champions

As the conspiracy grows, it must incorporate champions able to take the charter farther on its journey. The transformation process is like a relay race: Different runners with different skills are required at different points in the process. The organizational leader must anticipate the new focus, person, or skill necessary for getting to the next stage and must ensure that each is applied in the right format and at the right time to move the process along.

As in most conspiracies, movement toward the goal is not along a straight line. Backward or horizontal steps are occasionally required to refresh or expand the process. In addition, as progress occurs, the kind of champions needed often can be found at new locations. That is as it should be. The conspirators must celebrate any support that moves the transformation along to the next stage and increases its chance of success.

Ensure Small Successes Occur Early and Often

Successes must take place along the way to maintain momentum. Creating a plan for substantive change and getting the whole organization to embrace it are long, gradual processes, and people will remain unmotivated if they perceive their efforts as unlikely to make a difference. Even small accomplishments show that movement has occurred, and without some deliverables the organization is sure to lose interest before it gets very far. The accomplishments give the transformation process "legs" and ensure that the process's champions can overcome objections and opposition in a manner that allows them to incorporate new ideas into the process and convert possible opponents into supporters.

Make the Transformation the Mainstream Activity

The goal is to enable the whole organization to thrive well into the future. The conspiracy is simply a means of ensuring the organization's survival at a time when the organization appears to be missing an opportunity to prosper. Thus, the conspirators must always keep in mind that the purpose of their efforts is to benefit the organization, not themselves. They also must avoid becoming so committed to the conspiracy that their attention is diverted from the real end and their energies wind up misdirected. Once the conspirators have attained their objective—to make the transformation the central activity of the organization—the nature of their endeavors shifts toward initiating work processes related to the new reality. The conspirators must now fully embrace the character, context, and content of the new reality, which means redefining the work, retooling the workplace, and focusing on the conditions that allow the organization to thrive. In a sense, the conspiracy has now become the new reality.

Of course, the metaphor in this section of a conspiracy is merely a way of highlighting the focused commitment to fundamental change that leaders in an organization must have when options are limited or opportunities are being missed. It pinpoints the sense of urgency the leaders must impart to the entire organization to get everyone to make the kind of effort needed to ensure the organization's ability to thrive in a highly charged and changing set of circumstances. It also emphasizes the understanding that engagement and response to the demand for major change is a process with specific stages and points at which different stakeholders engage and accelerate their involvement in the journey of change. The leaders, acting as change agents, must stimulate the staff and other stakeholders to raise their own levels of energy and refocus their efforts. The conspiracy enlists them in an effort that is greater than they are as individuals, giving them a sense of meaning and purpose and generating the energy, emotion, insight, spirit, and commitment they need to adapt and grow. Focused commitment and strong motivation, along with appropriate processes, methodologies, and techniques, round out the requisites of revolutionary yet sustainable transformation.

Innovation Coaching

A team leader has the responsibility to create the right conditions for the team and its members to learn and grow. In fact, the main purpose of team leadership is to ensure the team members can develop and become what they must to thrive in shifting circumstances. The achievement of this goal, of course, requires the team leader to overcome existing obstacles to effective coaching (**Exhibit 12-4**).

To become successful in the new age, leaders and staff members must relate to the processes of transformation so that they see them as the essence of their work and not as mere responses to a demand to do things differently. Adaptability is as much an attitude as it is a way of doing business, and the goal of leaders should be to help everyone be different, not just perform new job activities. After all, in this era of revolution, it is not just the work that is changing, it is the very workplace itself—the conditions, elements, and technologies of work.

Exhibit 12-4   Impediments to Effective Coaching

Use of power
- Inadequate power
- Autocratic application of power
- Lack of empowerment
- Nonstrategic use of power

Self-image
- Poor self-esteem
- Unclear role
- Psychological flaws

Knowledge
- Undeveloped knowledge
- Learning needs
- Inexperience
- Lack of personal technique

Problem solving
- Inadequate worldview
- Intolerance of diversity
- No clear process
- Situational solutions

Because the working conditions are being substantially altered, leaders must ensure that the differences do not escape the attention of those who do the work. They need to help the workers revise their mental model of work and turn every worker into a revolutionary. In other words, they need to publicize the fact that innovation is now a way of life and help the workers develop the skills and attributes they require to live that way of life and become part of the transformation of the workplace (**Figure 12-3**).

To convert work into innovative effort, leaders need to follow several rules, discussed subsequently. They should also keep in mind that workers must figure out the emerging context for their work and relationships and create the structures and content for the journey itself.

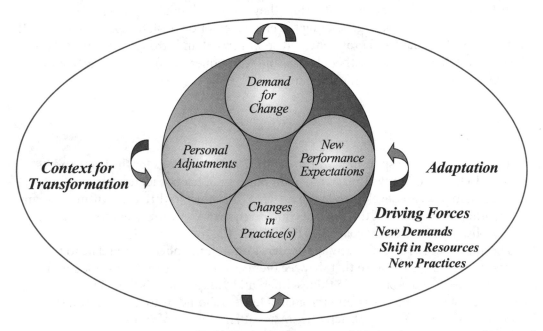

Figure 12-3 Innovative as a Way of Life. The leader focuses on the central components of personal transformation to ensure that each person can embrace change.

Set the Bar High

Leaders need to convince workers that expectations for their performance are high, but not so high they cannot be met. The challenge is to set expectations that prevent workers from falling back on old behaviors and practices but that also do not discourage them. The expectations should stimulate the workers to engage in different thinking and to change the very nature of the work.

Another way of saying this is that the transformation of work requires new models for thinking, a new context for work, and goals that demand new ways of working. The goals should not be so easily attainable that the workers can retain their old ways of doing things.

Be Clear About Who You Are

In the new world of work, people need to redefine who they are and their definition of success. For example, hospitals, which were originally defined as places where sick people were cared for, have been redefined as places where healthcare services are delivered. The range of services that falls under the rubric *health care* differs from the range that falls under the rubric *caring for the sick*.

Because the health services landscape is moving toward more accountable care models, healthcare leaders must highlight the changes in the context of work and the implications for its performance, including the new demands that have arisen. They must then revise the structures and processes of work to meet the new demands and to assist staff in adjusting their insights, attitudes, and behaviors appropriately. Staff members must live the image of the organization in all they are and do. Making sure that staff members see the shift and can live the new perspective in their work and relationships is a critical element in the journey into the future.

Treat Transformation as a Mission, Not a Job

The staff of an organization must not simply change the way they do their work but also change the way they live their work. Therefore, the organizational leader, acting as a coach, must be able to explain how to live and work differently using the broadest and clearest language possible. Transcending simple notions of labor, the leader creates an image of healthcare delivery as having a purpose beyond its immediate effects. By showing how work efforts can influence the world of health care, the leader transforms the performance of work by an individual into the pursuit of a mission. People want to support good and noble causes that take them outside of themselves and also want to view their efforts as having a profound value. The leader can help them take this leap from the mundane to the honorable and incorporate a sense of mission into the very fabric of their work activities.

Expose Staff to Different Messages and Different Messengers

To motivate staff members, the leader must give them encouraging messages that differ from those they have often heard in the past. The leader must also communicate new expectations and provide opportunities for staff members to learn what they need to know to meet these expectations. The encouragement and the expectations

> ## Key Point
>
> The leader must be so consumed by the organization's mission that transformation becomes second nature. In addition, by being committed to this mission, the leader presents a visible example of transformation in action that has the power to inspire others to transform themselves and their job activities.

communicated must be consistent with the transformation on which the organization has embarked. The goal is to stimulate staff members to think about how to do their work more effectively.

New voices should also be heard. Young workers, workers who are quiet and reserved, and workers from outside the particular work group should be included in the collective dialogue. The leader should do as much as possible to "push the walls" to move people out of their comfort zones to stretch into new ways of thinking and doing.

Create an Egalitarian Organizational Structure

Hierarchy should be minimized in times of great change. In fact, in the new age hierarchy has limited value. Horizontal relationships, defined not by position but by role, are the cornerstone of accountability. The leader of an organization must therefore facilitate relationships with those he or she depends on for planning and performing the organization's work.

In other words, the leader must value the work and the worker equally. Each worker has a contribution to make. Because the workers know best what produces results, the leader's job is to get each to offer innovative ideas on how to improve methods and processes. The leader therefore needs to make it safe and easy for workers to become part of the collective dialogue and put forth suggestions. Barriers to interaction, sharing, and challenging simply cannot exist if the spontaneous communication of ideas is to become the organization's modus operandi. Ideas are an important form of capital for any enterprise and can come from any place. For them to be released, the organization's culture must make it not only possible but routine.

Put Money Where the Ideas Are

For an idea to be implemented, some level of resource support is required. Although not every idea is worth supporting, funding for good ideas must be available because staff members need to know that their ideas have the potential to go somewhere and make a difference. If their ideas are ignored for lack of funding, they will eventually go back to old routines and refuse to contribute. If their ideas, on the other hand, are taken seriously and investigated, they will continue to make suggestions.

The funding or budgeting process must make it possible to explore ideas and innovations to an extent commensurate with their likely utility. Out of 1,000 ideas perhaps only 10 will ever be used, but those 10 could not have emerged unaccompanied by the rest. In short, the exploration of all ideas is critical to the discovery and application of the few that do become part of the organization's practice.

Let the Talented Experiment

It is impossible to apply new thinking by rote or through using a "straight line" approach. Talented people must be gathered together and supported. This means, among other things, allowing them to take risks. The outcomes of ideas are often unpredictable, and thus a certain amount of trial and error is necessary. Ideas must be tried and possibly modified before their worth can be known. If an idea is not shown to be beneficial after a trial period, it should be discarded.

Nothing should be set in cement. Strategies should be implemented and then modified as necessary. Structures and permanent processes should be avoided because they create barriers to necessary revisions. In addition, enough creative people must be included in the organization to ensure that innovative thinking occurs. Constant attention to bringing in and keeping such people is critical for sustaining the transformation. The leader must be comfortable with those who are bright and creative and come up with ideas that challenge the leader to think and act differently.

Allow People to Share in the Fruits of Their Creativity

This is perhaps the most challenging notion for healthcare leaders. For some unfathomable reason, the practice of rewarding people for their contribution has not become common practice within the healthcare arena. However, people own their creativity and ideas and lose interest and move on if their ownership is not honored. Keeping creative people means investing in them, and investing in them means rewarding them for their innovations.

> **Point to Ponder**
>
> Experimentation is critical to innovation and adaptability. An organization not willing to experiment is doomed to failure.

Creative people often do not seek to be compensated financially. For them, seeing their originality have an impact can be reward enough. Nonetheless, the leader should acknowledge contributions in a meaningful way. Although a bonus is the most recognized and established kind of reward and should be seriously considered, there is a host of other kinds of recognition, including public acknowledgment (celebrations and events), publishing the work inside or outside the institution, gain sharing (sharing the rewards), and shared ownership. Whatever rewards are defined by the organization, the reward granted to an individual for a given contribution should fit the needs of the person and the kind of contribution. Remember, highly creative people are looking not for long-term, permanent positions but for opportunities to express their gifts and talents. Keeping them on as employees depends on whether the organization's culture provides them with an ability to create, grow, and advance.

The leader is always attentive to the need to keep the organization moving and to respond to current demands (**Figure 12-4**). Creating the environment, structure, and processes necessary to ensure the organization's adaptability is the leader's single most important task. Because inventive people are essential to the organization's ability to respond to new demands, the leader is forever looking for, challenging, and rewarding such people in an effort to maintain a pool of creative talent (**Figure 12-5**).

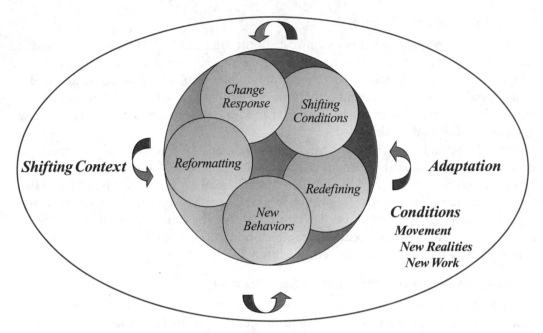

Figure 12-4 The Dynamics of Continuous Adaptation. The leader ensures that each element of adaptation is addressed by those whose work must be transformed.

Making Integration Work

Because of the systems-oriented dynamics of health care and the effort to create a seamless and population-based approach to ensuring health, making things fit together is very important. The leader of a healthcare organization must evaluate the fit between elements and improve it wherever possible (**Exhibit 12-5**). When a merger or alliance occurs, however, creating proper fit can be a great problem. People bring to the new entity their past ideas, commitments, cultures, and notions of how the work is to be done, and they resist or find it difficult to create the level of integration that is required. Much of the energy of the leader is devoted to making the new arrangements not just workable but productive.

Group Discussion

A common topic of discussion today in accountable care is the nature of true integration. As a group, brainstorm the basic elements of integration. Identify areas where group members disagree. Break into two debating teams of two or three members each and have each team take a position and argue for it. The remainder of the group will critique the debate and evaluate the arguments. After the debate, the group members should discuss how their view of integration has been altered or reinforced. Finally, identify three or four common elements of integration that can be used as criteria to determine whether integration has been achieved.

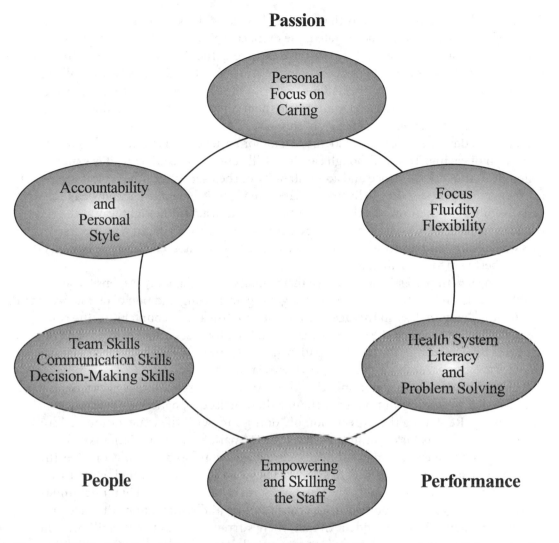

Passion

Personal
Focus on
Caring

Accountability
and
Personal
Style

Focus
Fluidity
Flexibility

Team Skills
Communication Skills
Decision-Making Skills

Health System
Literacy
and
Problem Solving

People

Empowering
and Skilling
the Staff

Performance

Figure 12-5 The Elements of Personal Transformation. Change is not complete until the cycle of transformation is complete. The leader brings personal passion to moving people to a new level of performance.

Exhibit 12-5   Elements of Integration

- Accountability
- Alignment
- Focus on the whole
- Goodness of fit
- Integrity
- Interdependence
- Orientation toward outcomes
- Role congruence

Perhaps the greatest concern is the speed with which things seem to happen today. Although time itself has not accelerated, the extra complexity of work has made it difficult to accomplish tasks at the pace once expected. The sheer complexity of the transformation processes currently under way in the American healthcare system challenges both pace and intensity. Because staff members find they no longer have enough time to do what they used to do, the leader must help them replace their focus on doing lots of activities with a focus on doing the right things.

In the old days, healthcare providers did a lot for patients. In fact, this reality drove the definition of caring. Today, although caring is still central to health care, it is expressed differently. The independence and accountability of the users of health services are now as important as the services delivered by care providers. People must acknowledge their responsibility for their own health and be empowered to act in the right way at the right time to ensure their own well-being. Providers consequently are faced with a different mix of activities and priorities and must recognize that doing everything for patients is not the best way to render needed assistance.

To many health professionals, the idea that patients are unilaterally responsible for their health borders on heresy. At the very least, it goes against a long tradition of provider-owned "doing for." Nonetheless, in this age of consumer control and accountability, the complexity of health care and the added demands on the providers' time require many of the tasks to be placed in the hands of patients. This transfer of responsibility, of course, changes the character of the patient–provider relationship.

The leader must ensure not only that the transfer of responsibility is carried out but also that providers and patients change their attitudes, beliefs, and practices accordingly. Replacing the expectation of "doing for" with the expectation of "doing with" is an arduous task, not just for staff but for patients as well. Patients, too, have grown up with a certain image of health care and certain expectations of what they should obtain from the healthcare system. They can feel disappointed when these expectations are not fully met. They, too, operate with a dependency model under which they surrender responsibility, accountability, and control to healthcare providers in return for being tended. In fact, their surrender sometimes facilitates their descent into conditions and lifestyles that contribute to the illnesses for which they seek treatment.

Today, part of the healthcare provider's role is to alter patient expectations of "being taken care of." Part of the healthcare leader's role is to work with providers in creating a new model of health care and revising the patient–provider relationship. The ultimate goal is to help providers use their time more effectively and appropriately in delivering care and providing services to those in need.

In particular, providers must focus on teaching and otherwise empowering patients to see more and do more in their own interest. They must also involve family members and significant others in the delivery of services and in counseling, supporting, and caring for loved ones in need of assistance. For these changes to occur, healthcare leaders need to focus on four important responsibilities, described subsequently.

Speeding Up Processes

Time is of the essence. Providers have less and less time to talk with patients about their healthcare needs and provide appropriate services, and therefore providers and patients must make better use of their time together. For example, follow-up now means making sure patients can gain access to the resources they need (i.e., connecting them to a network of resources, including sources of information that can guide their actions when they are no longer within the healthcare system).

> ### Key Point
>
> The healthcare system is changing in fundamental ways, so providers and patients need to act differently and "expect differently." The providers, in particular, need to change their behaviors and expectations and educate the patients to change theirs.

As noted, the locus of control is with patients (where it really belongs). Providers must make sure that it never shifts away from there and that patients have what they need to take care of their health. Healthcare leaders have the task of helping staff become comfortable with this reality and guiding them into practices that allow patients to make the best decisions and carry out those decisions. For the transition to the new patient–provider relationship to occur, both staff and patients must develop new skills and skill sets.

Orchestrating the Dynamics of Change

Making the shift to new ways and new roles is difficult for everyone. Complicating the situation is the fact that new rituals and routines must replace those that reinforce behaviors suitable to the older model of service. Staff members, having lived for so long with the more traditional dependent practices, now need approaches, tools, and skills to help them initiate and sustain new behaviors. Leaders must ensure that they develop and use these in ways that fit their culture and experience with change. By exchanging best practices, staff members can connect with others who are busy creating and constructing methods and models for improving services and changing their relationships with those they serve.

Building Relationships

Everything is built on good and sustainable relationships. The most important leadership task is to ensure that everyone is "singing off the same song sheet." Keeping an organization's staff on target and focused on its mission is difficult yet critical work. The leader continually tests, challenges, and extends personal and collective relationships with stakeholders throughout the process of changing behavior. When things get tough or stuck, the leader's only resource may be the personal relationships he or she has developed during this process. Identifying with the difficulties that staff members are experiencing and supporting them through the changes they encounter are critical to sustaining their efforts. Testing, stretching, evaluating, renewing, supporting, and challenging are steps in the normal cycle of action, relationship, and response that every leader needs to know how to do (**Figure 12-6**).

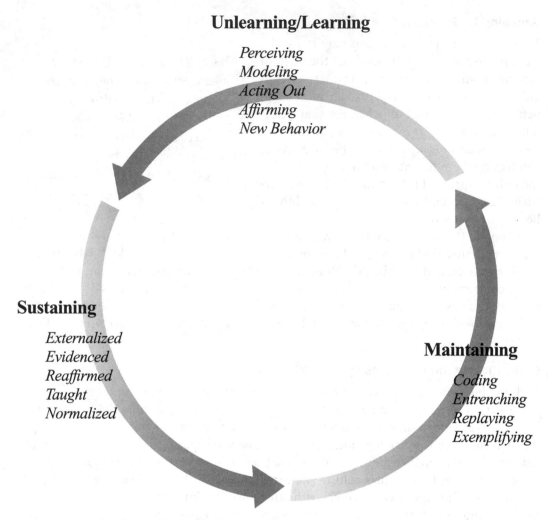

Figure 12-6 Cycle of Transformational Learning.

Putting Necessary Structure in Place

New behaviors are not sustainable without accompanying structural supports. Care providers for those with chemical dependency issues know that addressing an addict's behavior is not enough—the environment also must be changed. Creating a context for change means building an environment that leads to desired behaviors. When workers fully participate in creating their environment, chances increase that they will own the appropriate behaviors and achieve the desired outcomes.

Leaders often fail to pay close attention to the structural realities, allowing staff to fall back into old patterns of behavior. Creating structures that limit old patterns and foster preferred patterns, along with rewarding the performance of desired behaviors, can make the difference between an effective workplace and one that is unproductive and problematic. As an impetus for positive change, structure is at least the equal of behavior itself.

Addressing Problems Head On

People who do not approach problems proactively acquire a "firefighting" mind-set. Unfortunately, because of the large number of problems and issues that confront leaders daily, they often end up spending more time on daily skirmishes than on substantive issues. A focus on firefighting, by leaving their real responsibilities unattended, simply begets more fires to fight.

Some ways of dealing with problems allow leaders to do their transformational work. Indeed, problem solving can be a source of growth and can support a leader's transformational work. The trick is not to look at problems situationally and attempt to resolve them within the context of the situation but instead to investigate the circumstances in which they occur. Rather than filling holes in the staffing schedule on the spur of the moment, for example, a leader should identify and address the underlying causes; otherwise, the problem will occur again, often in a form more difficult to resolve.

Group Discussion

Tracy Polus, the head of the respiratory department, had a difficult time confronting behavior problems. She habitually used the third person when discussing such problems and could often be heard saying, "When a person does . . ." or "If someone would . . ." or "If people could . . ." The staff never really knew if she meant to refer to their behavior in particular or to the behavior of people in general. Eventually, they began to discount her comments, and because no one else was dealing with problematic behaviors, relationships in the department suffered. What recommendation would you give Tracy? How could she change her own behavior to make her a more effective manager? Is there a type of developmental program that she should undergo? Is it too late for her to establish new ground rules for her staff? What would some of the ground rules be?

A patchwork approach to solving problems creates more problems than it solves. It also creates problems in related but remote parts of the system. When a process is broken, other processes that interact with it pay the price. For instance, a delay in laboratory testing results in a delay in treating patients. In a complex system, problems can cascade through the system, causing difficulties for everyone.

Leaders, in dealing with problems, should follow a few basic rules. Although simple, they are often forgotten, to the detriment of the problem-solving process.

<table>
<tr><td>

Key Point

Not all problems can be solved quickly, so the leader of an organization must prioritize problems to make sure the critical ones are dealt with immediately. People problems always come first, relationship problems second, and external problems last. Structure and process problems are ongoing, as are the procedures for handling them.

</td></tr>
</table>

Solve Problems Selectively

It is unbelievable how many leaders take on, all at once, the full range of problems affecting their organization. Not all problems can be or need to be solved immediately. Leaders must approach problem solving like any other deliberative process. In particular, they must develop strategies for prioritizing problems and bringing order and focus to the effort of addressing problems critically.

Because problems are omnipresent and affect everything that people do, leaders must look at the relationships among problems, explore the way in which they interact, and then decide the order in which the problems are addressed. Not every problem has the same weight or the same ability to obstruct work and the achievement of desired outcomes. Setting up a list of problems to be dealt with first is a necessary step in the problem-solving process.

Work on the Fundamental Problems First

Many leaders believe they should work on the most urgent problems of the day. Yet problems that seem small can be the source of these seemingly more critical problems. If the root problems are not resolved, all others caused by them also do not get resolved. In addition, problems that appear to be critical to people in the midst of a crisis usually turn out to be mere symptoms of more fundamental problems. Thus, an important goal in problem solving is to determine which problem is a root cause and which is an effect.

Include People with the Necessary Skills and Power in the Resolution of Problems

Although it is best for people to assert ownership of the problems that concern them, it is not always possible for everyone affected by a problem to be part of the problem-solving effort. What is more important is that the right people be involved—those who have the skills to resolve the problem and the power to make the resolution permanent. In most cases, finding and implementing a solution to a problem requires the engagement of a broad range of players and stakeholders.

Be Accountable for Ensuring Problems Are Solved

Although leaders are obligated to see that problems are solved, they are not obligated to solve problems they do not own. The important consideration in determining who should deal with a problem is who owns it and who is best placed to resolve it (i.e., usually one and the same person or group). The role of the leader, in most cases, is merely to provide the proper people with everything they need. As a result, the leader's focus is not so much on the problem as on the process.

If the owners of a problem turf it outside of their locus of control, the problem is unlikely to remain fixed for long. Therefore, leaders must make sure that problem-solving skills and processes are embedded in the organizational culture and that those who are attempting to deal with a problem have the wherewithal to take care of it.

Counterproductive beliefs and practices are significant barriers to the permanent resolution of problems. For example, despite what many leaders believe, being committed to resolving problems is not nearly as important as being committed to using good problem-solving techniques and processes. These techniques and processes create the insights and skills necessary to deal with problems effectively and quickly enough to avoid long-term trauma.

Eliminating Firefighting Altogether

The best thing the leader of an organization can do is replace firefighting activities with much more productive behaviors. The research and work of Roger Bohm have been important in codifying what is wrong with most problem solving and in publicizing better methods (Savitch, 2008). To make problem solving truly effective, the leader needs to use analytic and tactical methods and strategic approaches and to alter the organization's culture (Schabracq, 2007; Zedeck & American Psychological Association, 2011).

> **Point to Ponder**
>
> Firefighting is not a good problem-solving approach because it keeps the focus off the root issues and on the symptoms. In fact, the more firefighting a leader does, the more firefighting the leader has to do.

Tactical Methods

The advantage of tactical methods of problem solving is that they can be put into place quickly to deal with problems in the short term while the infrastructure for the more lasting approaches is constructed. *Tactics* simply means making a change applicable and practical so that it can be successfully implemented. Tactics provide a means that is useful and can be replicated, evaluated, and changed when required. They are not cast in stone and can be readily adapted to new realities or necessary changes. The dynamic nature of tactics allows the leader to bring flexibility to bear on issues or problems and to introduce adaptability in the work process.

Getting Help from Outside the Circle

It is often wise to have someone from outside the service or unit help with the response to problems inside. A person from outside has a fresh view of the issues and is not invested in the issues or the solutions under consideration. Leaders often refrain from using outside resources because they are uncomfortable with others knowing their problems or simply because they have not attempted this maneuver in the past. Yet the more insight that can be obtained from those who do not own the issues, the more objective and effective the solutions are likely to be. In the new age, one of the expectations should be that leaders will call on each other as outside consultants in dealing with the deeper and more complex problems and issues that undoubtedly arise.

Trying Something New

People have a tendency to do the same things while expecting different outcomes. They become attached to rituals and routines that are inherently problematic and refuse to face the challenge of learning new practices. Most problems in organizations occur because the members hold on to old practices that have become barriers to smooth functioning and effective performance. The leader of an organization, acting as a change agent, must begin at the fundamental level—by creating a good fit between form and function and establishing a culture that supports changes in behavior. Here again, it is by creating the right context for change and creativity to occur that leaders can most help reduce the impact of habit and make it possible for people to let go of past practices.

Triaging Problems

Problems are always occurring. The goal is to solve them as soon as possible so that they do not incubate greater problems. It therefore makes sense to sort through current problems quickly to determine which are normal or trivial and which are pivotal and likely to cause other problems. A conflict between two practitioners, for example, might create a bottleneck in the flow of work, especially if they sabotage each other's efforts. Resolving their conflict would therefore prevent a range of difficulties down the road, and so the conflict would appear high on the list of problems to be tackled immediately.

Strategic Approaches

Strategic approaches, because they are embedded in an organization's way of working and doing business, take longer to plan and implement than do tactical methods.

Prioritizing Problems

Problems should be viewed as a normal part of organizational operations and their solution as a normal part of the leader's work. As much as possible, the leader should help the staff see problems as normal and develop categories for classifying problems according to their potential impact. Problems that affect staffing and the availability of clinical support resources, for example, would be treated as more urgent than office supply problems, and conflicts between departments would rank higher than conflicts between individuals on a given unit. Prioritizing problems is not intended to diminish the importance of any problem; it simply ranks them so that more critical issues are not left hanging.

Using Learning Scenarios

The leader of an organization is crippled if she or he is the only one to take on the responsibility of solving problems. The "mama" syndrome, in which problems are seen as exclusively within the leader's jurisdiction, prevents problem-solving processes from being built into the system. Everyone needs to develop problem assessment and problem-solving skills and the independence to take care of problems at the right time.

There is no way to avoid or eliminate all problems, and indeed problems are a sign of life in the universe. Once staff members understand this, the leader can use present or past problems as vehicles for teaching problem-solving skills. Through this kind of scenario learning, the leader can help staff members alter their attitudes toward problems and can change the locus of control for solving them. The staff can embrace problems as tools and develop the skills necessary to manage them to the organization's benefit.

Building a Problem-Solving Tool Chest

The solution of each problem should build the skill sets necessary to solve subsequent problems more quickly and easily. In a sense, each solution serves as a database for future problems. Codifying and recording approaches to specific kinds of problems increases the likelihood that recurrences will be solved in a similar fashion. Better still, it increases the likelihood that recurrences can be dealt with early enough to prevent a negative impact. In addition, banding together the strategies for dealing with particular types of problems creates a good framework for handling problems effectively.

Cultural Changes

An organization's attitude toward its own problems is as critical to their permanent resolution as any other single factor. If the organization refuses to see its own problems, nothing it does will ensure its ability to thrive in the long term.

Rejecting Patching as a Problem-Solving Approach

Focusing on situations instead of issues—or being sucked into situations and seeing the issues only from the inside—is sure to lead to failure. The best policy is to help the staff develop problem-solving skills so that they see clearly the problems that arise as part of their work and act as independent troubleshooters. Everyone who faces a problem wants the associated pain taken away. However, the pain is merely a symptom, and focusing solely on it ensures that the underlying issues never hit the table. In other words, the patching approach to problems must be challenged and eliminated from the set of permissible approaches.

Making Problem-Solving Deadlines Irrelevant

It is true that problems cannot be allowed to go on forever. Rather than set deadlines for solving problems, however, the leader should embed a problem-solving methodology into the work itself. If the methodology is effective and problem solving is fostered by the organization's culture, deadlines become moot. The problems that arise are not avoided or treated as belonging to "the other guy," but instead are viewed as opportunities for growth.

Refusing to Reward Firefighting

In health care, a premium tends to be placed on those who can make critical decisions quickly and correctly. Health professionals with this ability are treated as heroes by every medical soap opera and documentary. Heroes make poor citizens, however, and require a great deal of ego feeding. In fact, they are not necessarily good models except in war and can cause more problems than they are credited with solving.

It is better to implement good problem-solving methods and mechanisms than to have staff use individualistic approaches. It is better to build an organization committed to problem solving than to reward good firefighters. Waiting for problems to manifest means being a day late and a dollar short—by the time the problems are addressed, most of the damage has been done. The preferred strategy is to anticipate problems and incorporate their resolution into the life and work of every member of the organization.

TABLE 12-1   Personal and Group Stages on the Journey of Transformation

Stage	Personal	Group
Stage 1	Unlearning Letting go Reacting	Seeing change Acknowledging Resisting Mourning
Stage 2	Naming new skills Learning new skills Applying new skills	Discerning impact Finding meaning Experimenting Giving form
Stage 3	Reinforcing the new Evaluating behavior Teaching the new Extinguishing the old	Shifting expectations Relating in new ways Celebrating Taking ownership

Conclusion

For a leader, transformation can be a way of life. It is a journey consisting of logical stages made up of specific actions and processes. At its best, the journey is rational, progressive, and purposeful (**Table 12-1**).

Leaders who accept the role of transformational coach must embrace and cope with the vagaries of these changing times. Through role modeling and commitment to self-direction and growth, they create a context for new expectations and new behaviors. Through living the reality of change, they ensure that others can embrace their own changes and respond appropriately. In all their actions, they fulfill the aims of transformational coaching by remaining fully engaged with the staff and guiding them on the way to a productive future.

Case Study 12-1

Coaching for Growth

Casey is recognized in her organization as one of the most innovative and progressive leaders. The directors who report to her also seem to be more progressive than many of the other department directors, and they are frequently the leaders or chairs of various hospital councils. Casey's department is always on the leading edge of change, and they have the highest nurse, patient, and physician satisfaction scores when compared to other hospital departments. The entire department seems to run like a well-oiled machine.

Sandra is in her second year of a PhD program in executive leadership for nursing, and she has been assigned to Casey for her practicum experience. She is required to spend 100 hours with Casey for a semester as a participant observer to all that Casey does in her role as chief nursing officer (CNO) and vice president (VP) of Patient Services. Sandra's professor has told her about Casey's reputation for being a transformational leader not only in her hospital, but also in the entire community. The professor suggests that Sandra interview Casey to gain insight into how Casey has developed her own leadership skills, as well as the leadership skills of those who report to her. Sandra develops a list of questions that she wishes to discuss with Casey and her learning objectives for the practicum experience. Sandra will work with Casey and her directors over the semester and will accompany them to the group/council meetings and individual meetings with their direct reports. She plans to observe how the directors interact with one another as well as how they interact with Casey and other executives in the hospital.

It doesn't take Sandra long to recognize the differences between Casey and her colleagues at the VP level. In the nurse executive meetings, Casey is engaged and involved in the discussions and constantly looks for opportunities to expand her scope of responsibility and to demonstrate the accomplishments of her department. She frequently shares some of the innovations that have been developed by her directors to improve patient care outcomes, develop the clinical nurses, improve relationships with physicians, or ensure the best experience for patients and families. The other VPs don't seem nearly as engaged in the discussion and rarely come to the meetings as prepared as Casey is.

In a meeting with Casey, Sandra asks Casey, "What attributes do you desire in your directors as leaders of their units?" and "How have you developed the directors to be successful in their roles?" Casey explains that she looks for individuals who could develop their staff to reach their fullest potential. She looks for individuals who are risk takers and who are open to new ideas for innovation.

When observing Casey with the directors who report to her, Sandra observes a very dynamic and active team who obviously enjoy working together and who support each other as they present their challenges and successes.

During Casey's individual meetings with her directors, Sandra observes Casey constantly teaching and coaching each director and giving support and advice as needed. Casey often shares articles with the directors to expand their knowledge on leadership topics. She encourages the directors to assess the strengths of their direct reports and seek out individuals who could be groomed for future leadership positions. They discuss specific clinical nurses who could champion various changes and innovations on the clinical units. Casey also encourages each director to develop a succession plan with developmental goals for individuals who demonstrate leadership potential.

When possible Casey invites one or more of her directors to accompany her to meetings. She is transparent about issues that she deals with in her role, and she explains to Sandra that it is her philosophy to ensure that each of her directors is prepared to step into her role at a moment's notice if needed. Sandra marvels at Casey's personal commitment to mentoring her directors because some VPs might be threatened by strong direct reports, fearing that they might usurp authority or try to position themselves for the VP role. In contrast, Casey states, "If I stepped out of this role, I hope to be missed personally, but any one of my direct reports should be able to step into the role without even a ripple felt by the organization."

While accompanying Casey to her hospital-wide meetings, Sandra notices Casey is also very encouraging to her colleagues and frequently observes Casey "managing them up" to the chief operating officer. Casey spends time building her relationships with the VPs of other departments, which, she explains, is critically important as a foundation for times when challenges or problems might arise. She states, "Building positive relationships with others makes problem resolution much easier, and potential problems can be avoided with early discussions rather than waiting for the problems to escalate." Casey not only lives these principles, she also holds her own direct reports accountable for developing relationships with their peers as well.

Questions

1. What attributes of a transformational leader do you think that Casey exhibits in her role as CNO and VP of the nursing department?
2. How does Casey hold herself and her direct reports accountable for the department's outcomes and outputs?
3. How does Casey demonstrate the coaching aspect of her role as a leader?
4. If you were Casey, what might you do to develop your own team of directors?
5. In the *Future of Nursing Report*, there is a recommendation that every nurse be groomed to become a leader. With this in mind, what might you do, if you were Casey, to ensure that every clinical nurse is developed to become a leader?

Case Study 12-2

Mentoring Frontline Leaders

Andy has been the CNO of Whitefish Community Hospital for the past 5 years. He has done an excellent job of advancing the knowledge, skills, and self-confidence of his directors, and the hospital was recently awarded Magnet designation with special commendation for research and innovation. Andy considers this to be a major accomplishment because when he first came to Whitefish Community, the nursing department was led by a very authoritative leader in a hierarchical organizational structure. Andy has made many changes to the nursing organization and has won the respect of the executive team for all that has been accomplished. Physicians in the hospital have also commented on how nursing has improved dramatically over the past 5 years. Although Andy has every right to feel proud of nursing leadership and the clinical staff, he feels uneasy about the level of preparedness of the frontline leaders at the point of service.

The nursing organizational structure consists of directors who report to Andy, managers who report to the directors, and assistant managers who are shift leaders with responsibility for the day-to-day direction of staffing and the interface with the clinical nurses for their schedules and performance appraisals. In addition to the assistant managers, the more advanced clinical nurses are also designated as charge nurses, who are responsible for leading the clinical activities of the unit including the patient assignments for each shift.

What concerns Andy is that the least experienced "manager" has the greatest interface with the clinical nurses, other professional partners, and the patients and families. He recognizes a need to improve the knowledge and competencies of the frontline leaders to improve patient outcomes, increase nurse and physician satisfaction levels, and ensure that there are adequate numbers of prepared individuals for a viable succession plan should the need occur. Andy realizes that the frontline leaders who are unprepared for their roles could significantly affect the hospital's reputation for excellence.

Andy often states, "A good reputation is hard won, easily lost, and sometimes never regained." He encourages his direct reports to focus on the issues that define quality from the perspective of the patient, physician, and employees. "It matters significantly that our nursing-sensitive indicators and all other quality metrics meet and exceed our targeted goals, but it's also critical that we address issues that are perceived by our customers as quality indicators. A clean environment, meal trays delivered on time, medications given when requested, and a comfortable space for the families are all issues of quality for the patients. Having information and resources available, the presence of the nurse during rounds, and an efficient hospital visit are all issues of quality for physicians. Having needed resources, adequate staffing, and a healthy work environment are all issues of quality for the nursing staff. We as leaders need to ensure that our nurses have the resources that they need to do what they do best, and then we need to get out of their way and let them do it! We need to assure our physicians that we have the best, the brightest, and the most competent nurses in the world who can provide excellent care for their patients and their families. We need to provide a calm, pleasant, healing environment for patients and their families. The only way that we can accomplish these goals is to be authentic leaders who are physically and emotionally present in our support for our nursing staff and particularly for the frontline leaders who are the least prepared for their critically important role."

Andy shares his concerns with his directors and the other executives on the healthcare team. He gathers their ideas, and they develop a mind map of all possible ways that the frontline leaders can be developed in the most cost-efficient way. They decide to develop a Leadership Institute with an array of courses and classes offered online and in quarterly presentations. They design a leadership development program that includes lectures online and in class, reading materials, video presentations, and group discussions of actual case presentations. It is decided that after the participants earn 25 units of education, they will be given a leadership certificate and pin presented at a graduation ceremony. The graduation will include a national speaker and recognition of the new graduate in the Whitefish Community Hospital publication that is distributed to all employees, physicians, patients, friends of the hospital (financial donors), and the board of directors.

Andy is pleased that this plan provides an educational foundation for the frontline leaders who may not have had the opportunity for leadership education beyond their basic nursing education; however, he still feels that something is missing in advancing the leadership skills and competencies of the frontline leaders. During the budget season, Andy had the opportunity to review all of the programs and services offered by the nursing division and other hospital divisions to ensure their "worthiness" of being financially supported in the upcoming year. During this analysis of all programs, Andy reviewed the annual report for the New Graduate Residency Program, and the data clearly indicated the positive outcomes and cost efficiency of the program. Nested in the program was a strong and viable mentor program for the new graduate residence. Feedback from the new graduates indicated that the mentor program provided the social support that they needed to be acculturated on their units and provided a "safe resource" for them when they had questions, concerns, or frustrations they didn't feel comfortable sharing with their direct supervisors. When Andy read the annual report and the anecdotal comments, he had an "ah-ha!" moment. "Of course! This is the support that is missing for frontline leaders. We need to pair them with more prepared and experienced managers or directors who have clearly demonstrated success in their roles and who are willing and able to mentor the frontline leaders beyond the planned educational courses and sessions." Andy is excited about developing a leadership mentoring program not only for new leaders in the organization, but also for the existing less-experienced frontline leaders. He strongly believes that a mentor from another department would provide the social and experiential support that is often missing in formal education.

When Andy shared his vision with the directors and executive colleagues, they are also interested, particularly when he shares the positive outcomes of the mentor program for the new graduate residents. He mentions that he would be using that program as a pattern for the development of the leadership mentor program. He also shares how he would be evaluating the program's effectiveness with outcome metrics that he would report back to the executive team. He indicates that the program would be provided within existing budgeted educational funds, and the return on the investment would not only be measured in financial terms, but also in terms of patient, physician, and provider outcomes because the frontline leaders strongly influence these outcomes. Andy's next steps are to engage some of the directors, managers, selected frontline leaders, and the research nurses in the design, development, and measures of the leadership mentor program.

Questions

1. What is your opinion of Andy's plan to advance the knowledge and competencies of the frontline leaders?
2. What additional benefits, if any, do you see resulting from the development of a leadership mentor program?
3. What attributes of a transformational leader and coach does Andy demonstrate in his role with his direct reports, executive colleagues, and the nursing division as a whole?
4. Compare and contrast the similarities and differences between an authentic leader and a transformational leader.
5. In reviewing the attributes of quantum leader, how do these attributes intersect with the attributes of authentic and transformational leaders?
6. If you are in Andy's role, what would you do to advance the knowledge, skills, and competencies of frontline leaders and how would you measure whether you were successful in this endeavor?

References

Argote, L. (2013). *Organizational learning: Creating, retaining, and transferring knowledge.* New York, NY: Springer.

Argyris, C. (2006). *Reason and rationalizations: Capital limits to organizational knowledge.* New York, NY: Oxford University Press.

Brewer, G., & Sanford, B. (2011). *Decade of change: Managing in times of uncertainty*. New York, NY: Gallup Press.

Hickey, M., & Kritek, P. B. (2012). *Change leadership in nursing: How change occurs in a complex hospital system*. New York, NY: Springer.

Lencioni, P. (2008). *The five dysfunctions of a team*. New York, NY: Wiley.

Naylor, M., & Kurtzman, E. (2010). The role of nurse practitioners in reinventing primary care. *Health Affairs, 29*(5), 893–895.

Porter-O'Grady, T. (2007). *Implementing shared governance*. Atlanta, GA: Tim Porter-O'Grady Associates.

Porter-O'Grady, T. (2009). *Interdisciplinary shared governance: Integrating practice, transforming health care*. Sudbury, MA: Jones and Bartlett.

Porter-O'Grady, T. (2013). From tradition to transformation: A revolutionary moment for nursing in the age of reform. *Nurse Leader, 12*(1), 32–37.

Savitch, W. (2008). *Problem solving with C++*. New York, NY: Addison Wesley.

Schabracq, M. (2007). *Changing organizational culture: The change agent's guidebook*. New York, NY: Wiley.

Shomaker, T. S. (2011). Commentary: Preparing for health care reform: Ten recommendations for academic health centers. *Academic Medicine, 86*(5), 555–558. doi:10.1097/ACM.0b013e3182103443

Zedeck, S., & American Psychological Association. (2011). *APA handbook of industrial and organizational psychology* (1st ed.). Washington, DC: American Psychological Association.

Suggested Readings

Heibing, D. (2012). *Social self organization: Understanding complex systems*. New York, NY: Springer.

Northouse, P. (2012). *Leadership: Theory and practice*. New York, NY: Sage.

Sandberg, S. (2013). *Lean in: Women, work and the will to lead*. New York, NY: Knopf.

Quiz Questions

Select the best answer for each of the following questions.

1. Accountability always _____.
    a. Is externally generated
    b. Is delegated from above
    c. Is internally generated
    d. Moves from the bottom upward

2. Accountability differs from responsibility in which of the following ways?
    a. They measure different kinds of processes.
    b. Responsibility is more results oriented.
    c. Accountability is measurable and responsibility is not.
    d. Accountability is defined in terms of outcomes.

3. In confronting change, what do most people find is their first response?
    a. To personalize it
    b. To feel excitement
    c. To challenge the necessity for change
    d. To refuse to change

4. In transformative learning, how can theory-in-use be described?
   a. It consists of the conceptual foundations for an action.
   b. It is an automatic thought process related to an action.
   c. It is the theoretical validation of an action.
   d. It is a research-based response to a need.

5. What is the first step in gathering staff together for the purpose of learning and adapting?
   a. Identify a good methodology to use.
   b. Enumerate the rules of engagement.
   c. Understand the stages of the change process.
   d. Get to work on the problems immediately.

6. The issue of resources plays a critical role in all problem solving. In dealing with this issue, leaders should keep in mind which of the following rules of thumb?
   a. It is always possible to find more money if you look for it.
   b. Providing additional resources is not the way to reach a sustainable solution.
   c. Allocating more resources is necessary for solving problems.
   d. Budgeting adequate resources is part of all planning.

7. In problem solving, leaders must remember that which of the following is the one absolute unforgivable?
   a. To leave problems unresolved too long
   b. To create inadequate processes for resolving problems
   c. To lack a methodology for change
   d. To solve other people's problems for them

8. The coach is the chief _____.
   a. Facilitator
   b. Problem solver
   c. Learner
   d. Agent of change

9. When a coach is acting as a revolutionary, which of the following is the most important task?
   a. Get action under way quickly.
   b. Bring down existing structures as quickly as possible.
   c. Expand the circle of conspirators.
   d. Construct an individual plan of action.

10. In innovation coaching, risk is critical for success. What else is critical?
    a. Experimentation
    b. Planning
    c. Creating ideas
    d. Brainstorming

11. In undertaking tactical changes, which of the following is the first thing the leader does?

    a. Get out of the way.
    b. Outline a process for change.
    c. Direct the participants in their work.
    d. Create a set of priorities.

12. In managing strategic changes, what does the leader focus on?

    a. Processes, elements, and tasks
    b. Priorities, learning scenarios, and problem-solving tools
    c. Context, functions, and solutions
    d. Vision, solutions, and outcomes

13. In facilitating cultural change, what does the leader avoid?

    a. Fighting, opposition, and conflict
    b. Directing, controlling, and disciplining
    c. Patching, setting deadlines, and firefighting
    d. Narrowing, limiting, and refining

The Leader's Courage to Be Willing: Building a Context for Hope

Something unforeseen and magnificent is happening. Health care, having in our time entered its dark night of the soul, shows signs of emerging, transformed.
—*Barbara Dossey and Larry Dossey*

Chapter Objectives

At the completion of this chapter, the reader will be able to

· Review the sources of healthcare professional disenfranchisement.
· Describe the behavioral concept of willingness as it relates to the role of the leader.
· Describe a process for identifying and evaluating dogma in the healthcare system.
· Define the five essential qualities of will.
· Identify specific situations in which leaders can positively affect practice using the five essential qualities of will.

This chapter explores the concept of willingness and related concepts (e.g., will, the will, and willpower), the personal and organizational context in which willingness unfolds, and the factors that may erode its expression. It explains how the will of a person generally operates, how leaders can maximize their will, the evolutionary stages that a person's will goes through, and the purposes toward which a person's will can be directed. It also describes the five essential qualities of will (or willpower): courage, passion, energy, discipline, and trust. Finally, it presents nine strategies for facilitating willingness and associated assessment questions for leaders.

Why are healthcare workers, especially nurses, so discouraged? Where has all the hope gone? Job-related stress, emotional exhaustion, and feelings of depression, helplessness, hopelessness, and entrapment continue to fuel dissatisfaction and discouragement among all health professionals, even physicians and healthcare administrators. The combined assault of staffing shortages, excessive regulation, and reduced reimbursement has left a pall of apathy over the healthcare profession.

First, severe staffing shortages are challenging leaders to find quick solutions—a nearly impossible task. Second, state and federal regulations require healthcare leaders and workers to perform numerous procedural tasks to document compliance, with associated high costs in time and money. A recent article identified more than 30 regulatory bodies at the national level and a number of state licensing agencies (8 or more per state) that have jurisdiction over healthcare organizations. The complex laws and regulations generated by these agencies are often conflicting, and their benefit to the public is generally unknown.

The fact is that the regulation of health care would almost certainly be less extensive if health professionals were consistent in their practice and used value-based interventions exclusively. After all, it is not clear whether regulations passed to govern procedures are working as intended.

Yet, despite the problems in the nursing profession, the public has more regard for nurses than for any other type of health professional. Nurses have a powerful voice in their communities—perhaps even more powerful than they know. Consumers and politicians want to know what nurses think about prescription issues, ensuring access to care, and changing the health system to meet the needs of patients and their families.

Why are some leaders more successful than others in leading an organization through transformational change necessary to address staff shortages, reimbursement, consumer needs, and regulations? Why do some leaders fail to sustain their commitment to a change, letting it slowly subside or disappear altogether? Why can some people create an environment of hope and calm despite desperate or difficult circumstances? One answer can be found in the notions of will and personal willingness. Willing leaders are the co-creators of change. They recognize that no one person or situation can take away their personal peace, joy, and sense of competence, and they transmit these feelings to others.

Because of feelings of desperation, personal investment in the status quo, or a need for psychological preservation, some very knowledgeable leaders lose their willingness to take the initiative in making changes. Instead, they replace their willingness with an organizational mask, becoming what they believe the organization or a powerful other wants them to be. Such leaders may be incapable of seeing the whole and acting on their vision of it. Willing leaders not only see the whole but also claim responsibility for creating their personal experience of transformational change.

A Context for Hope

Leaders of quantum organizations can move only in one direction—toward building and sustaining the context for healthcare services and reinforcing expectations for a better future. These leaders behave in new and bold ways and see things from an optimistic and futurist perspective. Further, they are willing to do the work that needs to be done to meet patient needs, adhere to professional standards, and stay within the limits of available reimbursement. By their commitment to creating a hopeful context, they ensure that healthcare workers are better able to do the work of healing and health promotion.

The degree of a leader's willingness to lead can be explained by the extent to which he or she possesses courage, passion, energy, discipline, and trust. By possessing these qualities in abundance, the leader can engender in others not only hopefulness but a greater willingness to provide service.

> **Point to Ponder**
>
> Hope springs not from trying to remodel the past but rather from being willing to continually create the future with our colleagues to meet the changing needs of the community.

Will

Will (or willpower) has been defined as an inner power—a power over nature and over the self (i.e., self-control). Only the development of this inner power can offset the risk of our losing control of the tremendous forces at our disposal and becoming victims of our own achievements.

The terms *will* and *willpower* are typically used to refer to this inner power in the abstract, apart from the consideration of any individual person. The term *the will* is used when discussing willpower as evidenced by an individual person. In this usage, a person is said to have a will, and this will, typically viewed as the center of the person's self, is what exhibits willpower (or lack of willpower). Because the development of each person's will depends on the person's culture and the current circumstances, including political and economic factors, a person's will can be very powerful, very weak, or some degree in between these two extremes.

In coaching others, leaders should recognize that developed willpower has an enormous potential for creating and adapting to change. Once leaders gain an appreciation for how the qualities of willpower are expressed, they can comprehend the dynamics of those whose will is less strong and understand their rationale for pulling away. Reframing the work of leadership in terms of willpower can serve to create or rebuild hope and to redirect others toward greater achievement and satisfaction.

Discovery of Will

This section explores the view that a quantum leader's will is critical to his or her leadership success. The leader needs to discover the essence of his or her will and create the conditions for others in the organization to discover and honor their own will.

> **Key Point**
>
> Will is the self-directing capacity of human beings—the internal body of personal power.

For each person, the discovery of his or her will encompasses the following five phases:

1. Recognizing that willpower exists
2. Realizing that one has a will
3. Living one's personal will
4. Recognizing one's soulfulness (an awakening of the self resulting from insight and self-exploration)
5. Recognizing that awakening the will can be risky and can even threaten paralysis

517

The simplest and most frequent way in which a person discovers his or her will is through determined action and struggle. When a person makes a physical or mental effort or actively wrestles with some obstacle or opposing force, the person feels a power, or energy, rise up inside.

Self-exploration, particularly investigation of one's will, does not appear to be widely embraced by those in leadership positions. Overworked and sometimes taken for granted, leaders must struggle with a number of issues before they can embark on an examination of their will. These issues include the following:

- Leaders often have a Victorian conception of will, according to which it is associated with stern control over others.
- Most people are reluctant to change, particularly if it involves personal examination. Also, change requires time and patience—two commodities that are in short supply. It is easier to sit back and let others carry the ball.
- Leaders often do not want to pay the price for becoming more involved in change (or becoming less involved).
- Leaders are hesitant to discuss willpower and its characteristics with the executive team for fear of job loss.

Not surprisingly, the organization's culture strongly influences whether an exploration of willpower does in fact occur. The values, practices, and longevity of employees can facilitate or obstruct meaningful changes that foster a readiness to investigate the nature of willpower.

Initially, a person's will has a regulatory and directive function. Take the case of a rehabilitation patient. He knows what his legs are supposed to do and in which direction he is supposed to move, but in addition to the normal power he uses to propel his legs, he needs the encouragement of the physical therapist, giving him the willpower to act. Without this encouragement, the patient's willpower would be weak or sporadic and might disappear altogether.

When individuals discover that willpower exists within themselves and realize that the will and the self are intimately connected, they become more oriented toward the self and concomitantly less oriented toward others and the world. Recognizing that the power to make changes is located primarily in the self and not in others, they are now free to use their willpower to choose, relate, and bring about changes in themselves and others. They feel a new sense of unlimited potential for action, whether this involves altering themselves or acting on the outside world.

Consider the prevalence of noise in patient care areas. It is well known that noise prevents patients from relaxing and resting. Care providers know they should be less noisy and also remind others of the importance of quiet, but only rarely does an individual with a high degree of courage speak up about the need for a restful environment. In other words, the will to act is usually missing or is not sufficient for action. Although solving the problem of noise would seem to be simple, the fact is that noise in patient care areas continues to be one of the most common causes of patient complaints.

Another example concerns the resistance of workers to changes in their work routines. They may believe that the current work routines are the best way to achieve the desired goals, but often they are merely fearful of what will happen to them after the changes are implemented. Thus, their fear, rather than their will, drives their behavior. Overcoming resistance to change is a consistent theme in management literature, and efforts to guide leaders in developing the skills needed to foster change and innovation are well documented.

Given that any complex adaptive system exhibits self-organization, unpredictable interactions, and interdependencies, leaders need to learn to work with the natural energy of the system. They can learn this and overcome resistance to change more effectively by developing an understanding of will and willingness. It is helpful to note that will, despite the Victorian conception of it, is not about sternness but rather about the multidimensional directive and regulatory balances used by an individual.

It is not difficult to let the easygoing side of one's nature take control and to allow internal or external influences to dominate change when negative pressures exist. Such behaviors reinforce apathy and discouragement. Leaders need to take the trouble to oppose negative behaviors. They should not expect training of the will to be accomplished without the expenditure of energy and persistence required for the successful development of any other quality, physical or mental. Effort lies at the base of any worthwhile leadership activity and is a requisite for success.

Group Discussion

Identify at least two situations in which you thought about reacting to a problem situation but did not. Was your reluctance related to patient care, the behaviors of coworkers, organizational policy, or something else? Now that you have identified a situation that should be managed, how can each member of the group support you in summoning the courage to react in the future?

Nature of Will

Because will is embedded in the self, self-exploration and the astute observation of colleagues are starting points for gaining an appreciation of the significance of will for leadership. Self-exploration can help a leader

- Control his or her own will
- Identify areas that need to be developed
- Assess the application of willpower by others
- Intervene in cases of inappropriate use

Awakening of the self requires insight, self-absorption, and struggle. In the journey through transformational change, leaders discover the power to make choices, relate to others, and bring about changes in themselves and others. As a result of the new insights they gain during this journey, leaders could withdraw their support for certain projects or change priorities. Both positive and negative actions can be conscious or unconscious, depending on the degree of self-examination. When self-examination is a conscious process, the effect on the individual can be profound because the self shifts its orientation inward.

Unfortunately, there are obstacles to and dangers in self-exploration of the will. All too often, leaders work to become who they believe the organization wants them to be, preventing themselves from becoming who they really are. When this happens, they struggle and perceive themselves stuck in a persona that is not authentic, with the result that they feel impotent, apathetic, and insincere. The questions that leaders, not to mention other individuals, need to ask themselves are these: Are you willing to say yes—to act, think, and feel as you really are? Can you picture what this would be like? Would it not be joyful to do things because they reflect your will and are authentic rather than solely because the organization expects such behaviors?

> **Key Point**
>
> Are you willing to want what you get when it comes or to force yourself to get what you want? How strong is your will?

By developing their will, leaders are better able to make decisions intuitively and rationally. By integrating their personal heart and objective mind, they become more authentic individuals and increase their willingness to act. Alternatively, if they act solely for reasons and values outside of themselves, they will continue to suffer and be disinclined to participate in the changing environment.

Further, denying one's personal will is a way of avoiding personal accountability. Assuming accountability, on the other hand, means never experiencing anything that is not a product of one's vision, mental model, or emotions. The self, not the external world, is the source of experiences. It follows that nothing can take away one's peace, joy, or sense of adequacy—each of these must be given up voluntarily.

Types of Will

Characterizing the types of will that people have can help clarify what will is. For example, it is relatively common to hear people described as having a strong will, a skillful will, or a good will. A brief account of each type follows.

To say that someone has a strong will is to say that that person has significant power or determination. A typical mistake is to believe that strength of will is the essence of the whole will—that having a will means always attempting to get one's own way.

Someone who possesses a skillful will is able to achieve desired results with the least amount of energy. People who have this type of will must understand their own habits, goals, and desires, and the relationships among these, to use them skillfully.

A person with a good will is benevolent, has a high degree of integrity, and does not use his or her will to overpower or corrupt the will of others.

Essential Qualities

The notion that a person's will consists only of strength or weakness, or goodness or badness, is incorrect and can lead someone engaged in self-exploration in the wrong

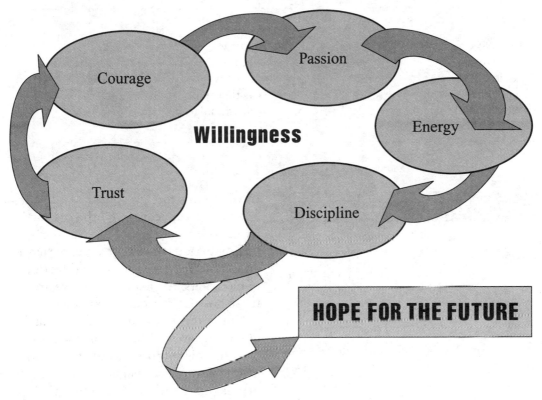

Figure 13-1 The Five Essential Qualities of Will Lead to Hope for the Future

direction. Instead, for individuals to exhibit will or willpower, they must possess a certain set of qualities, namely, courage, passion, energy, self-discipline, and trust (**Figure 13-1**). Leaders who are interested in increasing their expertise should use this set of qualities as a paradigm of will during periods of self-examination or when evaluating the behavior of others.

Courage

Courage is that quality of mind or spirit that enables individuals to face difficulty, danger, and pain without fear and to act in accordance with their beliefs. Courage is required to stay the course during the shaking and shuddering of the chaotic stage of change and to manage resistance to change to reach new levels of knowledge and performance. It is also required to tolerate paradox—to function while holding two competing forces inside. Courageous individuals also tend to be creative, daring, and trusting of their intuition, whereas individuals who lack courage are cautious, to put it politely (**Exhibit 13-1**).

Courage often does not emerge until the pain of not doing something exceeds the fear of doing it. The fear that we feel when we encounter an unfamiliar pathway and must enlarge our thinking is a signal that we are on the brink of learning. It is like

Exhibit 13-1   Qualities Associated with Willingness and Reluctance

Willingness	Reluctance
• Courage	• Fear
• Passion	• Apathy
• Energy	• Lethargy
• Self-discipline	• Self-indulgence
• Trust	• Skepticism

Point to Ponder

To know what is right and not to do it is the worst cowardice.

—Confucius

There is nothing more difficult to take in hand, more perilous to conduct, or more uncertain in the success, than to take the lead in the introduction of a new order of things.

—Machiavelli

traveling in a foreign country and being seized by a vague fear and the instinctive desire to go back home. Similarly, during periods of change we experience an instinctive desire for the protection of old habits. At that moment, we are tense but also porous to learning.

Numerous explanations for the lack of courage exist. Most point to fear of the unknown or discomfort with what is happening. Fear is paralyzing and brings out the worst in people—their most basic instincts, those for self-protection and survival. Yet healthy fear—the kind of fear that enhances the acquisition of new knowledge—needs to be valued, reinforced, and fostered.

To create a more hopeful culture, leaders need to assist others in finding the courage to deal with the type of fear that causes imperviousness to learning and shuts down the capacity for connectedness. Believing in others and remaining patient while they endure and experience the process further support their personal growth and accountability.

The Nike slogan "Just do it" calls individuals to jump out of the comfort zone and into the fringe of the unknown. Leaders need the same "just do it" attitude. This does not mean acting impulsively and without a plan, but instead doing the best that one can given what one knows and expects at that particular time.

As an example, although the perceived conflict between financial viability and professional standards will probably continue forever, decisions still need to be made. Leaders must often "just do it"—make a decision that balances standards and reimbursement. To develop the courage to make such decisions, you must let go of what others believe you should be and boldly show the world who you are. Courageous leaders

- Face their fears
- Explore their vulnerability
- Lean toward risk

Group Discussion

After reading the following case study, identify the presence (or absence) of courage, energy, trust, passion, and discipline in the behavior of the nurse.

A staff nurse admitted a terminally ill patient and reported to her supervisor that she believed she really had made a difference in the care of the patient and in the final outcome. She also stated that she had required a total of 2 hours for the admission process—an hour in excess of the allocated time. The supervisor, in response, showed concern about the extra time used in the admission process and the additional expense for this type of care.

The staff nurse then explained the situation more fully. A female patient with terminal cancer, accompanied by her husband, was admitted for pain management and relief of abdominal ascites. She was scheduled for a fluoroscopy-guided paracentesis to relieve the fluid and to receive IV pain medication. The patient was exhausted and wanted relief from her discomfort. Also, in the course of the admission, the patient informed the nurse that she was ready to die, that she had fought hard and long enough and knew nothing could be done to extend her life. Her husband agreed.

The nurse asked the patient if she knew that draining the fluids from her abdomen would relieve the pressure temporarily but would leave more space for the fluids to collect again. The patient was told that she could be kept comfortable without the paracentesis and could be assisted to die as comfortably as possible. This approach was discussed with the physician, who gave it his approval. The patient and husband chose to have pain management only. The patient died peacefully 2 days later.

In discussing the case with her supervisor, the nurse argued that use of 2 hours for the admission process resulted not only in a desirable outcome but in an economic savings. True, the admission cost the organization an additional hour of RN time, but eliminating a fluoroscopy-guided paracentesis avoided the addition of approximately $2,500 in charges to a DRG bill. The organization was saved this entire amount because the reimbursement for the patient was fixed. Thus, the nurse maximized the quality of the care while minimizing the organization's costs.

- Celebrate failures
- Never give up

Passion

Creating a sense of passion and willingness in employees requires leaders to institute employee incentives based on patient satisfaction and to empower employees to do what is right for the patients. The goal is to create an organizational culture that turns employees

Group Discussion

Reflect on a situation in which you were at your wits' end and finally reacted. At what moment and for what reason were you inspired or forced to respond? In the future, will you react more quickly? Why or why not?

and patients into thunderous evangelists for the organization. This type of culture is very different from the traditional organizational culture, in which

- The employees are expected to manipulate patients into using a select group of providers in a particular geographical region.
- Employee productivity is closely monitored.
- Policies are strictly enforced.

Energy

Energetic individuals are vigorous and active, with a capacity for serious effort. Such individuals also have an intensity of will capable of overcoming opposing forces, like an athlete in competition. This intensity of will is a form of power and needs to be recognized and used positively. The energy required for optimal willingness is never limitless; rather, energetic individuals learn to temper and manage their energy expenditure, balancing high-energy times with quiet times.

In contrast, low-energy individuals are apathetic, uninterested, or burned out. Some are fearful of getting involved or becoming too hopeful because of past disappointments. For these individuals, the lack of a clear defined sense of self is often at the root of their inaction. If they see themselves as disempowered, which many of them do, their stagnation is reinforced. What low-energy individuals need is assistance in reentering the unfolding processes of life. In particular, they need to assess their goals, focus on the future and on what is positive and working, and accept that human beings are inherently imperfect.

Self-Discipline

Self-discipline is personal willingness to adhere to standards and meet responsibilities. It is the ability to check impulsive actions while persisting in selected activities. Self-discipline is regulation of one's own behavior, not that of others. Without self-discipline, a leader with a strong will acts impulsively and unpredictably, negating the positive spirit of leadership willingness.

When leaders develop self-discipline, they are better able to focus their attention and minimize impulsive and scattered activities. Their inner concentration grows, allowing them the steady control and clarity of action and thought they need to gain the support of colleagues.

Trust

Developing trust between colleagues requires congruence of values, nonpossessive warmth, effective communication, and empathy (i.e., the ability to understand the

---

Exhibit 13-2   Attributes of a Willing Leader

- *Openness to change:* Willingness to approach changes in staffing, organizational structure, and roles with a positive attitude while maintaining a focus on patient care; willingness to be a co-creator of change rather than a defender of the past
- *Acceptance of diverse perspectives:* Willingness to look at multiple reasonable alternatives while giving up the role of patient advocate; willingness to acknowledge that some situations may not be acceptable but are a major part of one's work life and must be handled patiently
- *Focus on value:* Willingness to educate others to understand evidence-based approaches as the new context for providing healthcare services
- *Awareness of the larger system:* Willingness to move between micro and macro views of issues— from the patient to the team to the department to the organization to the community to the state to the world and back

---

perceptions and feelings of others). It also requires knowledge that the shared values are ethically sound and that the work of the care providers is truly intended to further the public's interest. The trust that has been built up between colleagues is reinforced when everyone consistently behaves in accordance with accepted patient care standards and uses resources wisely, shares information appropriately, and discusses new ideas openly.

A leader with a fully developed will, characterized by courage, passion, energy, self-discipline, and trust, creates a positive and encouraging context in which employees are expected to practice within professional standards and values. This type of leader also instills a sense of hopefulness in all members of the organization, increasing the chance that together they will bring about a better and more meaningful healthcare future (**Exhibit 13-2**).

Hope

Hope is the feeling that what is wanted can be had or that events will turn out well. People find it difficult to be hopeful if they do not believe things are going satisfactorily. They become less inclined to get involved and less willing to do the right thing because it does not seem to matter. When the qualities of will—courage, passion, energy, self-discipline, and trust—are present, a beacon of hope emerges to begin a positive cycle of behaviors. Discouraged and disenfranchised workers start to see new opportunities and develop a new willingness to focus on the present and future, leaving the past behind.

Strategies to Facilitate Willingness

Once leaders understand the nature of will, they are in a position to facilitate willingness as a means of achieving their goals. Following is a discussion of strategies that incorporate the qualities of courage, passion, energy, discipline, and trust. Note that these do not exhaust the strategies for increasing the willingness of employees, but constitute a beginning on which to build.

Group Discussion

The following questions are posed for reflection. Examine behaviors related to all five categories: courage, passion, energy, self-discipline, and trust. Are some behaviors more prevalent than others? How can you improve behaviors in each category? Finally, develop a plan to incorporate the desired behaviors into the interview process for new employees and in the annual performance review competency set.

Courage
- Is there evidence that members of the organization are able to share their values and ideas in a nonthreatening manner?
- Is there evidence that members are able to stand their ground in defending their values and ideas?
- Are the members brave enough to ask the right questions?

Passion
- Is there evidence in the organization of a strong and vocalized commitment to ideas? To projects?
- Is there evidence that all employees take great pride in their work?
- Are there groups or projects in which enthusiasm is lacking? If so, which are they?

Energy
- Does the organization's leader exhibit vigor and vitality when managing projects?
- Does the leader's opinion dominate the ideas or actions of others?
- Are employees willing to participate in organizational group activities, social events, and/or committees?

Self-Discipline
- Does the organization's leader regulate his or her activities appropriately?
- In managing projects, does the leader act impulsively?
- Are meetings or programs well thought out and implemented with little chaos?

Trust
- Is the organization's leader honest, forthright, and candid with others, or does the leader tell half-truths, damaging the trusting bond between leader and colleague?
- Are team members open and honest with each other?
- Do team members rely on each other?

Removing the Dogma Brick Wall

So much health care is done routinely and automatically, with little thought to its rationale. As science advances, new technologies and practices emerge and become popular. These and the older technologies and practices should be examined to ensure that the highest quality care is being provided at the lowest cost. Examining technologies and practices demands significant courage, for it can involve challenging the system and its players. It also requires openness to new ideas and the recognition that change is (i.e., change is inevitable and should not be avoided).

In surveying health care for the purpose of making improvements, leaders should not look first to see what additional products, services, and providers are needed in the future, but rather review the current situation to identify non-value-adding services for elimination. Or at best, they should review both the current and the proposed improvement simultaneously. This approach, besides helping to create excess capacity for future needs, revalidates what is important in health care. All too often, practices become integrated into the system and continue to be used long after their rationale is lost or forgotten. "We have always done it this way" is not a good reason to keep on using a nonbeneficial practice.

For one thing, we have not always done it this way. At one time, only physicians were allowed to take blood pressures, insert nasogastric tubes, administer IV bolus medications, and write prescriptions. Now aides, technicians, and nurses perform these same tasks. The fact is that health professionals, especially physicians, often hesitate to relinquish technical tasks that the state practice act does not really require them to perform. New research and evidence examining the value of the nursing history has challenged one of nursing's sacred cows (Ackman, Perry, Wolfard, Steckel, & Hill, 2012). The authors report in a performance improvement project that the nursing history was a one-time, non-value-added process.

This is also cause to wonder, for example, how and when the task of taking and recording blood pressure came within the purview of nursing assistants—or, better still, the responsibility of the patient! An individual somewhere, someplace was willing to question whether it was really appropriate for physicians to own this chore. Courage is needed to examine current practices, give up what is not appropriate, and retain what is. Further, this type of examination needs to be done with passion for the essence of the profession, not for personal recognition or benefit.

Unquestioning adherence to authority and tradition is a well-known barrier to the development of knowledge. Although authority and tradition provide a seemingly stable foundation, in fact blind faith is problematic and can be detrimental to survival. Continuing progress in nursing and other areas of health care thus warrants an examination of all dogmas and a release from those that are without foundation.

Dogmas pertain to professional roles as well as procedures and practices. Efforts to delineate the boundaries of each profession need to be ongoing. Those responsible for delineating the domains of the various health professions must look at the received wisdom (conventional beliefs) within each profession, the profession's knowledge base (science), and the profession's application of that knowledge (art). The practices of any professional

527

Group Discussion

Dogmas, or unquestioned beliefs, exist in every organization and in every culture. Following are three examples that might exist in a healthcare organization: (1) nursing is women's work, (2) nurses wear white, and (3) patient registration takes place at the front entrance of the facility.

Identify at least three practices based on dogma in your current organization. Begin with the policy and procedure manual in your department. Can you suggest any changes that would improve organizational efficiency?

healthcare worker go beyond science as traditionally conceived to include, for instance, the use of intuition and the therapeutic use of the self. Likewise, the emerging principles that pertain to building relationships and partnerships beg for inclusion into the healthcare disciplines.

The real work of quantum leaders is to deconstruct the dogmas of traditional Newtonian science and transform current organizational underpinnings to reflect the essence of complexity science. The realities of current organizations—the great number of connections and relationships among the many elements and the inherent capacity for change or adaptation—demand a better explanation than can be delivered by the linear thinking characteristic of Newtonian science. Once the non-value-added work is identified, the processes to engage nurses to actually change practice may in fact be more challenging than identifying the outdated work.

Unlike the mechanistic Newtonian paradigm, complexity science affirms that no leader is an island. In other words, the achievement of desired outcomes in a system is beyond the talents of any one individual. Instead, outcomes result from the relationships between individuals. Although the abilities of a single individual are important, they are not completely useful until the individual establishes relationships and works together with other individuals. Thus, the attention of leaders shifts from individual performance to appropriate patterns of interrelationship. Strategies for minimizing dogma include these:

- Examine and assess the value of at least three current practices each month. Retain or eliminate each practice depending on its value.
- Believe in the value of process so strongly that at least three employees gain the same appreciation each month.
- Approach difficult situations in which there is personal impact with the same enthusiasm as situations that do not affect you personally.
- No matter how long current practices have been used, be willing to examine others.
- Review prevalent dogmas in a patterned way. Commit to making no change impulsively. Instead, first talk with colleagues to ensure that every proposed change makes good sense.
- Know that colleagues share concerns about long-held practices and believe there are better ways as well but may not be quite ready to address the issues. Patience is needed.

Continuous Learning

High-quality healthcare services can be delivered only by educated, compassionate, and skilled care providers. Further, such providers need to maintain or increase their competence levels through continuing education. Following through on a commitment to professional growth, however, can be incredibly difficult in an organization steeped in reorganization. Everyone's energy is channeled into the redesign and maintenance of the new context, making continuing education hard to pursue. The quantum leader must therefore support the acquisition of new knowledge and skills by employees, while at the same time sustaining the reorganization efforts. According to Schein (Contu, 2002), learning and change that inevitably accompany new knowledge are part of a complex process that includes both the achievement of increased knowledge and the frustrations of the change dynamic. Following are some ways for a leader to ensure that continuous learning becomes part of the organization:

- Create and maintain a culture that fosters continuous learning.
- Recognize that new knowledge is essential for all to survive.
- Participate enthusiastically in continuing education, and share the knowledge you gain with colleagues.
- Support continuous learning consistently, namely, through every budget cycle and challenge throughout the year.
- Identify and trend performance measures that support the value of continuing education.

Minimizing Professional Antagonism

In hierarchical departmental organizations, the work groups tend to become competitive and adversarial. In healthcare organizations, for example, nursing and non-nursing departments continually battle for resources and position.

In addition, nurses have been reported to "eat their young." A recent panel of student nurses working in a particular healthcare organization identified the nurses who coached and mentored them in a positive way and those who reinforced their novice status in the presence of others. One student freely shared why she would not select that organization for employment: She had been assigned a preceptor who was a nationally recognized nurse expert but who was avoided by students because of her intimidating behaviors and perceived intolerance.

Antagonism exists among new employees often because of poor interpersonal skills of supervisors, preceptors, and colleagues. In nursing, the nurses (the staff and the nurse manager), not non-nurse coworkers, have the greatest impact on nurse stress. Thus, in this regard, nurses truly are their own worst enemies—and consequently the solution may lie within nursing rather than outside the healthcare system. Nurses need to care for each other—just as they do for their patients. They need to be their brothers' and sisters' keepers. The leader's role in reducing professional antagonism is to do the following:

- Bring issues into the open for discussion and minimize behind-the-scenes dialogue.
- Realize that relationships truly can be therapeutic. Expecting collaboration is the only way to develop the culture and context for high-quality, low-cost patient care services.
- Address issues as they arise.
- Stay focused and remain objective.

Group Discussion

The assumption that people working in health care are shallow, single-minded, materialistic, and socially unfettered is consistent with Newtonian science. These beliefs support the practice of attracting new employees by giving them sign-on bonuses. Do you agree or disagree with this rationale? What are the effects, positive and negative, of this approach to recruitment on quality, productivity, and cost? What types of reward and recognition practices would be consistent with complexity theory? What are the effects of these reward and recognition practices on quality, productivity, and cost?

Meeting the Needs of Employees

There are two categories of employees: those who have jobs and those who have careers. Those with jobs report to work, perform their duties as well as possible, and go home at the end of their tour of duty to get on with their lives. In contrast, those with careers not only do the necessary work but plan where they are going in their chosen profession and participate in professional activities outside of the workplace.

Not every person is seeking a career. Some individuals are satisfied with a job that is meaningful and fairly compensated. Expecting to motivate all employees to commit to a career is unrealistic. It is especially ill advised to dangle cash before professionals as a way of inducing desired behaviors and changes. This strategy is based on the assumption that people are motivated only by material gain and is likely to lead to a healthcare workforce that is indeed petty and greedy. It is also based on the assumption that individuals act independently of their social institutions and that social systems are nothing more than the sum of individual actions. This is a shallow notion of human decision making and ignores the way our values and actions are conditioned and constrained by social relations.

The world of work today is very different from what it was in the past. Workers stayed with one company or organization for a lifetime, whereas now workers may have several career pathways, and mobility rather than promotion is the symbol of advancement. The notion of loyalty needs to be redefined to reflect the marketplace of the twenty-first century. Loyalty to an organization may have been appropriate at one time, but now loyalty to one's core values is more suited to the way work is organized.

Leaders need the courage to recognize this phenomenon and ensure that both types of employees—job holders and career seekers—are valued and treated fairly. The organization must meet not only the needs of the customers, but also those of the individuals it employs. The presence of employees from different generations and with different values requires leaders to use multiple strategies:

- Create a compensation system that recognizes the multiplicity of employee values and needs. In addition, the system should support retention and guide employees to new opportunities when the organization's needs change, the required job skills change, or the employees' desires change. Become a partner with employees in managing their work and planning for the next position.

- Be vigilant and persistent when implementing and maintaining an appropriate compensation system and recognition and reward program.
- Stay focused and committed despite resistance from those who would like the current compensation system and recognition and reward program to remain unchanged.

Providing Value-Based Services

What one does and what difference it makes are the key issues for all providers. If an organization provides 1,000 services and only 25 make a difference, then the other 975 services must be considered for elimination—even if the 975 services have billing codes that render them reimbursable.

Provider accountability for contributions to patient care outcomes is a missing piece of health care. All professional care providers must focus their actions on achieving desired outcomes and implement only interventions that have a basis in science or a realistic chance of benefiting patients.

The measurement of healthcare outcomes is gradually becoming more meaningful and reflective of patient needs (Pappas, 2013). Unfortunately, indicators are often looked at in an order that fails to take into account the basic goal of health care—health improvement. For example, productivity measures are typically examined before clinical outcomes. If productivity targets are exceeded, increases in productivity are mandated without consideration of their potential impact on care provision.

Nonetheless, consumers of healthcare services expect that the services received are based on logic and scientific knowledge and that the intended outcomes are likely to occur. Further, they view the primary goal of healthcare organizations as providing effective clinical services, not making a profit. The problem for these organizations is how to provide value-based, high-quality care that is affordable and at the same time makes money (this is different from making as much money as possible).

Given the constraints caused by balanced budget initiatives, leaders are often caught in a cost–quality balancing act and are not always sure how to achieve value-based care. No clear solutions are on the horizon for the ailing healthcare system—certainly no financial relief of any significance. This raises the question whether we can afford to spend money on quality initiatives. Ethically, the answer is a resounding *yes!* And that is the public's expectation as well.

Perhaps it would be helpful to reframe the quality question as a value question. Value is determined by the three elements of cost, quality, and service (Malloch & Porter-O'Grady, 1999). Cost is driven by the available resources, which are currently very limited. Quality is partly determined by the outcomes of care. Service is a matter of the time and type of care provided. Thus, the following question becomes relevant: Are healthcare leaders obligated to provide value-based services to patients and family members? The issue of spending money on quality is now linked to both cost and service.

Achieving value-based health care faces an additional challenge: drawing conclusions about quality initiatives and return on investment when there are multiple factors involved. A further complication is the extensive use of a type of cost–benefit analysis that is not sensitive to healthcare objectives. If the benefits of a program can be priced in dollars, then a cost–benefit analysis can identify the alternative with the largest benefit-to-cost ratio. However, many decisions involve benefits that are not easily quantifiable in monetary terms or otherwise, such as psychological benefits and environmental benefits (clean air and water).

Healthcare leaders and providers are now required to examine services using the value equation and to make decisions accordingly. If resources are limited, leaders must ask whether every patient sign and symptom requires intervention, particularly if minimal or no improvement in the patient's clinical condition is the likely outcome. Paying close attention to the health improvement value of healthcare services is an incredibly difficult challenge for providers and leaders schooled in the doctrine that increasing access to health care and growth in the healthcare system were absolute goods. Unfortunately, accountability and control were absent from the cost-based payment system, and the results are well known—exhaustion of resources. Health professionals are currently challenged to move from "rich" care to "wise" care.

Another value-related issue of interest is productivity. Because business still operates under questionable assumptions regarding productivity—that the more hours employees work, the more productive they are; that the faster employees work, the more they accomplish; and that the more employees are paid, the more motivated they are to be productive—leaders are challenged to better understand the reality of employee productivity (**Exhibit 13-3**). Health professionals in this country are working more hours than ever before and getting less done. In fact, Americans have the dubious distinction of being first in the number of hours worked each year. The U.S. Department of Labor, Bureau of Labor Statistics, noted only a slight increase in productivity from 1960 to 1990, and the productivity increase in the last 10 years is attributed to technological advances, particularly the development of the Internet.

Exhibit 13-3   Myths and Truths About Employee Productivity

Accepted Notions
- If employees work more hours, they will be more productive.
- If employees work faster, they will be more productive.
- If employees are paid more, they will be motivated to work harder and produce more.

The Reality
- Employees perform optimally for 6 to 7 hours and may be able to work longer in a burst of energy or inspiration, but then they must rest.
- Employees need balance; they need a life outside of work.
- Slower, intuitive thinking is often more effective in solving problems than mental agility.
- Studies show that in Germany, where individual performance is not rewarded with pay increases, productivity is often higher than in the United States.
- Employees are most productive when their employers pay them equitably and then do everything possible to help the employees put money out of their minds.

Source: Data from Johnson, C. B. (2000). When working harder is not smarter. *Inner Edge, 3*(2), 18–21.

Healthcare employees are burning out faster than the replacements are coming in, yet they are still being pushed to become more productive. They are working 12-hour days, are commuting up to 2 hours a day, and are held by an electronic leash to the office. Their opportunity to relax is almost nonexistent.

Contrary to popular belief, we need to learn how to slow down our thinking, not speed it up. Time for reflection and contemplation of ideas and issues is sorely missing in health care. The never-ending checklist is always present and demanding attention. Further, experts report that pay is not the chief motivator for productivity. In general, employees desire to do meaningful work most of all, next they desire opportunities for collaboration through group decision making, and then they want equitable pay.

What drives people to work at their best? How can healthcare leaders revitalize the lost passion of employees? What retention strategies support the rebuilding of a hopeful culture? Interestingly, the answer is simple. When employees believe their work is meaningful—productive in the sense of producing beneficial results—they are motivated to work harder and experience a renewal of passion and hopefulness. Productivity is not only about quantity; it is also about quality.

Optimizing employee performance takes on a whole new meaning in this context. All human beings have a need to express their uniqueness and their talents in the work they do and be recognized for their contributions (**Exhibit 13-4**). Therefore, employees are typically motivated by jobs that develop their skills and expand their minds, demand individual initiative, involve working on teams, benefit others, and spark a desire to make a difference in the world. Jobs that have these characteristics possess what Cedric Johnson (2000) called fruitfulness—work flows from one person to another in a way that is both

---

Exhibit 13-4   Optimizing Performance: Productivity or Fruitfulness?

Productivity
- Productivity is mechanistic.
- In a productivity-driven organization, employees are treated like machines and judged on the quantity of their output.
- The predominant concern is getting more "bang for the buck."
- Efforts to increase employee motivation are dependent on external sources, pay, benefits, and so forth.

Fruitfulness
- Fruitfulness is humanistic.
- Fruitfulness involves a respectful, holistic view of each person that recognizes values, beliefs, and expectations.
- Fruitfulness honors the inner need of each person to express his or her uniqueness and talents and to develop and expand.
- Fruitfulness engages the inner selves of employees and causes them to grow and be sustained naturally and enduringly.

Source: Data from Johnson, C. B. (2000). When working harder is not smarter. *Inner Edge*, 3(2), 18–21.

respectful and valued. To ensure that healthcare work possesses fruitfulness, leaders need to do the following:

- Continually examine services, measures, and systems to assess their impact on patient outcomes. Retain those that improve patient outcomes, and eliminate those that have no effect or a negative effect.
- Believe that hope can be restored to care providers through restoring value to the work they do.
- Believe intensely that individuals give their best when treated like adults.
- Be committed to doing what is best for patients.
- Consistently expect only value-adding services to be delivered to patients. Publicly recognize individuals who focus on value, and guide those who require assistance in eliminating unnecessary and non-value-adding work.
- Believe that all healthcare providers intuitively know that restoring value to work is the right path but have not been able to translate their perceptions into practice. Believe that most, but not all, will eventually make the transition.
- Believe that the healthcare system will not only support but will require increases in the value of healthcare services. Know that colleagues support caring, healing work that makes a difference.

Becoming Mentally Fit

Some care providers appear to be tougher than others. In fact, their "toughness" might be a kind of mental fitness resulting from their sense of commitment, perception of control, and ability to view change as a challenge. Mental fitness involves taking responsibility for one's reactions to adversity. Through this kind of fitness, individuals can prevent emotional exhaustion and turn stressful events into meaningful challenges. Often, the expectations of altruism as a basic nurse value and behavior are different from societal values in which altruism is sometimes seen as not in the best interest of the patient (Guiffra, 2013).

Mental fitness is helpful for handling role modifications and reductions in the workforce. Employees who lack mental fitness often develop an attitude of learned helplessness. For example, if they are laid off, they react with anger, believe getting laid off is beyond their control, blame themselves, and generally feel helpless. Their helplessness triggers a downward spiral of self-defeat in which they see themselves as increasingly unable to get ahead.

Goal setting, mental imagery, emotional mastery, and positive thinking are all part of the mental conditioning that is necessary to overcome this helplessness and survive substantial changes. The mentally fit alter the perception of stress and mobilize effective coping techniques, lessening the trauma of stressful events. In fact, they transform these events into opportunities for increased meaning in life. Leaders who are mentally fit learn to manage the context of the work as well as the specific content of their discipline.

Mental fitness among leaders is associated with leadership resilience and leadership agility. As leaders become more mentally fit, they also become more resilient, decreasing the probability that they will experience burnout. Many leaders, particularly those at the vice-presidential level, work persistently to support and guide the chief executive

Exhibit 13-5   Planning for Position Elimination

- Recognize that no position is forever nor should it be if the work of the organization is changing to meet the needs of the marketplace.
- Consider other roles that might be of interest in the future and begin to develop skills in the relevant areas.
- Discuss your interests with your immediate supervisor, request assistance in continuing to meet current expectations, but also be prepared for changes. (Note: Although it may be difficult to discuss role changes, open and honest communication is always the best approach.)
- Retain control of your career—avoid letting other factors control you.

in clinical matters in addition to meeting their own responsibilities. The relationship between the head of the nursing department, for example, and the chief executive is not only intense but typically requires more from the nurse, who is likely to be continually providing feedback about the impact of decisions on patient outcomes and care provider satisfaction. Not surprisingly, the nurse leader, if lacking in mental fitness, will be prone to burnout

Leaders who are downsized experience a much greater emotional and psychological impact than typically has been acknowledged, and their ability to deal with such trauma is minimal at best. For one thing, the skills needed to handle disappointment are seldom taught in educational programs. Therefore, downsized leaders spend considerable time second guessing past decisions and become reluctant to make decisions for fear of further emotional insult. If they get follow-up counseling, it is directed toward helping them cope with their behaviors, rather than preparing them for future disappointments. Becoming mentally fit, on the other hand, is a matter of learning to expect, anticipate, and plan for job-related disappointments and defeats and taking a proactive approach to managing one's personal destiny (**Exhibit 13-5**).

Leadership agility is the ability to respond quickly and appropriately to input from employees and colleagues, the actions of competitors, and developing crises. Leaders with this ability are better able to manage the stress of situations and to calculate the odds of success or failure. Once they acquire agility, along with resilience and mental fitness, leaders are in a good position to handle their responsibilities without becoming exhausted and incapable of experiencing the pleasures of their work. They are also in a good position to appreciate the virtues of mental fitness and to understand its importance for the organization as a whole. To ensure that the organization's entire workforce is mentally fit, leaders should do the following:

- Create a culture that recognizes that good and not-so-good events occur, understand that employees need support when things do not go well, and provide the necessary support to those who require it.
- Develop a personal commitment to help others acquire mental fitness, resilience, and agility.
- Continually strive to increase their own mental fitness and create the culture that requires others to do the same.
- Extract hope and energy from the mission of health care.

- Establish a program of self-examination and self-renewal.
- Recognize that no individual is an island and that each person needs relationships, support, and feedback.

Balancing the Use of Time

The transition into the Information Age has left many people with far too many activities on the to-do list and too little time to accomplish them. Leaders must therefore guide employees toward looking at time use in a different way. No individual ever has enough time for all the things he or she would like to do. Time management strategies may assist employees in eliminating nonproductive or nonessential tasks, but the employees still need to find a good balance between the things that are truly important to them. More specifically, they need to achieve an equilibrium between the activities of work and personal activities so that they can find joy and pleasure in both.

Some progress has been made in creating more balance between work and personal life, but more needs to be done to minimize the burnout and keep employees from feeling discouraged and disenfranchised. When organizations identify balancing work and personal life as a goal, they tend to focus on the time at work. An organization might develop initiatives to help employees have flexibility in work hours, for example, but at the same time it might leave vacancies unfilled and ask employees to do more with less. It does not matter that the employees have flexible hours if they also have to work 5 or 10 more hours each week. Because they are not much better off as a result of the initiative, the employees view the message as ambiguous. In addition, management might then perceive the employees as ungrateful, causing the employees to feel that the executives just do not get it.

Achieving a balance between work and personal life is a never-ending process for both leaders and employees. Employees need tools to do their jobs well and to help them feel successful, and they need recognition and reward systems that measure and acknowledge their accomplishments. Leaders need to build a culture of respect for employees and their accomplishments. When people feel successful, leaving the workplace at the end of the day is easier both physically and mentally because the shadow of work is not hanging over their heads.

Leaders also should help employees feel successful in other aspects of their lives. Sometimes the support needed might seem like it falls outside the leader's jurisdiction. However, quantum leaders recognize that no individual ever enters the door of the organization and leaves all personal issues behind. They understand that personal issues have an impact on any employee's ability to work effectively and that assisting the employee might be critical to the team's success. Employees have a wide variety of needs that change as their lives change. Few have the personal skills to achieve and maintain balance. A strong mentoring program not only produces better employees but also can teach the skills needed to balance work and personal life.

Once employees feel supported and successful in the workplace, they are better able to reduce or eliminate time-wasting activities and behaviors, such as gossiping. Certain attitudes and emotional states can act as hidden consumers of time. These include defensiveness, selflessness, and boredom. Defensiveness is a common problem. Reacting to criticism by uttering sharp remarks or lashing out in defense of one's actions creates an atmosphere of irritability and anger and can affect everyone in the environment for some time to come. Time spent in angry rumination is wasteful at best.

Selflessness, not selfishness, can be a time waster as well. Saying yes to every request is not realistic. Learning to say no on occasion lets the individual take back some of the time he or she has been losing. The hardest part, of course, is getting beyond the guilt.

Boredom is another time waster that is not often recognized. Boring tasks often cause individuals to waste time procrastinating. If a task is extremely boring to an individual, it most likely could or should have been delegated.

The following strategies should be used by leaders to help themselves and employees balance their work and their personal life and avoid activities, behaviors, and emotions that consume time to no good purpose:

- Recognize that everyone has the capacity to balance his or her use of time better.
- Focus on balancing time use as an opportunity for increasing meaningfulness and not as an opportunity for increasing control and regimentation.
- Share the reality that time is short, desires are many, and every person engages in a never-ending struggle to close the gap.
- Be persistent in examining personal activities for balance and avoid the tendency to shift back to being task focused.
- Be persistent in coaching others in how to balance work and personal life.
- Believe that colleagues know that a good balance between work and personal life results in higher productivity and greater job satisfaction.

Increasing the Focus on Patients

It is no secret that the locus of control for healthcare services should be the patient, not the provider. Yet in spite of all the efforts to create patient-focused care delivery systems, few patients would agree that they are in fact the focus of services or in control of anything. In explanation, they could cite facts such as these:

- Providers continue to prescribe treatments without discussion with the patients.
- Visiting hours are still in effect.
- Appointment times for services are based on Monday through Friday schedules.
- Patient procedures and their scheduled times are determined by providers without input from patients or families.

Leaders have plenty left to do to transform the healthcare system into one that is truly based on the will of the patient. A good place to begin is the Internet, which should be pushed as a proactive means of assisting consumers in interpreting healthcare information. Other strategies leaders should use to increase the patient focus of health care include these:

- Find the courage to continue the journey to creating a better system. Avoid the tendency to believe that the system is as consumer focused as it can be.
- Recognize that personal experiences as a patient can be invaluable for learning the truth about healthcare service delivery.

- Remain committed and focused when complaints override positive feedback. Resist the temptation to retire from health care.
- Never stop asking patients to share their experience of the healthcare system. Learn from them and share the information gained with other health professionals to improve the system.
- Believe that every health professional possesses courage, passion, energy, and self-discipline but may need reassurance and encouragement to exhibit them fully.

Becoming Politically Competent

Political competence encompasses the ability to accurately assess the impact of public policies on one's domain of responsibility and the ability to influence public policymaking at both the state and the federal levels (Longest, 1998). Politically competent leaders are aware of relevant regulations, laws, proposed acts, and certification procedures and are able to remove or mitigate outside barriers to the delivery of services. They also work within the organization to define issues affecting the delivery of patient care services and identify internal policies or procedures that should be altered.

However, these are only the first steps. The leaders need to ensure that all members of the organization have a degree of political competence, can address concerns in a timely manner, and can suggest possible solutions. The point-of-service staff members experience the real concerns and successes that occur at the delivery of services, know when things do not go well, and can offer recommendations for change. Their input is needed not only in the executive suite but, in many cases, in the legislative arena as well. Strategies for increasing the political competence of the organization as a whole include the following:

- Develop the ability of all employees to share information about system effectiveness. Be aware that the empowerment of employees, if not guided, can result in chaos.
- Recognize that empowerment can light a fire throughout the organization. When a person's personal contributions are valued, the fire in that person's heart is fueled.
- Patiently guide employees to communicate and share information. Never give up trying to ensure that the information necessary for identifying and implementing improvements is available to the members of the organization.
- Pay close attention to the desired outcomes of care as well as to the processes used to achieve them. On the other hand, never circumvent necessary processes for the sake of efficiency.

Relighting the Lamp

Nursing and health care have always been hard work. But in today's healthcare environment, they are harder than ever. There are cutbacks in funding, difficult government regulations, and the worst nursing shortage in history. All these add up to challenges to work more effectively than ever and to achieve job satisfaction in an atmosphere of tremendous pressure and shrinking support. Cost-saving measures may be crucial to an organization's survival, but to caregivers, they mean stress, frustration, and attrition.

With job stress high and morale at an all-time low, interdepartmental tensions have grown to epidemic proportions. With fewer nurses on staff and with the budgetary scalpel cutting deep, nurses are expected to do more with less—work more shifts, attend to more and sicker patients, and perform a broader range of duties. And they are expected to do all this with greater sensitivity, patience, and empathy. It is ironic that the emphasis on patient satisfaction in health care comes at a time when the pressures are making high-quality care next to impossible—when safe care has become the motto of many nurses. (Buckley & Walker, 1989)

Although the preceding quotation was written more than 20 years ago, it is still applicable today, partly because of the cyclical nature of health care and the recurring need to create healthcare services that are congruent with the demands and resources of the marketplace. We have much to learn about the healthcare system's cycle, but the basic needs are always the same—to meet current challenges, to learn from the past, and to continue to create new and better methods to integrate technology, information, and the wisdom of providers and leaders.

Some days the work of leadership seems like more than a person can handle, yet dedicated leaders continue on through seemingly insurmountable challenges. Most likely, the work of leadership has become an internal calling. The calling to leadership or the urge to give away one's gifts and make distinct contributions to the world not only uncovers the joy that everyone seeks but also affirms one's life work and contributions to a better world. It is the calling to leadership that energizes, affirms, and sustains leaders in times of great challenge.

According to Leider (2004), engaged leaders not only know who they are and what they stand for but also are able to assist others to heed their own life callings. They are able to guide others to uncover their embedded destiny and to see beyond today to what they can become tomorrow. This is the ultimate coaching and mentoring process! Thus, the engaged leader with emotional competence can both identify personal destiny and assist others in the journey of discovery and commitment to their calling as a part of the larger design of the world. Not surprising, engaged leaders recognize their calling not as a destiny or goal, but as a wellness issue; leading is doing what needs to be done, and not doing the work of leadership would be frustrating and stress producing. The calling of leadership guides the leader in integrating the internal personal self with the outer world—a struggle that is continuously present in many leaders. Knowing from the internal self what needs to be done and living those beliefs and values in the real world marks the leader's journey. The leader must role-model the integration of the personal, authentic self with the real, external world. The journey starts with the self and moves toward others and the needs of the world. The fully engaged leader emulates a high level of consciousness or spiritual connection with those in the world. The leader is fully present in each situation, listens carefully with an open mind, and, on the basis of core values, interacts assertively and honestly.

The words of Florence Nightingale offer hope and gentle reminders for all healthcare workers. Her perceptions are consistent with the public and political consciousness of today, namely, that public health and human caring are supremely important. Further, as in her time, many are now calling for reform of basic social and healthcare practices. In our era, for example, there are many critics of our society's response to the needs of the homeless, the medically indigent, those who are HIV positive, those who are living with AIDS or another incurable or chronic illness, and those who are relatively powerless or neglected, including pregnant women, children, and older adults.

Consider these themes from Nightingale's writings:

- Basic caring and healing practices must be restored.
- The moral, the spiritual, and the metaphysical must be reintegrated.
- The knowledge and values of women—the sacred feminine healing spirit—must be allowed to play an essential role in health care.
- Healing professionals must recapture their sense of "calling."
- The public's requirement of personal and professional caring competencies and commitments must be honored.
- The wisdom of connected oneness and wholeness—the interrelationship among person, nature, environment, and health—must also be honored.

Aren't these same themes relevant today? Is there any doubt that the transformative journey we are on dates back at least to the nineteenth century? As Watson (1999) noted, our work should be about relighting the lamp and helping our colleagues to reintegrate and reconnect to restore the professional wholeness that was wounded during the recent modern era.

Group Discussion

> In our rush to reform education, we have forgotten a simple truth: Reform will never be achieved by renewing appropriations, restructuring schools, rewriting curricula, and revising texts if we continue to demean and dishearten the human resource called the teacher on whom so much depends. Teachers must be better compensated, freed from bureaucratic harassment, given a role in academic governance, and provided with the best possible methods and materials. But none of that will transform education if we fail to cherish—and challenge—the human heart that is the source of good teaching. (Palmer, 1998)

The preceding comments by Parker Palmer, noted educator, are about the current state of the education system. With these words in mind, answer the following questions: In what way is the state of health care similar to the state of education? Is it possible that health care already has enough financial resources and that the solution to the problems in the healthcare system is to rearrange funding, reduce bureaucracy, and increase involvement? Are there other important strategies that need to be part of the solution? How do the concepts of will and willingness apply to the current situation in health care?

Conclusion

The Age of Complexity encompasses exponential increases in information, technology, and interaction between diverse people and cultures, confirming that our world is truly global. In addition, despite the fear that many people feel today, the complexity of this new age can be a source of hope. The speed of change, the blurring of work and home life, and the new global relationships enrich each one of us directly or indirectly.

In this next era, leadership thinking will be more humanistic and more sensitive to the complex interrelationships in the world. Hope in the future and willingness to transform bureaucracies into self-renewing organizations are other aspects of the journey of leaders into and beyond the millennium. To accomplish their goals, leaders require courage to do the right thing, passion for the work of healing, energy to stay the course, self-discipline to remain focused, and trust that others are partners in the process. Finally, they must be steeped in the belief that the future will indeed be better because they have designed it.

Case Study 13-1

Managing Pressure to Decide

Al has noticed that two of his directors are exact polar opposites of each other in their leadership style, skills, and competencies. He often thought to himself that they are classic textbook pictures of leadership skills on a continuum. Pete is a strong thinker and is full of innovative ideas to improve his department and the hospital as a whole. He doesn't perceive traditional lines of authority or regulations as a barrier to his innovative ideas, but views them as a potential challenge, as a chess master would regarding his opponent. Pete was full of ideas and energy and was constantly changing, fixing, and moving things forward in his departments. Al had personally witnessed Pete discussing his ideas with the president of the organization with such confidence and courage that even Al did not possess. It seemed that Pete was fearless and disregarded the commonly understood rules of organizational hierarchy. He spoke to the president as if they were best friends or individuals who worked together frequently. Al secretly coveted Pete's ability to be "out there" or "in your face" on issues that Pete was passionate about.

In contrast Caroline was a very quiet but effective leader. She had been in her role for more than 25 years and had 35 years of seniority in the organization. She was highly regarded as an expert in her clinical area and as a soft, compassionate leader with her staff. Caroline was nearing retirement and probably would have retired a few years ago had it not been for the sudden death of her husband. Caroline had shared with Al that she was not retiring now because of her fears and concerns about her financial stability in the present economy. Al noticed that Caroline rarely brought forth any new or innovative ideas, but rather her departments seemed to hum along without much controversy, crisis, or change. Although Caroline was open to new ideas, she certainly put forth no effort to promote innovation or change in her departments. She seemed quite content with the status quo.

When reflecting on these two individuals and their strengths and areas needing development, Al would have characterized Pete as a strong-willed and an engaged individual who was like a "dog with a bone" when he felt strongly about a proposal or situation. In contrast, Caroline simply and quietly got the job done and changed things when necessary. Caroline could be characterized as a person with a soft, good will who exuded caring and compassion for others but had little energy or will to change the status quo. Al's boss, the chief operating officer (COO), once mentioned to Al that they needed to develop a strategy to deal with the "walking retired," and Al silently wondered if he was referring to Caroline along with some of the others whom they both knew were no longer effective in the roles. Al felt protective of Caroline because of her long years of service and because her performance was essentially good. She met all of the performance goals required of her, her staff seem to be satisfied with her as a leader, and the patient and satisfaction scores were also within expected limits. It was just her quiet and unengaging demeanor that caused others to perceive her as low energy and ineffective. In some ways Al thought she was a good balance to Pete's constant whirlwind of energy, excitement, and passion and eagerness to put forth his agenda and to please others. Caroline on the other hand had shared with Al that she no longer felt the need to impress others and that she had no desire to move up in the organization to promote herself for other positions. She stated that "my performance speaks for itself, so why do I need to behave differently just to impress others."

Al was under constant pressure from the COO to do "something" with Caroline—reassignment to a less visible position or encouragement to retire. Al was a bit concerned about his boss's perception of his own skill incompetency in his role if he didn't do something with Caroline. He was saddened that she was perceived as "burned out" when she met all of the performance requirements and was positively perceived by her staff and physicians. He realized that the organization valued high-energy, quick-thinking, innovative individuals who not only got the job done but also were constantly moving the organization forward into new service lines, care delivery methods, and strategies to improve the workplace environment for staff and physicians. What a quandary! Al was absolutely conflicted about what he should do with Caroline. He knew with certainty that there would be chaos among the clinical nurses and physicians if he should encourage her to move to a new position or to retire. He knew that Caroline did not want to retire, and therefore he could expect a backlash from his actions to encourage her to do so. In his mind he questioned the COO's intentions and the congruency with the organization's values. Looking at it differently, however, Al realized the potential benefits of having an individual in the role who was more energetic and innovative. Such a person might propose new programs and services that would accelerate the department's success and make changes to improve patient care, physician satisfaction, and employee engagement (although these metrics were already within expected ranges). It was more of a "decision of potentiality" than "necessity," which made Al all the more unsettled about pressure to make a change in Caroline's role.

Questions

1. What is your perception of Al's personal conflict in this case?
2. How would you describe Al's level of courage in facing the COO's pressure for Al to make a change in Caroline's role when Al clearly feels conflicted about the fairness and appropriateness of the change given that she meets expectations in assigned organizational goals?
3. What do you think Al's best strategy should be in meeting the COO's agenda, being fair to Caroline, and making the best decision for the overall good of his departments and hospital?
4. If you were Al, how would you perceive the political correctness of Pete's informal interactions with the president of the organization given the circumstances described in this case?
5. What qualities does Al demonstrate that may characterize him as being a willing leader, and which attributes might he continually develop to improve his own authenticity as a leader?
6. If Al determines that Caroline should stay in her role, what methods might he consider to "relight her lamp" as described earlier in this chapter?

Case Study 13-2

Courageous, Tenacious, and Resilient

Susan has been in her role as executive director of Women's Services for nearly 7 years. During this time, she is witnessed tremendous growth in the annual volume of deliveries, women surgeries, and neonatal intensive care admissions. The phenomenal success of the department has led to her managing issues related to the tremendous growth in volume and a lack of an adequate number of beds to place newly delivered mothers, neonatal admits to the ICU, and even surgical admits for preoperative and postoperative services. It's clear that Community Memorial Hospital needs to expand its building for maternal-newborn services and women's surgery services or build a new building on an adjacent site. Susan has been to a number of national conferences and talked with other leaders of freestanding women's hospitals who have shared stories of how the new hospital has positioned them well as market leaders and provided opportunities to expand services for patients. When sharing her observations with her physician colleagues, they agree that a proposal for a freestanding women's and newborn's hospital should be developed for the executive team to consider. Susan meets with the Market Research department to acquire data about the patient catchment areas and projections for potential growth in the women's service line. She also meets with the director of finance to review the current financial data and requests assistance in developing the projected pro forma with growth assumptions built into the financial scenarios.

The executive team at Community Memorial Hospital is well aware of the burgeoning growth of the women's service line. The planning committee reviewed options for expanding the existing building on campus but quickly determined that an expansion would not be a viable option because the current building had many deficiencies that would also need replacement or repair. The building no longer meets current patients' requests for private rooms and space for mother–baby couplet care, and the normal newborn nursery and neonatal intensive care unit are completely undersized for the obstetrical volume. Although most of the gynecological surgeries are performed in the department, the patients have to be moved to a different building for postoperative care because all available beds are used for maternity patients. Not building new space soon would result in loss of market share.

Susan and the medical directors for Perinatal Services and Neonatal Services worked with the financial department to develop a feasibility analysis proposing a new free-standing women's hospital with a new birthing center, private postpartum rooms, private rooms for high-risk maternity patients, a large neonatal intensive care unit, a 10-room surgical center, and a women's postoperative unit. Once the feasibility analysis was prepared, Susan and the medical directors presented the concept proposal to the executive team at Community Memorial Hospital. They asked for resources and financial support to hire a hospital planning company to do a preliminary space program outlining the departmental needs and overall space requirements so that the project costs could be correctly estimated and entered into the pro forma equations to determine the return on investment and internal rate of return.

Susan could never have anticipated the initial pushback that she received from some of the members on the executive team who previously acknowledged that the women's and newborn service line had outgrown the current facility. Discussion ensued about the need to build a new facility for the cardiovascular service line, which was also growing exponentially and had a greater revenue base than that of the women's and newborn service line. The proposal was sent forward to the board of directors, who were also split in their support for either the new women's hospital or the cardiovascular pavilion. When Susan attended the meetings, she was often the brunt of jokes by some board members who scoffed at the need for women's hospital. Some of them asked, "Why don't we just build a men's hospital as well?" Susan had carefully scripted responses to such questions and reiterated the importance of appealing to women because the evidence supported that women were often the healthcare decision makers for families. Susan explained that market research information validated that the women in the family often guided decisions related to choosing healthcare plans during open enrollment periods and in choosing physicians. By providing a women's hospital, Community Memorial Hospital could position itself well as a market leader in women's health for both inpatient and outpatient services.

The executive director of the cardiovascular service line also had a compelling rationale for building a new cardiovascular pavilion instead of a women's hospital. Many advances in technology, interventional radiology, and the medical and surgical care of cardiovascular patients supported the need for more space for these patients. Because there was only enough resources for one new facility or expansion, the executive team and the board of directors had to decide which of the two options would provide the greatest value and position the hospital for future growth, financial stability, and recognition for excellence.

Susan was passionate about the vision for a new women's hospital, and she spent many hours discussing the vision with potential donors, community organizational leaders, hospital executives, and the board of directors. She believed so strongly in the vision that she was willing to meet with anyone who could assist in moving the vision to reality. Susan also realized that the executive director for cardiovascular services was equally passionate about his vision for a new cardiovascular service line and was also aligning supporters for his vision as well. Both were articulate in expressing how patient outcomes could be positively influenced with the new buildings and that the hospital would be viewed positively in the community with the new facility. Susan presented the story of her vision over and over and was courageous in "the line of fire" when people challenged the need for a new women's hospital. In the end her persistence was fruitful, and she successfully persuaded the executive team and board of directors to allocate resources for the planning of a new women's hospital. Although Susan was triumphant with this news, she was also sensitive to her colleague's dismay that his vision for a cardiovascular pavilion would be put on hold for a few years.

Questions

1. How did Susan show courage when proposing the new women's hospital?
2. In what ways did Susan demonstrate her tenacity and resilience in proposing the women's hospital?
3. How would you strategize to propose your vision of a new building in the face of a competing proposal that also has great value to the success of the organization?
4. Healthcare executives rarely have the resources to fund all the needs for capital equipment, operational expenses, and facility improvement, so resources must be carefully allocated based on the merits of the proposal in adding value to patients and to the organization. With this in mind, how would you weigh the merits of the two proposals in this case study for a new women's hospital or the cardiovascular pavilion?

References

Ackman, M., Perry, L. A., Wolfard, E., Steckel, C., & Hill, C. (2012). Changing nursing practice: Letting go of the nursing history on admission. *Journal of Nursing Administration, 42*(9), 435–441.

Buckley, C. D., & Walker, D. (1989). *Harmony: Professional renewal for nurses.* Chicago, IL: American Hospital Publishing.

Contu, D. L. (2002, March). The anxiety of learning: An interview with Edgar Schein. *Harvard Business Review,* 100–106.

Guiffra, M. J. (2013). Letter to the editor: Altruism is the heart of our story. *Nursing Outlook, 61,* 67–69.

Johnson, C. B. (2000). When working harder is not smarter. *Inner Edge, 3*(2), 18–21.

Leider, R. (2004). Is leading your calling? *Leader to Leader.* 31(36-40).

Longest, B. (1998). Managerial competence at senior levels of integrated delivery systems. *Journal of Healthcare Management, 43,* 115–135.

Malloch, K., & Porter-O'Grady, T. (1999). Partnership economics: Nursing's challenge in the quantum age. *Nursing Economics, 17,* 299–307.

Palmer, P. J. (1998). *The courage to teach: Exploring the inner landscape of a teacher's life*. San Francisco, CA: Jossey-Bass.

Pappas, S. H. (2013). Value, a nursing outcome. *Nursing Administration Quarterly, 37*(2), 122–128.

Watson, J. (1999). *Postmodern nursing and beyond*. New York, NY: Churchill Livingstone.

Suggested Readings

Berenson, R. A., & Docteur, E. (2013). Doing better by doing less: Approaches to tackle overuse of services. RWJ/ The Urban Institute. Retrieved from http://www.rwjf.org/en/research-publications/find-rwjf-research/2013/01/doing-better-by-doing-less—approaches-to-tackle-overuse-of-serv.html

Buerhaus, P. (1998). Milton Weinstein's insights on the development, use, and methodologic problems in cost-effectiveness analysis. *Image: Journal of Nursing Scholarship, 30*, 223–227.

Drucker, P. F. (2006). What executives should remember. *Harvard Business Review, 84*(2), 145–152.

Gifford, W. A., & Davis, B. (2008, Fourth Quarter). Doing the right things to do things right: A commentary on leadership and the use of evidence in practice. *Worldviews on Evidence-Based Nursing*, 170–171.

Gordon, S. (2005). *Nursing against the odds: How health care cost-cutting, media stereotypes and medical hubris undermine nurses and patient care*. Ithaca, NY: Cornell University Press.

Hamel, G. (2009). Moon shots for management. *Harvard Business Review, 87*(2), 91–98.

Huber, C. (1998). *The key: And the name of the key is willingness*. Murphys, CA: Keep It Simple Books.

O'Malley, M. N. (2000). *Creating commitment: How to attract and retain talented employees by building relationships that last*. New York, NY: Wiley.

Rauen, C. A, Vollman, K., Arbour, R. B., & Chulay, M. (2008). Challenging nursing's sacred cows. *American Nurse Today, 3*(4), 23–25.

Williams, L. L. (2006). The fair factor in matters of trust. *NAQ, 30*(1), 30–37.

Zimmerman, B., Lindberg, C., & Plsek, P. (1998). *Edgeware: Insights from complexity science for health care leaders*. Irving, TX: VHA.

Quiz Questions

Select the best answer for each of the following questions.

1. Which of the following is not among the reasons that healthcare workers report disenfranchisement?
   a. Staff shortages
   b. Excessive regulations
   c. Loss of patient respect
   d. Job stress

2. Which of the following characterizes the fully developed will?
   a. The fully developed will creates an enormous potential for change.
   b. The fully developed will requires significant coaching and mentoring.
   c. The fully developed will is inherent in all leaders.
   d. The fully developed will avoids expressing authentic feelings.

3. From the perspective of a leader, the will emerges through several phases of discovery. In the most important of these phases, what does the leader do?

   a. Evaluates colleagues' perceptions of the leader's degree of willingness
   b. Informs his or her supervisor of the intention to explore the concept of will
   c. Makes an attempt to identify areas in which personal growth is needed
   d. Recognizes the will as a unique and describable phenomenon

4. Among the obstacles to a leader's exploration of his or her will, which of the following is the most common?

   a. Peer pressure to avoid additional work
   b. Organizational pressure to conform to established practices and norms
   c. Lack of time
   d. Lack of knowledge about exploration of the will on the part of the leader's supervisor

5. Passion as an essential quality of will is expressed in which of the following ways?

   a. Employees share their values and ideas in a nonthreatening manner.
   b. People in the organization take pride in their work.
   c. In decision making, the leader's opinion dominates the opinions of others.
   d. Power is distributed equally among all loaders.

6. Dogmas obstruct the transformation of the healthcare system for which of the following reasons?

   a. Policies require too much time to review.
   b. Employees are allowed to retain jobs that no longer are needed.
   c. The boundaries between professions continue to remain unclear.
   d. The use of resources is not always related to patient outcomes.

7. Regaining balance between work and personal life requires courage to do which of the following?

   a. Create new compensation systems to recognize the differing values of employees.
   b. Pursue change with zeal until satisfactory human resources policies are created.
   c. Accept that employees are interested in the recommendations of the leader.
   d. Remain focused on creating change.

8. Value-based services differ in several ways from the kind of services most commonly delivered. Which of the following would not be affected by the transformation to value-based services?

   a. Quality of the services
   b. Research base of the services
   c. License of the provider
   d. Available reimbursement for the services provided

9. Leaders who are mentally fit are better able to manage the complexity of the healthcare system. Which of the following is not a benefit that mental fitness bestows on leaders?

   a. Ability to handle the disappointment of not being selected for a position
   b. Ability to take responsibility for one's actions and one's reactions to adversity
   c. Increased sensitivity to the situation of employees who have been laid off
   d. Ability to avoid confrontations and the discussion of pertinent issues

CHAPTER FOURTEEN

Sustaining the Spirit of Leadership: Becoming a Living Leader

I am being driven forward into an unknown land. The pass grows steeper, the air colder and sharper. A wind from my unknown goal stirs the strings of expectation. Still the question: shall I ever get there? There where life resounds, a clear pure note in the silence.

—*Dag Hammarskjöld, "Markings"*
With kind permission from Springer Science & Business Media, Analecta Husserliana XCIV edited by Anna-Teresa Tymieniecka, 125-136. (c) 2007 Springer.

Chapter Objectives

At the completion of this chapter, the reader will be able to

- Describe the personal needs that relate to self-care and development as a leader and as a person.
- Construct a personal plan for self-direction and self-development that addresses professional, personal, and spiritual needs.
- Distinguish between the various competing aspects of life as a leader and understand the creative skills necessary to manage the leadership role and make a difference.
- Understand how to set time aside in a format that permits deepening of the spiritual journey.
- Enumerate 10 spiritual rules for personal growth that incorporate the principles of chaos and complexity.

In the midst of what seems to be an endless sea of change, it becomes obvious that leadership requires great energy. The intensity of focus and attention of the leader's role draws a great deal from the spirit and energy of the leader. Without a sense of spiritual centering and integrity, leaders do not have adequate support because much of the needed support must come from within. Leaders must have self-discipline, resolve, insight, and a sense of direction to prepare for the tough experience of empowering others to manage their own lives. Leaders

Point to Ponder

The spiritual and consciousness-centered leader focuses each eye separately: one eye focuses on the close-up realities and vagaries that must be addressed now, and the other focuses on the farthest horizon of the future.

must also focus on their resources and enter into a process of self-reflection, centering, and nourishing the spirit. This chapter describes the elements and processes associated with leadership self-care and support, including spiritual and personal routines.

Leadership is more than a set of learned skills. Effective leaders possess a deep comfort with themselves and an engagement with life that is generative and harmonizing. They exhibit an excitement and a way of embracing life that are encouraging and hopeful to those they lead. They have a depth of commitment and a reservoir of spirit and energy that are inspiring, along with a sense of being fully in touch with who they are and what moves them. At the same time, effective leaders appear never fully content, as though on a journey or in search of something still just out of their reach that drives them on.

Leaders who are more than just effective—who qualify as great leaders—have an understanding or acceptance that some deep force runs through all existence, giving it form and life and direction, yet at its center the universe remains mysterious. This force comes in many forms and goes by an unlimited number of names, but it operates regardless of what it is called. Great leaders sense, indeed, feel, this force and at some point are driven by an awareness of its movement within. In the lives of most great leaders, a question arises about what they would do in response to the call deep within, and they respond by moving in concert with this inner force and by making out of it whatever they can. In short, they commit to the great "yes" of their lives and as a result are driven to do great and meaningful things.

This "call" is not just reserved for the great of the world; it is actually part of the greatness that is in each of us. Regardless of the place we occupy in society, moments of opportunity, risk, and commitment surround us. We all experience the sense that a call is being made to our own greatness. We all possess gifts and strengths that determine our uniqueness and that, when fully expressed, can have a valuable impact on our lives and, at least by reflection, on the lives of others. We each simply need to be aware of the stirrings of the force within and to act in concert with it. Our awareness of the force does not simply happen, however; it comes out of the insight born of a spiritual discipline (**Figure 14-1**). Spiritually grounded leaders undergo a cycle of interactions that demonstrates their ongoing commitment to personal growth and development.

Chaos and the Call to Leadership

In these times, it is difficult to find enough moments of peace to think reflectively about anything. Days seem filled with activity, change, and movement, responses to ever-increasing demands for the new and different. As we more fully move into the Information Age, we can sense the significance of the changes in understanding, work, relationships, and life itself. All the science fiction we have read appears to be coming to life before our very eyes.

The pace of change has in fact picked up during the past 20 years as we close in on leaving the old age behind forever. Our movement into this new digital age tempts us with the loss of all the beliefs and practices that characterized the Industrial Age, especially the linearity and vertical orientation of our thinking, which had a defining influence on all our social institutions and practices, from science to government and religion.

The unidirectional and linear notions associated with the Newtonian view of the universe have now been significantly eclipsed. The quantum theorists, for example, proved

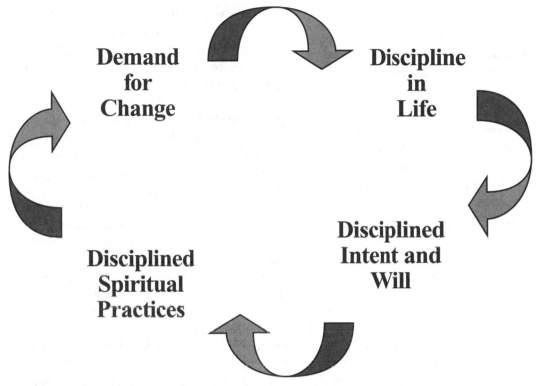

Figure 14-1 The Cycle of Spiritual Discipline.

that life cannot be understood in terms of unilateral and vertical action. The chaos of the universe has a rhythm and flow that move multidirectionally, and through the cloud of chaos a discrete and elegant simplicity can be seen that defies the chaos that created it.

These realities confound and confuse us. They disrupt our sensibilities and our rituals and routines. They create incongruities in our beliefs and understanding. The uncertainty they cause makes us disquieted and anxious. The confidence we garnered from settling on a set of practices and beliefs that brought order to our lives has been undermined. Yet we are not sure with what to replace those practices and beliefs. We hunger for some certitude and some sense of the absolute that can guide our thinking and acting, but finding these tools of life is turning out to be extremely difficult.

Group Discussion

Recall a serious tragedy or overwhelmingly painful experience you thought you would never recover from. Then, discuss with the other participants what it was that moved you on, got you past the pain, and enabled you to reengage with life and make a difference once again.

> ### Key Point
>
> Chaos and the loss of certainty provide an opportunity to let go of those things that are inherently changing and passing. Chaos is a fundamental element of the spiritual discipline, severing us from our false certainty about what can never be certain, refocusing us on the journey, and allowing us to hear the journey's call to adapt and grow.

There is a tremendous backlash associated with the loss of certainty. Groups on the political extreme express a high level of anger and anxiety and call for a return to fundamental beliefs and historical practices as a solution to the loss of certainty. However, this approach does not engage with the facts recently revealed by science and research—facts that will not disappear because they are disconcerting and incongruous with what we believe should be true.

Change is always a challenge to human beings. It presents us with the task of confronting ourselves and everything that defines our lives. It reminds us that life is forever in movement and is more journey than event. Truth is also more journey than event. We want truth to be immutable to avoid the discomfort, uncertainty, and ambiguity associated with change and to keep from questioning the premises of our actions. Absolutism removes control over our lives from our hands and puts it someplace outside of us. It frees us from the obligation to own what we know and how we must change, and it limits the experience of "noise" that accompanies all aspects of life. The surrender of control to an external absolute eliminates the pain, challenge, risk, and suffering that arise out of the struggle to cope with the vagaries of existence.

It is into this fray that the leader enters, attempting to engage with the vagaries of life and to incorporate the uncertainties of the experience into the work of adaptation and growth. The leader finds comfort not in the safe haven of an unchanging external reality, but in staying the course and deepening his or her personal journey. The spiritually aware leader recognizes that being available to the challenges and opportunities embedded in the endless process of change is critical to personal growth. By connecting to the experience of change and demonstrating growth within his or her life, the leader encourages others to continue on their own journey of discernment and development.

Chaos is pervasive throughout the universe. Yet, to understand the chaos, it is important to visualize the simplicity that lies at its center. Touching that center brings confidence and order to an individual's life and encourages experimentation and engagement. It is hard work, however, to move through the clouds and shrouds of the chaotic experience to land at the center—the place where the elements of chaos converge and create the mosaic that represents—at the same time—mystery and order. Endeavors to get to that place make up much of the work of personal leadership.

Certain principles can illuminate the conditions of participation in change and help to explain the proper role of leadership in a world defined by chaos and complexity:

- The universe is a work in progress, still unfolding, yet in creation, moving everything in it forward in a web of energy and understanding.
- Chaos and complexity are the essential characteristics of the universe. The universe cannot be understood independent of its own complex reality.

- Everything in the universe is self-organizing. The patterns, webs, and intersections of life create a mosaic of intense goodness of fit that reveals the ultimate connection among all the elements of the universe.
- People, too, are part of the universal network of relationships and are co-creators in the ever constant unfolding and self-organizing activity.
- Organizations (systems), as smaller reflections of the universe, are self-organizing, complex, and adaptive entities in which people purposefully express their creativity, energy, and meaning together.

Quantum science revealed many of these principles in its attempt to understand the physics of the universe. From the moment of the "Big Bang" (itself a complex uncertainty) to the present, all aspects of the universe, including those that involve life, operate within the context of the principles of chaos and complexity.

The leader's role is to apply these principles to the organization. This includes showing a willingness to act in concert with quantum design—that is, to engage with chaos and harness its implications. The traditional institutional and vertical views of work and relationship are inadequate for understanding how to lead and implement changes. Instead, a "whole systems" view must underpin the work of the leader and inform the actions and priorities of the organization's members.

Leaders of organizational units, such as services, departments, and divisions, must recognize that, rather than merely leading their units, they lead the whole organization from the perspective of their units. Most leaders see their primary responsibility as making their units operate as effectively as possible. Although this is a laudable goal, no unit can thrive if the other units do not. Thriving requires an intersection of actions, each advancing the others and together ensuring the health of the whole. All the leaders of units are working to harmonize the efforts of everyone in the organization in an array of connections that together advance the organization's mission. Chaos and complexity are simply the normal context for all work and relationships, and therefore leaders must use their understanding of chaos and complexity in every element of their work.

Self-Management and Creativity

There are those who suggest that the universe is a cold, mechanical process and that life is harsh, hierarchical, accidental, and beyond the ability of human beings to affect. This view of the universe as mechanistic and indifferent or even hostile is inaccurate (Wheatley, 2009). Work by quantum scientists reveals that the universe is an exploring, experimenting, adapting process that is continuously and endlessly in the act of creation. Potential, change, adjustment, and becoming represent the character of existence, indicating that life is more challenging and dangerous than previously imagined. Because all things are essentially related, no action is without a wide-ranging influence. In particular, each person's behavior has an effect on the processes of life everywhere. The well-known fact that small events can have large effects far away—encapsulated in the notion that the gentle flapping of a butterfly's wings in China can influence the unfolding of a hurricane in the Atlantic—is a reminder of the interconnectedness of everything.

Group Discussion

Reflect on three words that describe your fundamental beliefs about life. Then, present your words to the group, spending no more than 2 minutes to explain what they mean. Write all the words from all participants randomly on a flip chart. At the end of the session, look at the composite of words, and on a second flip chart write the one word that best describes what each participant sees or feels about all the words on the first flip chart. When all the participants have finished, that page represents the prevailing spiritual culture of the group.

Point to Ponder

Rather than being harsh and unforgiving, life is full of opportunity. All it asks is that you desire it enough, work at it the right way, patiently build your personal resources, and then grab it when it calls. Whether good things happen to you depends more on you than on the good things.

For leaders, the implications of these newer notions are profound. Leaders, by the smallest of their actions, can have a significant impact on others at every level in the organization. By their behavior, which is under constant scrutiny, they create the organization's culture and build the framework for responding to the challenges and uncertainties of a world forever in flux. They exemplify the normalcy of change by embracing and engaging with it and responding with acceptance and adaptation.

It is important for leaders to fully live up to the expectations of their role. If a leader is not personally disposed to live in the potential, he or she cannot ask others to live there either. Leaders must demonstrate in their leadership practices a personal pattern of response to life's calls. For example, the universe delights in exploration and transformation, and leaders must exhibit in their behavior the enthusiasm of experimentation, challenge, and engagement (**Figure 14-2**). Indeed, they must be the living representatives of this dynamic. In this section, we discuss some issues that leaders need to consider to live and lead in accordance with the realities of life.

Life is joyful. If the leader of an organization is not excited, neither are the other members. The leader creates the context for work and relationships. If the mental model of the leader implies that life is hard and treacherous, it will be hard and treacherous in that organization. The leader must believe that life is exciting and full of adventure so that everyone feels they are being invited on a journey of discovery and transformation. Otherwise, the environment is rife with the fallout of what the leader does believe about work and relationships.

Time must be allowed for reflection. Leaders need to spend time thinking about their role and the context of their role. No leader can be in touch with what is influencing his or her work if there is no room in the day for personal reflection. Call this activity what you will—meditation, deliberation, or some other term—it leads to renewal, insight, engagement, and reenergizing response. Both the external and internal elements of life's

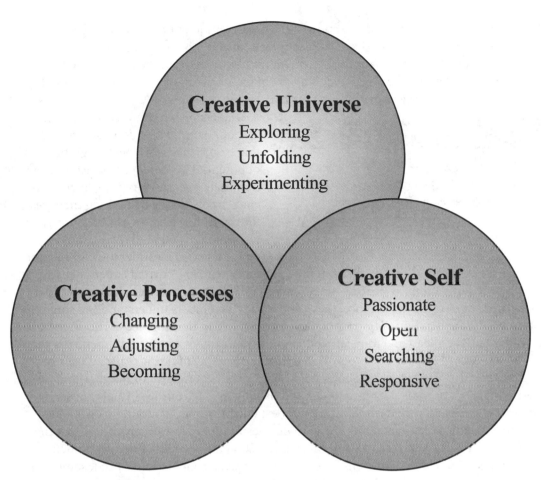

Figure 14-2 The Creative Spirit.

changes are considered in a way that has meaning for the leader. The focus is on the person of the leader and that individual's own life issues, priorities, challenges, and growth.

Leaders are co creators. Leaders know that things do not simply happen by accident or without meaning. They are always seeking to discern the relationship between specific actions and their significance. Sorting through the vagaries of change to find its prime movers and intersections is a part of the work of transformation. People do not make change. Change is. People give change the form it takes and link it to all the elements that either constrain it or facilitate it. By "seeing" the inner life of change and identifying what it is trying to reveal, leaders attach to it the factors that give it form and meaning for those it affects. Knowing this, leaders act as co-creators, operating in concert with the change, digging for its meaning and impact, and working with others to determine the most appropriate response.

Chaos is always the route to order. Leaders know that chaos is a constant. They also know that order is generated out of chaos. Looking at the simplicity that lies at the center of complexity, leaders search for the connections that the chaos is breaking up or reformatting on a way to the very next stage of the change journey. They tie the forces at work to the mission, purposes, and direction of the organization to fit the pieces together to converge around the change. Leaders recognize that chaos is a requisite of order and are thus better able to accept chaos as an element in their own lives. They also recognize that chaos is normal and to be welcomed as a part of life. Further, they embrace chaos before expecting others to engage with their own experience of chaos.

> ### Point to Ponder
>
> If leaders have no idea what drives them, how can they expect anyone else to know? Self-knowledge is the beginning point of self-direction.

Leadership is a contract with possibility and opportunity. Leaders understand that experience is simply the application of potential to present circumstances and that their role is to give substance to the changes occurring by making them real for those they lead. In other words, they translate the potential reality into language that has meaning for staff members in their present situation. In addition, they put staff members' current experience into a much broader context by treating it as a stage, a milepost, on a longer journey. By operating with this frame of reference, they can help staff members understand the context of their work and actions. Here again, leaders must live in the embrace of the potential, always seeing it ahead and translating its implications into language staff members can understand. As has been repeatedly noted, leading is a way of life, not just a skill set.

Life gets messy before order shows up. Living with mess is hard for many people. We desire logical, rational, and visual order and usually manage our lives to obtain such order. The problem is that while we are busy establishing and maintaining order, life is getting ready to put sand in its gears. In our desire for order, we sometimes treat the journey of life as a stationary condition that can somehow be fenced off by an unchanging set of self-created parameters. The journey, however, soon reasserts itself, sometimes dramatically, as when it brings down our neatly constructed world of supposed impervious order. This type of disruption reminds us of the impermanence of order and the essential character of the journey that is life, which is to move from where we currently are through a process of change, challenge, and, hopefully, growth. The movement does not occur in a straight line, however, and messiness is one of the reminders that we need to continuously adapt.

Leaders must preserve their identity. All living things seek to preserve their identity and sustain themselves. Leaders are no different. Yet leading is demanding work and can lead to burnout and damage to one's personal integrity. Living in the world means finding a place in the world. For leaders, it means recognizing that they occupy a space that is influencing all the surrounding spaces. How well they live in their own space, respond to the demand for movement, address personal issues, and confront the challenges to growth determine their ability to affect others through their personal leadership. Leaders cannot help others adapt to that which they cannot adapt. The paradox of identity is that persons must change to maintain their identity. Leaders must adapt to assist others in becoming reconciled to their own changes.

We all participate in each other's evolution. We all have an impact on others—there are no foreigners on life's journey. Everything everywhere ultimately connects to facilitate change at every level. The rules, processes, and conditions of growth are ever changing and cannot be counted on to act in the same way at different times and places in the change cycle. The leader knows this, understanding that synthesis rather than analysis, fluidity rather than solidity, principle rather than law, and focus rather than function are the real operating conditions of life. Discernment is a more valuable gift than definition. Direction is more important than location. These truths merely indicate how different the workings of change are from our linear expectations. We confront the patterns and movements of change in our responses to life, but change continues regardless of our responses. Our success in the journey of life depends mostly on the congruence of our responses and our recognition that we are fundamentally interdependent (Bakker, 2013).

Leadership work is important and influential, and thus requires care and concerted effort. The personal engagement of leaders in their own journey, for example, is a means of demonstrating that they have an obligation to confront the challenges presented by change and also a means of guiding them in their attempts to adapt to change (Bodaken & Fritz, 2006; Hickey & Kritek, 2012). On the other hand, leaders who have not attended to the personal issues of adaptation and have failed to sustain their insights, courage, and creativity probably will be unable to help others gain the self-understanding and discernment they need to meet their own challenges successfully.

Creativity and Innovation

We are born creative. No matter what else or who else we perceive the spiritual force in our lives to be, this spirit is the source of creativity. Artists, musicians, writers, creators of every type all make reference to some deep source of power from which flows the energy of creativity. Yet, although creativity is inextricably linked to the life force in each of us, many of us talk of creativity as something we can own or control and manipulate. We treat it as external to ourselves and profess to believe we could do so much more if we only could get hold of it. We fail to realize that we all have it—it is a part of who we are. We do need, however, self-awareness and discipline to access it and to give it form and direction.

There is a direct relationship between creativity and discipline. Creativity needs its own time. We need to allow it the space to take form and to have expression. Although accidents of creativity and innovation regularly occur, rarely are they accidentally refined and developed. If it is visible, it is because it was made visible, disciplined by the action that brought it forward and molded it into a format that could be experienced and then shared with the world, for all to marvel at and enjoy (**Figure 14-3**). For its expression, creativity demands a format and also a context. By setting a specified time and place for its expression, we provide the discipline necessary for the elements of creativity to converge and

> **Key Point**
>
> We are all creative. We are, however, naturally creative in different ways. Although creativity is deeply hardwired within each of us, it is malleable enough to be expressed in almost any way we choose. The only requirement is that we do decide to do something with it because it can wither and die if left unattended.

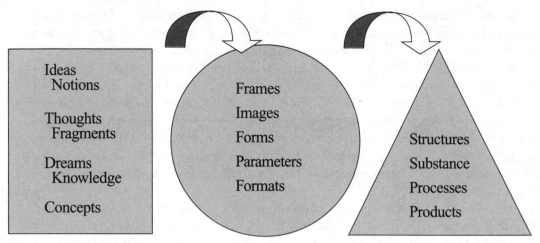

Figure 14-3 Requisites of Creativity.

produce something of value. The products of creativity could not exist without the work of creativity, requiring that we appreciate the latter as much as the former.

At the same time, creativity demands release from the slavishness of routine and the straightjacket of habit, rote, and ritual. Only within the chaos of experience can the elements of creativity converge. Further, the format for its expression must be allowed time and space to emerge. Forcing creativity into prescribed structures of expression limits its ability to take shape. This does not mean that no format is required. There is no pottery without the potter's wheel, no painting without a canvas.

It is difficult to live creatively. There is always some reason not to. We have all made comments about creative people who seem eccentric, even weird. Because they appear to live fully in their own world or to walk their own way, they make us feel uncertain or uncomfortable. In general, we experience uncertainty and unease if people fall outside our definition of what is appropriate, and because creative people tend to operate outside the parameters of normal behavior, we wonder whether getting in touch with the creative in ourselves will make us become like them. The answer, of course, is that creativity does not have a look and a walk and that we can connect with our creativity without changing in every way possible.

It is important to recognize that leaders cannot get the best out of those they lead if they cannot touch the best in themselves. This means they need to develop an awareness of who they are and how their essential self is expressed in the normal course of living each day. Leaders must understand that their spiritual part is frequently expressed in their most creative moments. Getting in touch with one's own creative center means discerning the spiritual values that lie within as well. For creativity to find expression, of course, requires discipline and habit and the meeting of certain conditions.

Finding the Source of Creativity

A person's creativity does not simply appear on demand. The person has to search for it and then develop ways to give it expression. The best way of getting in touch with it is to

Group Discussion

Getting in touch with the unrestrained child within is critical to touching our own creativity. Take a moment to reflect on a childhood episode in which you did something that was different or even unique (at the time)—in a word, creative. Those who wish to can tell their story to the rest of the participants. During each story, the listeners write down what each perceives as the key elements of the story. The group then discusses these elements and considers whether they are present in creativity regardless of age or time. Finally, the participants identify ways in which they can incorporate these elements into their own efforts at touching their individual creativity.

set aside a regular time during the day to focus on nothing but the inner self. Journaling is a helpful tool in this endeavor because regularly writing down one's thoughts establishes the habit of focusing on the creative and bringing it out into the open. The process need not be complicated or demanding. The goal is to write from one to three pages about whatever comes to mind at the moment. No one need see what was written because the purpose is merely to make sure that something has been done. In time, the act of writing begins to touch a deep part of the self, and expressing what lies within becomes easier. How long it takes to achieve fluency depends on how many blocks are standing in the way.

Everyone possesses an internal auditor who judges what is written or spoken or thought as appropriate or not. Often the auditor appears just as an individual is about to get in touch with his or her creativity and prevents the expression of ideas on the grounds that they are, for example, inappropriate, not right, not good, or not normal. This review and approval function is the person's own creation. A good way to bypass it is to commit to the process of daily writing and go wherever it leads. In time, the auditor will disappear and be replaced by a sense of freedom and openness, which is the groundwork for creative expression.

Journaling is a way of meditating that is often easier than the more defined forms of meditation. What often happens is that the wisdom that lies deep within emerges through the process and finds expression in a language that can inform, inspire, and guide. It is a chance for the inner voice to assume an outward form, deepening the meaning of our lives and perhaps moving us in a new direction.

Spending Time with the Child Within

As Jung and many contemporary psychotherapists revealed, we each have a child embedded deep within us that resides there throughout our lives. This child is the enthusiastic, joyful, excited part of ourselves that embraces life fully and without reservation. It is only when we are wounded by the behavior of others or by negative experiences that our inner child loses touch with the primordial joy that typifies the experience of the spirit. And even when the child loses touch with the joy of life, it continues to seek it until it finds joy again, renewing itself in the process.

The creative process often, if not always, meets up with this inner child. Many say it is impossible to get in touch with one's creativity without confronting this inner child and giving it a voice. Indeed, it is this voice that is the expression of creativity. Further, because the inner child, by its very nature, is not bound by the rules and parameters of adulthood, these are rendered powerless to limit the expression of creativity. However, whatever the child is feeling, whether pain or joy or some other emotion, will emerge as a part of the journey to the place of creativity, and until these feelings are expressed and dealt with in a meaningful way, the creative expression will remain blocked at the very place where it resides. That is why we must take up our unfinished business with this child (the pains and hurts of our life experiences and journey to adulthood) to free the creativity within.

Through the process of journaling, a person typically arrives at the door of creativity but is prevented from entering by the remnants of past pain. In verbalizing these on the daily pages of the journal, the person can get them out of the way and open the route to creative expression. In some circumstances, working on the issues with a professional or other trusted person may be a necessary step in the journey to freeing the inner child and releasing the creativity residing within.

Opening the Gates of Creativity

When we complete the journey to the center of our being, we find a deep well of creativity—a place filled with things that can be used as vehicles for creative expression (Leonard-Barton, 2011). We are all artists of one kind or another. Some of us are creative with our hands, some with our heads, some with our hearts—all of us with something. By using our regularly set aside time to explore different avenues, we can find that form of creative expression that most resonates with our inner self. Some people, of course, may discover more than one form. In any case, to give shape to our creativity we need to release the energy that lies within the urge to create. Creativity always seeks a way out into the world, and once touched and released it cannot be contained and must find expression, enriching the lives of everyone it touches and connecting all of us in ways we cannot even imagine.

Creativity is expressed in symbols and images. Even the wordsmith has a vision before forming that vision into words. Leaders also express their creativity through the construction of a vision. They then present this vision to others as evidence of their commitment to make some difference, to cause something to happen that enhances the life experience of everyone.

In this dynamic, leaders recognize that the critical ability is to be available to the creative force without attempting to master it. Creativity is very much a mystery and requires awareness instead of readiness. The creative force must first be seen before it can be expressed. Further, to give it form the creative mind must be attentive to what it might be saying. Form comes as a product of good discernment and the discipline of translating the creative force into words or substance.

Creativity leads each of us inward and then onward. We must spend time in the

> ### Point to Ponder
>
> The creative leader recognizes that what is critical is being available to the creative force, not mastering it.

"inward place." As Georgia O'Keeffe and Brenda Ueland caution us, we must spend time watching the flowers, puttering around in the imagining, idling, seeing, forming stuff that lives within. Leaders must identify the activities that guide them to the creative place within. Each of us can recall where we got our best ideas. For some it is the shower stall; others, the car; still others, the bathroom. From wherever the ideas come, the creative force is always seeking expression; we need only be aware of where and how it operates.

Overcoming the Fear of Being Wrong

Many artists and psychologists have noted that the opposite of love is not hate but fear. Fear closes off access to the creative—indeed, to most of life. Fear is a mental door that keeps the spirit imprisoned and unaware. How much faith is an expression of fear and as a result narrow, ritualistic, and rigid? How many people neurotically seek the spiritless road, comfortable in their own rightness but devoid of life and joy?

Fear, like a trap from which there is no escape, imprisons the heart and keeps it from experiencing the fullness of life. It closes the mind and shuts the door on life. It is the ultimate indicator of nonengagement. It keeps people from reaching out toward those very things that advance their experience and reduce the chance that fear will rule them. It is all too common to see people failing to confront fears that affect their expression of life—or to see someone struggling to avoid something infinitely less painful than the life of fear the person is living.

There is virtually nothing redeeming about fear. Yet much of the relationship that so many people have with life is tinged by their accommodation of their own fears. In addition, the structures of twentieth-century organizations were largely grounded in the concept of fear. In hierarchical organizations pervaded by the culture of "bossism," the negative power of the boss is what keeps people in line, and the power that managers wield is often articulated in the language of control and punishment. It is no wonder that changing the way the leadership role is perceived and expressed is so difficult. To make the necessary changes and remove fear from organizational life, leaders must therefore confront the history of the role and people's perception and experience of it.

> ### Key Point
> Being wrong is not a defect. We learn as much from our errors (Stewart, Corneille, & Johnson, 2006) as we do from our successes. The critical issue is to learn the specific point from any error so that we do not repeat it or stay imprisoned in a never-ending cycle of repetition and decline.

Being wrong is an essential constituent of creativity. In fact, creative people spend more time being wrong than being right. The road to rightness is paved with experimentation, innovation, mistakes, and "re-dos." In fact, in systems language success of any kind is simply the culmination of sufficient error. When the right amount of error has occurred and a sufficient amount of learning in relationship to the error has been obtained, then success emerges. Mistakes are the signposts of the journey toward achievement. The only error that is untenable is the same error repeated. An error repeated indicates that no learning occurred and the error's lesson was missed.

Exhibit 14-1   Overcoming Fear

Sources of Fear	Means of Identifying Fear	Ways of Overcoming Fear
• Parents	• Self-awareness	• Meditation
• Teachers	• Therapy	• Risk-taking
• Peers	• Reflection	• Therapy
• Self	• Input from others	• Focused action
• Authorities	• Trauma	• Confrontation
• Religion		• Surrender–embrace
• Events		• Medication

Mistakes are to be embraced by the organization as the tools of growth. The more fully an error is incorporated into the expectations of work, the fewer errors are present and the more certain the leader is that the right errors will emerge. By celebrating error, the leader takes the fear out of it and puts it into the right category—the category of devices for determining where people are on the journey toward their goals.

Confronting personal fear and fear in the workplace is a challenging process (**Exhibit 14-1**). So much of human experience is defined by fear that it becomes nearly impossible to push it out of people's lives. From regulation to accreditation, there are plenty of opportunities to be afraid of something or someone in a way that limits creativity and engagement with life. So many folks worry about whether they will "get in trouble" because of projects or activities with which they might be associated. For example, instead of thinking about how their behavior enables the organization to deliver high-quality services, healthcare workers waste their time worrying about whether they will offend someone, or do the wrong thing, or even cause a patient's death.

Of course, the probability of any one person doing sustainable damage is very low. People in an organization are generally incapable of permanently jeopardizing its integrity and functioning unless they have that goal as their evil intent. Of late, much work has been written on fear in the workplace and how unnecessary it is, not to mention detrimental to performance and even dangerous. One of the main goals of leadership should be to drive fear-based behavior out of the workplace and replace it with the commitment to relationship and creativity.

So many people in the professional workplace spend much of their time concentrating on the "floor" of their practice. Establishing standards, maintaining standards, benchmarking, developing protocols, and establishing routines are all names for the mechanism of focusing on the foundation, or the floor, of work and practice. Although it is essential to establish and use evidence-based standards, the leader must keep in mind that these standards represent the ground upon which practice builds. Excellence is never achieved simply by maintaining standards. Excellence is achieved after standards have been established and as people climb from these foundations toward the "ceiling" of their work and practice. Excellence occurs when people and organizations aim for the ceiling, moving beyond the floor of their practice in a way that advances and transforms it into higher levels of value, meaning, and impact on others. This pattern of behavior eclipses fear, which limits perspectives and keeps people focused merely on avoiding error instead of advancing excellence.

How much of the fear present in the workplace is there because of the fear of management? If leaders have not resolved their own fear issues, do these issues affect their relationships with others and affect the organization as a whole? If their language is laced with fear-based terminology, are they helping to create an atmosphere of anxiety and suspicion?

Fear-based behaviors—judging, blaming, pointing fingers, complaining, and so on— kill innovation. In the new age, there is simply no place for them to emerge. The job of the leader is to eliminate fear-based behaviors by giving them no room. Leaders begin this process by making sure that their own fear issues have not tainted the environment. By focusing on fear issues and grappling with their presence in each individual's life journey, leaders have a good chance to create a workplace of trust and joy and creativity.

In addition, leaders need to be aware of the importance and vitality of transparency in the expression of their own humanity and challenges in their leadership journey. Perhaps one of the most significant personal characteristics of excellent leadership is the capacity to demonstrate personal vulnerability and openness regarding the individual journey of development and change. This vulnerability demonstrates the capacity of the leader to engage and embrace openly in the vagaries of risk, error, experimentation, and adaptation and serves as a visible template for staff to emulate, model, and replicate in their own journey of transformation and change. The leader's vulnerability gives individual staff members permission to demonstrate and express their own experiences and challenges of growth and adaptation in a way that provides advantage to each organizational member, the service unit or department, and, ultimately, those they serve.

> **Point to Ponder**
>
> Fear kills all creativity.

Confronting the Core Negativity Within

As we move through life, we collect flawed mental models, negative stereotypes, and unsupported generalizations. These become deeply embedded in our consciousness and are reflected in our attitudes and behaviors. They often surface in our self-talk and our conversation with those closest to us. Although the generalities we use are typically inaccurate, even groundless, we still fall back on them in the midst of stress or during periods of difficulty. Following are a list of examples (to which each of us could add):

- I always do this.
- No one likes me.
- I'm going to die of . . .
- I'll always be poor.
- I can't study.
- I've never been able to . . .
- I'm just not good at . . .
- It's too late for me to do . . .

How many of these phrases have we caught ourselves saying at some time or other? Most people are surprised that this type of language is so pervasive. Think about how limiting and just plain incorrect these statements are. The challenge for every leader is to look carefully at his or her own language and assess the extent to which it is laced with negativity. The fact is that most leaders use (and hear) more negative language in a day than any other type.

Most of our negative ideas and images are untrue, including those that pertain to our own abilities. If we really could not do most of what we imagine cannot be done, we could not do what we have already done. Most of our core negatives come from outside ourselves—from parents, friends, religion, society. On top of these we add other negatives based on our experience. Eventually we have so many that they cannot help but impair our relationships and degrade other aspects of our lives.

What is important to remember is that negative beliefs are just that—beliefs. They are also obstacles blocking the enriched experience and the creative endeavors everyone is capable of. They shut the door on awareness and limit the places where talent or opportunity can make a positive change in our lives. Further, they give us all an excuse not to address challenges: No matter what we do, we will not succeed anyway.

Sitting on the sidelines of life, we can join others in spreading negativity. When we see others struggling to be creative, we can assure them that they will not succeed and thus need not strain themselves. The most threatening person to a negativist is the person who has agreed to engage with his or her negatives, take on a creative task, and follow wherever it leads. This person creates a risk that the negativist will see someone achieve all that the negativist has failed to do and thereby make the role of negativist very uncomfortable.

Leaders struggling to fight their own negatives should remember that affirmation is the enemy of negativity, that affirmative beliefs are just as viable and powerful as negative beliefs, only they have more mileage. They also need to replace the negative terminology they have used in the past with affirmative language, demonstrating their commitment to a different set of images and mental models, raising the level of the dialogue in the organization and creating a healthier organizational culture. Here are some examples of affirming language:

- I am very good at . . .
- I've always been able to . . .
- You're an excellent . . .

Group Discussion

Discuss the content of your self-talk with the group—the things you say to yourself when you are alone. What are the words used? What are the themes? Are the comments primarily positive or negative? Then, share your self-talk words with each other. Taken as a whole, is the group's self-talk supportive and encouraging or negative and punishing?

- I am a brilliant . . .
- I am challenged by . . .
- It's great fun to . . .

If leaders fight the urge to blurt out a negative comment and substitute an affirming statement, they will notice the different results. Language and behavior are themselves strong change agents. Contemporary research shows that positive statements, even when untrue, can become true through changing behavior over time (de Bono, 2007).

The transition to a more positive culture does not happen overnight. The bombardment of negative images and generalizations that most of us have undergone eventually turns negativity into our second nature. Leaders therefore have to make the overcoming of negativity a focused part of their leadership work. To not get sucked into the drama of constant negativity, they must have a way of exploring the sources of their own negativity and lack of creativity, past and present (Simons & Havert, 2012).

For leaders, getting in touch with their own journey means looking squarely at themselves and at how their nature affects their relationship with and leadership of others. How much do they understand about negativity and what causes it? What overwhelms their creativity? What affects their ability to embrace innovation? What personality characteristics keep them from relating to the elements of life that challenge or frighten them? How can they help others reflect on their attitudes and behaviors if, as leaders, they have no mechanism for doing that in their own lives?

Leaders cannot ask others to go to places they themselves are not willing or able to go. They thus need to routinely engage in reflection to gain essential insights about themselves, including whatever internal obstacles block their own creativity, engagement, and courage and decrease their ability to guide others and help them overcome the many challenges they face on their individual journeys.

Equally important to the leader is the willingness to demonstrate vulnerability and openness to what the personal journey teaches and reveals to each of us. Good leadership and mentorship require that leaders share the personal reflections that come with the struggle to grow and become effective leaders with others to inform others' personal journeys. No secrets or mystical unmentionables are imbedded in the leadership journey. Every leader's story is food for another's journey and can be fodder for new learning and advancing others' experiences of leadership.

Exercising the Spirit

We all know how important it is to exercise the body. Almost all medical literature about longevity tells us that exercise is an essential part of our lives. Regular exercise leads to good health and lifelong productivity, and failure to exercise is one of the major causes of untimely death (**Exhibit 14-2**).

Stretching the Spirit Within

Each person's spirit of consciousness—the source of creativity, energy, and engagement and seat of the self—has precisely the same need for exercise. When the spirit of

Exhibit 14-2   Exercising the Spirit Within

Requisites	Obstacles
• Setting aside time daily	• Fear
• Exercising regularly	• Tiredness
• Being self-disciplined	• Distractions
• Using a specific format or method	• Laziness
	• Excuses
	• Other commitments
	• Family responsibilities

consciousness is not exercised, it becomes weak and flabby and fails to grow. A weak spirit cannot provide the meaning that people need and look for in their lives. In the case of leaders, a weak spirit limits their effectiveness and causes them to lose direction. When that happens, their enthusiasm is diminished and they cannot motivate others to embrace the challenges of change. They then become depressed and subject to all and any of the diseases of the spirit. Without exercise, both the muscle (spiritual strength and creativity) and the immune system (moral courage and focus) of the spirit cease to operate effectively. They become susceptible to spiritual infections, such as evil intent, lack of direction, poor decision making, depression, and lack of focus.

Most leaders who want to pursue self-development read motivational or spiritual books. Reading these books can pique their interest in spiritual matters, even to the point of moving them to discuss spiritual topics with others. It does not, however, ensure that they grow spiritually or deepen their connection to their consciousness. In fact, reading often prevents people from growing spiritually by keeping them at a certain level of interest. Reading never calls people to do the deeper task of stretching their spirits in a way that actually changes their lives. Touching the spiritual energy within requires regular discipline—and focus!

Developing an Exercise Routine

Every leader needs regular spiritual workouts every day. The stress caused by confronting so much change requires a regular recess for recentering and refocusing on the meaning that drives the work of leading. This daily period of reflection and connection to one's spiritual energy should last at least 15 minutes. Of course, each leader must adjust the routine and time based on his or her individual needs and circumstances. The length of the period can be extended as the leader develops more skill and as the spirit increases its tone and strength. It is recommended that the leader gradually work up to spending 30 minutes on spiritual exercises each day.

A large body of research indicates that a spiritual/psychodynamic-conscious and intentional workout should encompass five specific steps: deep breathing, a spiritual warm-up, spiritual stretching, spiritual strengthening, and a spiritual cool-down. The following paragraphs demonstrate one of many different suggested approaches to establishing a regular routine of reflection and spiritual centering (**Exhibit 14-3**). Leaders are advised to find the discipline to allow the approach to be unique to their own personal needs and

---

Exhibit 14-3   A Spiritual Exercise Routine

Deep breathing. Transitioning from a high energy level to a lower one.

Spiritual warm-up. Reading a selection from a source that has special relevance.

Stretching the spirit. Reflecting on an incident or theme.

Strengthening the spirit. Applying knowledge and experience to gain wisdom.

Spiritual cool-down. Breathing, letting go, and choosing a thought to keep for the day.

---

capacity for reflection and discernment. The method they choose is not nearly as important as is the regular, consistent discipline of time spent in self-reflection.

Deep Breathing

At the beginning of every exercise routine, you need to transition from one level of energy to another lower level. You also need to move from a primarily external focus to looking inward. Deep breathing is a technique that helps you make the necessary journey.

Deep breathing facilitates the transition from a high level of energy to a lower level. In a relaxed position, slowly but continuously breathe deeply through your nose. After each inhale, hold your breath for a second and then let it go fully out through your mouth all at once. You need to do 10 to 20 of these before you begin to feel the relaxation unfold. The routine should be slow and continuous, completely unrushed, allowing you to peacefully and quietly relax yourself and refocus your attention on yourself and the reflective work you are about to undertake. Every time you sit down to do your reflective work, you should begin with deep breathing because it sets you up for the steps to follow.

Spiritual Warm-Up

The next step is to read a brief selection from a source that has relevance to your own life or experience. The reading is meant to move your spirit and mind into a reflective mode. By making the transition to a quieter, more peaceful perspective, you become ready to begin the journey to an intensive internal experience. This exercise should last anywhere from 3 to 5 minutes.

Stretching Your Spiritual Energy

You can use a real-life event or situation to center your attention on a particular theme or aspect of life. For example, you might choose an event that exemplifies the theme of the selection read during the warm-up. Using an actual incident or circumstance as a focal point is designed to narrow the reflective work so that it fits within the workout period but is still illuminating. This exercise, like the warm-up, should last 3 to 5 minutes.

Strengthening and Focusing the Spirit Within

During reflection, a question or series of questions arises. These might concern an aspect of your life or experience or a component of your role, relationships, or work. At this point you apply your knowledge and experience to learn about yourself—about your issues, relationships, problems, and concerns—and gain wisdom.

> **Key Point**
>
> Spending time with ourselves is the most valuable and most difficult thing we can do in life.

This is where the heavy exercise occurs. Your response to your insights has an important impact on your choices, approach, method, and focus for the day. The insights you obtain during this strengthening exercise may accumulate over a number of days and eventually come together to clarify what course you should take in dealing with a challenge, problem, or issue. You should spend 5 to 10 minutes (and no more than 10 minutes) on this part of the workout.

Cooling Down

The spiritual workout is concluded with a brief period of breathing and letting go. This exercise brings the workout to a close and transitions you back into your daily activities. You should choose an important thought or moment in the reflection to remember and keep with you for the rest of the day. You might even write it on a small card. Writing down important thoughts or memorable moments allows you to recollect them at any time during the day and to apply them whenever and in whatever way appears right. This finishing exercise should take between 2 and 3 minutes. Please keep in mind that the effort here is to provide an opportunity for quiet reflection as a vehicle for providing the kind of directed discernment related to your person as a leader and to deepen your capacity for insight, self-reflection, purposefulness, and intentional personal transformation.

Quiet, Please

A quiet place is necessary for proper exercise of the mind and spirit. Unlike the body, which can be toned by exercising to vigorous music and enthusiastic encouragement, the spirit needs quiet to be stretched and strengthened. The quieter it is during spiritual exercises, the better the results.

Finding and maintaining quiet can be difficult. Some people even feel initial anxiety in a quiet place. Today, distraction is the name of the game, and we have become conditioned to continuous assaults on our consciousness. For leaders, the very work of leading forces them into a host of relationships, conversations, processes, and problems that leaves no time for consideration and reflection.

Focusing on our spiritual resources is inner exercising. The better we get at it, the deeper we go and the more we desire the joy and peace that come from going deeper.

> **Key Point**
>
> In developing self-awareness, the discipline of regular reflection can make an important difference. Progress is always variable, but no progress will be achieved if the process is not a regular habit.

Regular spiritual reflection leads to a surprising yet extremely satisfying calm, accompanied by a deep sense of peace and contentment. The secret to discovering this place is the quiet and calm that surrounds us when we undertake our exercise routines. Each workout should be done in a quiet place and at an available time (i.e., a time free of other commitments), and preferably the same time and place should be used for all the workouts.

A wide variety of mental and spiritual resources has emerged over the history of humankind. The warm-up exercises, for example, can be drawn from a broad selection of spiritual or reflective works. The goal of reflective exercising is to stretch the spirit through a variety of growth experiences and challenges that fall inside and outside of the person's usual life context. These experiences and challenges instigate growth by pushing the person to use a diverse set of learning resources as a tool kit.

> **Key Point**
>
> A leader is never off duty while in the leadership role. Leaders are under constant scrutiny of others while they try to turn every moment, every interchange, every experience into an opportunity to make a difference in the lives of those they lead.

The notes written during the spiritual cool-down act as "memory joggers" to help connect our experiences to the wisdom gained through the exercises. In the midst of daily activities, our consciousness periodically generates windows or moments of perception that affirm the insights that arose from that day's reflection. The notes from a particular exercise session can also serve as a doorway back to the work done during that session, allowing the wisdom gained to continue to play a role in meeting life's challenges.

Importance of Exercising Every Day

Regularity is the key to good spiritual work. It is recommended that these exercises be done first thing in the morning or as early as possible in the day. Although morning is best, exercising the spirit is valuable any time it is done. As mentioned, exercising for 15 to 30 minutes a day is enough for the benefits to accrue.

If a leader does the exercise routine daily, he or she will begin to see a difference in the areas of feeling, acting, and thinking. The leader will have more energy, experience more enthusiasm, exhibit more creativity, and feel more centered. As a result, the leader's work relationships will improve, among other positive consequences. As the spirit uses better strategies to handle stress, anger and tension will ease and then dissipate, sleep will come more easily, and worry will begin to lessen. After faithfully completing a full 100 days of regular workouts, the leader will almost certainly see dramatic changes in his or her life.

The First 100 Days

The leader commits to a set of daily exercises for 100 days. This commitment is meant to help the individual continue the workouts long enough to experience some of the benefits of reflection and seek out other sources and methods of spiritual strengthening. The spiritual energy of every person matures in its own fashion, and by the time the workout routine is well established the leader's spirit will thirst for further spiritual experiences. Indeed, the leader will come to find that he or she cannot live without them.

Spiritual Intelligence: Ten Rules of the Road

Leadership is not simply a set of skills but a whole discipline. As such, it requires a commitment to constant growth and self-development. Leaders, in living the role, not only direct the process of change and adaptation but also exemplify adaptability, modeling it for others. This means that personal change, maturation, and development make up a fundamental part of the life of any leader. Consequently, leaders are always involved in reaching for the potential within the self.

Following is a discussion of 10 basic themes that thread through the life of a leader. These themes underscore the fact that leaders, in virtue of their role, are on a journey of exploration and growth (**Exhibits 14-4** and **14-5** and **Figure 14-4**).

1. *The leadership role demands courage.* For leaders, risk is a pervasive fact of life. Leaders live in the potential, by definition a place of great risk. They have a responsibility to translate the potential into real experiences in a way that helps others see how the journey of transformation affects their own roles. Leaders alert staff members to the meaning and requisites of their work and the direction it must ultimately take to have value. Thus, they are sometimes required to live on the cutting edge, pushing against the walls of reality, forcing staff members to confront their own perceptions and behaviors, and challenging them to create their own futures. Leaders frequently appear to be running counter to the prevailing sensibilities and must confront the noise that their actions create, holding strongly to what is right and necessary in a way that advocates for these things in the face of the noise—certainly a challenging reality but a requisite of the role.

2. *Caring for the self is the first priority.* Leaders are not self-sacrificing, long-suffering, passive personalities who mindlessly implement the organization's directives. Instead, they have a strong sense of self and are fully in touch with their own motives and intentions. They are clear where they are in relationship

---

Exhibit 14-4   Ten Spiritual Rules of the Road

1. The leadership role demands courage.
2. Caring for the self is the first priority.
3. Setting a few focused goals and achieving them are preferable to setting and failing to achieve a broad range of goals.
4. Prayer is a tool of leadership.
5. Challenge and change are normal features of the universe.
6. The universe is full of creative and transforming energy as well as mystery.
7. Leaders need to seek out others who are committed to change and growth.
8. The goal of leadership is to connect to the journey of transformation.
9. Judgment is an enemy of the spirit within.
10. You can't love your creation if you don't love the creator.

Exhibit 14-5   Requisites of the Spiritual Journey

- A desire for truth
- Self-love
- Creativity
- The support of others
- A disciplined process
- Ability to see life itself as a journey

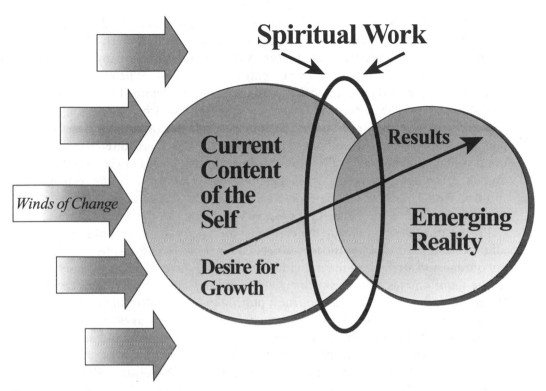

Figure 14-4 The Journey of Spirit.

to what motivates action and response, and they always act on the basis of their understanding of this. They also recognize that they cannot address the needs of others if their own neediness is greater. Therefore, they realize that they require time for reflection, opportunities for self-development, and the skills necessary for dealing with critical growth issues. It is only through self-understanding that leaders can help meet the needs of others.

3. *Setting a few focused goals and achieving them is preferable to setting and failing to achieve a broad range of goals.* There is nothing more debilitating than setting a host of goals and not meeting them. Thus, it is wise to set a small number of goals and commit to achieving them. Being less ambitious ensures that the focus does not get lost and that significant progress can be made. Personal development is a work in progress and requires a lifetime commitment.

Focusing only on key issues of self-development makes it possible to resolve them and move on. Not every behavior or habit can be altered at the same time. Leaders need to be kind to themselves and not expect progress on every front. Small successes can serve as the foundation for significant change and as the means for attaining ultimate goals.

Leaders need to be similarly kind to those they are helping to change. They should assist them in setting priorities so that they can better succeed in revising their behaviors and practices. By being realistic and not expecting too much, leaders can turn success into a way of being. Success does much to alter attitudes and reenergize performance, changing both the milieu and the spirit of the work.

4. *Prayer can be a powerful tool of leadership.* Although there are as many religious traditions as there are leaders, prayer is central to all of them. Whatever their convictions, leaders should know that prayer has been determined to have a great impact on the quality of decisions and the comfort with which challenges are faced. Prayer is simply a reflection of a reality beyond one's own. It harnesses the spiritual forces within and without to help create the stamina required to carry on. It centers the mind and calls it to focus in a way that leads to new insights and deep, strong relationships. This reflective capacity has value for the secular mind as well. Time set aside in deeply reflective activity has demonstrated psychobiological benefits that affect positive well-being.

   Prayer and reflection ensure the constancy necessary to any meaningful effort and link the effort to the forces needed for something to happen. They encourage and strengthen the individual, realigning the individual's energy to fit the requirements of the task. They help keep things in perspective and pull the mind and heart back to the journey, putting the work into a life framework rather than an event model. In prayer, the issue or situation takes on broader and deeper implications and gets connected to a whole range of intersections that give it meaning and call people back to the larger picture. Prayer renews, strengthens, encourages, and connects people in a way that ensures their faithfulness to the effort and to each other.

5. *Challenge and change are normal features of the universe.* Stability is equivalent to death. Change is the normal state of existence. The role of leaders is to walk the tightrope between stability and chaos, with a tendency to favor the latter. Chaos is a sign of life in the universe and pervades human experience. Realizing this, leaders do not expect stability to last for long. Any stability they find is simply a resting point on the journey to the next place.

   Opposition, including the clash between differing interests, is part of change. Thus, leaders are always prepared for opposition and contrary arguments, practices, and behaviors. Indeed, the techniques of managing relationships encompass ways of challenging people's mental models. Leaders begin by clarifying their own perceptions, roles, and commitments and then challenge others to make their own commitment to fostering change and meeting the challenges that arise on the journey.

> **Key Point**
>
> Sometimes all that is possible is to embrace the mystery, the unknown, of a situation and allow it to be beyond reach or understanding for a while. Going with the flow of an experience helps position the leader to discern something different or new and advances the leader's insight and experience in a way that simply cannot be controlled or managed.

6. *The universe is full of creative and transforming energy as well as mystery.* Regardless of their personal belief traditions and perceptions, leaders need to understand what this means at the individual level because they must

harness the internal energy of the staff and the external energy embedded in all transformation. This combined energy reflects a resonance with change that itself can keep people focused and directed. Leaders need to appreciate that influence and the wisdom that is often evident in the demand for change.

Because everything is always in motion, everything that the leader does and creates somehow reflects change and adaptation. A particular change does not happen for its own sake. It is a reflection of a grand concert of changes that, when connected together, co-create the next stage of the universe. Leaders, along with everyone else, are participants in this universal dance or exchange of energy, and by understanding this fact they can deepen the meaning of their work and change efforts. Becoming aware of the wisdom deeply embedded in the action of the universe is the first step in discerning a deepening level of meaning and value in the individual efforts of all who are contributing to the transformation.

7. *Leaders need to seek out others who are committed to change and growth.* Companionship on the journey of leadership is a great gift—but only if the companions are of the right kind. There are those who, for some reason, are committed to making the journey of life difficult and rocky. They want others to be in their condition. They obstruct the processes of transformation and suck the life out of the experience of leadership.

These people should be carefully managed in the leader's life. Leaders need as much support as they can get in doing the work of leadership. They should expect colleagues and friends to be as committed to personal and organizational transformation as they are. The work of leadership takes a lot of energy and demands the support of good people who can clarify the work and stimulate the person doing it. Leaders must seek out those who are themselves well motivated and can act to advance, rather than limit, the leadership role. Likewise, they must break their relationships with people who are somehow driven to try to discourage them or deflate their energy. The work is tough enough as it is.

8. *The goal of leadership is to connect to the journey of transformation.* When surrounded by the challenges of leadership, leaders can lose sight of the fact that change is normal and that people cannot keep from changing. The issue, thus, is not whether they will transform but how they will change and what condition they will be in at the end of the change cycle.

People can change by design or by default, and it is part of the leadership role to help them change by design—to guide them on the journey of transformation rather than letting them be carried down the rapids. Working with people through their own tough times, however, can skew a leader's perceptions and obscure the fact that change is unavoidable. Therefore, leaders need to get away from their work occasionally or talk to colleagues to reaffirm their commitment to leading change and reestablish their connection with the journey and their vision of the future. Indeed, this is an essential part of leadership—staying grounded in transformation.

9. *Judgment is an enemy of the spirit within.* How many people have been sacrificed on the altar of judgment? Other than in courts of law, judgment is usually destructive. The appraisals that people make of their own activities

Group Discussion

As a group, brainstorm the ways in which judgment obstructs progress. Then, brainstorm impeding judgments and place these on a flip chart. Next, discuss possible approaches to use to prevent the various mechanisms of judgment from taking control of a leader's consciousness. Finally, enumerate the characteristics of the judgment process, identify clues that someone is habitually making judgments and acting on them, and discuss ways in which the tendency to make judgments might be managed or avoided.

are usually negative and have the effect of suppressing their creativity. The appraisals of others can be just as negative and just as counterproductive.

> **Point to Ponder**
>
> Judgment is always finally destructive. It puts up a barrier in our consciousness that prevents leaders from seeing the potential at their disposal. It keeps them stuck in the present and the superficial, unable to dig to a deeper place where meaning resides and truth can be found.

People's judgments reflect their feelings about what they are judging, and their judgments obviously are formed by their values and prejudices, fears and uncertainties. People rarely see things as they really are but instead make what they observe into shadows of their own biases. In addition, judgments about actions are often more concerned with the agents than with the actions themselves. An action or performance, for example, might be condemned just because the person who did it was assumed to be unskilled or inept or lacked the right to do it. Everything has value when seen in a valuable way. Even negative behavior can have meaning if it is understood.

Leaders should avoid making judgments, about themselves or others, and should not seek out or pay attention to the judgments of others. They should instead try to see things within their actual context and from a perspective generated from

> **Point to Ponder**
>
> You simply cannot love another for long if you cannot love yourself first.

within that context (Hosmer, 2006; Massaro, Bardy, & Pitts, 2012). Judgments are generally loaded with fear content, and fear disables and limits human responses and kills the creative urge. Leaders must do everything in their power to eliminate judgment to allow others to respond inventively to the demand for change.

10. *You can't love your creation if you don't love the creator.* No person can love another in a healthy way if the person feels unloved or even without the right to be loved. This is as true for leaders as for anyone else. How many people have aspired to hold formal leadership positions because they are still seeking from others the

love they could not get from their parents? How many actual leaders have a greater neediness than those they lead? How many are looking for satisfaction in the adulation and dependencies that can accompany the leadership role? How many leaders keep a tight rein out of the fear they will lose control and no one will love them because they failed to do their job or cannot own the glory?

Many seek the leadership role not solely out of a desire to make a difference. Instead, they seek it because of their own need to shine, to be noticed, and to get from their position what they could not get elsewhere: recognition, reward, and love. They do not realize that if they cannot find satisfaction within themselves, they will not find it in the leadership role either. Also, they do not understand that they must first love themselves before they can expect to get from the role what it truly has to offer. Unfortunately, others often have to pay the price for their ignorance.

These 10 themes are the givens around which the leadership role is built. Consequently, they can serve as a personal template for leaders as they struggle to make sense of their role and to find the center within that informs each of them about their own issues. In addition, leaders who embark on a spiritual exercise regimen of the sort described previously can incorporate a personal assessment of the individual implications of these themes into their initial workouts (or periods of reflection).

Becoming Self

All creation is good. There is simply no other way to evaluate it. Life appears because it wants to. Life wants life. Life seeks fullness, expression, identity, emergence, and flowering. In every aspect of creation, it appears as though life wants to live. The evidence is to be found in all of its acts of self-creation, change, adaptation, and growth.

Life's drive toward self-organization is a fundamental feature of the universe, and it has operated from the beginning of existence as we know it. We simply needed the right science, the right moment, and the right perceptions to grasp these facts.

Francisco Varela, a famous biologist, coined a term for life's creation of more life out of itself. He named this process autopoiesis, which means "self-formation." He affirmed that life is unique in having the ability to create itself—to continue to generate more life.

> ### Key Point
>
> Life wants life. Life seeks fullness, expression, identity, emergence, and flowering. In every aspect of creation, it appears as though life wants to live. The evidence is to be found in all of its acts of self-creation, change, adaptation, and growth.

The process of autopoiesis is continuous and cyclical. And it is generative in that life enlarges itself, growing the options and the potential and the fullness that make it what it has become at any moment in time. Life cannot stay the same. It complicates and diversifies itself, constantly becoming something more than it was.

The journey of life is an experience without boundaries. It moves in all directions and offers choice without limit. Once a selection has been made, however, boundaries emerge, forcing the selection to take form, to be lived fully in the form that it takes, expressing the reality that the selection now represents. Yet, paradoxically again, the boundaries themselves, while disciplining the selection into form and action, allow choice to move in a new direction and seek options that could not have arisen without the discipline imposed by the boundaries.

Each person must find the way into this mosaic of simplicity and complexity that best exemplifies the person's own journey. This self-referencing process, in which the discipline of choice requires living consistently with any selection made, operates at every level of the universe. For instance, the patterns or "habits" of role can appear anywhere, from the operation of scientific laws to the simplest routines of human behavior. This self-referencing also influences how we see the world because it affects what our eyes see and what form our seeing takes in our lives. Our self-perception informs our world, not usually the other way around. We begin to create what makes sense to us, and the limits and permissibles embedded in our personal worldview create boundaries around whatever it is that supports our worldview.

Self-referencing tells us a lot about how we change, grow, and adapt at every level, from the personal to the societal to the systematic to the universal. As Teilhard de Chardin, the famous Jesuit paleontologist, eloquently pointed out, we are co-creators of the universe, working in concert with the energies and forces of creation to engage with the requirement to keep creating. Each component of life is working within its parameters, intersecting with others, and interacting with the components it most directly touches. Together, all the components operate in a way that ultimately changes everything in an endless cycle of creativity and growth.

This paradox of boundary and intersection is critical to the role of the leader. Nothing in life operates outside of this paradox. Each boundary intersects and interacts in a dynamic way with every other boundary in a dance that ultimately causes each of them to change. The energy of life comes out of this complex interaction of intersecting boundaries moving in a constant flux of relationship that transforms each of them singly and collectively. Such are the physical laws of the universe and conditions under which leaders must act out their role.

Life evolves in a context of co-creation. No one acts independently of anyone else. Indeed, there is no real independence but only interdependence, and this fact gives both form and direction to the role of the leader. Leaders are always working to understand the interdependence of situations, circumstances, and people. They know that in the workplace everything has an impact on everything else. Yet every person is acting out of his or her own space, doing the work that is expected. It is the aggregation of all the elements of the work and the efforts of the workers that, when brought together, makes something sustainable happen.

Leaders live life in the white spaces—the boundary land—between people, places, and processes. They do their work in the context of the potential future to which the confluence of their efforts ultimately leads. They read the signposts of the journey by identifying the elements of the journey and the forces that, when aggregated, tell the story of direction and process. At the same time, they are working to evolve, to respond to the demand for personal change. In short, they are managing both the journey and their personal experience of it.

Each member of the organization must do the same thing. The main leadership task is to make it possible for all members to have an awareness of this work, know its implications for their personal journey and the collective journey, and respond to the demand for change by applying their creativity.

The leaders of an organization must also see the undercurrent of linkage that exists every place in the organization. To achieve this goal, they need to be highly receptive and to hear the sounds of the universe in the language of persons, movement, and self.

Listening for the Sounds of Change

Perhaps the most important and, at the same time, difficult skills for a leader to obtain are listening skills, including those needed to hear the sounds of direction and change. We are always getting ready to speak or respond even as we listen to someone else talk. In short, much of the time we are not really listening.

To exercise good leadership, leaders must listen from the very core of their being. They must listen to the sounds of change and to the more spiritual sounds of life, hearing themes as well as words, seeing intent as well as message, determining direction as well as impression. Listening deeply is essential for adapting to the vagaries of the journey and meeting its challenges. By hearing themes and undercurrents, leaders can anticipate events and take the right action at the right time.

No one can listen deeply without preparation and development of listening skills. Leaders must assess their level of attention to the words and actions of others, as well as their focus on the ebbs and flows of the work. They must ask themselves about their readiness to respond to the issues affecting health care and their ability to detect the trends, including economic trends, that will affect its future.

Deep listening comprises contextual listening and content listening (**Exhibit 14-6**). Both are critical. The purpose of contextual listening is to become aware of the surrounding circumstances—the external events that affect what work people do and what resources are available to them. The purpose of content listening is to hear what people are saying, understand what it means, and grasp its implications. The deep listener listens to content while maintaining an awareness of the context, at the same time recognizing that what people say is always influenced by their beliefs, experience, perspectives, and prejudices. Listening with a broad frame of reference provides the listeners with an accuracy gauge—a way of placing what they see and hear within a context that validates, challenges, or alters its meaning.

Leaders develop an inner ear through reflection and self-awareness. They must understand their own perspectives and perceptions—those things that might skew their ability to hear with openness and acuity—to hear the voices of others accurately. If leaders cannot hear their own notions, values, fears, and prejudices and give them a language and a

---

Exhibit 14-6   Contextual and Content Listening

Contextual Listening	Content Listening
• Circumstances	• The message
• Conditions	• Components
• Framework	• Players
• Environment	• Truth
• External factors	• Perception
	• Issues

---

place in the journey, they will be unable to incorporate incoming information into their knowledge base, undermining their ability to lead effectively.

Leaders who have not yet done deep spiritual and personal work still have filters in place that adjust messages from the outside to their comfort level or even block messages that are not congruent with their beliefs and values. By modifying what is heard, these filters reduce the leaders' ability—and the ability of the entire organization—to respond appropriately and effectively to the messages.

By using their inner ear to access their beliefs and attitudes, leaders can become alert to the same dynamic going on in others. They can then perceive more completely the struggles, uncertainty, barriers, and challenges embedded in the utterances they hear and also understand better how information is received and used by the staff as they attempt to deal with the realities affecting their own work and relationships.

Spending time in quiet self-reflection is a proven way of enhancing one's ability to listen deeply. If leaders can get past their self-constructed barriers to self-knowledge, they can see behind the words, read into the language, and look beyond the present, all gifts that, among other things, help them create a more accurate profile of the issues they face.

Finding Spirit in the Chaos

Art and nature have always had an impact on the human spirit. The culminating beauty of a mountain vista or a symphony orchestra has the power to move the spirit and bring great contentment. Yet each of those is the fractal image of smaller units of what would otherwise be seen as chaos. Imagine looking at the tangle of infrastructure of a forest or listening to each individual instrument play its own music. Clearly, only when the elements of the forest or the symphony aggregate can the beauty of the collective intersections be revealed and fully enjoyed.

It is the ability to see the whole and recognize its beauty that inspires the spirit and deepens the character. Further, although the art of Mandelbrot sets (mosaics created when aggregated chaos reveals the order within) can be enjoyed to a degree, the addition of human consciousness, as occurs in the art of the human spirit, intensifies the experience and raises the level of appreciation.

The human story and the art and spirit of life are filled with metaphors, contradictions, challenges, myths, and created scenarios. Using patterns of self-similarity and self-discord, artists and mystics create in ways that stimulate, challenge, and resonate with our humanity. By experiencing these convergent and divergent realities, we can fathom our connection to each other and to the universe and can grow in ways that intensify and enrich our lives.

The art of chaos can also have an impact on the way in which leaders address uncertainty, diversity, and variability. Leaders must come to prize divergent and convergent realities at the

> **Key Point**
>
> It is important not only to listen to the words of the message but also to listen for the intent, value, passion, focus of the message, and the speaker's relationship to what he or she is communicating. By listening deeply, the listener gets the message and the meaning as well.

same time. Suspending the expectation to see order right away is the first step toward appreciating what complexity has to offer. By looking broadly at problems and opportunities, leaders can understand what they are and what they entail, whereas examining them too closely would obscure their meaning. Standing on the balcony of experience gives leaders the chance to observe both actions and their context and to perceive a reality that might otherwise make no sense.

The ability to see things broadly, one of the foundations of wisdom, takes time to acquire. Only after observing enough from the balcony can leaders develop the depth of insight and understanding needed to put everything into its proper context. Leaders, like other people, frequently get stuck in their own experience and are co-opted by their attachment to it, making it impossible for them to place it in a broader frame. By keeping unattached to any particular position, leaders can see every event, situation, or issue from outside and also can link it to other elements of the system invisible from inside. There is no indictment intended here of the perspective of those inside an issue, for example. The point is to celebrate the distance and wisdom of the leader coming from the outside and thus the leader's ability to place the issue into a context that gives it meaning.

The ability of leaders to operate in this manner of appreciative inquiry is enhanced by personal work directed toward putting life in perspective—that is, seeing it as part of a chaotic and complex world (**Figure 14-5**). Spending time reflecting on the mystery of life and integrating this fact into their lives gives leaders a firm center and inspires confidence and composure.

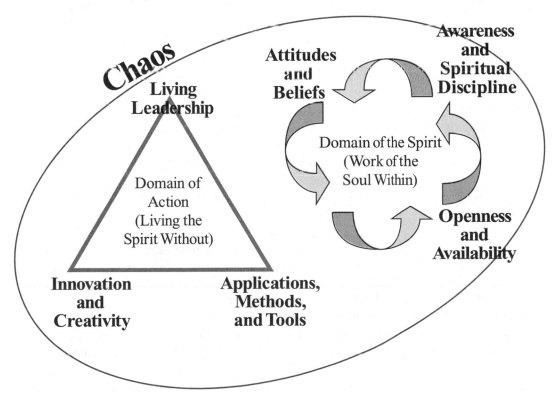

Figure 14-5 The Realms of Spirit Within the Chaos.

We have, all of us, seen leaders of this type and observed with interest and not a little awe how balanced they appear, even in the midst of a notable crisis. Their ability to see around, through, or beyond the crisis inspires us, especially when their insight stands the test of time. Having gained a deeper perspective (really, a broader one), these leaders show how everything, even a crisis, fits into the multiplicity that is life and experience.

The Compensations of Ignorance

Paradoxes are forever there to challenge each of us in our certainty. There is clearly more we do not understand than there is that we know. Much of what is written in this book, although true at our current level of understanding, soon enough will no longer be true. The authors can recall the commitment they brought to previous books and the energy with which they articulated the truth of the time, only to note how much has changed and how little of what was written 30 years ago is as true today.

> **Point to Ponder**
>
> Truth is a journey, not an event. Honor those who are seeking truth; avoid those who have found it.

Still, every generation, through its work, builds the foundation for the next. No work is an end in itself; no process or experience simply comes to a dead halt. Each piece is part of the mosaic of revelation that got us to today and will get us to tomorrow. This longer-term perspective must inform the leadership role. Even in the midst of a vital crisis or critical life event, leaders must use the fabric of complexity to put the circumstances in a larger frame of reference because this frame of reference better reflects the reality of the time than do the experiences and stresses of the event itself. It is so easy for leaders to get sucked into an event and allow it to become the center of their reality, losing all sense of its place in the course of events.

Koans, in the form of a riddle, which Buddhists use to focus the mind in a way that heightens understanding and intuition, keep us from putting temporal and spatial boundaries around our lives and experience. They invalidate our parameters. The minute something makes sense to us or becomes clear, the intersections of our clarity take us back into the chaos to the next level of intellectual or perceptual challenge. Rather than a negative, this feature of reality keeps us always on the edge of creativity and discovery. It also reminds us that there is no place to rest (at least for very long) and that nothing is an end in itself. For the leader, the journey of discernment is always deepening and broadening understanding and informing its translation into practice and application in the role of leadership and in the lives of others.

> **Key Point**
>
> For leaders, the issue is not how much information they have but how much they need to act. No amount of information eliminates all risk, and beyond a certain point gathering more information does not reduce the risk but the timeliness of any action taken.

The challenge for leaders and others lies in the engagement with the flow of life. If religious or intellectual beliefs become strongly entrenched, they can serve as the barriers to subsequent discoveries, insights, or revelations. As has been said, truth is a journey, not an event. It is a lived dynamic, not simply a fact of life.

None of us can know everything. Even those of us who are well educated come to understand how little we know of all that is knowable. Further, our quest for knowledge is a delusion if we think of knowledge as a thing. Knowledge is not a thing but rather a dynamic—a revelation bound up in the time and circumstances that make it available. Although it is valuable, knowledge is not an end in itself. Nor is it ever complete. In mathematics, when equations are carried out to the third decimal, they reveal a particular product. When carried out to the sixth decimal, they reveal a different product. This process can continue ad infinitum.

In decision making, the issue is not the total quantity of information possessed but whether there is enough information to make a decision. In no case will more information eliminate all the risk associated with choosing. Indeed, the collection of information can be pursued for so long that any action that would have been effective becomes untimely. Leaders must recognize that the leadership role is rife with risk, just like every other aspect of life. The demands of the time are part of a broader canvas that resists comprehension, and every decision sends into motion effects that can never fully be known.

In considering a particular decision, leaders need to be concerned about two things: Is it the right decision for the time, and does it set a direction that fits the circumstances of the journey? In short, do the signposts appear to validate the decision? If they do, that is the best indicator that the decision is the correct one. After all, the overarching goal is to make decisions that, over time, take the organization and everyone in it to a better place where knowledge and the quality of life are advanced. Thomas Edison made more than 1,000 attempts before the light bulb went on. After which failed attempt should he have stopped? All 999 were necessary for the journey to light, and we can be thankful for every one of them.

Mystery

Perhaps the most notable need of leaders today is to be reenchanted by a sense of mystery. In every area of life, the more questions get answered, the more questions get raised. Indeed, the explicit lesson of chaos and complexity is the profound inscrutability of it all.

Despite the advances of science and the discoveries of medicine, we still are largely in the dark about the nature of the universe and the things that it contains. The billion-dollar effort to decipher the human genetic code was a seminal event in the course of human history. Of course, besides finally revealing the code, what it did was open the door to a whole new project: identifying the billion or so proteomes that do the work of the genes and discovering how the genes perform their myriad tasks through these proteomes. Collating and codifying the proteomes are tremendous undertakings, yet it is the work demanded by the revelations of the genome project. One level of complexity leads to an even deeper and broader level of complexity.

Wherever there is progress, there is a temptation to become arrogant and controlling. We are easily lured into believing that what we are doing is magnificent and grand—that we are creating the future of humanity. Because we know so much, we become deluded by our knowledge, giving it more credence and more importance than it merits. If history has taught us anything, it is that we are forever learning. That is to say, what is unknown is infinitely greater than the combined knowledge we humans have garnered on our short journey through time.

In the United States, our enthusiasm and egotism often insulate us from the depths of our ignorance. Being so busy making discoveries and applying them in different and exciting ways, we have little time to set aside for contemplating the fathomless mysteries that remain and feeling awe at the very small part we play in the unfolding of the universe. It is this awe for the unknown, this respect for the mystery of life, that is so important to leaders in the midst of the chaos of transformation. Leaders need to put their efforts into perspective as the Industrial Age gives way to our current age—one filled with promise but, as of yet, lacking much substance.

> ### Point to Ponder
>
> The wonderful thing about mystery is that it relieves us of the obligation to know everything. It allows us to appreciate the uncertain, the unformed, indeed, the journey of life. Mystery opens us up to discernment and discovery and moves us away from definition and control. It deepens our appreciation for the experience of life rather than the management of life.

Leaders today, besides regaining a sense of mystery themselves, face the additional challenge of deepening the appreciation of staff for the chaos and complexity that pervade the universe. They can do this by engaging with change directly and exemplifying in their behavior an awareness of the mystery in all movement. By not knowing, by not having all the answers, by being uncertain and exploring alternatives, leaders demonstrate their vulnerability to the effects of complexity. They also create a safe space for staff members to express their own uncertainty, discomfort, anxiety, and excitement. A further consequence is that leaders and staff together, through their appreciation for the mystery of their journey, will come to realize that they are about important things—that they are all participating in a larger project as co-creators and that what they do makes a difference, sometimes apparent, at other times unknown, but an inexorable difference nonetheless. And this is the centerpiece of the mystery.

Synthesis and Synergy

Finally, leaders need to be reminded that the work of leadership itself is filled with mystery. We have all done apparently inconsequential things that, we later discovered, had a profound impact on someone else. In some secret way, quietly and steadily, our words or actions thoroughly changed that person's life. Caught up in the moment, a leader might see an act as unimportant—and as a single act it might be. When connected to some other reality, it can take on a new form and new dimensions and have a significant impact on another's life.

Unseen forces are embedded in all reality, and mystery is present in all aspects of life. Everywhere, unknown influences, relationships, and intersections exist just beneath the surface of the actual and operate synergistically to continue the movement of change. Because some of these have no form or are not yet perceived, their effects can sometimes be traumatic. As part of their role, lead-

> ### Point to Ponder
>
> The imagery of complexity pervades the world, from artwork to zebras. The order embedded in complexity—an order made visible as a mosaic of intersections and interactions—reflects the synthesis and seamlessness of creation and the connections within and among all things.

ers are always looking for the unseen, the intersections, the goodness of fit among the elements of chaos and change. By looking for the linkages and connections, reading the signposts of the journey, looking within or behind motives, they are able to give language to the experience and the journey. Being disciplined to see the whole and to distinguish the contribution that the whole makes to the parts and vice versa, they are in a position to appreciate the greater mystery to which everything relates, to be awed by its implications and moved by its inscrutability.

There are always missing pieces. We may be tempted to believe that by discovering those pieces we can unravel the ultimate secrets of the universe and know everything we need to know. Of course, this is just plain foolishness. Every secret unlocked reveals a host of new secrets not yet addressed—meaning that the process of discovery is endless. Understanding this, leaders see

> ### Key Point
>
> Any knowledge that we gain forms the foundation for the next mystery. Inscrutability outruns understanding as long as there is life.

and experience their role as the journey it really is. All parts of the journey intersect in visible and invisible ways, and the array of interactions and intersections necessary to the experience of life is also the work of life and the raw material for the work of leadership.

Operating within the context of their own journey, facilitating the experiences of others, and finding and defining the relationships among the elements and forces of movement and change, leaders are faced with the challenge of seeking and seeing the synergies that allow them to pursue their work and support the collective work of the organization. In harnessing these synergies, they represent for everyone in the organization the action of creation, complete engagement with life, and the full embrace of the mystery of complexity.

Case Study 14-1

Want Should I Do for an Encore?

Sarah just celebrated her 60th birthday, and this milestone in her life has caused significant self-reflection. Sarah has been a nurse consultant for the past 15 years and the president of her own consulting firm, Nursing Leaders Consulting Group (NLCG). NLCG has 10 employees, including Sarah, an executive assistant, a part-time chief financial officer (CFO), a part-time data analyst, a part-time writer/editor, and a part-time marketing/promotions person. The rest of the employees are all master's-prepared or PhD nurse consultants with various clinical backgrounds. NLCG provides strategic planning, operational improvement, professional development, and organizational culture transformational services to hospitals and healthcare organizations throughout the United States and internationally.

Reflecting on the last 15 years, Sarah is proud of the tremendous growth and reputation of the organization that she has built with her expertise and that of her colleagues. The consultants for NLCG have not only conducted numerous on-site consultations but also have made presentations at national and international conferences, written articles for professional journals, prepared their own booklets, and presented webinar conferences for various audiences for continuing education units (CEUs). Although Sarah has truly enjoyed the consulting experience, the rigorous travel schedule and on-site consulting demands have made her physically and emotionally weary. It has been difficult to schedule time away from her work because, as a principal member of the firm, she typically fields all of the calls inquiring about their consultation services. Once she speaks to the prospective client and determines the client's specific needs, she either delegates the consultation to one of the nursing specialists or takes the lead herself on the project. Lately, there has been a tremendous demand for the services of the nurse consultants at NLCG, and the consultants have been spread thin trying to meet the needs of numerous clients, maintaining contact with existing clients, and marketing their services to prospective clients through speaking engagements and writing for publications.

Sarah and the other consultants have enjoyed the independence and autonomy that consulting affords them as contrasted to being employees for a major organization. Sarah often comments that she is "engaged in many of the nation's leading healthcare organizations," which gives her a very unique perspective in contrast with an individual who has worked for the same organization for most of the individual's career. Sarah states, "I have truly seen the good, the bad, and the ugly in healthcare organizations." Overall, she is extremely satisfied and fulfilled with the work and feels that she and her colleagues have made a tremendous difference in the growth and development of leaders nationally and internationally. The consulting role has allowed her to be extremely creative and innovative in the work that she does and in mentoring and coaching nursing leaders to manage the complexity of their organizations.

Although Sarah feels great pride with her work and career accomplishments, she also feels that she will be unable to keep the current pace for much longer. She feels that few understand how difficult it is to be a consultant. Considering all of the complexity of travel, trying to rest or sleep in different hotels night after night, and managing the long consulting hours with few breaks during the day have taken their toll. Sarah recalls many examples of starting the consulting day at 7 o'clock in the morning over a breakfast meeting, consulting with groups all morning, making a presentation over lunch, meeting with groups again in the afternoon, and attending dinner meetings or even evening meetings before the day ends and she can return to the hotel or catch a flight home. On many such days, she hardly has time allotted for a bathroom break. Being a consultant means being "on stage" all during the engagement. Sarah also realizes that although she has developed many professional relationships with her clients and colleagues, these relationships are very different from personal friendships, and it would be inappropriate to share her feelings with her clients.

Reflecting on her career and the options for the future, Sarah feels perplexed and wonders, "What shall I do for an encore?" She is at the top of her game, and she wants to end her consulting career at her peak, instead of becoming resentful of all of the hours it took to be a successful consultant. She thinks about selling the firm to one of the other nurse consultants or to an outside interest, but she fears leaving her consulting life and her own firm. She still needs a steady income, benefits, interaction with colleagues, and outlet for her sense of creativity. At times her head is filled with negative self-talk because she feels that it would be a mistake to do anything other than consulting. On the other hand, she has visions that there must be a way that she could give back to the nursing profession, to her community, and to emerging and developing leaders in the sunset years of her career. She just needs to take that first step of faith and explore the possible opportunities for a career change despite her overwhelming success as a nurse consultant and business owner.

Sarah explores many options available to her. She could apply for a chief nursing officer (CNO) role at a local hospital, interview for a tenure-track faculty position at the university near her home, or relocate to another city for a position in professional development in a large multihospital healthcare system. All of these alternatives have merit and would provide a steady income, benefits, and an opportunity to "make a difference." Not entirely sure of the direction she should take in designing her future, Sarah decides to sell her firm to her colleagues. She offers her assistance to ensure the smooth and successful transition to the new ownership and to continue to market and promote the expertise of her colleagues.

Realizing that she is completely exhausted mentally, emotionally, and physically, Sarah gives herself permission to "not make a decision" immediately. She decides to take some time off and take care of herself. She takes a trip to a sunny location to sit on the beach, to read some fun books instead of professional material, and to share experiences with a close, long-time friend who has been always accepting of Sarah and honest in her assessment of situations and recommendations when asked. Upon returning home, Sarah takes time to meditate, take long walks, and enroll in a yoga class. She does many of the things that she didn't have time for when she was working as a consultant. She buys season tickets to the symphony, attends several plays, and joins a literary group that reads and discusses literature.

After a few months of getting in touch with her self again, Sarah applies for the tenure-track faculty position at the local university. She feels that she wants to "give back to the community" and teach and mentor emerging leaders in the graduate nursing program. Although the transition from complete independence and autonomy to a more structured position is challenging, Sarah finds that she really enjoys the intellectual stimulation that she receives from the inquisitive students who are eager to learn. She has lots to share, not only about nursing theories but also about practical applications and case studies that she experienced as a nurse consultant in many different types of healthcare organizations. At first her new life seems very chaotic with trying to keep up with the readings to make her courses current and practical, preparing innovative methods for teaching and delivering course content, and reading, editing, and advising students in their written work. It doesn't take long for Sarah to say, "I love this new life that I have planned for myself, and it is a healthy transition for me in the last chapters of my fantastic nursing career!"

Questions

1. Sarah had a very satisfying career and successful business enterprise. How do you feel about her decision to leave that behind and pursue other career opportunities? What other changes could she have made to continue as a consultant?
2. We are often confronted with a personal "fork in the road," with both opportunities and challenges in either direction that we might choose. Describe the forks in the road that Sarah faced and the potential opportunities and challenges of each.
3. What are your thoughts about Sarah's personal journey to renew herself spiritually and physically?
4. What might you do if you were making such a large decision and feeling the internal conflict and the physical and emotional exhaustion that Sarah was feeling?
5. Describe how innovation and creativity are affected by emotional and physical exhaustion and possible solutions to energize the creative spirit again.
6. How did Sarah manage the negative self-talk that she experienced? How do you manage both negative and positive self-talk?

Case Study 14-2

Lifelong Learning and Striving for What Is Around the Corner

Brook has had quite a nursing career! As he reflects on the past 15 years, Brook is surprised at himself for having accomplished so much in such a short period of time and at such a young age. He graduated at 21 with a bachelor's of science in biological sciences, and then decided that he had wasted the last 4 years of his life earning a degree in an area that he did not want to work. Considering all of his possible career options and dabbling for a year in pharmaceutical sales, Brook decided to apply to a second degree nursing program to become a nurse. He had always been interested in the healthcare field and assumed that after he received his BS he might return to graduate school in pharmacy, public health, or healthcare administration. He hadn't really considered nursing before, but the idea became more and more intriguing to Brook. Perhaps he was influenced by the recent illness and death of his mother, and observing the compassionate care that she had received sparked an interest in his soul. He watched the nurses and admired their knowledge and competence coupled with sincere compassion when caring for his mother and other patients. He hadn't realized before how much science that nurses are exposed to in their education, but in talking with them he realized that his own background in biological sciences would be a great platform for a new career in nursing. It was a great choice for Brook, and he not only obtained a master's degree in nursing in the second degree program, but he also made a firm decision that he would continue on in his education.

His first job as a nurse was not only stimulating but also absolutely invigorating to his spirit. He loved every minute working with the patients, his colleagues, and the physicians. He worked as a clinical nurse in the surgical intensive care unit initially, but after a year, he asked to be transferred to the emergency department (ED). He loved the pace and the constant challenge of the ED, and he recognized and appreciated the physical and emotional challenges that his patients faced as they came into this unknown and often threatening environment. Every day he left work feeling that he'd made a positive difference for his patients, and he felt good about himself. Yes, life was good . . . but he yearned for something more. He asked himself, "Am I crazy, or what?"

Brook enrolled in a doctor of nursing practice (DNP) program, and although he thoroughly enjoyed exposure to the class content, he also found it challenging to be a full-time student and a full-time clinical nurse. The hours were long, and he had to make every minute count to keep up with the volumes of reading material, long practicum hours, and his work in the ED. At times he was completely and utterly exhausted and spent emotionally and physically.

Brook took every opportunity during the semester breaks to take paid leave from the hospital and to travel. He went hiking in the Grand Canyon, spent a week on the beach in Hawaii, and took a fun trip with friends backpacking around Europe. After these excursions he felt refreshed and renewed, eager for school to start, and ready return to work. He asked himself, "Am I crazy, or what?"

It didn't seem long until Brook graduated with his DNP. The degree opened several new career opportunities, and Brook landed a phenomenal position in the San Francisco Bay area as the director of research and professional development for the emergency services of a large healthcare system with hospitals throughout northern California. It was a great position with many challenges but strong leadership and resources to ensure his success in such a role. Brook had the opportunity to work with other directors to lead one hospital on its Magnet journey and to facilitate meaningful evidence-based practice projects and research studies to improve patient outcomes in the emergency service experience. It was an exciting time in Brook's personal and professional life for a few years, but it wasn't long until he felt restless again. He couldn't believe that he felt motivated to go back to school to earn his PhD in nursing. He asked himself, "Am I crazy, or what?"

Brook admires several of his PhD-prepared colleagues and their depth of knowledge about research. Although the DNP prepared him to use research evidence in practice, he yearns for a greater depth of understanding about research, statistics, and the entire qualitative and quantitative research processes and theory development. So, Brook applies and is accepted into the PhD program, and he continues his career while earning his PhD. Reflecting back, he never would have guessed that this would be the path his nursing career followed; yet he appreciates all that he had learned about himself in his formal educational experiences and in his real-life experiences caring for patients and their families in his nursing role. Brook realizes that he arrived at this point in his life and career by living in the potential as well as the reality of his life. It hasn't been an easy path, but he feels that he is a better person for having taken the journey. He can honestly say that he feels inner peace with the decisions that he made and the path that he chose.

Questions

1. What are some examples of self-talk that you could find in this story about Brook and his career path?
2. Going to school while working full time is not easy for anyone. What did Brook do that rejuvenated his spirit and refreshed him physically? What do you do to refresh yourself and rejuvenate your spirit?
3. What were some of the challenges that Brook faced in his journey, and what inner strength did he employ to meet these challenges?
4. What might have been the consequences if Brook had taken a different course when he realized that he was unfulfilled with his BS degree in biological sciences?
5. How do our life's experiences shape and influence our personal and professional decisions?
6. How can we know when we have made the right decision for our self and our career?

References

Bakker, A. B. (2013). *Advances in positive organizational psychology* (1st ed.). Bingley, England: Emerald.

Bodaken, B., & Fritz, R. (2006). *The managerial moment of truth.* New York, NY: Free Press.

de Bono, E. (2007). *Tactics.* New York, NY: Profile HarperCollins.

Hickey, M., & Kritek, P. B. (2012). *Change leadership in nursing: How change occurs in a complex hospital system.* New York, NY: Springer.

Hosmer, L. T. (2006). *The ethics of management* (5th ed.). Boston, MA: McGraw-Hill/Irwin.

Leonard-Barton, D. (2011). *Managing knowledge assets, creativity and innovation.* Hackensack, NJ: World Scientific.

Massaro, M., Bardy, R., & Pitts, M. (2012). Supporting creativity through knowledge integration during the creative processes: A management control system perspective. *Electronic Journal of Knowledge Management, 10*(3), 258–267.

Simons, M., & Havert, M. L. (2012). Using appreciative inquiry to support a culture shift in transition. *Technical Services Quarterly, 29*(3), 207–216.

Stewart, R., Corneille, M., & Johnson, J. (2006). Transparent and open discussion of errors does not increase malpractice risk in trauma patients. *Annals of Surgery, 243*(5), 645–651.

Wheatley, M. (2009). *Turning to one another: Simple conversations to restore hope to the future.* San Francisco, CA: Berrett-Koehler.

Suggested Readings

Brown, J. (2012). *The art and spirit of leadership.* London, England: Trafford.

Cordeiro, W. (2009). *Leading on empty: Refilling your tank and renewing your passion.* Ami, MI: Baker Publishing, Bethany House.

McKee, A., Boyatzis, R., & Johnston, F. (2008). *Becoming a resonant leader: Develop your emotional intelligence, renew your relationships, sustain your effectiveness.* Boston, MA: Harvard Business School Press.

Palmer, S. (2012). *Digital wisdom: Thought leadership for a connected world.* New York, NY: York House Press.

Rothwell, W. (2012). *Becoming an effective mentoring leader: Proven strategies for building excellence in your organization.* New York, NY: McGraw-Hill.

Wheatley, M. (2006). *Leadership and the new science: Discovering order in a chaotic world.* San Francisco, CA: Berrett-Koehler.

Quiz Questions

Select the best answer for each of the following questions.

1. Most great leaders can recall a time when _____.
   a. Situations made them what they became.
   b. All greatness was simply chance and mystery.
   c. They felt a deep call within to leadership.
   d. They thought that leadership was simply learned.

2. The spiritually focused leader emphasizes the importance of which of the following?
   a. The here and now
   b. The longer and more distant road
   c. Keeping focused on the emerging issues
   d. Only focusing on the future

3. Chaos is always the route to _____.
   a. Order
   b. Complexity
   c. Uncertainty
   d. Mystery

4. We all participate in each other's evolution because of which of the following?
   a. All things are ultimately interconnected.
   b. The universe acts independently on all other creation.
   c. We have been made masters of creation.
   d. Genomics shows that we are essentially the same.

5. Creativity is expressed in which of the following ways?
   a. Art and music only
   b. The scientific process
   c. Symbols and images
   d. All of the above

6. There is virtually nothing about fear that is _____.
   a. Unnecessary
   b. Redeeming
   c. Invalid
   d. Just

7. Exercising the spirit requires which of the following?

   a. Prayer
   b. A fixed approach
   c. A regular routine
   d. A guru

8. According to the 10 spiritual themes of leadership, which of the following must leaders have the ability to do?

   a. Point in the proper direction.
   b. See all issues with clarity.
   c. Embrace the needs of others.
   d. Take risks.

9. Which of the following is a major enemy of the spirit within?

   a. Anger with others
   b. The tendency to make judgments
   c. Lack of regular reflection
   d. Lack of strong relationships

10. Which of the following is a fundamental tenet of the universe?

    a. All life is self-organizing.
    b. All things can ultimately be understood.
    c. All action is rational.
    d. All change is impermanent.

11. There is no more important ability for leaders to develop than the ability to

    _____.

    a. Direct
    b. Act
    c. Listen
    d. Take risks

12. To those they lead, what do leaders represent?

    a. The respect for the mystery that is present in all aspects of life
    b. The hardships that attend every action
    c. The challenges that arise out of all action
    d. The internal logic that guides all creation

APPENDIX

Quiz Answers

Chapter 1: A New Vessel for Leadership: Changing the Health Landscape in an Age of Reform 1(d), 2(b), 3(a), 4(b), 5(a), 6(d), 7(c), 8(c), 9(a), 10(b)

Chapter 2: Ten Complexity Principles for Leaders for Thriving in the Quantum Age 1(d), 2(b), 3(a), 4(a), 5(c), 6(d), 7(b), 8(c), 9(c), 10(a), 11(b), 12(d)

Chapter 3: Evidentiary Leadership: An Expanded Lens to Determine Healthcare Value 1(a), 2(c), 3(b), 4(c), 5(a), 6(c), 7(d), 8(d), 9(b), 10(c)

Chapter 4: Innovation as a Way of Life: Leading Through the White Water of Change 1(c), 2(d), 3(a), 4(b), 5(c), 6(b), 7(a), 8(d), 9(b), 10(c)

Chapter 5: Innovative Leadership 1(b), 2(d), 3(a), 4(c), 5(a), 6(b), 7(d), 8(d), 9(a), 10(d)

Chapter 6: Leadership and Normative Conflict: Managing the Diversity of a Multifocal Workplace 1(c), 2(b), 3(a), 4(d), 5(c), 6(b), 7(a), 8(a), 9(d), 10(d)

Chapter 7: Leading Constant Movement: Managing Crisis and Change
1(True), 2(False: cataclysmic events are just one stimulus for crisis), 3(True), 4(False: crises and conflicts cannot be prevented; they can be well managed), 5(False: humans shape organizations; organizations do not shape humans), 6(True), 7(False: the complexity of the organization has a direct impact on crisis and conflict), 8(True), 9(True), 10(False: good crisis plans are always developed with both management and staff), 11(False: crises are always generated at the intersections between external and internal forces in organizations), 12(True)

Chapter 8: Living Leadership: Vulnerability, Risk Taking, and Stretching 1(d), 2(a), 3(d), 4(b), 5(b), 6(c), 7(c), 8(a), 9(b), 10(c)

Chapter 9: Healing Brokenness: Error as Opportunity 1(c), 2(c), 3(d), 4(c), 5(a), 6(d), 7(b), 8(d), 9(a), 10(a)

Chapter 10: The Fully Engaged Leader: Integrated Capacity for Success 1(b), 2(a), 3(d), 4(b), 5(c), 6(a), 7(d), 8(a), 9(d), 10(a), 11(c)

Chapter 11: Toxic Organizations and People: The Leader as Transformer
1(a), 2(a), 3(b), 4(d), 5(b), 6(c), 7(a), 8(d), 9(d), 10(a), 11(a), 12(b)

Chapter 12: Coaching for Unending Change: Transforming the Membership Community
1(c), 2(d), 3(a), 4(b), 5(b), 6(b), 7(d), 8(c), 9(c), 10(a), 11(a), 12(b), 13(c)

Chapter 13: The Leader's Courage to Be Willing: Building a Context for Hope
1(c), 2(a), 3(d), 4(b), 5(b), 6(d), 7(a), 8(c), 9(d)

Chapter 14: Sustaining the Spirit of Leadership: Becoming a Living Leader
1(c), 2(b), 3(a), 4(a), 5(d), 6(b), 7(c), 8(d), 9(b), 10(a), 11(c), 12(a)

INDEX

Note: Page numbers followed by exhibit, *f* and *t* indicate material in exhibits, figures, and tables, respectively.

A

Abrahamson, E., 315
absolutism, 552
abuse of power, 440
   intolerance toward diversity, 441
   mandatory overtime, 441
accident, defined, 361
accountability, 472, 473
   conflict resolution and, 232
   for error management, 358
   expect, 459–460
   fiscal, 365
   in healthcare system, 101
   horizontal relationships and, 494
   individual *vs.* system, 361 (exhibit 9-6)
   internal, moving from external oversight to, 370–371
   living, 370
   personal will and, 520
   from responsibility to, 470–474, 471 (exhibit 12-1)
   shared, for learning, 380–381
   systems evaluation and, 298
accountability-based organizations, 472
acting as agent of transformation principle, 458
acting out, conflict and, 214
action
   learning tools, 482 (exhibit 12-3)
   risk and, 29
action (ARIA format), 230–232
active listening, 246, 454
active team members, conflict resolution and, 213–214
actual reality, 7, 53
   potential reality *vs.*, 53, 53 (exhibit 2-1)
acuity, 380, 384
adaptation, 73, 78. *See also* flexibility
   borderland of chaos and, 266
   dynamic, 481
   effective, 479
   error and, 69
   leaders and requirements for, 483
   as more important than anticipation, 273
adaptive capacity
   change and, 261-262
   in human organizations, 264–265
adaptive effectiveness
   crisis preparedness and, 296
   DCTM details of components for assessing, 293*f*

Adner, R., 189
advanced beginner stage
   in emotional competence development, 414, 415 (exhibit 10-3)
   team emotional competence, 418–419, 418 (exhibit 10-4)
advancing the organization, rational risks and, 318
adverse event, defined, 361
advocacy leadership, 450
Age of Accountability, 471
Age of Complexity, 451
Age of Enlightenment, 7
Age of Health Reform, 6, 19
Age of Technology, 8*f*
agendas, for action, 231
Ages, transition between, 7–9
aggregation, across systems, 66*f*
agility, leadership, 535
agreement, interest-based conflict resolution and formalizing of, 244
alignment, innovation and, 137–142, 157, 157*f*
Alzheimer's disease, 16
ambidextrous organizations, 182
ambiguity
   conflicts and, 220
   evidence in healthcare system, 101–104
   messages, 447
American College of Physicians, 259
anger, unresolved, 436
anomaly, recognizing value of, 187
antagonism
   identity-based conflict and, 223–225
   professional, minimizing, 529
anticipation, adaptation more important than, 273
antisocial behavior, tolerance of, 444–445
apprenticeship model, of training, 3
Argyris, Chris, 144, 477
ARIA format (for conflict resolution), 223–232
   action, 230–232
   antagonism, 223–226
   invention, 228–230
   resonance, 226–228
art, of chaos, 578
artifact, change and, 84
authentic leader, 312
authority
   effects from unquestioning adherence to, 527
   systems evaluation and, 298